General Anatomy and
Musculoskeletal System

THIEME Atlas of
Anatomy
Second Edition

Authors

Michael Schuenke, MD, PhD
Institute of Anatomy
Christian Albrecht University, Kiel

Erik Schulte, MD
Department of Anatomy and Cell Biology
Johannes Gutenberg University, Mainz

Udo Schumacher, MD
FRCPath, CBiol, FIBiol, DSc
Institute of Anatomy II: Experimental
Morphology
University Medical Center, Hamburg-
Eppendorf

Consulting Editor

Lawrence M. Ross, MD, PhD
Department of Neurobiology and Anatomy
The University of Texas Medical School at
Houston

Illustrations by

Markus Voll

Karl Wesker

Thieme Medical Publishers, Inc.
333 Seventh Avenue
New York, New York 10001

Vice President and Editorial Director, Educational Products:
Anne T. Vinnicombe
Editorial Assistants: Shira Kaye, Huvie Weinreich
Senior Vice President, Editorial and Electronic Product Development:
Cornelia Schulze
Senior Vice President and Chief Financial Officer: Sarah Vanderbilt
President: Brian D. Scanlan

Translators: Terry Telger and Judith Tomat

Illustrators: Markus Voll and Karl Wesker

Compositor: Agnieszka & Martin Waletzko, Leonberg, Germany
Printer: Everbest Printing Company, Hong Kong, China

Library of Congress Cataloging-in-Publication Data is available from
the publisher.

Printed in China
5 4 3 2 1

ISBN: 978-1-60406-922-8
eISBN: 978-1-62623-084-2

WinkingSkull.com *PLUS*

Your study aid for must-know anatomy

...ngSkull.com *PLUS* –
...tomy with this
...online learning tool.

...gister for **WinkingSkull.com** *PLUS*
...strations and radiographs from
...nd radiology publications. After
...bank, you can quiz yourself on key
...ore instantly to check your progress
...results.

...rything you need for course study

...omy illustrations
...navigation
...n that makes studying easy and fun
...results
...uding MRIs and CT scans with paired

...ull.com and follow these
...ed today.

...ve a free WinkingSkull.com
...kingskull.com, click on
Register Now," and complete the registration form.
Enter the scratch-off code below.

If you already have a WinkingSkull.com account,
go to the "My Account" page and click on the
"Enter WinkingSkull PLUS Access Code" link.
Enter the scratch-off code below.

*This product cannot be returned if the
access code panel is scratched off.*

General Anatomy and Musculoskeletal System

THIEME Atlas of Anatomy
Second Edition

Foreword

Each of the authors of the single volume *Thieme Atlas of Anatomy* was impressed with the extraordinary detail, accuracy, and beauty of the illustrations that were created for the *Thieme* three volume series of anatomy atlases. We felt these images were one of the most significant additions to anatomic education in the past 50 years. The effective pedagogical approach of this series, with two-page learning units that combined the outstanding illustrations and captions that emphasized the functional and clinical significance of structures, coupled with the numerous tables summarizing key information, was unique. We also felt that the overall organization of each region, with structures presented first systemically - musculoskeletal, vascular, and nervous – and then topographically, supported classroom learning and active dissection in the laboratory.

This series combines the best of a clinically oriented text and an atlas. Its detail and pedagogical presentation make it a complete support for classroom and laboratory instruction and a reference for life in all the medical, dental and allied health fields. Each of the volumes - *General Anatomy and Musculoskeletal System, Neck and Internal Organs, and Head and Neuroanatomy* - can also be used as a stand-alone text/atlas for an in-depth study of systems often involved in the allied health/medical specialty fields.

We were delighted when *Thieme* asked us to work with them to create a single-volume atlas from this groundbreaking series, and we owe a great debt to the authors and illustrators of this series in as much as their materials and vision formed the general framework for the single volume *Thieme Atlas of Anatomy.*

We thank the authors and illustrators for this very special contribution to the teaching of anatomy and recommend it for thorough mastery of anatomy and its clinically functional importance in all fields of health care-related specialties.

Lawrence M. Ross, Brian R. MacPherson, and Anne M. Gilroy

Preface to the Second Edition

Six years have passed since the first edition of the *Thieme Atlas of Anatomy: General Anatomy and Musculoskeletal System* was published. It has passed its first test and met the needs of students and practitioners everywhere, as evidenced by the many letters and e-mails we have received. We thank you for your praise and constructive criticism, which helps us keep improving this atlas.

Clinical knowledge presented in conjunction with anatomy is increasingly important earlier and earlier in the study of medicine. This has been further strengthened in this edition with the inclusion of about 30 new two-page spreads across the book devoted to

- osteoarthritis of the hip joint,
- compression syndromes of peripheral nerves,
- conduction anesthesia of peripheral nerves,
- shoulder arthroscopy and degenerative changes of the shoulder joint,
- functions of individual muscles and the symptoms associated with shortening or weakening of these muscles, and
- diagnostic imaging of the large joints, such as the shoulder, elbow, and wrist, and the hip, knee, and ankle.

In addition, we have added spreads on important foundational information on the common imaging planes for plain film, MRI, and CT scans, the structure of skeletal muscle fibers, the structure and chemical composition of hyaline cartilage, and the regeneration of peripheral nerves.

We have also checked, corrected, and updated all the information in this atlas.

With these improvements, this atlas is even better suited to students of medicine in what the World Health Organization (WHO) is again calling the "Decade of Bones and Joints" (first 2000 to 2010 and now 2010 to 2020) to draw attention to the continuing prominence and dramatic rise of diseases of the musculoskeletal system with the rise in average life expectancy worldwide. Today over half the chronic diseases of those over 60 involve the bones (e.g., osteoporosis) and joints (e.g., osteoarthritis), with tremendous economic consequences. One of the main reasons WHO is publicizing this is so that the world's universities appropriately prepare physicians, physical therapists, and other health care workers to address the growing global burden of these diseases due to the aging population.

This atlas emphasizes the correlations between physiologic changes in the course of life, the frequency of certain pathologic phenomena, and effective diagnostics while teaching the anatomy, better preparing students to treat patients with musculoskeletal diseases when they meet them in the clinic or in practice. When an elderly person suffers a fracture, it is not sufficient to just address the fracture. The doctor must learn why the fracture happened and address the underlying cause. Does, for example, the patient have osteoporosis, or is he or she so inflexible that any unexpected need to move leads to a fall? Interdisciplinary cooperation is needed to address these causes and provide appropriate preventive and rehabilitative care. The older we get, the more important it is for us to keep the musculoskeletal system in motion to curb degenerative disease and prevent injury.

This atlas, we hope, continues to meet your needs in the classroom and clinic, helps you attain a more nuanced understanding of the anatomy of the musculoskeletal system, and brings the fascination of anatomy in motion home to you.

Our special thanks to Prof. Dr. Cristoph Viebahn, Georg-August University, Göttingen, and Prof. Dr. Thilo Wedel, Christian-Albrechts University, Kiel, for their commitment to and constructive help on the new edition.

Michael Schünke, Erik Schulte, Udo Schumacher,
Markus Voll, and Karl Wesker
Kiel, Mainz, Hamburg, Munich, and Berlin in September 2011

Preface to the First Edition

When Thieme started planning this atlas, they sought the opinions of students and instructors in both the United States and Europe on what constituted an "ideal" atlas of anatomy —ideal to learn from, to master extensive amounts of information while on a busy class schedule, and, in the process, to acquire sound, up-to-date knowledge. The result of our work in response to what Thieme learned is this atlas. The *Thieme Atlas of Anatomy*, unlike most other atlases, is a comprehensive educational tool that combines illustrations with explanatory text and summary tables, introducing clinical applications throughout, and presenting anatomic concepts in a step-by-step sequence that includes system-by-system and topographical views.

Since the *Thieme Atlas of Anatomy* is based on a fresh approach to the underlying subject matter, it was necessary to create an entirely new set of illustrations for it—a task that took eight years. Our goal was to provide illustrations that would compellingly demonstrate anatomic relations and concepts, revealing the underlying simplicity of human anatomy without sacrificing detail or aesthetics.

With the *Thieme Atlas of Anatomy*, it was our intention to create an atlas that would guide students in their initial study of anatomy, stimulate their enthusiasm for this intriguing and vitally important subject, and provide a reliable reference for experienced students and professionals alike.

"If you want to attain the possible, you must attempt the impossible"
(Rabindranath Tagore).

Michael Schünke, Erik Schulte, Udo Schumacher,
Markus Voll, and Karl Wesker

Acknowledgments

First we wish to thank our families. This atlas is dedicated to them.

We also thank Prof. Reinhard Gossrau, M.D., for his critical comments and suggestions. We are grateful to several colleagues who rendered valuable help in proofreading: Mrs. Gabriele Schünke, Jakob Fay, M.D., Ms. Claudia Dücker, Ms. Simin Rassouli, Ms. Heinke Teichmann, and Ms. Sylvia Zilles. We are also grateful to Dr. Julia Jürns-Kuhnke for helping with the figure labels.

We extend special thanks to Stephanie Gay and Bert Sender, who prepared the layouts. Their ability to arrange the text and illustrations on facing pages for maximum clarity has contributed greatly to the quality of the atlas.

We particularly acknowledge the efforts of those who handled this project on the publishing side:

Jürgen Lüthje, M.D., Ph.D., executive editor at Thieme Medical Publishers, has "made the impossible possible." He not only reconciled the wishes of the authors and artists with the demands of reality but also managed to keep a team of five people working together for years on a project whose goal was known to us from the beginning but whose full dimensions we only came to appreciate over time. He is deserving of our most sincere and heartfelt thanks.

Sabine Bartl, developmental editor, became a touchstone for the authors in the best sense of the word. She was able to determine whether a beginning student, and thus one who is not (yet) a professional, could clearly appreciate the logic of the presentation. The authors are indebted to her.

We are grateful to Antje Bühl, who was there from the beginning as project assistant, working "behind the scenes" on numerous tasks such as repeated proofreading and helping to arrange the figure labels.

We owe a great debt of thanks to Martin Spencker, managing director of Educational Publications at Thieme, especially to his ability to make quick and unconventional decisions when dealing with problems and uncertainties. His openness to all the concerns of the authors and artists established conditions for a cooperative partnership.

Without exception, our collaboration with the entire staff at Thieme Medical Publishers was consistently pleasant and cordial. Unfortunately, we do not have room to list everyone who helped in the publication of the *Atlas*, and we must limit our acknowledgments to a few colleagues who made a particularly notable contribution: Rainer Zepf and Martin Waletzko for support in all technical matters; Susanne Tochtermann-Wenzel and Manfred Lehnert, representing all those who were involved in the production of the book; Almut Leopold for the index; Marie-Luise Kürschner and her team for creating the cover design; to Liesa Arendt, Birgit Carlsen, and Anne Döbler, representing all those who handled marketing, sales, and promotion.

The Authors

As consulting editor I was asked to review, for accuracy and appropriateness, the English translation of the *Thieme Atlas of Anatomy: General Anatomy and Musculoskeletal System*, second edition. My work involved a review and edit of the translation, conversion of nomenclature to terms in common usage in English, and some small changes in presentation to reflect accepted approaches to certain anatomic structures in North American anatomy programs. This task was eased greatly by the clear organization of the original text. In all of this, I have tried diligently to remain faithful to the intentions and insights of the authors and illustrators, whom I wish to thank for this outstanding revision.

I would also like to thank the team at Thieme Medical Publishers who worked with me. First, I wish to thank translators Terry Telger and Judith Tomat for their work with the new and altered text and Anne Vinnicombe, editorial director for Educational Products, and editorial assistants, Shira Kaye and Huvie Weinreich, for their work with the translator and for checking and correcting my work and preparing this volume with care and speed.

Finally, heartfelt thanks go to Cathrin E. Schulz, M.D., editorial consultant, for her invitation to work on the first edition of this series and her assistance and constant encouragement at that time.

Lawrence M. Ross

Contents

General Anatomy

Trunk Wall

Upper Limb

Lower Limb

23   Neurovascular Systems: Topographical Anatomy

General Anatomy

1.1   Human Phylogeny

A Brief overview of human phylogenetic development

To better understand the evolution of the human body, it is helpful to trace its phylogenetic development. Humans and their closest relatives belong to the **phylum Chordata**, which includes approximately 50,000 species. It consists of two subphyla:

- Invertebrata: the tunicates (Tunicata) and chordates without a true skull (Acraniata or Cephalochordata)
- Vertebrata: the vertebrates (animals that have a vertebral column)

Although some members of the chordate phylum differ markedly from one another in appearance, they are distinguished from all other animals by characteristic morphological structures that are present at some time during the life of the animal, if only during embryonic development (see **G**). Invertebrate chordates, such as the cephalochordates and their best-known species, the lancelet (*Branchiostoma lanceolatum*) are considered the *model of a primitive vertebrate* by virtue of their organization. They provide clues to the basic structure of the vertebrate body and thus are important in understanding the general organization of vertebrate organisms (see **D**).

All the **members of present-day vertebrate classes** (jawless fish, cartilaginous fish, bony fish, amphibians, reptiles, birds, and mammals) have a number of characteristic features in common (see **H**), including a row of vertebrae arranged in a *vertebral column*, which gives the subphylum its name (Vertebrata). The evolution of an *amniotic egg*, i.e., the development of the embryo within a fixed shell inside a fluid-filled amniotic cavity, was a critical evolutionary breakthrough that helped the vertebrates to survive on land. This reproductive adaptation enabled the terrestrial vertebrates (reptiles, birds, and mammals) to live out their life cycles entirely on land and sever the final ties with their marine origin. When we compare the embryos of different vertebrate classes, we observe a number of morphological and functional similarities, including the formation of branchial arches (see **B**).

Mammals comprise **three major groups:** monotremes (egg-laying mammals), marsupials (mammals with pouches), and placentals (mammals with a placenta). The placental mammals, which include humans, have a number of characteristic features (see **I**), including a tendency to invest much greater energy in the care and rearing of their young. Placental mammals complete their embryonic development inside the uterus and are connected to the mother by a placenta. Humans belong to the mammalian order of **primates**, whose earliest members were presumably small tree-dwelling mammals. Together with lemurs, monkeys, and the higher apes, human beings have features that originate from the early adaptation to an arboreal way of life. For example, primates have movable shoulder joints that enable them to climb in a hanging position while swinging from branch to branch. They have dexterous hands for grasping branches and manipulating food, and they have binocular, broadly overlapping visual fields for excellent depth perception.

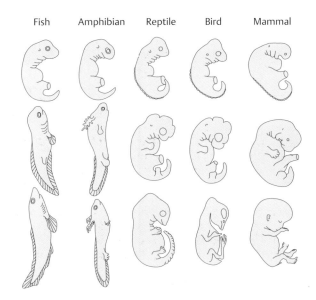

Fish   Amphibian   Reptile   Bird   Mammal

B Different stages in the early embryonic development of vertebrates

The early developmental stages (top row) of fish, amphibians, reptiles, birds, and mammals (as represented by humans) present a series of striking similarities that suggest a common evolutionary origin. One particularly noteworthy common feature is the set of branchial or pharyngeal arches in the embryonic regions that will develop into the head and neck. Although it was once thought that the developing embryo of a specific vertebrate would sequentially display features from organisms representing every previous step in its evolution ("Ontogeny recapitulates phylogeny," the "biogenetic law" of Ernst Haeckel [1834–1919]), subsequent work has shown that the vertebrates share common embryonic components that have been adapted to produce sometimes similar (fins and limbs) and sometimes radically different (gills vs. neck cartilages) adult structures.

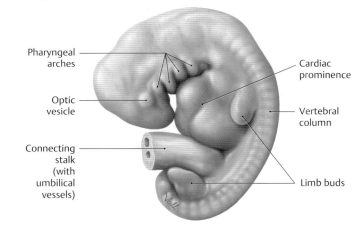

Pharyngeal arches — Optic vesicle — Connecting stalk (with umbilical vessels) — Cardiac prominence — Vertebral column — Limb buds

C Formation of the branchial or pharyngeal arches in a 5-week-old human embryo

Left lateral view. The branchial or pharyngeal arches of the vertebrate embryo have a *metameric* arrangement (similar to the somites, the primitive segments of the embryonic mesoderm); this means that they are organized into a series of segments that have the same basic structure. Among their other functions, they provide the raw material for the species-specific development of the visceral skeleton (maxilla, mandible, middle ear, hyoid bone, and larynx), the associated facial muscles, and the pharyngeal gut (see p. 11).

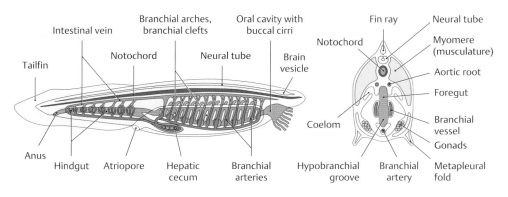

D Basic chordate anatomy, illustrated for the lancelet *(Branchiostoma lanceolatum)*
The vertebrates (including humans) are a subphylum of the chordates (Chordata), of which the lancelet is a typical representative. Its anatomy displays relatively simple terms of structures common to all vertebrates. The characteristic features of chordates include the development of an axial skeleton called the *notochord*. The human body still has remnants of the notochord, such as the nucleus pulposus of the intervertebral disks. The notochord is present in humans only during embryonic life, however, and is not a fully developed structure. Its remnants may give rise to developmental tumors called *chordomas*. Chordates have a *tubular nervous system* lying dorsal to the notochord. The body, particularly the muscles, is composed of multiple segments called *myomeres*. In humans, this myomeric pattern of organization is most clearly apparent in the trunk. Another distinguishing feature of chordates is the presence of a closed circulatory system.

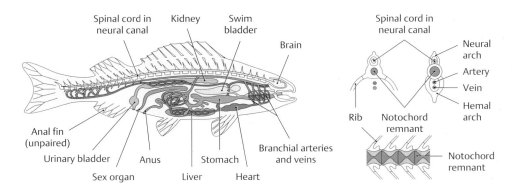

E Basic vertebrate anatomy, exemplified by the bony fish
The vertebrates are the *subphylum of chordates* from which humans evolved. With the evolution of fish, the notochord was transformed into a vertebral column (spinal column). The segmentally arranged bony vertebrae of the spinal column encircle remnants of the notochord and have largely taken its place. Dorsal and ventral arches arise from the vertebral bodies. The dorsal arches (vertebral or neural arches) in their entirety make up the neural canal, while the ventral arches (hemal arches) form a caudal "hemal canal" that transmits the major blood vessels. The ventral arches in the trunk region are the origins of the ribs.

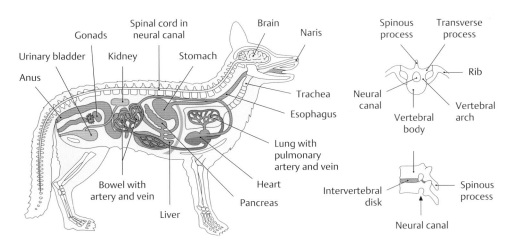

F Basic vertebrate anatomy, the dog

G Characteristic features of chordates

- Development of an axial skeleton (notochord)
- Dorsal neural tube
- Segmental arrangement of the body, particularly the muscles
- Foregut pierced by slits (branchial gut)
- Closed circulatory system
- Postanal tail

H Characteristic features of vertebrates

- Nerve cells, sensory organs, and oral apparatus concentrated in the head (cephalization)
- Multipart brain with a pituitary gland
- Replacement of the notochord by the vertebral column
- Generally, two pairs of limbs
- Development of branchial arches
- Presence of neural crest cells
- Closed circulatory system with a ventral, chambered heart
- Labyrinthine organ with semicircular canals
- Stratified epidermis
- Liver and pancreas always present
- Complex endocrine organs such as the thyroid and pituitary
- Complex immune system
- Sexes almost always separate

I Characteristic features of mammals

- Highly glandular skin covered with true hair (terminal hair)
- Females always have mammary glands for nursing offspring, which are usually born live (viviparous)
- Well-developed cerebrum
- Well-developed cutaneous muscles
- Diaphragm is the major respiratory muscle and separates the thoracic and abdominal cavities
- Heterogeneous and specialized teeth
- Four-chambered heart with a (left-sided) aortic arch
- Constant body temperature (homeothermy)

3

1.2 Human Ontogeny: Overview, Fertilization, and Earliest Developmental Stages

Besides gross and microscopic anatomy, the developmental history of the individual organism (ontogeny) is of key importance in understanding the human body. Ontogeny is concerned with the formation of tissues (*histogenesis*), organs (*organogenesis*), and the shape of the body (*morphogenesis*).

A 5- to 8-week-old human embryos
Streeter (1942) and O'Rahilly (1987) classified early human development and the embryonic period into 23 stages based on specimens from the Carnegie Collection. The Carnegie stages are defined by morphological characteristics that can be closely correlated with specific age (postovulatory days or weeks) and size (measured as the greatest length, excluding lower limb [GL], or crown–rump length [CRL], see **C**).

Stage 14: 5th week, GL 5–7 mm, future cerebral hemispheres become identifiable
Stage 17: 6th week, GL 11–14 mm, digital rays become visible.
Stage 20: 7th week, GL 18–22 mm, upper arms bent at the elbow, hands in a pronated position.
Stage 23: 8th week, GL 27–31 mm, eyelids fuse, external genitalia begin differentiation.

B Longitudinal growth and weight gain during the fetal period

Age (weeks)	Crown–rump length, CRL (cm)	Weight (g)
9–12	5–8	10–45
13–16	9–14	60–200
17–20	15–19	250–450
21–24	20–23	500–820
25–28	24–27	900–1300
29–32	28–30	1400–2100
33–36	31–34	2200–2900
37–38	35–36	3000–3400

C Timetable of antenatal human development
(The Carnegie stages are shown in parentheses.)

Weeks 1–3:	Early development
Week 1:	Tubal migration, segmentation, and blastocyst formation (stages 1–3)
Week 2:	Implantation and bilaminar embryonic disc, yolk sac (stages 4–5)
Week 3:	Trilaminar embryonic disc, start of neurulation (stages 6–9)

Weeks 4–8:	Embryonic period
Week 4:	Folding of the embryo, neurulation concluded, axial organs, basic body shape (stages 10–13)
Weeks 5–8:	Organogenesis (formation of all essential external and internal organs, elongated limb buds) (stages 14–23)

Weeks 9–38:	Fetal period
Weeks 9–38:	Organ growth and functional maturation (sex-specific differentiation of the external genitalia)

Length of gestation

- p.o. = postovulatory age — 266 days = 38 weeks
- p.m. = postmenstrual age — 280 days = 40 weeks

Size

- GL = greatest length, excluding lower limb — simplest, most consistent ultrasound measure
- CRL = crown–rump length — similar to GL in embryonic period, used in most descriptions of the fetal period

Fertilization → Early development (weeks 1–3) — Low rate of malformations, high rate of spontaneous abortion → Embryonic disc

Early embryo — Primitive streak → Embryonic period (weeks 4–8) — High sensitivity; every organ system has its own sensitive phase → Embryo

Fetus in utero — Placenta, Amniotic cavity → Fetal period (weeks 9–38) — Decreasing sensitivity, functional maturation

D Stages sensitive to teratogenic influences (after Sadler)

Oogenesis   **Spermatogenesis**

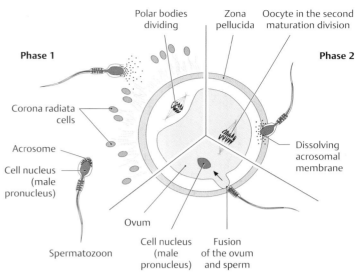

Phase 3

F Schematic representation of the fertilization process
(after Sadler)
In *phase 1*, the spermatozoon penetrates the corona radiata cells. In *phase 2*, the acrosome dissolves, releasing enzymes that digest the zona pellucida. In *phase 3*, the cell membranes of the ovum and sperm fuse, and the spermatozoon enters the egg.

E Formation of the ovum and sperm (after Sadler)
During the formation of the gametes (sex cells), two successive cell divisions occur (the first and second meiotic maturation divisions). This results in cells having a chromosome set that is reduced by one half (haploid). When fertilization occurs, a diploid (full) chromosome set is restored. During meiosis, extensive chromosomal rearrangement occurs, thus recombining the internal genetic information into new and different subsets.

Oogenesis: The initial oogonia first undergo a mitotic division to form primary oocytes, which still have a diploid chromosome number (44XX). Later the primary oocytes undergo a first and second maturation division by meiosis, resulting in four haploid cells (22X): one mature ovum and three polar bodies.

Spermatogenesis: Diploid spermatogonia undergo mitosis to form primary spermatocytes (44XY). These cells then divide meiotically to form four haploid spermatids, two of which have an X chromosome (22X) and two a Y chromosome (22Y). The spermatids develop into motile spermatozoa (spermatohistogenesis).

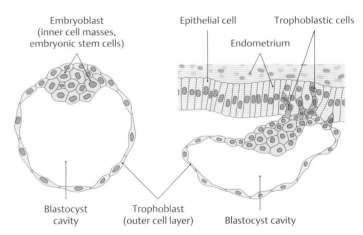

G Implantation of the blastocyst in the uterine mucosa on postovulatory day 5–6 (after Sadler)

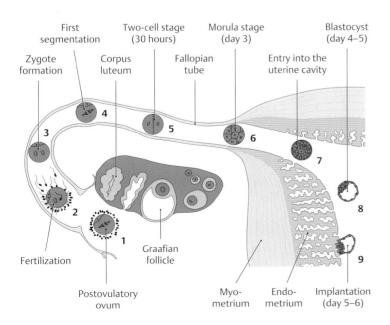

H Developmental processes during the first week of development
(after Sadler)
1. Ovum immediately after ovulation
2. Fertilized within approximately 12 hours
3. Male and female pronucleus with subsequent zygote formation
4. First segmentation
5. Two-cell stage
6. Morula stage
7. Entry into the uterine cavity
8. Blastocyst
9. Early implantation

5

1.3 Human Ontogeny: Gastrulation, Neurulation, and Somite Formation

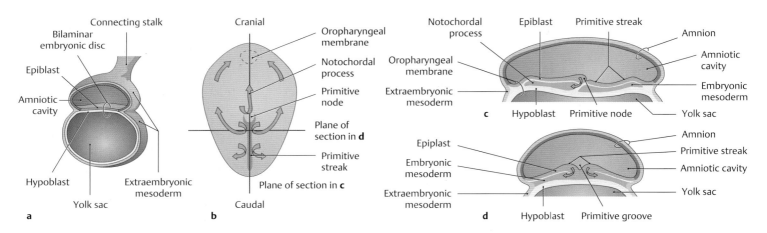

A Formation of the trilaminar human embryonic disc (gastrulation) at the start of the third postovulatory week (after Sadler)
As a result of gastrulation, the cell layers become differentiated into an *ectoderm*, *endoderm*, and *mesoderm*, from which all structures of the human body are derived (e.g., the endoderm gives rise to the central nervous system and the sensory organs). Gastrulation also establishes the primary axes of the body (ventral–dorsal, cranial–caudal, and left–right).

a Sagittal section through a conceptus at 2 postovulatory weeks. The embryonic disc is *still bilaminar* and is stretched between the amniotic cavity and yolk sac. The extraembryonic mesoderm, whose formation commences at the posterior pole of the embryonic disc, already covers the entire conceptus, which is attached to the chorionic cavity by a connecting stalk.

b Dorsal view of a human embryonic disc at the start of gastrulation. The amnion has been removed. At the start of gastrulation, the epiblast develops a primitive streak, where the embryonic mesoderm is generated and migrates between epiblast and hypoblast. Shortly afterward, at the level of the primitive node (the cranial tip of the primitive streak), epiblast cells migrate cranially to form the notochordal process and radially to form the definitive endoderm. In the process, the definitive endoderm sequentially replaces the hypoblast, while the notochordal process only temporarily fuses with the hypoblast layer. The notochordal process expands cranially from the primitive node to the oropharyngeal membrane.

c Sagittal section: embryonic disc along the notochordal process.

d Cross section: embryonic disc at the level of the primitive groove (arrows in **c** and **d**: direction of gastrulation movements by the mesoderm).

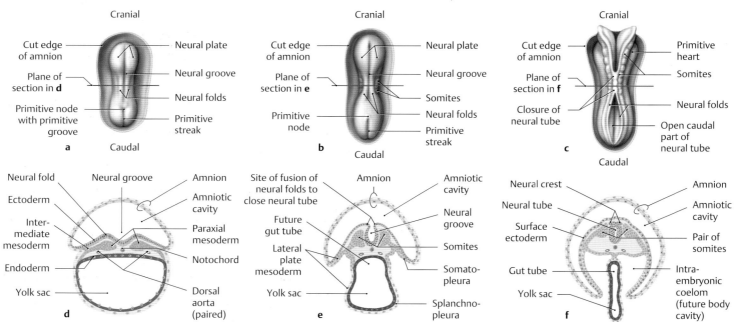

B Neurulation during early human development (after Sadler)
a–c Dorsal view after removal of the amnion.
d–f Schematic cross sections of the corresponding stages at the planes of section marked in **a–c**. Age in postovulatory days. During neurulation, the neuroectoderm differentiates from the surface ectoderm due to inductive influences from the notochord.
a, d Embryonic disc at 19 days. The neural tube is developing in the area of the neural plate.

b, e Embryonic disc at 20 days. The first somites have formed, and the neural groove is beginning to close to form the neural tube, with initial folding of the embryo.
c, f Embryo at 22 days. Eight pairs of somites are seen flanking the partially closed neural tube, which has sunk below the ectoderm. At the sites where the neural folds fuse to close the neural tube, cells form a bilateral neural crest that detaches from the surface and migrates into the mesoderm.

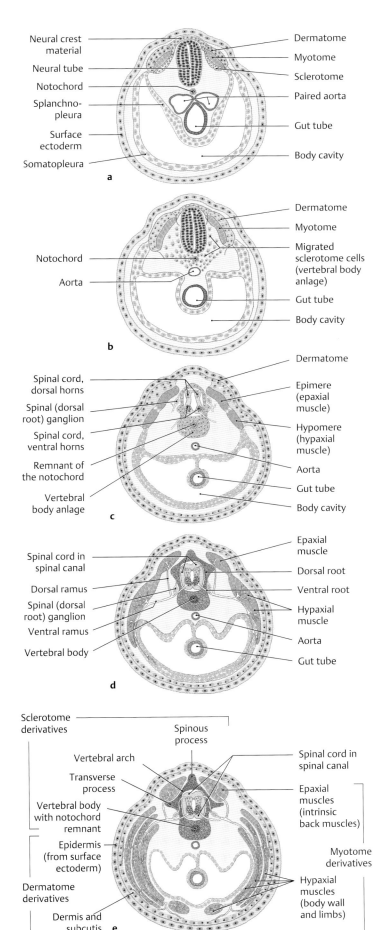

Neural crest material
Neural tube
Notochord
Splanchno-pleura
Surface ectoderm
Somatopleura

Dermatome
Myotome
Sclerotome
Paired aorta
Gut tube
Body cavity

a

Notochord
Aorta

Dermatome
Myotome
Migrated sclerotome cells (vertebral body anlage)
Gut tube
Body cavity

b

Spinal cord, dorsal horns
Spinal (dorsal root) ganglion
Spinal cord, ventral horns
Remnant of the notochord
Vertebral body anlage

Dermatome
Epimere (epaxial muscle)
Hypomere (hypaxial muscle)
Aorta
Gut tube
Body cavity

c

Spinal cord in spinal canal
Dorsal ramus
Spinal (dorsal root) ganglion
Ventral ramus
Vertebral body

Epaxial muscle
Dorsal root
Ventral root
Hypaxial muscle
Aorta
Gut tube

d

Sclerotome derivatives
Vertebral arch
Transverse process
Vertebral body with notochord remnant
Epidermis (from surface ectoderm)
Dermatome derivatives
Dermis and subcutis

Spinous process
Spinal cord in spinal canal
Epaxial muscles (intrinsic back muscles)
Myotome derivatives
Hypaxial muscles (body wall and limbs)

e

C Somite derivatives and spinal nerve formation during the embryonic period (weeks 4–8), shown in schematic cross sections (after Drews)

D Differentiation of the germ layers (after Christ and Wachtler)

Ectoderm	Neural tube		Brain, retina, spinal cord
	Neural crest	Neural crest of the head	Sensory and parasympathetic ganglia, intramural nervous system of the bowel, parafollicular cells, smooth muscle, pigment cells, carotid body, bone, cartilage, connective tissue, dentin and cementum of the teeth, dermis and subcutaneous tissue of the head
		Neural crest of the trunk	Sensory and autonomic ganglia, peripheral glia, adrenal medulla, pigment cells, intramural plexuses
		Ectodermal placodes	Anterior pituitary, cranial sensory ganglia, olfactory epithelium, inner ear, lens
	Surface ecto-derm		Enamel organ of the teeth, epithelium of the oral cavity, salivary glands, nasal cavities, paranasal sinuses, lacrimal passages, external auditory canal, epidermis, hair, nails, cutaneous glands
Mesoderm	Axial	Notochord, prechordal mesoderm	Extraocular muscles
	Paraxial		Spinal column, ribs, skeletal muscle, connective tissue, dermis and subcutis of the back and part of the head, smooth muscle, blood vessels
	Intermediate		Kidneys, gonads, renal and genital excretory ducts
	Lateral plate meso-derm	Visceral (splanchno-pleura)	Heart, blood vessels, smooth muscle, bowel wall, blood, adrenal cortex, visceral serosa
		Parietal (somato-pleura)	Sternum, limbs (cartilage, bones, and ligaments), dermis and subcutaneous tissue of the anterolateral body wall, smooth muscle, connective tissue, parietal serosa
Endoderm			Epithelium of the bowel, respiratory tract, digestive glands, pharyngeal glands, eustachian tube, tympanic cavity, urinary bladder, thymus, parathyroid glands, thyroid gland

(For clarity, the surrounding amnion is not shown.) The first pairs of somites appear at approximately 20 postovulatory days. All 34 or 35 of the somites ("primitive segments") have formed by day 30.

a When differentiation begins, each of these somites subdivides into a dermatome, myotome, and sclerotome (i.e., a cutaneous, muscular, and vertebral segment).

b At the end of 4 weeks, the sclerotome cells migrate toward the notochord and form the anlage of the spinal column.

c The neural tube—the precursor of the spinal cord and brain—differentiates to form a rudimentary spinal cord with dorsal and ventral horns. Cells within the ventral horn differentiate into motor neurons that sprout axons that form the *ventral root*. The neural crest has multiple derivatives, including sensory neurons that form dorsal root (spinal) ganglia, which send central processes into the spinal cord via the *dorsal root*. The myotomes become segregated into a dorsal part (epimere = epaxial muscles) and a ventral part (hypomere = hypaxial muscles).

d Each pair of dorsal and ventral roots unites to form a spinal nerve, which then divides into two main branches (a dorsal ramus and a ventral ramus). The epaxial muscles are supplied by the dorsal ramus, the hypaxial muscles by the ventral ramus.

e Cross section at the level of the future abdominal muscles. The epaxial muscles become the intrinsic back muscles, while the hypaxial muscles develop into structures that include the lateral abdominal muscles (external and internal oblique, transversus abdominis) and the anterior abdominal muscles (rectus abdominis).

1.4 Human Ontogeny: Development of the Fetal Membranes and Placenta

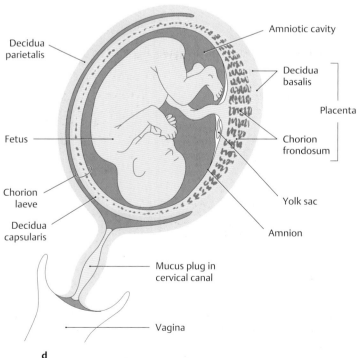

A Development of the fetal membranes and placenta (after Sadler and Drews)

a, c, and **d** Schematic sections through a pregnant uterus at different points in gestation.

b Detail from **a**.

a **Embryo at 5 weeks:** After the blastocyst has implanted in the uterine mucosa, the embryo initially derives its nutrition through the developing trophoblast and chorionic mesoderm. Chorionic villi are formed that surround the entire chorionic sac and embryo. They develop from primary to secondary villi and finally to tertiary villi (see close-up in **b**).

b **Detail from a:** The mainstem villi of the chorionic plate are attached on the maternal side to the basal plate of the decidua basalis by compact columns of trophoblastic cells. Like the small villous trees that sprout and branch from them, these mainstem villi have a syncytial covering (syncytial trophoblast), which in turn rests on a continuous layer of trophoblastic cells. Inside the villi, capillaries develop in the chorionic mesoderm and communicate with the vessels in the connecting stalk. Maternal blood flows through spiral arteries into the intervillous spaces.

c **Embryo at 8 weeks:** While the chorionic villi continue to grow and arborize at the embryonic pole, forming the chorion frondosum, the villi outside of this zone begin to regress, forming the nonvillous chorion laeve directly below the decidua capsularis. The amniotic cavity has enlarged at the expense of the chorionic cavity, and the amnion fuses with the chorion.

d **Fetus at 20 weeks:** The placenta is fully formed and consists of two parts: a fetal part formed by the chorion frondosum and a maternal part, the decidua basalis.

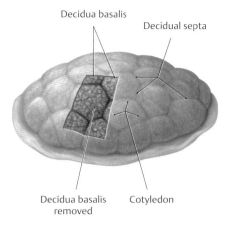

B Schematic cross section of a mature human placenta

The mature placenta is shaped like a frying pan, the maternal decidua basalis (basal plate) forming the base of the pan and the fetal chorionic plate forming the "lid." Some 40 arborizing villous trees containing fetal vessels project from the chorionic plate into the portions of the placenta that are filled with maternal blood (intervillous spaces). The maternal blood flows through approximately 80 to 100 spiral arteries into the intervillous spaces, which are divided into cotyledons by incomplete decidual septa. After the blood has bathed the villi, it is collected by irregularly distributed venous openings in the basal plate and returned to the maternal circulation.

C The postpartum placenta (after Sadler)

View of the maternal side of the delivered placenta (with a piece of the decidua basalis removed). The bulging cotyledons on the maternal surface are separated from one another by decidual septa.

E Characteristics of a mature human placenta

Size:	18–23 cm in diameter
	2–3 cm in thickness
Weight:	450–500 g
Total placental volume:	approximately 500 mL
Volume of the intervillous spaces:	approximately 150 mL
Villous surface area:	approximately 11–13 m^2
Blood circulation on the maternal side:	500–600 mL/min

Structure of the placental barrier

- Endothelium of the fetal capillaries and basal lamina
- Fibrous villous stroma
- Syncytiotrophoblast and basal lamina
- Continuous trophoblast cell layer (becomes discontinuous after 20 weeks of gestation)

  Diffusion distance approx. 5 μm (initially approx. 50 μm)

Primary functions of the mature placenta

1. *Transport of substances and exchange of metabolic products*

   Mother-to-fetus
   O_2, water, electrolytes, carbohydrates, amino acids and lipids, hormones, antibodies, vitamins and trace elements, but also drugs, toxins, and certain viruses

   Fetus-to-mother
   CO_2, water, electrolytes, urea, uric acid, bilirubin, creatinine, hormones

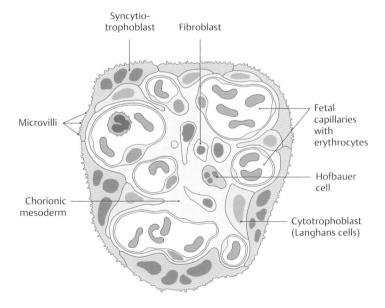

D Cross section through a terminal villus from a mature human placenta (after Kaufmann)

2. *Hormone production (syncytiotrophoblast)*

   - Human chorionic gonadotropin (HCG)
     → maintenance of the corpus luteum
   - Estrogens
     → growth of the uterus and breasts
   - Progesterone
     → inhibits uterine muscle contractions

Clinical note: The HCG formed in the syncytiotrophoblast prevents premature breakdown of the corpus luteum and sustains the pregnancy. HCG can be detected in the maternal urine at an early stage, providing the basis for early pregnancy testing.

1.5 Development of the Pharyngeal (Branchial) Arches in Humans

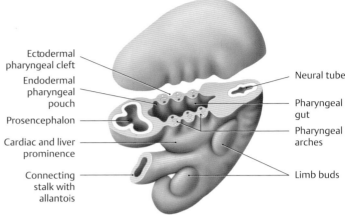

A Head and neck region of a 5-week-old human embryo, demonstrating the pharyngeal arches and clefts

Left lateral view. The pharyngeal arches are instrumental in the development of the neck and face. In *fish* and *amphibians*, the branchial arches develop into a respiratory organ (gills) for exchanging oxygen and carbon dioxide between the blood and water. *Land-dwelling vertebrates* (including humans) have *pharyngeal arches* rather than true branchial arches. Development of the pharyngeal arches begins in the 4th week of embryonic life as cells migrate from the neural crest to the future head and neck region. Within 1 week, a series of four oblique ridges (first through fourth pharyngeal arches) form that are located at the level of the cranial segment of the foregut and are separated externally by four deep grooves (pharyngeal clefts). The pharyngeal arches and grooves are prominent features of the embryo at this stage. Although the human embryo has no equivalent to the fifth and sixth branchial arches of other vertebrates, some of their components are incorporated into the human fourth pharyngeal arch.

B Cross section through a human embryo at the level of the pharyngeal gut (after Drews)

Left superior oblique view. Due to the craniocaudal curvature of the embryo, the cross section passes through the pharyngeal arches and pharyngeal gut, as well as the prosencephalon and spinal cord.

The pharyngeal gut is bounded on both sides by the pharyngeal arches (see also **A**), which contain a mesodermal core. They are covered externally by ectoderm and internally by endoderm. Ectodermal pharyngeal *clefts* and endodermal pharyngeal *pouches* lie directly opposite one another. Because the embryo is curved craniocaudally, the pharyngeal gut and pharyngeal arches overlie the prominence of the rudimentary heart and liver.

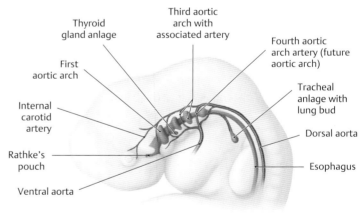

C Structure of the pharyngeal arches (after Drews)

View of the floor of the pharyngeal gut and the transversely sectioned pharyngeal arches. The typical components of a pharyngeal arch are easily identified: the aortic arch, musculature and associated nerves, and a cartilaginous skeletal element of each pharyngeal arch. The derivatives of these structures are of key importance in the formation of the face, neck, larynx, and pharynx. Because the developmental transformation of pharyngeal arch structures is complex, it is readily disrupted, causing malformations that may involve a cluster of related derivatives. Defects in pharyngeal arch development result in branchial and lateral cervical cysts and fistulas and in a group of "first arch syndromes" involving mandibulofacial deformities.

D Location of the aortic arch and pharyngeal pouches (after Sadler)

The aortic arches (branchial arch arteries) *arise* from the paired embryonic *ventral aorta* and run between the pharyngeal pouches. They *open* dorsally into the *dorsal aorta*, which is also paired. The definitive aortic arch develops from the fourth aortic arch on the left side (the development of the aortic arch is described on p. 12). The pharyngeal pouches are paired, diverticula-like outpouchings of the endodermal pharyngeal gut. A total of four distinct pharyngeal pouches develop on each side; the fifth is often absent or rudimentary.

Note: The pouch protruding from the roof of the oral cavity is called *Rathke's pouch* (precursor of the anterior pituitary). Note also the *lung bud* extending ventrally from the pharyngeal gut and the anlage of the *thyroid gland*.

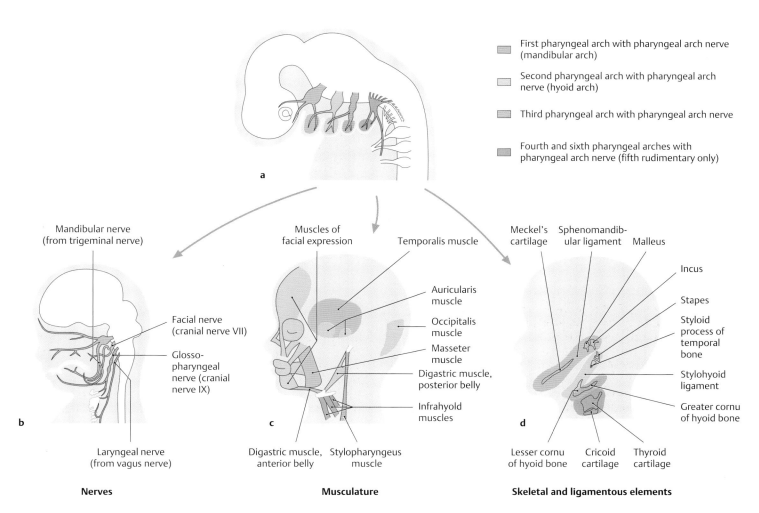

First pharyngeal arch with pharyngeal arch nerve (mandibular arch)

Second pharyngeal arch with pharyngeal arch nerve (hyoid arch)

Third pharyngeal arch with pharyngeal arch nerve

Fourth and sixth pharyngeal arches with pharyngeal arch nerve (fifth rudimentary only)

a

Mandibular nerve (from trigeminal nerve)

Facial nerve (cranial nerve VII)

Glosso-pharyngeal nerve (cranial nerve IX)

b

Laryngeal nerve (from vagus nerve)

Nerves

Muscles of facial expression

Temporalis muscle

Auricularis muscle

Occipitalis muscle

Masseter muscle

Digastric muscle, posterior belly

Infrahyold muscles

c

Digastric muscle, anterior belly   Stylopharyngeus muscle

Musculature

Meckel's cartilage   Sphenomandibular ligament   Malleus

Incus

Stapes

Styloid process of temporal bone

Stylohyoid ligament

Greater cornu of hyoid bone

d

Lesser cornu of hyoid bone   Cricoid cartilage   Thyroid cartilage

Skeletal and ligamentous elements

E The system of pharyngeal or branchial arches (after Sadler and Drews)

a Anlage of the embryonic pharyngeal arches with the associated pharyngeal arch nerves.

b Definitive arrangement of the future cranial nerves V, VII, IX, and X.

c Muscular derivatives of the pharyngeal arches.

d Skeletal derivatives of the pharyngeal arches.

F Derivatives of the pharyngeal (branchial) arches in humans

Pharyngeal arch	Nerve	Muscles	Skeletal and ligamentous elements
First (mandibular arch)	Cranial nerve V (mandibular nerve from the trigeminal)	Masticatory muscles – Temporalis – Masseter – Lateral pterygoid – Medial pterygoid Mylohyoid Digastric (anterior belly) Tensor tympani Tensor veli palatini	Malleus and incus Portions of the mandible Meckel's cartilage Sphenomandibular ligament Anterior ligament of malleus
Second (hyoid arch)	Cranial nerve VII (facial nerve)	Muscles of facial expression Stylohyoid muscle Digastric muscle (posterior belly) Stapedius	Stapes Styloid process of the temporal bone Lesser cornu of hyoid bone Upper part of hyoid body
Third	Cranial nerve IX (glossopharyngeal nerve)	Stylopharyngeus muscle	Greater cornu of hyoid bone Lower part of hyoid body
Fourth and sixth	Cranial nerve X (superior and recurrent laryngeal nerve)	Pharyngeal and laryngeal muscles	Laryngeal skeleton (thyroid cartilage, cricoid cartilage, arytenoid cartilage, corniculate and cuneiform cartilages)

1.6 Early Embryonic Circulation and the Development of Major Blood Vessels

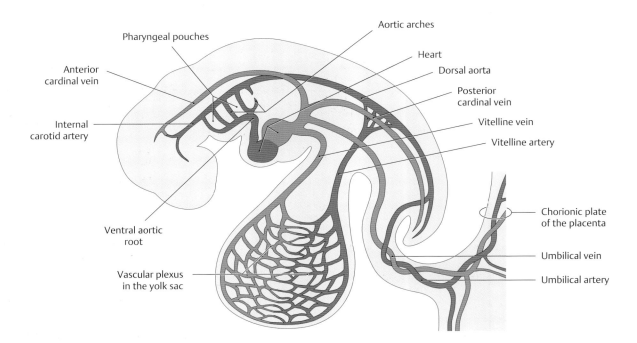

A Circulatory system of a 3- to 4-week-old human embryo
(after Drews)
Lateral view. The cardiovascular system of a 3- to 4-week-old human embryo consists of a well-functioning two-chambered heart and three distinct circulatory systems:

1. An **intraembryonic systemic circulation** (ventral and dorsal aorta, branchial arch and aortic arches, anterior and posterior cardinal veins)
2. An **extraembryonic vitelline circulation** (omphalomesenteric arteries and veins)
3. A **placental circulation** (umbilical arteries and veins)

The vascular pathways still show a largely symmetrical arrangement at this stage.

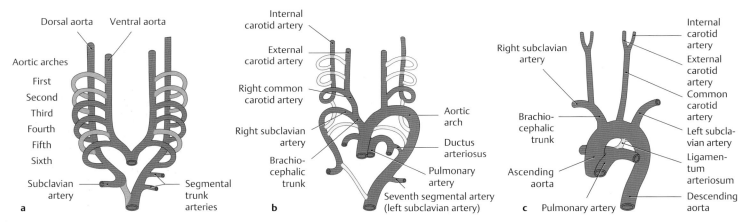

B Development of the arteries derived from the aortic arch
(after Lippert and Pabst)

a Initial stage (4-week-old embryo, ventral view). An artery develops in each of the pharyngeal arches, proceeding in the craniocaudal direction. These arteries arise from the paired ventral aortic roots, course through the mesenchyme of the pharyngeal arches, and open into an initially paired dorsal aorta. These vessels give rise to segmental trunk arteries. The six aortic arches are not all present at any one time, however. For example, while the fourth arch is forming, the first two arches are already beginning to regress. The development proceeds in such a way that the original symmetry is lost in favor of a preponderance on the left side.

b Structures that regress or persist: The first, second, and fifth aortic arches on both sides regress with continued development. The third

aortic arch gives rise to a common carotid artery on each side and the proximal portion of the internal carotid artery. The left fourth aortic arch later becomes the definitive *aortic arch*, while the artery on the right side becomes the proximal right subclavian artery. The left subclavian artery is derived from the seventh segmental artery. The trunk of the pulmonary arteries and the ductus arteriosus are derived from the sixth aortic arch.

c Variants in the adult: Besides the typical case pictured here (77%), there are numerous variants of the brachiocephalic trunk that occur with different frequencies. In the second most common pattern (13%), the left common carotid artery also arises from the brachiocephalic trunk. A right-sided aortic arch and a duplicated aortic arch each occur with a frequency of about 0.1%.

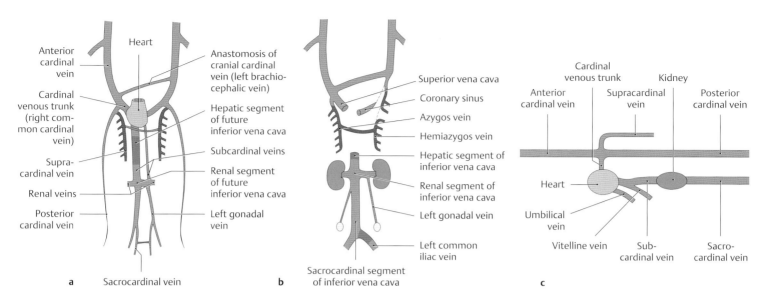

C Development of the cardinal venous system from weeks 5–7 to birth (after Sadler)

a At 5–7 weeks (ventral view), **b** at term (ventral view), **c** lateral view at 5–7 weeks.

Up until the 4th week of development, three paired venous trunks return the blood to the heart: the vitelline, umbilical, and cardinal veins. The cardinal venous system at this stage consists of the anterior, posterior, and common cardinal veins. The following additional cardinal venous systems are formed between weeks 5 and 7:

- **Supracardinal veins:** These vessels replace the posterior cardinal veins and receive blood from the intercostal veins (future azygos system: azygos and hemiazygos veins).
- **Subcardinal veins:** These vessels develop to drain the kidneys—the right subcardinal vein becoming the middle part of the inferior vena cava, and the transverse anastomosis becoming the left renal vein. The distal segment of the left subcardinal vein persists as a gonadal vein (testicular vein or left ovarian vein).
- **Sacrocardinal veins:** These vessels develop during the formation of the lower limbs, their transverse anastomosis becoming the left common iliac vein.

Characteristic transverse anastomoses are formed between the individual cardinal venous systems. These connections transfer blood from the right to the left side, channeling it to the inflow tract of the heart. The transverse anastomosis between the anterior cardinal veins, for example, forms the future left brachiocephalic vein. The future superior vena cava develops from the right anterior and common cardinal veins, while the left common cardinal vein contributes to the venous drainage of the heart (coronary sinus).

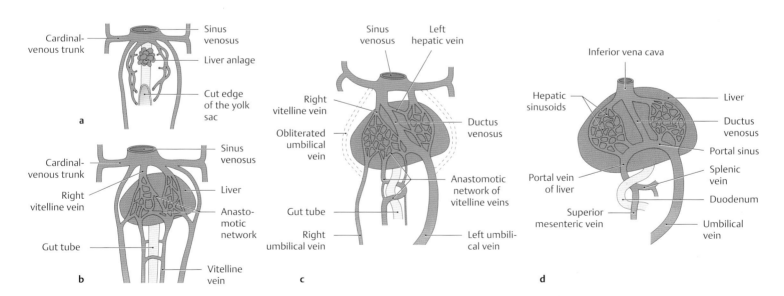

D Development of the vitelline and umbilical veins (after Sadler)

a 4th week, **b** 5th week, **c** 2nd month, **d** 3rd month (ventral view).

Before the vitelline veins (omphalomesenteric veins) open into the venous sinus, they form a venous plexus around the duodenum, perfuse the embryonic liver anlage, and form the first hepatic sinusoids. At this stage the two umbilical veins still course on both sides of the liver anlage. With further development, however, they establish a connection with the hepatic sinusoids. While the right umbilical vein regresses completely during the 2nd month, the left umbilical vein assumes the function of transporting all blood back from the placenta to the fetus. The blood flows through a shunt (ductus venosus) into the *proximal* trunk of the right vitelline vein (the future posthepatic part of the inferior vena cava) and back to the sinus venosus. The *distal* portion of the right vitelline vein develops into the future portal vein, by which blood is conveyed from the unpaired abdominal organs to the liver (superior and inferior mesenteric veins, splenic vein).

1.7 Primordial Skeleton, Prenatal Skeletal Development, and Ossification Centers

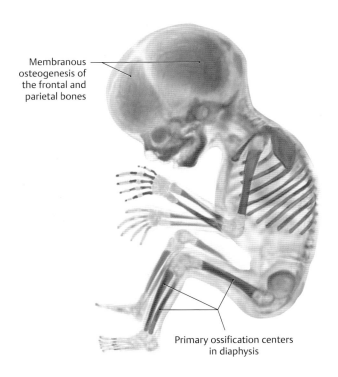

Membranous osteogenesis of the frontal and parietal bones

Primary ossification centers in diaphysis

Pharyngeal arches

Optic vesicles

Connecting stalk (with umbilical vessels)

Cardiac prominence

Vertebral column

Limb buds

a

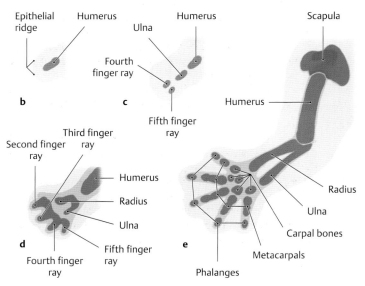

Epithelial ridge

Humerus

Ulna

Humerus

Fourth finger ray

Scapula

b

c

Humerus

Fifth finger ray

Third finger ray

Second finger ray

Humerus

Radius

Ulna

d

Fourth finger ray

Fifth finger ray

e

Carpal bones

Metacarpals

Phalanges

Humerus

Radius

Ulna

A Primordial skeleton, prenatal skeletal development, and ossification centers

(Transparent specimen of an 11-week-old fetus's ossification centers stained with alizarin red; after Starck and Drews). The supporting tissue of the human skeleton (mainly cartilage and bone tissue) arises from embryonic connective tissue (= mesenchyme), derived from the middle germ layer (= mesoderm, see p. 7, **D**). Mesenchymal cells initially differentiate into chondroblasts (endochondral osteogenesis), which form a miniature model of the skeleton in its final form (primordial skeleton) from hyaline cartilage. It is only at a later developmental stage that the hyaline cartilage is replaced by bone tissue. Endochondral osteogenesis leads to the formation of the largest part of the human skeleton (torso, limbs, and skull base). The ossification of the primordial skeleton begins at the end of the embryonic period (8th week). It extends from the secondary ossification centers in the diaphyseal region of the long bones (perichondral ossification = bone formation directly from the mesenchyme, thus desmal osteogenesis). Soon after, with the start of endochondral ossification (= bone formation around the cartilage, thus endochondral osteogenesis), the formation of primary ossification centers in the diaphysis begins. By the 12th week, there are ossification centers in all long bones. In the epiphysis, endochondral ossification (secondary ossification centers) only begins some time after birth (exception: distal femur and proximal tibial epiphysis, which already exist at birth). At birth, many short bones, e.g., most of the tarsal bones and all of the carpal bones, consist entirely of cartilage and form an ossification center only in the ensuing months and years. Only the bones of the cranial roof, parts of the facial bones, and the collar bone (clavicle) ossify directly (membranous osteogenesis, which means mesenchyme cells develop into osteoblasts [see p. 17]).

B Development of the limbs illustrated for the arm

At the end of the 4th week of embryonic development, the limb anlage (primordia) appear as paddle-shaped outpouchings around the lateral trunk regions (**a**). These limb buds consist of mesenchymal cells (so-called limb bud blastema, see p. 145) and an ectoderm covering with an apical epithelial thickening, the epithelial ridge (**b**). The growth and arrangement of the limb buds occurs within a three-dimensional coordinate system, which has both proximal-distal and cranial-caudal axes of differentiation. The humerus of the upper arm develops first, followed by the ulna and adjacent skeletal elements of the carpal roots (**c**). The ulna and the fourth and fifth finger rays are referred to as the postaxial (caudal) section; the radius and first, second, and third finger rays, as the preaxial (cranial) section (**d**). The finger and foot rays, for example, form when the cells of the epithelial ridge divide into five segments through programmed cell death (interdigital apoptosis [**e**]). In case of a disruption of apoptosis, adjacent fingers or toes fuse together (syndactyly). The absence of entire limbs is called *amelia*; the absence of parts of the arm or leg is called *meromelia*.

Note: Achondroplasia is a genetic disorder that causes a disruption in the endochondral ossification and is one of the most frequent causes of disproportionate short stature (short limbs, short trunk, too large of a skull relative to the rest of the body). Due to a disruption in cell division and maturation of the chondrocytes in the growth plates, all bones generated by endochondral osteogenesis remain too short. Membranous osteogenesis, however, proceeds normally.

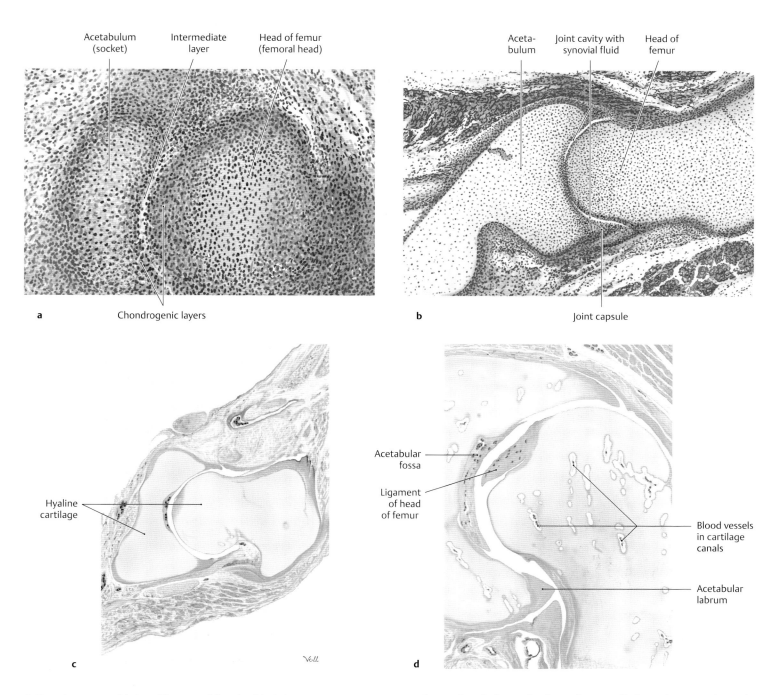

a — Acetabulum (socket) — Intermediate layer — Head of femur (femoral head) — Chondrogenic layers

b — Aceta-bulum — Joint cavity with synovial fluid — Head of femur — Joint capsule

c — Hyaline cartilage

d — Acetabular fossa — Ligament of head of femur — Blood vessels in cartilage canals — Acetabular labrum

C Development of joints illustrated for the hip joint (after Uhthoff)

a In the 6th week of embryonic development, cell condensation occurs where the joints will eventually develop. A three-layered joint interzone forms. It consists of two chondrogenic layers covering the cartilage anlage (primordia) and an intermediate layer containing fewer cells.

b Around the 8th week of embryonic development, programmed apop-topic cell death leads to the formation of the joint cavity around the intermediate layer. The joint capsule arises from the peripheral region of the joint interzone and begins to produce synovial fluid.

c After the joint cavity has been formed, hyaline cartilage develops in chondrogenic layers. At the end of the 12th week of embryon-ic development, the development of joints is complete. The final structure of the joint is determined by functional loads (e.g., mus-cle force), although the joint has a genetically predetermined shape.

d The joint continues to grow (interstitial and appositional growth). With the start of the 13th week of embryonic development, nutri-tion through diffusion from both the perichondrium and synovia of the joint cavity is no longer sufficient, which leads to the formation

of intrachondral vessels along the so-called cartilage canals. Only one area close to the joint cavity remains blood vessel-free. The vas-cularization of the cartilaginous epiphysis, however, stands in no relation to the development of the secondary ossification center. At the femoral head of the hip joint, for instance, there is a delay of about 12 months between the first vascularization (3rd month of embryonic development) and the appearance of the ossification center in the proximal femoral epiphysis (6th postnatal month).

Note: There are essentially two ways in which joints can develop:
• Through segmentation (most common form), meaning cleavage of a continuous skeletal condensation (applies to almost all joints: hip joint, shoulder joint, elbow joint, etc.).
• Through appositional growth, meaning two initially separate skel-etal elements grow toward one another (e.g., temporomandibular, sternoclavicular, and iliosacral joints). First, a synovial bursa forms at the junction between those elements, which then transforms into the joint cavity. In addition, intra-articular disks are typical for this type of joints (exception: iliosacral joint).

15

1.8 Bone Development and Remodeling

Bone development and bone remodeling are closely interrelated. During growth, for instance, bone undergoes a constant remodeling process in which immature woven bone tissue is replaced by "mature" lamellar bone. Continual remodeling also occurs in the mature skeleton, particularly in cancellous bone (called also trabecular or spongy bone, see **F**). In this way, on average, approximately 10% of the entire adult skeleton is remodeled each year, meaning that the skeleton is completely renewed over about a 10-year period. This process is basically a functional adaptation of the bones to the dominant stress patterns to which they are exposed (and which vary over time). It also serves to prevent material fatigue, repair microinjuries to bone, and provide a rapidly available source of calcium.

A Development of a long bone

The long bones (humerus, tibia, etc.) are mainly a product of *indirect* bone formation i.e., they form by replacing a preexisting cartilaginous model of the bone (*endochondral osteogenesis*). But portions of the long bones (the perichondrial bone collar, which allows the bone to grow in thickness) are a product of *direct* bone formation i.e., they form from the direct transformation of condensed mesenchyme (*membranous osteogenesis*, see **E**).

a Cartilaginous model of a bone in the embryonic skeleton. **b** Formation of a perichondrial bone collar (directly from mesenchyme). **c** Differentiation to hypertrophic chondrocytes and mineralization of the cartilaginous extracellular matrix. **d** Ingrowth of a diaphyseal vessel and formation of a primary ossification center. **e** Development of the proximal and distal growth centers (epiphyseal plates). **f** Appearance of the proximal epiphyseal ossification center (secondary ossification center). **g** Formation of the distal epiphyseal ossification center. **h** Closure of the distal epiphyseal plate. **i** Closure of the proximal epiphyseal plate (occurs at the end of skeletal growth, between about 18 and 23 years of age for most tubular bones).

Note: Osteogenesis = the formation of an individual bone; ossification = the formation of bone tissue.

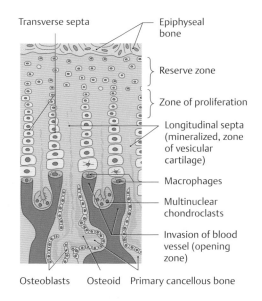

B Structure of the epiphyseal plate
a Blood supply, **b** detail from **a**: zones of the epiphyseal plate.

C Schematic representation of cellular processes within the epiphyseal plate

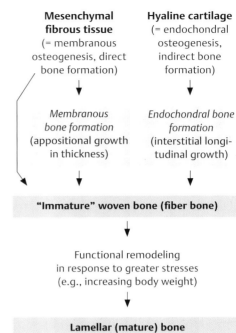

D Development of an osteon (after Hees)

The process of functional remodeling (see upper left page) begins with the invasion of blood vessels and accompanying osteoclasts ("bone-eating cells") into woven bone. They burrow through the woven bone like a drill, cutting a vascularized channel (resorption canal or cavity) that is equal in diameter to the future osteon.

a Longitudinal section through a resorption canal.
b Cross section at the level of the resorption canal.
c Transformation zone: osteoprogenitor cells (a kind of precursor for bone-forming cells) are transformed into osteoblasts.
d Osteogenic zone (osteoblasts produce bony lamellae).
e Newly formed osteon.

E Types of bone development (osteogenesis)

Note: Most bones are formed by *indirect* osteogenesis (the few exceptions include the clavicle and certain bones of the calvaria). But portions of these bones still develop from the direct transformation of mesenchyme, i.e., by *direct* osteogenesis.

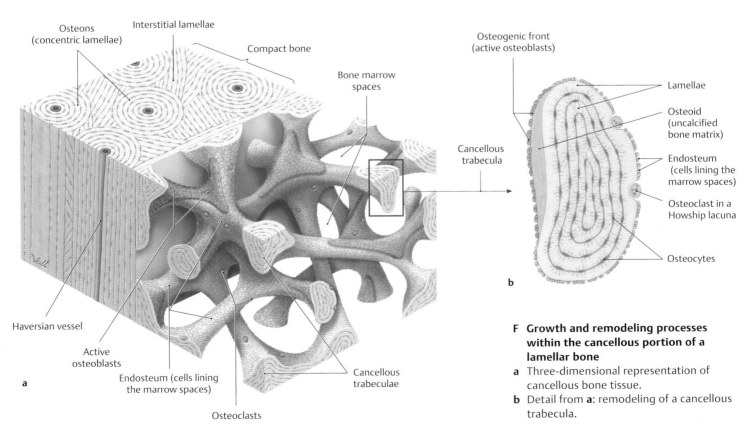

F Growth and remodeling processes within the cancellous portion of a lamellar bone

a Three-dimensional representation of cancellous bone tissue.
b Detail from **a**: remodeling of a cancellous trabecula.

1.9 Ossification of the Limbs

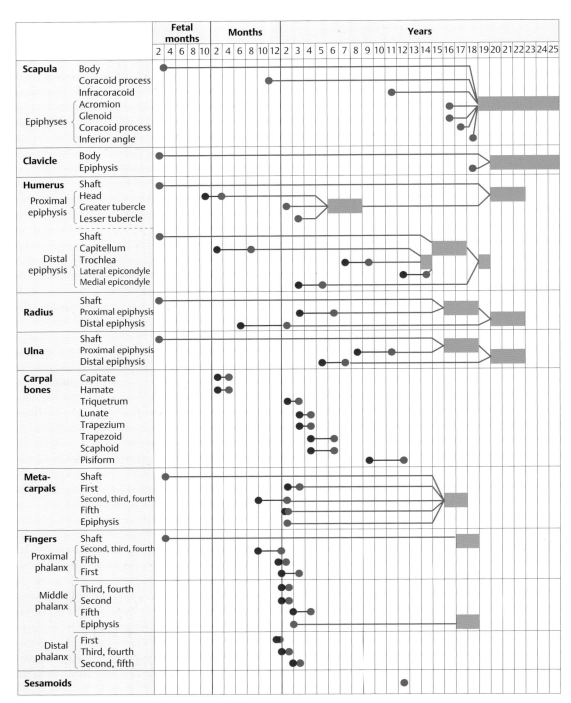

A Fetal months and first year of life are set off from the rest of the table.

Times of appearance of ossification centers:
- ● Female
- ● Male
- —— Period of ossification
- � Period of synostosis

a

b

B Ossification of the skeleton of the upper limb
- **a** Location of the epi- and apophyseal ossification centers.
- **b** Location of the epi- and apophyseal plates.

A and C Timetable of regional bone growth in the upper limb (A) and lower limb (C)
(from Niethard: *Kinderorthopädie* (Pediatric Orthopedics). Thieme, Stuttgart 1997)
The current stage of skeletal development, and thus the individual skeletal age, can be estimated from the times of appearance of the ossification centers. *Primary ossification centers*, which generally appear in the shaft region of bones *during the fetal period* (diaphyseal ossification), are distinguished from *secondary ossification centers*, which form *after birth* within the cartilaginous epiphysis and apophysis (epi-

and apophyseal ossification). Longitudinal growth ceases with the closure of the epiphyseal plate (synostosis). The greater tubercle of the humerus, for example, begins to ossify at 2 years of age. A period of synostosis follows from 6 to 8 years of age, and after that the greater tubercle shows only external, appositional growth. With the cessation of longitudinal growth, the ossification centers disappear and are no longer visible on X-ray films. The relationship between maturation and the appearance of secondary ossification centers is most clearly demonstrated in the bones of the carpus (see also **B**). The eight car-

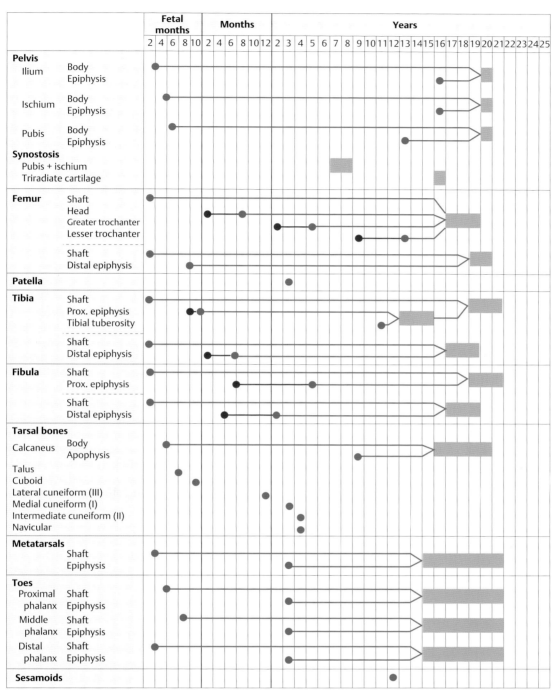

Table C — column headers: Fetal months (2 4 6 8 10), Months (2 4 6 8 10 12), Years (2 3 4 5 6 7 8 9 10 11 12 13 14 15 16 17 18 19 20 21 22 23 24 25)

Row labels:
- **Pelvis**
  - Ilium — Body / Epiphysis
  - Ischium — Body / Epiphysis
  - Pubis — Body / Epiphysis
- **Synostosis**
  - Pubis + ischium
  - Triradiate cartilage
- **Femur** — Shaft / Head / Greater trochanter / Lesser trochanter; Shaft / Distal epiphysis
- **Patella**
- **Tibia** — Shaft / Prox. epiphysis / Tibial tuberosity; Shaft / Distal epiphysis
- **Fibula** — Shaft / Prox. epiphysis; Shaft / Distal epiphysis
- **Tarsal bones**
  - Calcaneus — Body / Apophysis
  - Talus
  - Cuboid
  - Lateral cuneiform (III)
  - Medial cuneiform (I)
  - Intermediate cuneiform (II)
  - Navicular
- **Metatarsals** — Shaft / Epiphysis
- **Toes**
  - Proximal phalanx — Shaft / Epiphysis
  - Middle phalanx — Shaft / Epiphysis
  - Distal phalanx — Shaft / Epiphysis
- **Sesamoids**

C Fetal months and 1st year of life are set off from the rest of the table.

Times of appearance of ossification centers:
- ● Female   — Period of ossification
- ● Male   ▓ Period of synostosis

D Ossification of the skeleton of the lower limb

a Location of the epi- and apophyseal ossification centers.

b Location of the epi- and apophyseal plates.

pal bones ossify gradually over a period of approximately 9 years. The first ossification center is that of the capitate bone, which appears during the 1st year of life; the last is that of the pisiform bone, which ossifies at 9 years of age. It is standard practice to use the left or nondominant hand for radiographic examinations. The skeletal age reflects the biological maturity of the organism more than chronological age. The estimation of skeletal age, and thus of growth potential, is of key importance, for example, in the prognosis and treatment of orthopedic diseases and deformities in children. Also, given the relationship that exists between skeletal maturity and body height, the definitive adult height can usually be predicted with reasonable accuracy after 6 years of age based on the skeletal age and longitudinal measurements.

1.10 Basic Skeletal Structure and Development and Position of the Limbs

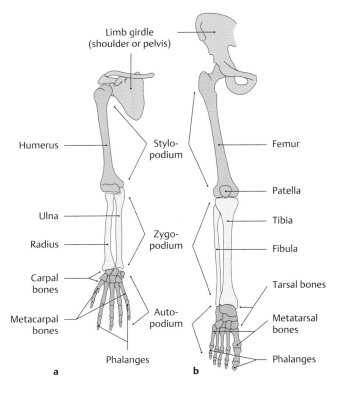

A Basic skeletal structure of a five-ray (pentadactyl) tetrapod limb (after Romer)

Both the forelimb and hindlimb of a free-ranging terrestrial verte-brate have the same basic, three-part structure consisting of a proxi-mal, middle, and distal segment (called the *stylopodium*, *zygopodium*, and *autopodium*). The elbow or knee joint is placed between the stylo-podium, which consists of a single bone (humerus or femur), and the zygopodium, which consists of two bones (the radius and ulna or the tibia and fibula). The five-ray autopodium (hand or foot) is also made up of proximal, middle, and distal units (called the *basipodium*, *metapo-dium*, and *acropodium*; see **C**). Additionally, there are some vertebrate classes that depart from this basic structure by showing a reduction or fusion of various bony units.

B Basic skeletal structure of the human limbs

Anterior view. **a** Right upper limb, **b** right lower limb.

The skeletal elements of the human upper and lower limbs have been colored to show how they are homologous with the tetrapod limb seg-ments shown in **A** (stylo-, zygo-, and autopodium). Congenital malfor-mations such as polydactyly or syndactyly (the presence of supernu-merary fingers or toes or their fusion) are not uncommon.

C Bony constituents of the pentadactyl tetrapod limb

Segments	Paired forelimbs	Paired hindlimbs
Limb girdle	Shoulder girdle – Scapula and clavicle	Pelvic girdle – Hip bone
Free limbs		
Stylopodium	Arm (brachium) – Humerus	Thigh (femur) – Femur
Zygopodium	Forearm (antebrachium) – Radius – Ulna	Leg (crus) – Tibia – Fibula
Autopodium	Hand	Foot
– Basipodium	Carpus – Proximal row: radiale, intermedium, ulnare – Central group: centralia I–IV – Distal row: carpals I–V	Tarsus – Proximal row: tibiale, intermedium, fibulare – Central group: centralia I–IV – Distal row: tarsals I–V
– Metapodium	Metacarpus – Metacarpals I–V	Metatarsus – Metatarsals I–V

– Acropodium	Fingers
	– Digits I–V
	  (with different numbers of phalanges)
		Toes
		– Digits I–V
		  (with different numbers of phalanges)

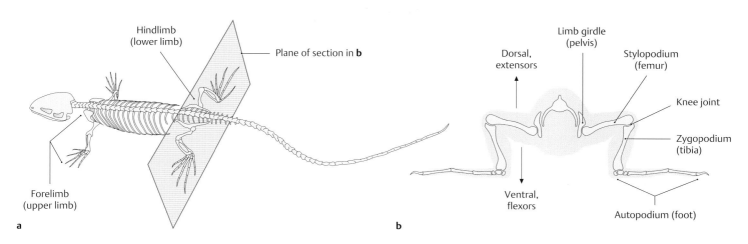

a

b

D Limb positions in a primitive terrestrial tetrapod (the lizard *Lacerta viridis*)

a Dorsal view, **b** cross section at the level of the hindlimbs.

In amphibian and reptilian tetrapods (e.g., salamanders, turtles, and lizards), the trunk is slung between the limbs and frequently touches the ground. The limbs are set almost at right angles to the body, so that the arm and thigh are nearly horizontal, and the elbow and knee point outward. The radius and ulna and the tibia and fibula are flexed at right angles at the elbow and knee. The volar surface of the hand and the plantar surface of the foot are in contact with the ground. The axes of all the joints are directed parallel to the spinal column (see **E**). *Note* that the *extensor* muscles are placed *dorsally*, while the *flexor* muscles are *ventral*. Thus, the location of the extensors and flexors relative to the bone does not change with evolution—the bone merely assumes a different alignment (see also **F**).

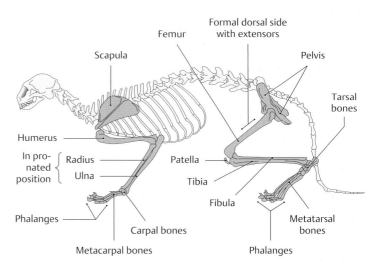

E Rotation of the limbs in mammalian evolution

a Before rotation, **b** after rotation.

An important feature of mammalian evolution involved *rotation* of the tetrapod limb. The limb was reoriented, placed parallel to the body, and moved closer to or beneath the body. This improved locomotion and supported the body more efficiently. The hindlimb rotated *forward* (with the knee pointing cephalad), while the forelimb rotated *backward* against the body (the elbow pointing caudad). As a result, both sets of limbs assumed a sagittal orientation under or alongside the trunk (see **F**).

F Skeleton of a cat (*Felis catus*)

Left lateral view. In order for the volar surfaces of the forelimbs to rest on the ground despite the backward angulation of the elbows, the forearm bones must cross to a pronated position. In the hindlimbs, there is no need for pronation of the leg bones because the thigh is rotated forward.

This arrangement of the skeletal elements in the various limb segments is essentially preserved in humans. Because the lower limb has been rotated forward, the *former dorsal side* of this limb faces *forward* in a human standing upright. As a result, the extensors of the thigh and leg (the genetically "dorsal" muscles) are on the anterior side of the limb, placed in front of the corresponding limb bones. This is one reason why the terms "anterior" and "posterior" are preferred over "dorsal" and "ventral" in the human lower limb. By contrast, the extensors and flexors of the arm and forearm have maintained their original dorsal and ventral positions, respectively.

2.1 The Human Body: Proportions, Surface Areas, and Body Weights

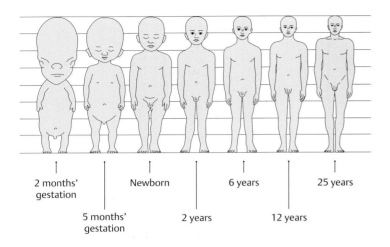

2 months' gestation   Newborn   6 years   25 years

5 months' gestation   2 years   12 years

A Change in body proportions during growth
While the head height in embryos at 2 months' gestation is equal to approximately half the total body length, it measures approximately one fourth of the body length in newborns, one sixth in a 6-year-old child, and one eighth in an adult.

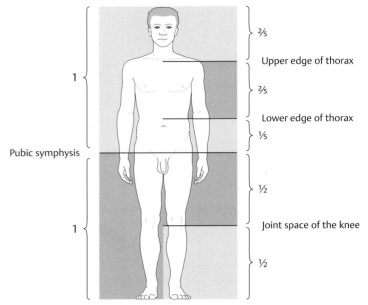

Pubic symphysis

⅖   Upper edge of thorax
⅖   Lower edge of thorax
⅕
½
Joint space of the knee
½

B Normal body proportions
In an adult, the midpoint of the total body height lies approximately at the level of the pubic symphysis; i.e., there is a 1:1 ratio of upper to lower body height at that level. The pelvis accounts for one fifth of the upper body height, the thorax for two fifths, and the head and neck for two fifths. The lower body height is distributed equally between the thigh and leg (plus heel) at the joint space of the knee.

C Span of the outstretched arms
The arm span from fingertip to fingertip is slightly *greater* than the body height (approximately 103% in women and 106% in men).

D Selected body measurements in the standing and sitting human being (unclothed, 18–65 years of age) after DIN 33402-2 (from Ergonomie—Körpermaße des Menschen—Teil 2: Werte. Berlin: Beuth; 2005)
The percentile values indicate what percentage in a population group are below the value stated for a particular body measurement (in this case, all those living in Germany, thus including migrants in the years 1999–2002). For example, the 95th percentile for body height in males 18 to 65 years of age with a body height of 185.5 cm means that 95% of this population group are shorter than 185.5 cm, and 5% are taller.

Measurements (in cm) (points 9, 10, 20, and 21 not shown)	Male 5th	Male 50th	Male 95th	Female 5th	Female 50th	Female 95th
1 Forward reach	68.5	74.0	81.5	62.5	69.0	75.0
2 AP body thickness	26.0	28.5	38.0	24.5	29.0	34.5
3 Overhead reach (with both arms)	197.5	207.5	220.5	184.0	194.5	202.5
4 Body height	165.0	175.0	185.5	153.5	162.5	172.0
5 Ocular height	153.0	163.0	173.5	143.0	151.5	160.5
6 Shoulder height	134.5	145.0	155.0	126.0	134.5	142.5
7 Elbow-to-floor distance	102.5	110.0	117.5	96.0	102.0	108.0
8 Hand-to-floor distance	73.0	76.5	82.5	67.0	71.5	76.0
9 Shoulder width	44.0	48.0	52.5	39.5	43.5	48.5
10 Hip width, standing	34.0	36.0	38.5	34.0	36.5	40.0
11 Sitting body height (trunk height)	85.5	91.0	96.5	81.0	86.0	91.0
12 Ocular height while sitting	74.0	79.5	85.5	70.5	75.5	80.5
13 Elbow to sitting surface	21.0	24.0	28.5	18.5	23.0	27.5
14 Height of leg and foot (height of sitting surface)	41.0	45.0	49.0	37.5	41.5	45.0
15 Elbow to gripping axis	32.5	35.0	39.0	29.5	31.5	35.0
16 Sitting depth	45.0	49.5	54.0	43.5	48.5	53.0
17 Buttock–knee length	56.5	61.0	65.5	54.5	59.0	64.0
18 Buttock–leg length	96.5	104.5	114.0	92.5	99.0	105.5
19 Thigh height	13.0	15.0	18.0	12.5	14.5	17.5
20 Width above the elbow	41.5	48.0	55.5	39.5	48.5	55.5
21 Hip width, sitting	35.0	37.5	42.0	36.0	39.0	46.0

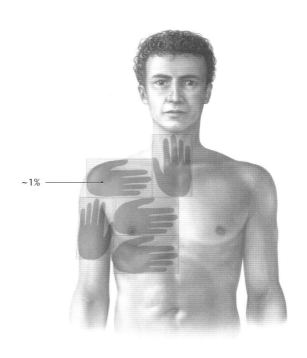

E Distribution of body surface area in adults, children, and infants

According to the "rule of nines" described by Wallace (1950), the body surface area of adults over about 15 years of age (**a**) can be divided into units that are a *multiple* of 9%: the head and each arm account for 9% each, the front and back of the trunk and each leg account for 18% (2×9) each, and the external genitalia comprise 1%. In children (**b**) and infants (**c**), the rule of nines must be adjusted for age.

Note: The rule of nines can be used in burn victims to provide a quick approximation of the area of skin that has been burned.

F Hand area rule

The percentage of the body surface affected by burns can be accurately estimated with the hand area rule, which states that the area of the patient's hand is approximately 1% of the patient's own total body surface area. The hand rule also applies to children, whose hands and total surface area are both proportionately smaller than in adults.

G Dependence of relative body surface area (skin surface area) on age, and consequences

For progressively larger solid bodies, the surface area increases as the square of the radius, but the volume increases as the cube of the body's radius. Because of this basic geometrical relationship, smaller animals generally have a larger relative surface area than larger animals. A higher ratio of surface area to volume causes smaller animals to radiate relatively more body heat. As a result, small animals, such as mice and children, tend to have a higher metabolic rate than larger animals, such as elephants and human adults.

Age	Body weight (kg)	Body surface area (cm²)	Body surface area over body weight (cm²/kg)
Newborn	3.4	2100	617.6
6 months	7.5	3500	466.7
1 year	9.3	4100	440.9
4 years	15.5	6500	419.4
10 years	30.5	10,500	344.3
Adult	70.0	18,100	258.6

H Body mass index

In anthropometry, the body mass index (BMI) has become the international standard for evaluating body weight because it correlates relatively well with total body fat. BMI is defined as the body weight in kilograms divided by the square of the height in meters:

$$BMI = \frac{kg}{m^2}$$

2.2 The Structural Design of the Human Body

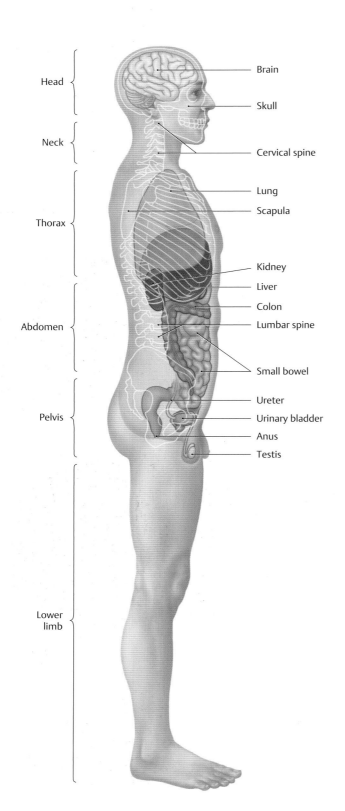

Head
— Brain

— Skull

Neck
— Cervical spine

Thorax
— Lung

— Scapula

— Kidney

— Liver

— Colon

Abdomen
— Lumbar spine

— Small bowel

Pelvis
— Ureter

— Urinary bladder

— Anus

— Testis

Lower limb

A Location of the internal organs
Lateral view.

B Regional subdivisions of the body

Head

Neck

Trunk
- Thorax (chest)
- Abdomen
- Pelvis

Upper limb
- Shoulder girdle
- Free upper limb

Lower limb
- Pelvic girdle
- Free lower limb

C Functional subdivisions by organ system

Locomotor system (musculoskeletal system)
- Skeleton and skeletal connections (passive part)
- Striated skeletal musculature (active part)

Viscera
- Cardiovascular system
- Hemolymphatic system
- Endocrine system
- Respiratory system
- Digestive system
- Urinary system
- Male and female reproductive system

Nervous system
- Central and peripheral nervous system
- Sensory organs

The skin and its appendages

D Topography of body cavities, serous cavities, and connective-tissue spaces

Organs and organ systems are embedded either in serous cavities or in connective-tissue spaces of varying size. A serous cavity is a fully enclosed potential space that is lined by a shiny membrane (serosa) and contains a small amount of fluid. The serosa consists of two layers that are *usually* apposed (both layers are not *necessarily* in direct contact, as in the abdominal cavity): a visceral layer that directly invests the organ, and a parietal layer that lines the wall of the serous cavity.

Enclosed serous cavities
- Thoracic cavity:
  - Pleural cavity
  - Pericardial cavity

- Abdominal cavity
  - Peritoneal cavity of the abdomen
- Pelvic cavity
  - Peritoneal cavity of the pelvis

Connective-tissue spaces
- Space between the middle and deep layers of cervical fascia
- Mediastinum
- Extraperitoneal space with
  - the retroperitoneal space (retroperitoneum) and
  - the subperitoneal space
- Bursa and synovial cavities

Note: The peritoneal cavities of the abdomen and pelvis are connected.

Cranial cavity

Pericardial cavity

Pleural cavity

Retroperitoneal space

Extraperitoneal space

Thoracic cavity

Abdominal cavity

Pelvic cavity

E Selected planes of section through the human body Superior view

a Midsagittal section.
b Cross section at the level of the head.
c Cross section through the thorax.

d Cross section through the abdomen.
e Cross section through the lesser pelvis (see also Terms of Location and Direction, Cardinal Planes and Axes, p. 26).

3.1 Terms of Location and Direction, Cardinal Planes and Axes

A General terms of location and direction

Upper body (head, neck, and trunk)

Cranial	Pertaining to or located toward the head
Cephalad	Directed toward the head
Caudal	Pertaining to or located toward the tail
Caudad	Directed toward the tail
Anterior	Pertaining to or located toward the front
	Synonym: Ventral (used for all animals)
Posterior	Pertaining to or located toward the back
	Synonym: Dorsal (used for all animals)
Superior	Upper or above
Inferior	Lower or below
Medius	Located in the middle
Flexor	Pertaining to a flexor muscle or surface
Extensor	Pertaining to an extensor muscle or surface
Axial	Pertaining to the axis of a structure
Transverse	Situated at right angles to the long axis of a structure
Longitudinal	Parallel to the long axis of a structure
Horizontal	Parallel to the plane of the horizon
Vertical	Perpendicular to the plane of the horizon
Medial	Toward the median plane
Lateral	Away from the medial plane (toward the side)
Median	Situated in the median plane or midline
Central	Situated at the center or interior of the body
Peripheral	Situated away from the center
Superficial	Situated near the surface
Deep	Situated deep beneath the surface
External	Outer or lateral
Internal	Inner or medial
Apical	Pertaining to the tip or apex
Basal	Pertaining to the bottom or base
Occipital	Pertaining to the back of the head
Temporal	Pertaining to the lateral region of the head (the temple)
Sagittal	Situated parallel to the sagittal suture
Coronal	Situated parallel to the coronal suture (pertaining to the crown of the head)
Rostral	Situated toward the nose or brow
Frontal	Pertaining to the forehead
Basilar	Pertaining to the skull base

Limbs

Proximal	Close to or toward the trunk
Distal	Away from the trunk (toward the end of the limb)
Radial	Pertaining to the radius or the lateral side of the forearm
Ulnar	Pertaining to the ulna or the medial side of the forearm
Tibial	Pertaining to the tibia or the medial side of the leg
Fibular	Pertaining to the fibula or the lateral side of the leg
Palmar (volar)	Pertaining to the palm of the hand
Plantar	Pertaining to the sole of the foot
Dorsal	Pertaining to the back of the hand or top of the foot

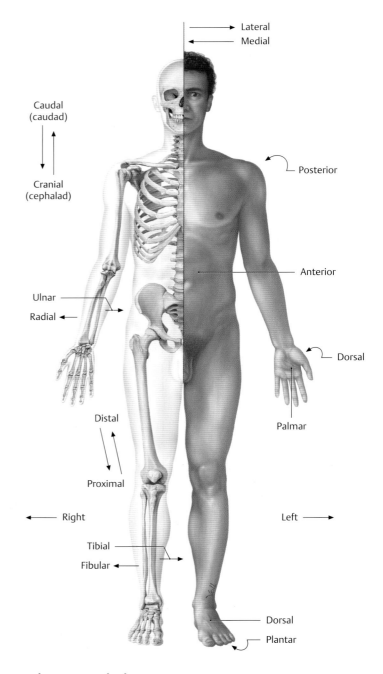

B The anatomic body position

The gaze is directed forward, the hands are supinated. The *right* half of the body is shown in light shading to demonstrate the skeleton.
Note that the designations "left" and "right" always refer to the patient.

C Abbreviations

a. artery (aa. = arteries)
v. vein (vv. = veins)
m. muscle (mm. = muscles)
lig. ligament (ligs. = ligaments)
l. n. lymph node(s)

D Cardinal planes and axes in the human body (neutral position, left anterolateral view)

Although any number of planes and axes can be drawn through the human body, it is standard practice to designate *three cardinal planes and axes*. They are perpendicular to one another and are based on the three spatial coordinates.

The cardinal body planes:

- **Sagittal plane:** Any *vertical* plane that is parallel to the sagittal suture of the skull, passing through the body from front to back. The *midsagittal plane* (= median plane) divides the body into equal left and right halves.
- **Frontal (coronal plane):** Any plane that is *parallel to the forehead* or to the coronal suture of the skull. In the standing position, it passes vertically through the body from side to side.
- **Transverse plane (axial plane):** Any *horizontal*, cross-sectional plane that divides the body into upper and lower portions. It is perpendicular to the longitudinal body axis.

The cardinal body axes:

- **Vertical or longitudinal axis:** In the standing position, this axis runs through the body *craniocaudally* and is perpendicular to the ground. It lies at the intersection of the coronal and sagittal planes.
- **Sagittal axis:** This axis runs *anteroposteriorly* from the front to back surface of the body (or from back to front) and lies at the intersection of the sagittal and transverse planes.
- **Transverse or horizontal axis:** This axis runs from side to side and lies at the intersection of the coronal and transverse planes.

E Axis deviation of upper and lower limbs

Joint deformities at the limbs can lead to axis deviation in the two articulating bones in both frontal and sagittal planes. In accordance with international guidelines, axis deviation in the frontal plane is called varus or valgus deformity and recurvation or antecurvation in the sagittal plane. A varus deformity in the knee joint exists if the axis deviation is concave to the vertical body axis or if the distal bone (the tibia) points to the median line (e.g., genu varum = bow-leggedness). In a valgus deformity of the knee joint, the axis deviation is convex to the vertical body axis, or the tibia points away from the median line (e.g., genu valgum = knock knee).

F The whole-body center of gravity and the line of gravity

a Anterior view. The line of gravity is directed vertically along the midsagittal plane, passing through the whole-body center of gravity below the sacral promontory at the level of the second sacral vertebra.

b Lateral view. The line of gravity passes through the external auditory canal, the dens of the axis (second cervical vertebra), the anatomic and functional junctions within the spinal column, the whole-body center of gravity, and through the hip, knee, and ankle joints (after Kummer).

3.2 Location and Designation of Imaging Planes

A Radiographic planes, illustrated for the skull

a Just as there are three standard anatomic sectional planes (frontal, sagittal, and transverse planes, see p. 27), certain standard sectional planes have been defined for the most important imaging techniques (computed tomography [CT] and magnetic resonance imaging [MRI]).

Radiographic plane		Anatomic plane
Coronal plane	=	Frontal plane (along or parallel to coronal suture)
Sagittal plane	=	Sagittal plane (along or parallel to sagittal suture)
Axial plane	=	Transverse plane (at the head, parallel to the Frankfurt horizontal plane, or at the trunk and limbs, vertical to the corresponding longitudinal axes)

b The Frankfurt horizontal plane (transverse plane) extends from the upper margin of the external auditory canal to the lower margin of the orbital cavity.

c u.d As a general rule, CT scans of the skull or the brain are slanted at a 19-degree angle from anterior to posterior (along the so-called canthomeatal line). This line extends from the upper margin of the external auditory canal to the canthus (corner of the eye) and protects the contents of the orbit from heavy X-ray exposure.

B Standard planes in MRI shoulder examination

The patient lies on his or her back with the arm of the shoulder joint that is to be examined positioned parallel to the body in arm outward rotation or neutral (null) position.

a Position of the axial (transverse) plane of the left shoulder, anterior view.

b Position of the angled coronal plane (parallel to the supraspinatus and vertical to the glenoid cavity), superior view.

c Position of the angled sagittal plane (parallel to the glenoid cavity), superior view.

Thanks to the imaging of the body in multiple sectional planes (or multiplane imaging) and the particularly good differentiation of the periarticular soft tissues, MRI is very well suited for joint exams. Depending on the sectional plane selected and the relaxation time (T1- and T2-weighted scans), the tissues can be differentiated according to their anatomic position and their fat and water percentages. *Note:* Axial (transverse) planes (see **D**) are always viewed from below (distal).

C Optimal MRI planes to show important anatomic structures of shoulder joint

MRI plane	Important visible anatomic structures
Axial (transverse) plane	• Supraspinatus • Glenoid labrum • Joint capsule • Glenohumeral ligaments • Tendon of biceps femoris, long head
Angled coronal plane	• Supraspinatus • Infraspinatus • Subacromial bursa • Acromioclavicular joint • Upper and lower glenoid labrum
Angled sagittal plane	• Rotator cuff • Coracoacromial ligament • Acromion • Glenohumeral ligament • Subacromial space

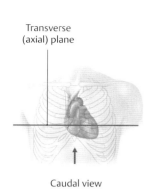

Transverse
(axial) plane

Caudal view

a

b

c

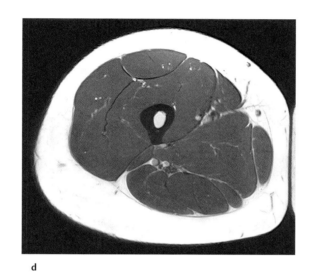

d

D Examining axial images
a u. b trunk; c–e lower limb.

a Anterior view of thorax and location of the transverse (axial) plane at the level of T8.

b Axial CT of thorax (inferior view) in the so-called soft-tissue window, which means the soft tissue (the heart) can be evaluated in high resolution; the lungs, however, because they are filled with air, are overexposed (black), and the bones are underexposed (white).

c Right upper thigh, anterior view, and position of the transverse (axial) plane.

d Axial, T1-weighted MRI of right thigh, distal view.

e Anatomic cross section with description of truncated structures.

Axial (transverse) CT and MRI images are viewed from below and distally for limbs: the patient lies on his or her back. Thus, axial images always show the posteriorly positioned spinal cord pointing downward, the anteriorly positioned skeleton of the thorax pointing upward. Correspondingly, the front of the upper thigh points upward and the back, downward; structures on the right side are displayed on the left side, and structures on the left side are displayed on the right side. *Note:* Coronal (frontal) cross sections are viewed as if the patient stands in front of the examiner.

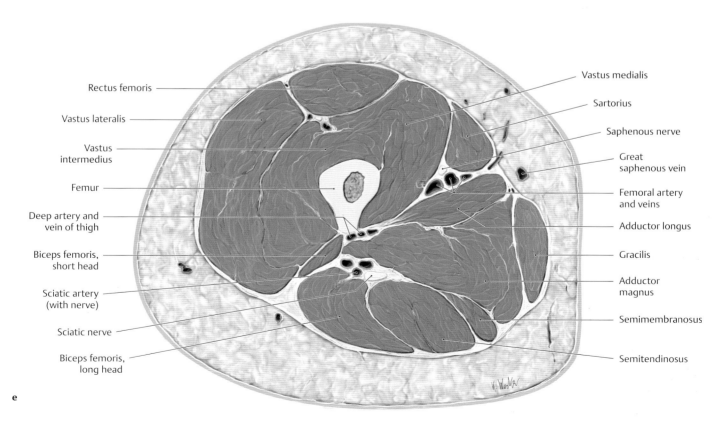

Rectus femoris

Vastus lateralis

Vastus intermedius

Femur

Deep artery and vein of thigh

Biceps femoris, short head

Sciatic artery (with nerve)

Sciatic nerve

Biceps femoris, long head

Vastus medialis

Sartorius

Saphenous nerve

Great saphenous vein

Femoral artery and veins

Adductor longus

Gracilis

Adductor magnus

Semimembranosus

Semitendinosus

e

29

3.3 Body Surface Anatomy

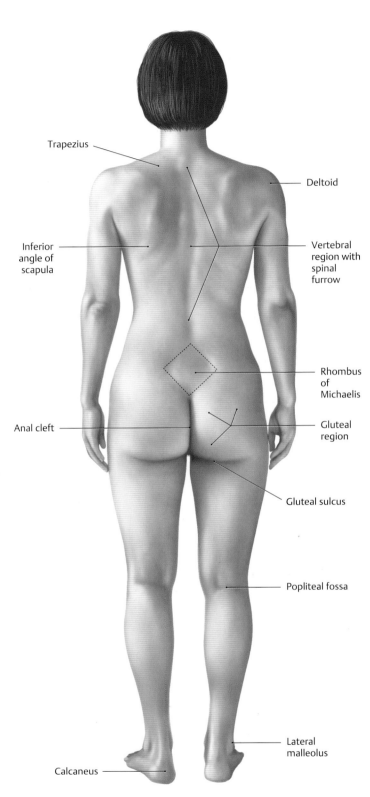

A Body surface anatomy of the female
Anterior view. Body surface anatomy deals with the surface anatomy of the living subject. It plays an important role in classic methods of examination (inspection, palpation, percussion, auscultation, function testing), and so it has particular significance in clinical examination courses. To avoid repetition, identical structures such as the olecranon have not been labeled on both the female and male bodies.

B Body surface anatomy of the female
Posterior view.

Larynx

Acromio-
clavicular
joint

Sternocleido-
mastoid

Supraclavicular
fossa

Pectoralis
major
muscle

Linea
alba

Tendi-
nous
in-
scriptions

Costal
margin

Semilunar
line

Umbilicus

Penis

Scrotum

Glans penis

Quadriceps
femoris

Head of fibula

Tibial
tuberosity

Dorsum
of foot

Vertebra
prominens
(C7)

Trapezius

Scapular
spine

Medial
border of
scapula

Olecranon

Iliac
crest

Intrinsic
back
muscles

Sacral
triangle

Styloid
process
of ulna

Semimembra-
nosus

Gastrocnemius
and soleus
(triceps surae)

Calcaneal
(Achilles')
tendon

C Body surface anatomy of the male
Anterior view.

D Body surface anatomy of the male
Posterior view.

31

3.4 Body Surface Contours and Palpable Bony Prominences

Palpable bony prominences are important landmarks for anatomic orientation in the skeleton, as it is not always possible to palpate articulating skeletal structures (e.g., the hip joint). In these cases, the examiner must rely on palpable bony prominences as an indirect guide to the location of the inaccessible structure.

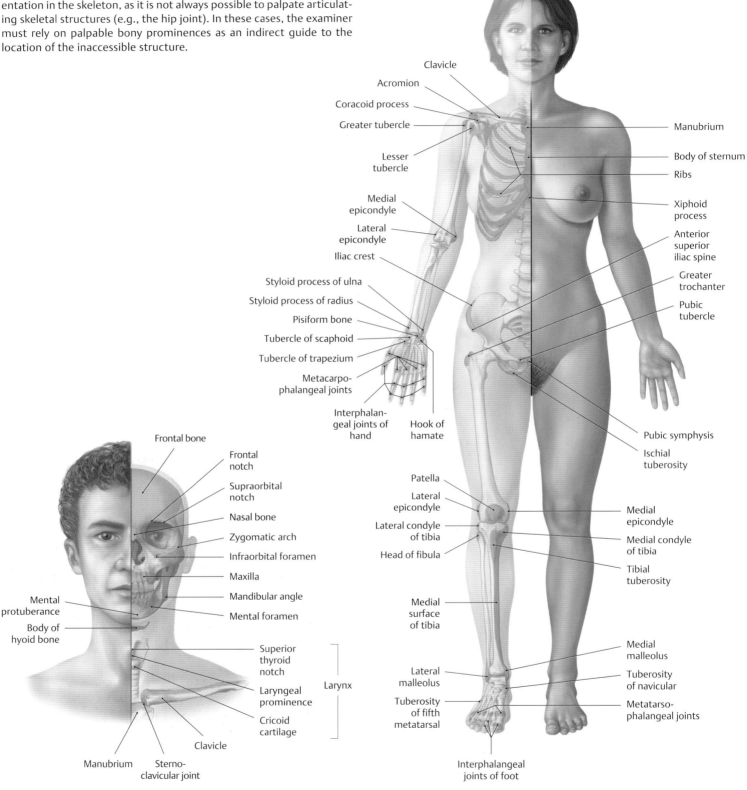

A Surface contours and palpable bony prominences of the face and neck
Anterior view.

B Surface contours and palpable bony prominences of the trunk and upper and lower limbs in the female
Anterior view.

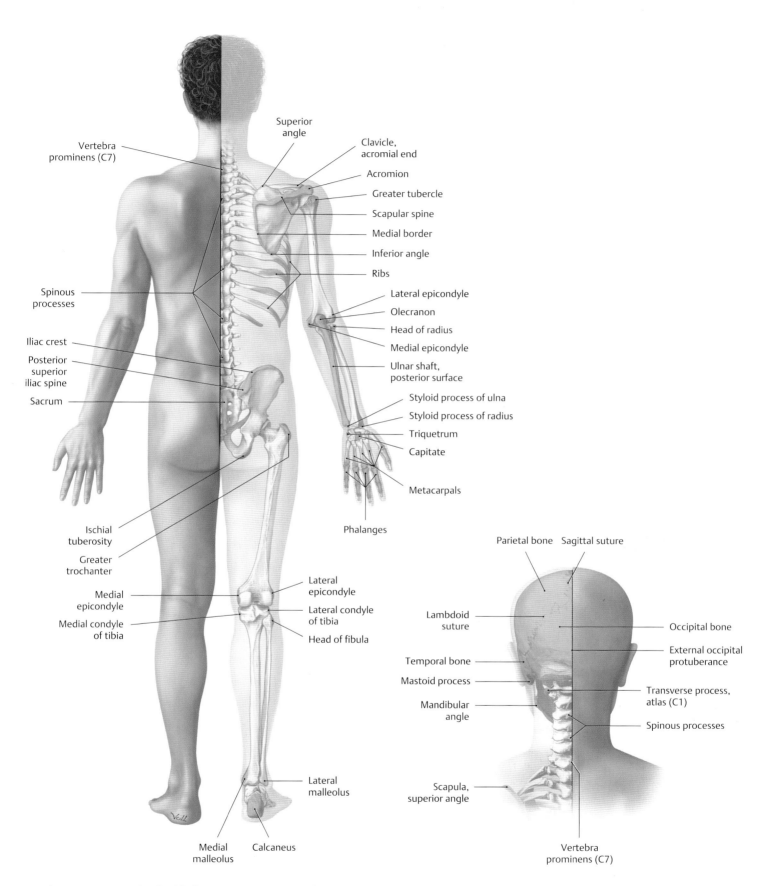

Vertebra prominens (C7)

Superior angle

Clavicle, acromial end

Acromion

Greater tubercle

Scapular spine

Medial border

Inferior angle

Ribs

Lateral epicondyle

Olecranon

Head of radius

Medial epicondyle

Ulnar shaft, posterior surface

Styloid process of ulna

Styloid process of radius

Triquetrum

Capitate

Metacarpals

Phalanges

Spinous processes

Iliac crest

Posterior superior iliac spine

Sacrum

Ischial tuberosity

Greater trochanter

Medial epicondyle

Medial condyle of tibia

Lateral epicondyle

Lateral condyle of tibia

Head of fibula

Lateral malleolus

Medial malleolus

Calcaneus

Parietal bone   Sagittal suture

Lambdoid suture

Temporal bone

Mastoid process

Mandibular angle

Scapula, superior angle

Occipital bone

External occipital protuberance

Transverse process, atlas (C1)

Spinous processes

Vertebra prominens (C7)

C Surface contours and palpable bony prominences of the trunk and upper and lower limbs in the male
Posterior view.

D Surface contours and palpable bony prominences of the head and neck
Posterior view.

33

3.5 Landmarks and Reference Lines on the Human Body

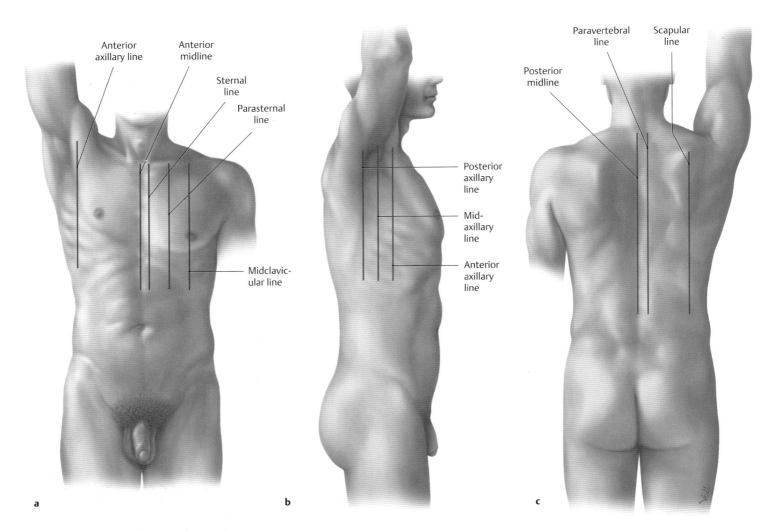

A Vertical reference lines on the trunk
a Anterior view, **b** right lateral view, **c** posterior view.

Anterior midline	Anterior trunk midline passing through the center of the sternum
Sternal line	Line along the sternal margin
Parasternal line	Line midway between the sternal line and midclavicular line
Midclavicular line	Line through the midpoint of the clavicle (often identical to the nipple line)
Anterior axillary line	Line at the level of the anterior axillary fold (pectoralis major muscle)
Midaxillary line	Line midway between the anterior and posterior axillary lines
Posterior axillary line	Line at the level of the posterior axillary fold (latissimus dorsi muscle)
Posterior midline	Posterior trunk midline at the level of the spinous processes
Paravertebral line	Line at the level of the transverse processes
Scapular line	Line through the inferior angle of the scapula

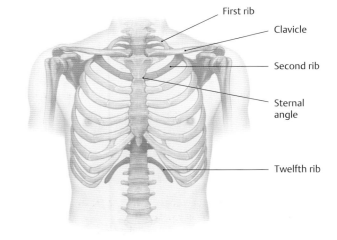

B "Rib counting" for anatomic orientation in the thorax
The first rib is covered by the clavicle. The first palpable rib is the second rib; therefore, the count begins at that level. The second rib attaches to the sternum at the level of the sternal angle. At the lower end of the rib cage, it is best to start at the twelfth rib, which is palpable only in its posterior portion.

34

C Standard transverse planes through the abdominal cavity
(see also p. 199)
Anterior view.

Transpyloric plane	Transverse plane midway between the superior borders of the symphysis and manubrium
Subcostal plane	Plane at the lowest level of the costal margin (inferior margin of the tenth costal cartilage)
Supracrestal plane	Plane passing through the summits of the iliac crests
Intertubercular plane	Plane at the level of the iliac tubercles (the iliac tubercle lies approximately 5 cm posterolateral to the anterior superior iliac spine)
Interspinal plane	Plane at the level of the anterior superior iliac spine

D Spinous processes that provide useful posterior landmarks
Posterior view.

C7 spinous process	Vertebra prominens (the projecting spinous process of C7 is clearly visible and palpable)
T3 spinous process	At the level of the line connecting the two scapular spines
T7 spinous process	At the level of the line connecting the inferior angles of both scapulae
T12 spinous process	Just below the twelfth rib
L4 spinous process	At the level of the line connecting the summits of the iliac crests
S2 spinous process	At the level of the line connecting the posterior superior iliac spine (recognized by small skin depressions directly over the iliac spines)

E Lithotomy position (supine with the legs, hips, and knees flexed and the thighs abducted)
The position of choice for proctological examinations. Clock-face notation is used for anatomic orientation (e.g., to describe the location of a lesion):

- Top = toward the pubis = 12 o'clock
- Bottom = toward the sacrum = 6 o'clock
- Right = 3 o'clock
- Left = 9 o'clock

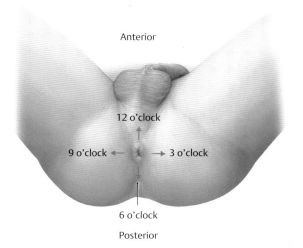

3.6 Body Regions (Regional Anatomy)

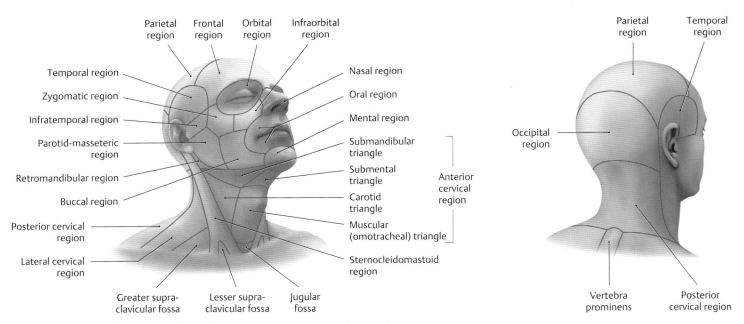

A Regions of the head and neck
Right anterolateral view.

B Regions of the head and neck
Right posterolateral view.

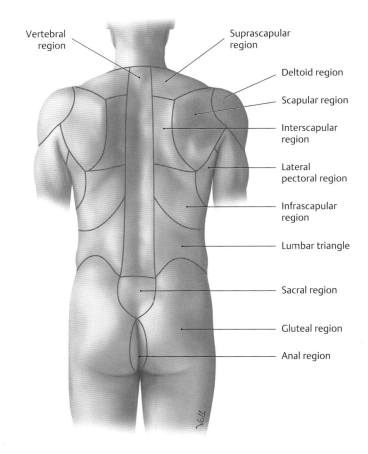

C Regions of the thorax and abdomen
Anterior view.

D Regions of the back and buttocks
Posterior view.

Deltoid region

Scapular region

Posterior arm region

Posterior cubital region

Posterior forearm region

Posterior carpal region

Dorsum of hand

E Regions of the upper limb
Posterior view.

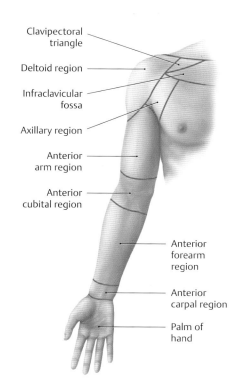

Clavipectoral triangle

Deltoid region

Infraclavicular fossa

Axillary region

Anterior arm region

Anterior cubital region

Anterior forearm region

Anterior carpal region

Palm of hand

F Regions of the upper limb
Anterior view.

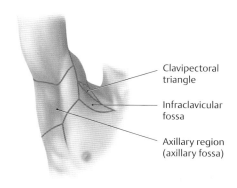

Clavipectoral triangle

Infraclavicular fossa

Axillary region (axillary fossa)

G Regions about the axilla
Anterior view.

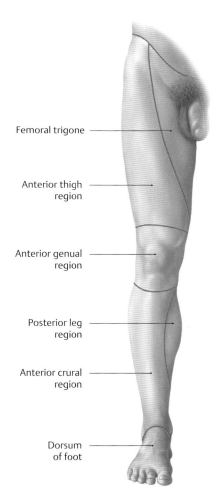

Femoral trigone

Anterior thigh region

Anterior genual region

Posterior leg region

Anterior crural region

Dorsum of foot

H Regions of the lower limb
Anterior view.

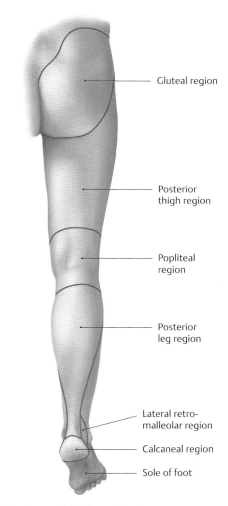

Gluteal region

Posterior thigh region

Popliteal region

Posterior leg region

Lateral retro-malleolar region

Calcaneal region

Sole of foot

I Regions of the lower limb
Posterior view.

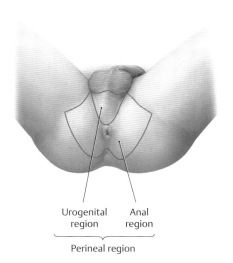

Urogenital region

Anal region

Perineal region

J Perineal region (lithotomy position)

37

4.1 The Bony Skeleton and the Structure of Tubular Bones

A Human skeleton from the anterior view
The left forearm is pronated, and both feet are in plantar flexion.

B Human skeleton from the posterior view
The left forearm is pronated, and both feet are in plantar flexion.

C Types of bone

- **Long bones,** e.g., tubular bones of the limbs
- **Short bones,** e.g., carpal and tarsal bones
- **Flat bones,** e.g., scapula, ilium, and bones of the calvaria
- **Irregular bones,** e.g., vertebrae anomalous, supernumerary bones not consistently present, as in the skull base

- **Pneumatic bones** (containing air-filled spaces), e.g., bones of the facial skeleton and paranasal sinuses
- **Sesamoid bones** (bones incorporated in tendons), e.g., the patella
- **Accessory bones** (anomalous, supernumerary bones), as in the calvaria and foot (generally result from the failure of fusion of certain adjacent ossification centers)

D Structure of a typical tubular bone, illustrated for the femur

a Coronal saw cuts have been made through the proximal and distal parts of an adult femur (without sectioning the midshaft region).

b Detail from **a**: The sectioned areas display the lamellar architecture ("lamellar bone") of the cancellous trabeculae. The lamellae are arranged in contiguous plates, similar to plywood. Since the cancellous trabeculae do not have an actual vascular supply and are nourished by diffusion from the adjacent medullary cavity, the trabeculae attain a thickness of only about 200–300 μm.

c Detail from **a**: Three-dimensional representation of compact bone, whose structural units consist of vascularized osteons approximately

1 cm long and 250–350 μm in diameter. The haversian canals, which tend to run longitudinally in the bone, are connected to one another by short transverse and oblique Volkmann canals and also to the vessels of the periosteum and medullary cavity.

d Detail from **c**, demonstrating the microstructure of an osteon. The haversian canal at the center is surrounded by approximately 5 to 20 concentric lamellar systems composed of osteocytes and extracellular matrix. The osteocytes are interconnected by numerous fine cytoplasmic processes.

e Detail from **c**, showing the structure of the periosteum.

4.2 Continuous and Discontinuous Joints: Overview and False Joints (Synarthroses)

A Different types of joints

False joints	True joints
(Synarthroses; continuously connected by connective tissue, cartilage, or bone; low to moderate degree of mobility; see right side)	(Separated by a joint space; mobility is variable, depending on the attached ligaments = discontinuous connection)

• **Syndesmoses** (fibrous joints, e.g., newborn fontanelles)
• **Synchondroses** (cartilaginous joints, e.g. spinal disks; if the intervening tissue is mostly fibrocartilaginous, the joint is called a symphysis, e.g., pubic symphysis)
• **Synostoses** (sites of bony fusion, e.g., sacral bone)
	• **Diarthroses** (joints with varying degrees of freedom, see p. 42); classified according to
	  – Shape and arrangement of articular surfaces (spheroidal, ellipsoidal, and saddle joints)
	  – Number of joint axes
	  – Number of degrees of freedom
	• **Amphiarthroses** (stiff joints, e.g., iliosacral joint)

B Short glossary

- **Pseudarthrosis:** So-called false joint (instability due to missing wedge of bone) after abnormal fracture healing (see p. 53).
- **Ankylosis:** Abnormal bony fixation of a true joint (see **C**).
- **Arthrodesis** (called spondylodesis in the spinal cord): Surgically induced joint ossification by performing osteosynthesisis procedure (see p. 53 bottom **D**).
  - Main indicators: infectious arthritis, post-traumatic joint destruction, degenerative joint diseases, and paralytic instability.
  - Principle: loss of mobility in favor of absence of pain and stability.
  - Important for good joint motion postsurgery: stabilization in mode of function, which means in the position that is crucial for the most important joint functions, such as grasping for the arm and standing and walking for the leg.
- **Arthrotomy:** Surgical opening of a joint.
- **Arthrography:** Examination of the joint cavity using x-rays with the aid of a contrast agent (has increasingly lost relevance after rise in the use of MRI).
- **Arthroscopy:** Endoscopic examination of the joint, often associated with ensuing endoscopic therapy, e.g., arthroscopic reconstruction of injured ligament and capsule structures, removal of loose bodies, and treatment of joint cartilage defects (e.g., osteochondrosis dissecans).
- **Synovectomy:** Removal of the synovial membrane, e.g., in chronic polyarthritis.
- **Joint puncture** (intra-articular injection): Puncture of a joint space to remove fluid (e.g., in an articular effusion) or application of substances (medication).
- **Joint endoprosthesis:** Joint replacement surgery through total or partial endoprosthesis in advanced joint disease (arthritis) (see p. 46).

C Ankylosis of the knee joint

Illustration based on a specimen from the anatomic collection of the University in Kiel. Following the complete loss of cartilage, bone gradually fills the joint cavity, resulting in complete stiffness of the joint.

a   b

D T-arthrodesis after Lambrinudi for treatment of a club foot deformity (after Niethard and Pfeil)

Right foot before (**a**) and after (**b**) arthrodesis treatment, lateral view. The surgical goal is to repair the club foot position caused by stiffness (arthrodesis) to achieve a plantigrade foot (lower leg and foot form a 90-degree angle) while at the same time maintaining mobility in the upper ankle joint. Since three joints (subtalar, talonavicular, and calcaneocuboid joints, see p. 454) are fused or stiffened, the procedure is called T-arthrodesis for "triple arthrodesis." It involves resecting the talar head and interlocking it with the navicular bone by performing osteosynthesis.
Note: In case of instability and ankle joint misalignment, arthrodesis is the safest treatment method.

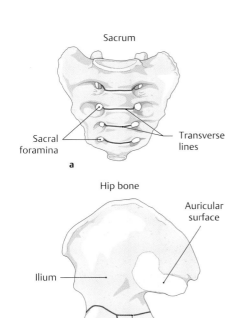

E Syndesmoses (fibrous joints)
a Interosseous membrane.
b Tibiofibular syndesmosis.
c Fontanelles.

d Gomphosis (immovable articulation).
e Ligamentum flavum, interspinous ligament, and supraspinous ligament.

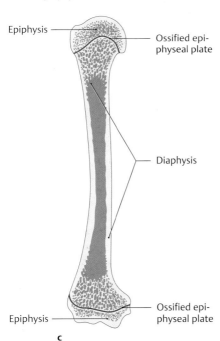

F Synchondroses (cartilaginous joints)
a Epiphyseal plates prior to closure.
b Hip bone before closure of the growth plates.

c Costal cartilage.
d Pubic symphysis and intervertebral disks (intervertebral symphysis).

G Synostoses (sites of bony fusion)
a Sacrum (fused sacral vertebrae).
b Hip bone (fusion of the ilium, ischium, and pubis).
c Closed and ossified epiphyseal plates.

41

4.3 True Joints: Components and Intra- and Extra-articular Structures

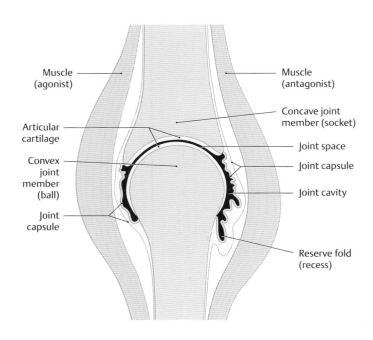

A Structure of a true joint

In true joints, the articulating joint surfaces are separated by cavities measuring no more than a few millimeters in width (diarthroses), unlike false joints, in which the joint surfaces are connected (synarthroses). True joints are also called synovial joints, as the joint capsule produces synovial fluid. In addition to the cavity, true joints have the following characteristics:

- Variously shaped articular surfaces covered by hyaline cartilage
- Joint cavity with articular recesses, the width of which vary
- All-around closed joint capsule increased by variously shaped alar folds, synovial folds, and synovial villi
- Highly viscous synovial fluid produced by joint capsule
- Intra-articular components to improve joint congruency and increase force-absorbing surface, e.g., articular menisci, disks, and labra
- Various forms of ligaments, with intra- and extracapsular ligaments acting as primary joint stabilizers
- Joint crossed by muscles that move it in opposite directions (agonist/antagonist)
- Synovial bursa, often located near the joint and thus articulating with the joint cavity
- Not all of the above are present in all true joints.

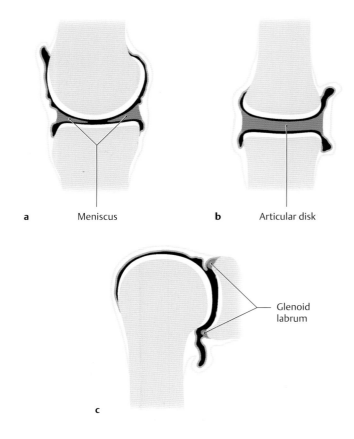

B Intra-articular structures and their importance to functional integrity of joints

Some joints contain intra-articular structures that ensure stability and function. For example, they increase the force-transmitting surface by balancing out incongruencies between the different parts of the joint, thus considerably reducing the compressive force on the cartilage. By definition, intra-articular structures are located in the articular cavity and float within synovial fluid, which means they are in direct contact with the synovial fluid through which they are primarily nourished (menisci, disks, articular labra).

a **Menisci:** Crescent-shaped structures, wedge-shaped in cross section, which are formed regularly in the knee only. They consist of collagen fibers, connective tissue, and fibrous cartilage. While their peripheral components are supplied by blood vessels of the joint capsule with which they are conjoined, the interiorly located fibrocartilaginous components are nourished by the synovia.

b **Articular disks** partially consist of connective tissue and fibrous, cartilaginous, disk-like structures, which divide the joint into two separate chambers. Articular disks are regularly found in the jaw, sternoclavicular joint, and proximal wrist joint (see p. 287).

c **Articular labra** are wedge-shaped structures at the outer margins of the osseous hip and shoulder joint sockets (glenoid and acetabular labra, see pp. 266 and 430). They consist mainly of fibrocartilage, and their outer layer is composed of connective tissue, the fibers of which are joined to the capsules. The articular labra enlarge the articulating surfaces of the shoulder and hip joint.

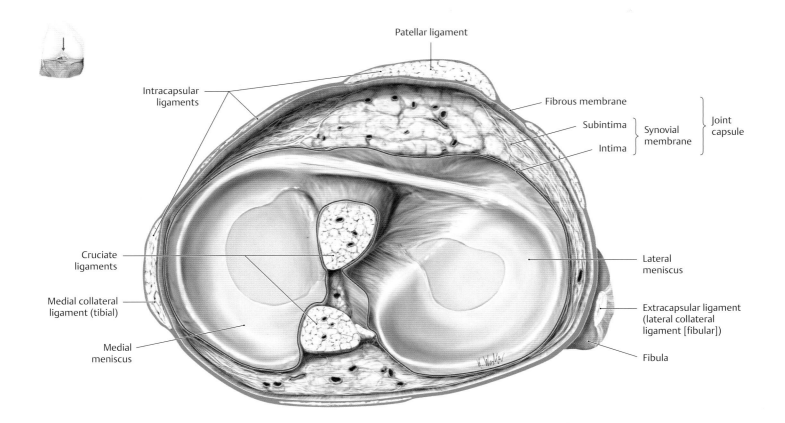

Patellar ligament

Intracapsular ligaments

Fibrous membrane

Subintima
Intima
Synovial membrane
Joint capsule

Cruciate ligaments

Lateral meniscus

Medial collateral ligament (tibial)

Extracapsular ligament (lateral collateral ligament [fibular])

Medial meniscus

Fibula

C The joint ligaments: extra-articular structures, which are usually located intracapsular (inside the joint capsule)

Intracapsular ligaments can run along both in the subintima (cruciate ligaments) and in the fibrous membrane (e.g., iliofemoral, ischiofemoral, and pubofemoral ligaments of the hip joint). They strengthen the capsule and thus serve mainly mechanical functions. For example, they are responsible for stabilizing and guiding the joint (guiding ligaments) or, to varying degrees, limiting or restricting motion (restraining ligaments). Occasionally, the joint ligaments extend without any direct contact to the actual joint capsule (extracapsular ligaments), such as the fibular collateral ligament in the knee joint. Often, ligament structures, which at first seem to run in the articular cavity (e.g., the cruciate ligaments in the knee joint, see p. 444, and the ligament of the head of the femur in the hip joint), are incorrectly called intra-articu-lar ligaments. However, unlike the meniscus and the articular labrum, they are always covered by a thin synovial intima and thus run subintimally. Strictly speaking, they are located inside the capsule, which means they are intracapsular, and thus outside the actual joint capsule, which means they are extra-articular (see p. 44).

Note: Ligaments must have the "right" length in order to be able to guide and stabilize the joint. If they are overstretched or tear (as a result of chronic overuse or injuries, e.g., as sprains or dislocation), the joint becomes unstable. If ligaments shorten because the joint is not moved or held permanently in an unfavorable position (e.g., knee joint in bent position, proximal phalanges in stretched position), the joint becomes more or less immobile (joint contracture).

D Composition and function of synovial fluid

Synovial fluid is a clear, slightly yellowish, viscous fluid (product of secretion of the synovial cysts; pH value 7.4–7.7). Even in large joints, such as the knee joint, its volume is only 3–5 mL (less than 1 mL in small joints).

Compositon	Function
• Hyaluronate (or hyaluronic acid), lubricin (mucin-like glycoprotein), and phospholipids • Blood plasma components (mainly blood proteins and glucose) • Defense cells 60–150/μL (mainly macrophages and lymphocytes)	① Nourishing the hyaline cartilage, which is devoid of blood vessels, through diffusion and convection ② Lubricating the cartilaginous articular surfaces, thus enabling frictionless motion ③ Functioning as a buffer by evenly distributing pressure across the articular surfaces

4.4 True Joints: Structure of Joint Capsule and Hyaline Cartilage

A Sructure of joint capsule and hyaline cartilage

The joint cavity of true joints is fully enclosed by a joint capsule, the two layers of which differ morphologically from one another and serve different functions:

Joint capsule

Fibrous membrane – WALL
(firm, collagenous connective tissue; fibers extend to the periosteum). Thickness varies both within one joint and in different joints, in many joints reinforced by ligaments (intracapsular ligaments), see p. 43

Synovial membrane – WALLPAPER
(attached to the margin of the joint capsule)

Synovial intima – lining cells (1 to 3 layers of epithelial-like [not epithelial cells because no basal membrane] covering cells); **production and resorption of synovial fluid.**

Type A synoviocytes (boundary layer to the joint capsule): macrophage-like cells with vacuoles, Golgi apparatus, mitochondria, lysosomes; resorption of used synovial fluid and phagocytosis of bacteria and cell debris

Type B synoviocytes (underneath the type A synoviocytes): fibroblast-like cells with rough endoplasmic reticulum, secretory granules; mainly production of synovial fluid

Synovial subintima (connective tissue with blood and lymph vessels, pain receptors [free nerve endings], and mechanoreceptors [Pacini and Ruffini bodies = proprioceptors], which react to changes in lengths or tension in the joint capsule = **helps guide joint movement sequences**), structure differs based on topography

- **Areolar synovial membrane** (loose, richly vascularized connective tissue)
- **Adipose synovial membrane** (mainly fat cells in connective tissue)
- **Fibrous synovial membrane** (vessel-poor and collagen-rich connective tissue)

Note: The **synovial membrane** can regenerate into old age, even after complete removal (= synovectomy; necessary, e.g., in cases of chronic arthritis due to rheumatism).

The synovial membrane reacts to stimuli by increased secretion, which appears as articular effusion and swelling in the entire joint region. Depending on the type of stimuli (mechanical, allergic, infectious), the effusion is either clear and thin or turbid and pus-filled. A true bloody effusion (hemarthrosis) develops in the wake of injuries (e.g., cruciate ligament rupture). The ensuing pain is the result of overstretching the joint capsule and the release of inflammatory mediators (e.g., prostaglandins, histamines, bradykinin, and cytokines). With the exception of the jaw and sternoclavicular joint, which are covered by fibrous cartilage, all articular surfaces are covered by **hyaline cartilage**. It is malleable and reacts to pressure (elastic compression). Depending on the amount of pressure, its thickness varies—ranging from 1–2 mm in the phalangeal joints to 5–7 mm in the femoropatellar joints. Hyaline cartilage consists of extracellular matrix (ECM) and chondrocytes (approximately 5% volume fraction).

Note: While the synovial membrane can regenerate through the adjoining connective tissue, the hyaline cartilage (except in the primordial skeleton) does not have any surrounding connective tissue (perichondrium) and thus can hardly regenerate. In addition, it is devoid of vessels. The cartilage cells (chondrocytes) must exclusively be nourished by synovial fluid (diffusion and convection, see **D**, on the right).

Hyaline cartilage can be divided into zones. They are determined by the arcade-like course the collagen fibrils follow (**a**). From zone IV (deepest zone, where the collagen fibrils are connected to the bone underneath the cartilage), the collagen fibrils extend almost vertically (radially) to the articular surface (zone III), then turn to follow a course parallel to the surface (zone II), and again after a short tangential course extend downward (zone I).

The collagen fibrils are visible only under the transmission electron microscope. In a light microscope image, they are "masked" as they break the light just as their surroundings do. After enzymatically liberating chondrocytes and proteoglycans using hyaluronidase, looking through the transmission electron microscope creates the impression of empty "cartilage holes" that are surrounded by a thick mesh of collagenous fibrils (for composition of collagen fibrils, see **d**). Proteoglycans, a component of the extracellular matrix, however, are clearly visible under the light microscope because they carry many negative charges, which can be visualized by using dyes such as hematoxylin (see **c**).

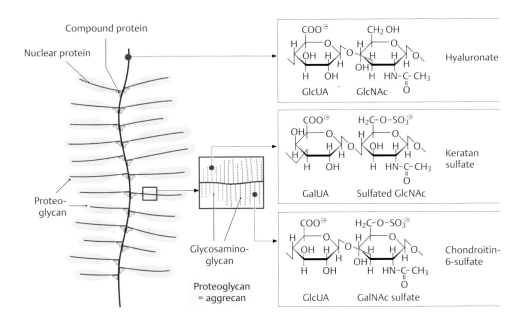

B Structure and function of extracellular matrix (ECM)

The extracellular matrix (all macromolecules that are secreted by cartilage cells and immobilized when interacting with other molecules in the extracellular space) primarily consists of

- Collagen fibers or fibrils (mainly collagen type II, IX, and XI)
- Proteoglycans (mainly aggrecan) with glycosaminoglycans (e.g., hyaluronate, chondroitin, and keratan sulfate), as well as core and compound proteins
- Glycoproteins (e.g., adhesion proteins such as chondronectin)
- Interstitial fluid (water) and electrolytes (mainly cations, Ca^+, K^+, Na^+)

The collagen fibrils (diameter of 15–130 nm) consist of collagen molecules, each of which are formed by three polypeptide chains (α-chains) and have the shape of a right-handed screw (triple helix). Individual triple helices (tropocollagens) are cross-linked by covalent connections, which give them their extraordinary tensile strength.

C Aggrecan, the most important proteglycan of the hyaline cartilage (after Koolman and Roehm)

Proteoglycans such as aggrecan are very large molecular complexes that consist of more than 100 glycosaminoglycan chains. They look like a bottle brush, with the individual glycosaminoglycan molecules as "bristles," affixed to a central hyaluronate molecule through so-called compound proteins. Disaccharide units, which mostly consist of a uric acid (e.g., glucuronic acid, GlcUA) and a type of amino sugar (e.g., *N*-acetylgalactosamine, GalNAc) and usually carry two negative charges (one each on the carboxyl and on the sulfate groups), form the basic structure of the glycosaminoglycan chains. For reasons of electroneutrality, the proteoglycans bind cations, which thanks to osmosis can reversibly bind a lot of water. Due to their strong water-binding capabilities, proteoglycan molecules take up huge volumes of water and thus create large, space-filling structures. GalUA, galacturonic acid; GlcNAc, *N*-acetylglucosamine.

D Biphasic viscoelastic model of the joint cartilage (after Mow and colleagues)

Firmness and elasticity during compression of the cartilage are crucial for the proper functioning of the joints. They are both ensured by the swelling pressure (the principle of the elastic spring). It arises from the interaction of proteoglycans and collagen fibrils in the extracellular matrix (ECM), where they collaborate to carry out particular functions. The extraordinary tensile strength of the collagen fibrils allows for mechanical stability and structural integrity of the joint cartilage. The polyanionic proteoglycans ensure its physiochemical properties (e.g., reversible water-binding capacity). In free, watery fluid, proteoglycans, which are negatively charged, would normally greatly expand by repelling each other. They are prevented from doing so only by the tensile strength of the collagen fibrils, so they can take up only one fifth of the space they actually require. There is only a limited possibility for further compressing the proteoglycans. If cartilaginous tissue is subjected to mechanical pressure (normal pressure), interstitial fluid and cations escape into the joint cavity, and the ECM increasingly thickens. As a result, it is harder for fluid to drain from the cavity, the hydrostatic pressure in the tissue rises (viscid components of the viscoelastic model), until the hydrostatic pressure from inside and mechanical pressure from outside are in balance, and no further compression occurs. With the thickening of the ECM, the negatively charged glycosaminoglycans approach each other, leading to an increased repulsion force as a result of which negative pressure builds up. When the pressure is relieved, the tissue swells up to its original size due to proteoglycans repelling each other, and interstitial fluid and free cations migrate anew into the tissue (elastic component of the viscoelastic model) until the collagen network again puts a stop to it. The flow of interstitial fluid is also called *convection*. It is a crucial precondition for the nourishment of the joint cartilage, which does not contain blood vessels.

4.5 Degenerative Joint Diseases as Exemplified by Hip Joint Arthrosis

A Etiology and pathogenesis of osteoarthritis

For many years now, degenerative joint diseases—mainly osteoarthritis—have been the top cause of disability worldwide. Due to the high cost of treatment and the large number of days employees are absent at work, osteoarthritis represents a major economic problem. Elderly people are particularly affected. The seeming increase in cases of this disease over the past few decades is due to people reaching ever higher ages, which allows them to actually experience their osteoarthritis (higher age and degenerative joint disease don't necessarily go hand in hand).

The main cause of osteoarthritis is an imbalance between the load and the capacity of the articular cartilage. Secondary osteoarthritis (in contrast to primary osteoarthritis, the cause of which is not pathologic) develops almost exclusively due to suboptimal biomechanics, e.g., in cases of incongruencies of the articulating surfaces. Over- or incorrectly loaded joints play a major role, e.g., caused by post-traumatic deformities, joint dysplasia, axis deviation, and instabilities. In particular, an increasing number of sports injuries lead to osteoarthritis. Excess weight, lack of exercise, and bad nutrition further contribute to the development of osteoarthritis. Early detection and correction of axis deviations or osteotomies to correct joint incongruencies are of particular significance for the prevention of osteoarthritis. If osteoarthritis has already developed, and conservative therapies have been exhausted, in addition to performing arthrodesis (joint stiffening, see p. 40), there is a possibility to replace the joint (endoprosthesis, see **C**).

One of the main causes of the disease is the gradual attrition, meaning the wear and tear and destruction, of the articular cartilage (see **D**). If the hyaline cartilage is too heavily loaded over the long term (see etiology), it disrupts the regular flow of interstitial fluid into the articular cartilage (see p. 40). This affects not only the elasticity but also the nourishment of the bradytrophic cartilage (no blood vessels), which, due to its limited metabolism and a missing perichondrium, is barely able to regenerate (see p. 44). As a result of increased mechanical overload of articular cartilage areas, both cartilage matrix and chondrocytes are damaged (see **D**). This damage is irreversible; complete restoration or repair is not possible. There are, however, endogenic compensatory mechanisms, which are supposed to make up for the loss of cartilage in the early stages (I and II, see **D**) and the increased pressure in the subchondral bone in the late stages (III and IV). The body's attempts to repair itself explain the shift between pain-free periods and periods marked by heavy pain. Heavily loaded joints such as hip or knee joints or the intervertebral joints of the spinal column are per se affected by osteoarthritis (see **B**).

* Synonyms: osteoarthrosis—in contrast to arthritis, in the process of which the cartilage disappears only secondarily as a result of inflammation of the articular cartilage.

Shoulder joint

Vertebral joints

Hip joint

Thumb basal joint

Proximal interphalangeal joints

Distal interphalangeal joints

Knee joint

B Preferred locations for degenerative joint diseases

Socket

Ball

Bone cement

Prosthesis stem

a Cemented TEP　　　**b** Noncemented TEP

C Total endoprosthesis (TEP) of the hip joint

Endoprosthetic joint replacement has become a possibility for almost all joints. The best results, particularly in terms of long-term success, have been achieved in the hip joint (replacement of head and socket). The implants—usually made of metal, synthetic material, or ceramic—are either attached to the joint with a special cement or implanted "cement free." The cemented TEP is immediately stressable postsurgery; the noncemented TEP requires a little more time (several weeks) to firmly connect with the surrounding bone tissue. However, a noncemented prosthesis is easier to replace should it be necessary if it becomes loose, since there is no cement to remove. Which prosthesis to implant depends on several factors, such as age, primary bone stability, and possible preexisting bone diseases (osteoporosis). Complications of artificial joint replacement are foremost loosening of the joint and infection. Both cemented and noncemented prostheses currently have a 90% probability of lasting significantly longer than 10 years.

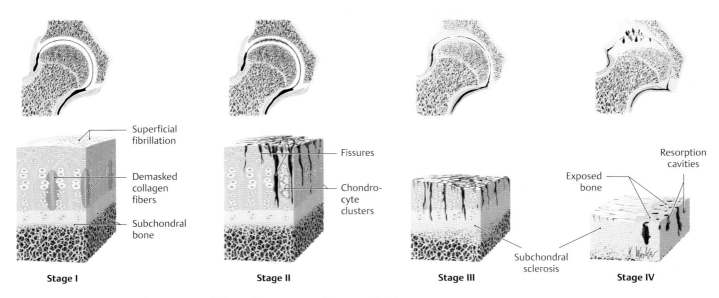

D Stages, compensatory mechanisms, and clinical symptoms of osteoarthritis

Stage I	Stage II	Stage III	Stage IV
• Articular surface is roughed up and begins to fray (surface fibrillations) • In the deeper lying cartilaginous layers, collagen fibers are exposed (demasked) by decreased proteoglycan synthesis	• Development of fissures that extend deep into the cartilage • Loss of cartilage matrix • In the fissure area, individual cartilage cells divide again (chondrocyte clusters develop)	• Increasing density of the subchondral bone as a result of increasing cartilage attrition • First osteophytes appear at the bone bridge • Inflammatory response at the articular capsule (reactive synovitis, usually with effusion) as a result of increased accumulation of deposits caused by cartilage wear	• The bone is entirely exposed; the bone surfaces rub on each other • Collapse of the subchondral bone roof (bone necrosis) • Development of large resorption cavities in the articulating joint surfaces (see **E**) • Increasingly strong growth of osteophytes

Compensatory mechanisms in the early stage	Compensatory mechanisms in the advanced stage	Goal of the compensatory mechanisms
• Limited proliferation (cell division) of the previously post-mitotic cartilage cells • Formation of so-called chondrocyte clusters, or brood capsules, with newly developed extracellular matrix	• Activation of mesenchymal progenitor cells in opened subchondral cavities within the spinal cord (subchondral cysts) • Followed by formation of a new articular surface through metaplastic fibrocartilage	Compensate for cartilage loss
Reactive thickening of the subchondral bone with increasing bone density (subchondral sclerosis)	Enlargement of the articular force–transmitting surface through formation of marginal osteophytes (so-called marginal exostosis)	Equalize pressure in the subchondral bone

Clinical symptoms: After an asymptomatic early stage of the disease (so-called latent arthrosis) that can last for years, patients initially report discrete pain, which gets worse with increased joint load and is accompanied by the first signs of referred muscle pain. In a more advanced stage of the disease, in addition to stress-related pain, patients experience pain when in neutral position (so-called activated osteoarthritis). Its cause lies in the inflammatory response of the articular capsule to the increased accumulation of deposits caused by cartilage wear. The reactive synovitis is almost always accompanied by effusions. As the disease progresses, symptoms intensify, with simultaneous increased joint instability. The final stage is characterized by constant pain, heavily limited load-carrying capacity, strong muscle contraction, drastic malalignment, and stiffening of the joint.

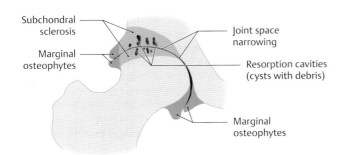

E Synopsis of the results of X-ray examination coxarthrosis of hip joint arthrosis

Schematic representation showing the radiologic changes seen in advanced of hip joint arthrosis. The destruction band degeneration of the hyaline articular cartilage leads to typical signs in the conventional X-ray, including narrowing of the cartilage gap in the joint parts that are most heavily loaded as a result of increasing loss of cartilage, the subchondral thickening (subchondral sclerosis) and lightening (subchondral cyst formation) of the bone, and the presence of osteophytes (from reactive bone changes) both in loaded and unloaded areas.

4.6 Basic Principles of Joint Mechanics: Movements

A Joints as functional units

In order to understand joints as functional units, it is best to draw on physical laws, for although joints primarily enable motion, at the same time they guarantee stability of the musculoskeletal system and assist in transmitting force between the articulating bones.

- Movements are changes of location in space (translational and rotational motion), which have both temporal (uniform or nonuniform motion in time) and spatial aspects (variable capacity for motion along the three axes) (see **B–D**).
- In order to balance the body and stand erect against gravity, almost every joint, according to their location relative to the body's center of gravity, has to be stabilized mainly through ligaments, muscles, and tendons (see p. 60).
- The forces acting on a joint (muscle and ligament force, body weight, or gravity) create joint pressure and cause movement to occur (via the torsional moment) if they are applied outside the center of rotation, e.g., via a lever arm (see p. 51).

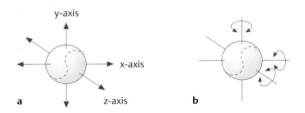

B Degrees of freedom, illustrated for the possible movements of a tennis ball in space

a Three degrees of freedom in *translation* (one each along the x-, y-, and z-axis).
b Three degrees of freedom in *rotation* (one each around the x-, y-, and z-axis).

With its similarity to a tennis ball, the spheroidal joint (see **Fc** and **Fd**) has the greatest freedom of movement.

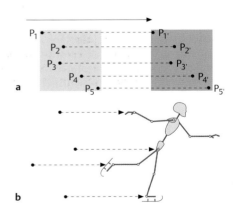

C Translation

Translation means that a body is sliding on a straight or curved path *without rotating*. As a result, all points on the moving body travel an *equal distance* in the same direction.
a All the points move in parallel lines.
b The gliding ice skater illustrates movement in translation.

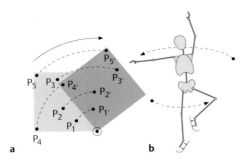

D Rotation

When a body is rotating, different points on the body move in concentric circles and travel *different distances*.
a All the points move in circular arcs. **b** The spinning ice skater illustrates movement in rotation.

E Sliding and rolling in rotational motions

When rotating, articular surfaces can glide onto each other or roll off each other. In most cases, however, it is a combination of both (roll-slide).
Note: The more congruent the articular surfaces (roughly the same radius of curvature, e.g., shoulder joint; **a**, **b**), the better they slide onto each other; the less congruent the articular surfaces, the more they roll off each other (e.g. knee joint; **c**, **d**). Rolling and sliding differ in relation to the path gain of the axis of rotation.

a, b Rotation without path gain of the axes of motion (= sliding), meaning one point of the articular surface successively touches different points on the other articular surface (**a**), as happens with abduction (= rotational motion) in the shoulder joint (**b**).

c, d Rotation with path gain of the axes of motion (= rolling), meaning the surface of the rotating body rolls off the articular surface of the other body, and so each point of the articular surface touches one point of the other surface, with the distance covered being the same for both joints. An example is flexion in the knee joint (**d**): rotation here is a combination of rolling and sliding, because the femur and the condyles of the tibia have markedly different radii of curvature. Thus, when rolling, the axis of motion moves back on a particular path (evolute), indicating only where the movement of flexion occurs at that instant. Such an axis is also called an instantaneous axis.

F Correlation between form and movement capabilities of a joint

The movements a joint can perform are most notably determined by the form, meaning the geometry, of the articulating surfaces. In general, there are two basic movements:

- Translational movement (**a**, **b**) and
- Rotational movement.

Whereas translational movements in the joints are usually limited to one or two axes of motion (e.g., femoropatellar joint in the knee [**a**], vertebral joints [**b**] in the spinal column), rotational movements that occur, for instance, in spheroidal joints (**c**, **d**) have up to three axes of motion. In the femoropatellar joint, for example, when bending the knee, the patella slides up or down in the femoral groove, meaning the joint has one degree of freedom in translation with, accordingly, two main movements. In vertebral joints with their mostly flat surfaces, translational movements usually occur along one straight line, albeit in different directions (often two degrees of freedom in translation with four main movements). A spheroidal joint, however, has three degrees of freedom in rotation relative to the number of axes of motion and thus six main movements (abduction/adduction, flexion/extension, internal/external rotation). In joints with rotational movements, depending on the form of the articulating surfaces, the number of axes of motion and thus the number of degrees of freedom can be limited, e.g., ellipsoidal or saddle joint (two axes of motion, thus four degrees of freedom, **e**, **f**), hinge or pivot joint (one axis of motion, thus two degrees of freedom, **g**, **h**).

a Femoropatellar joint

b Vertebral joint

c Spheroidal joint
A joint with three mutually perpendicular axes of motion, resulting in six primary movements (i.e., hip joint with deep socket).

d Spheroidal joint
A joint with three mutually perpendicular axes of motion, resulting in six primary movements (i.e., shoulder joint with shallow socket).

e Ellipsoidal joint
A biaxial joint with four primary movements (i.e., the radiocarpal joint).

f Saddle joint
A biaxial joint with four primary movements (i.e., the carpometacarpal joint of the thumb).

g Hinge joint
A joint with one axis of motion and two primary movements (i.e., parts of the elbow joint).

h Pivot joint
A uniaxial joint with two primary movements (i.e., the proximal radioulnar joint).

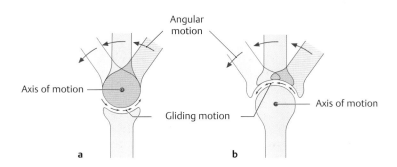

Angular motion

Axis of motion

Gliding motion

Axis of motion

a   **b**

G Convex-concave rule

The convex-concave rule describes the sliding motion in dependence of the angular rotation motion.

a If the convex joint partner moves in an angular direction around the axis of motion, its rotation motion inside the joint is in the opposite direction of the angular motion.

b If the concave joint partner moves in an angular direction around the axis of motion, its rotational motion inside the joint is in the same direction as the angular motion.

4.7 Basic Principles of Joint Mechanics: Stability and Transmission

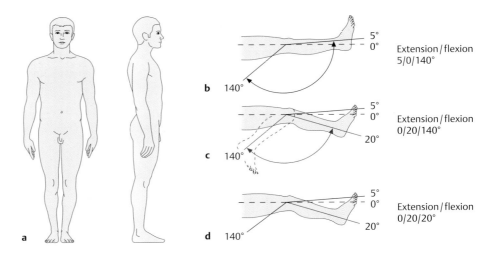

B The neutral zero method
The neutral zero method is a standardized method for measuring the range of joint motion.

a Zero-degree starting position, viewed from the anterior and lateral aspects.
b Range of motion of a normal knee joint.
c Limitation of motion caused by a flexion contracture.
d Ankylosis of the knee joint in 20° of flexion.

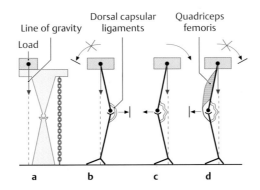

C Active and passive joint stabilization as demonstrated in the knee joint
The knee joint is actively stabilized by the quadriceps femoris and passively stabilized by the anterior ligaments (oblique popliteal and arcuate ligaments).

a Mechanical model: A load (body weight) causes a torsional moment in the joint as the line of gravity is in front of the middle of the joint. To prevent the upper joint partner from tilting forward, a chain acts as a counterforce.
b Passive stabilization through the popliteal and arcuate ligaments: The knee joint needs to shift behind the line of gravity posterior to the capsular ligaments so that the ligaments can stabilize the knee joint.
c If the line of gravity extends behind the knee joint, the ligaments are useless; the body tilts backward, and the knee joint gives way.
d Active stabilization of the knee joint by the quadriceps femoris extending on its front side.

A Constraints on joint motion
The range of joint motion depends not only on the shape of the bony joint members (see **D**, left) but also on the muscles, ligaments, and soft-tissue envelope that surround the joint. Accordingly, all of these factors determine the total range of joint motion:

a Bony constraint.
b Muscular constraint.
c Ligamentous constraint.
d Soft-tissue constraint.

D The most important groups of muscles and ligaments responsible for the maintenance of erect posture

Muscles	Ligaments
• The lower leg muscles, mainly triceps surae and tibialis anterior, stabilize the upper ankle joint in the sagittal plane • The upper leg muscles (quadriceps femoris) stabilize the knee joint • The gluteal muscles stabilize the hip joint in the sagittal plane • The smaller gluteal muscles (glutei medius and minimus) stabilize the hip joint in the frontal plane • The intrinsic back muscles stabilize the spinal column	• The anterior ligaments stabilize the knee joint • The iliofemoral ligament stabilizes the hip joint • The collateral ligaments stabilize the knee joint and the upper ankle joint in the frontal plane

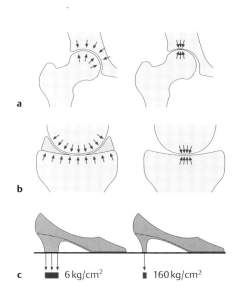

E One- and two-arm levers

a One-arm lever (elbow joint), **b** two-arm lever (hip joint).

Joint mechanics is based on the principles of the lever. The amount of force that a muscle can transmit to a joint depends on the length of the associated lever arm. This depends on the perpendicular distance from the muscle and its tendon to the center of rotation (= *force arm*) and is opposed by the force of the *load arm*. In the case of the elbow joint in **a**, the load arm is the distance from the joint axis (center of rotation) to the load. The *magnitude of each of the three active forces* is determined by multiplying the force by the force arm and the load by the load arm. This product is called the *torque* (= moment of rotational force) because the active forces produce a rotational movement of the associated lever. If the product of the load times the load arm equals the product of the force times the force arm, both torques are identical, and the joint is at rest. The lever in **a** is classified as a *one-arm lever* because the muscular force and load act *on the same side*—in this case, to the left of the center of joint rotation. The lever in **b** is a *two-arm lever* because the muscular force acts to the left of the center of joint rotation, while the force of the body weight acts to the right of the joint center.

F Dependence of joint load on the size of the force-transmitting surface on the joint load

The larger the force-transmitting surface, the more evenly the force is distributed and the lower the joint pressure, or joint load, per unit area.

a Normal and limited covering of the head of the femur.
b Knee joint with and without meniscus.
c Example of a square stacked heel and a stiletto heel: if body weight is the same, but the force-transmitting surface is less, the load on the bottom of the foot is many times higher.

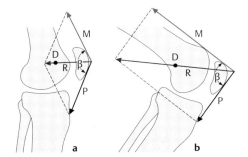

G Dependence of magnitude of the resultant force vector on the net joint force

a The resultant force vector (red) of the femoropatellar joint runs through the center of rotation of the joint (D) and is the summation of individual muscle force vectors (M) (quadriceps femoris) and the ligament force vector (P) (patellar ligament). It creates the joint pressure and is a measure of the forces acting on the joint.
b Due to the increased intensity of contraction of the quadriceps femoris when bending the knee, the resultant force in the bend position is significantly higher than in the stretching position, which means that with increased bending, the joint load in the femoropatellar joint increases.

H Load on the right hip joint in the support phase

Anterior view. In a one-legged stance or while walking in the support phase, the partial-body center of gravity (S) shifts, which results in a

turning moment of the load, which tends to tilt the body above the joint toward the supporting leg. In order to remain stable, the turning moment has to be balanced by a counter-force (e.g., a muscle or ligament force). In the hip joint, it is provided by the muscle force (M) of the hip abductors (glutei medius and minimus). However, unlike the force of the partial-body weight (K) at the hip joint, it acts at a lever arm that is three times shorter, which means the ratio between the lever arm of the muscle force (**a**) to the lever arm of the partial-body weight is 1:3. The muscle force needed to stabilize the hip therefore is approximately three times that of the partial-body weight when standing on one leg. From this it follows that based on the different length of the lever arms, the compressive force that the hip joint has to withstand when walking, (resultant force R) has to be four times higher than the partial-body weight (after Pauwels). That means that the hip joint has to be able to permanently withstand extreme loads and is thus very often affected by osteoarthritis.

4.8 Fractures: Classification, Healing, and Treatment

A Fracture classification

Fractures can be classified according to different characteristics; those mentioned below are practical and have proven successful in daily use:

- According to **formation and injury mechanism:**
  - Traumatic fracture caused by direct force (transverse or comminuted fracture, see **Ba** and **Bg**, e.g., as a result of being hit while walking) or indirect force (lever arm and rotational motion directed away from the force effect, e.g., torsion fracture to the lower leg as a result of a ski crash, see **Bf**).
  - Nontraumatic fracture ("spontaneous fracture") as a result of preexisting localized or generalized bone disease, such as tumors, osteomyelitis, or osteoporosis (= pathologic fracture, can occur without any external forceful impact) or as a result of microtrauma, which is caused by repeated moderate application of force at the same spot over and over again eventually leading to a fracture (= fatigue fracture, e.g., metatarsal fracture such as a so-called march fracture).
- According to **fracture morphology** (e.g., degree of break in continuity [fissure or fracture]), course of fracture lines, number of fragments, see **B** and **C**).
- According to severity of **soft-tissue damage:**

- Closed fracture or
- Open fracture: generally, it can be assumed to give direct access to germs; however, what is important in the end is the severity of soft-tissue damage, meaning to what extent muscles, vessels, or nerves have also been damaged.

Furthermore, with regards to long bones, when considering the location of the fracture (epiphyseal, metaphyseal, and diaphyseal), a distinction is made between proximal fractures, fractures of the long bones, and distal fractures with or without joint involvement. In addition to pain, clinical symptoms of a bone fracture include obvious deformation, abnormal mobility, and palpable and distinguishable crepitus (creaking, crackling as a result of crepitation).

Note: Fractures suffered during childhood show distinct characteristics and have to be disinguished from those suffered in adulthood. The most important anatomic difference involves the growth plates and the periosteum, which is thicker and more robust in children. If, for example, a fracture causes damage in the proliferative zone in the growth plate, cellular demise and callous bridges can lead to a premature closure of the epiphyseal plate. In so-called greenstick fractures, the cortex fractures on one side while maintaining the thick periosteal tube (intraperiosteal fracture).

B The most important types of fractures
a Transverse fracture; **b** oblique fracture; **c** shearing fracture (e.g., fracture of the femoral neck); **d** avulsion fracture (e.g., avulsion fragment in the intra-articular ligament of the medial malleolus); **e** bending fracture with bending wedge as third fragment; **f** torsion, or spiral, fracture; **g** comminuted fracture with more than six fragments.

C Typical fracture dislocations
Fractures can be primarily (by acting force) or secondarily (by a disrupted muscle balance, e.g., muscular traction at the fragments) more or less distinctly displaced or dislocated.
a Sideways dislocation; **b** axial dislocation; **c** angular malalignment; **d, e** shifting direction axis and overlapping.

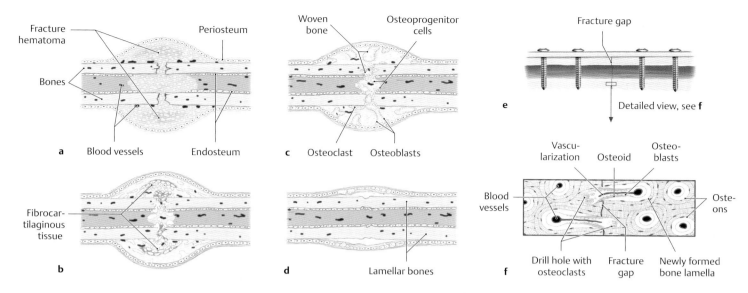

a Fracture hematoma / Periosteum / Bones / Blood vessels / Endosteum

b Fibrocartilaginous tissue

c Woven bone / Osteoprogenitor cells / Osteoclast / Osteoblasts

d Lamellar bones

e Fracture gap / Detailed view, see **f**

f Vascularization / Osteoid / Osteoblasts / Blood vessels / Osteons / Drill hole with osteoclasts / Fracture gap / Newly formed bone lamella

D Fracture healing

Preconditions for optimal fracture healing are repositioning and retaining the bone fragments of the fracture. In principle, this can be achieved both conservatively (e.g., with a cast) and surgically (see **E**). In addition, fracture healing requires cells with osteogenic potential, sufficient vascularization, and absolute mechanical rest in the fracture area. During the healing process, active movement therapy is crucial in order to prevent muscle atrophy, due to osteoporosis inactivity, stiffening of the joints, and circulatory disturbances. Endochondral and membranous ossification are part of the healing process. Thus, these processes, which occur in the course of the normal growth and the development of the skeleton, are repeated.

- **Indirect (natural or secondary) fracture healing (a–d),** which has the following physiologic stages:
  - Development of a fracture hematoma (inflammatory phase, **a**) and organization of the fracture hematoma with the help of loose, vessel-rich connective tissue (granulation stage)
  - Development of a fibrocartilaginous cartilage while involving cells of the periosteum and the endosteum (so-called fibrocartilaginous callus or fixation callus, **b**)
  - Mineralization of the cartilage (callus hardening within 6 to 8 weeks after fracture occurrence; so-called osseous callus or fracture callus; at first thick and bulky)
  - Loss of cartilage substance and new bone formation (woven bone) with the help of osteoprogenitor cells (**c**)
  - Bone restructuring in the lamellar bone, which takes months (**d**)

- **Direct (or primary) fracture healing (e, f).** In this case, no chondral fracture callus develops, but ideally (though only rarely) direct angiogenic ossification occurs, meaning the sprouting osteons grow directly from one fragment into another (**e, f**). However, this requires surgical osteosynthesis and that the fracture gap is no more than 0.5-mm wide (contact healing). Conservative stabilization using synthetic dressing will not result in direct fracture healing.
Note: Pseudarthrosis (failure of bone formation after 6 months) is among the most common complications of fracture healing. It arises due to both excessive mechanical load on the regenerating bone and absence of callus formation as a result of poor circulation.

E Basic principles of osteosynthesis

Surgical osteosynsthesis creates a temporary mechanical bone union using screws, plates, wires, or nails. The procedure neither replaces nor expedites bone healing. However, there are a number of **advantages compared to a conservative cast treatment:**

- Exact repositioning of bone fragments in joint fractures
- Immediate mobilization (prevents thrombosis, emboli, decubitus, and fracture disease, e.g., edema and dystrophy)
- Timely stabilization exercises (mobilization of joints without load) and partial load-bearing capacity to allow for healing

Disadvantages include the risks associated with anesthesia and surgery, as well as the possibility of infection. There are five different osteosynthetic procedures (which can be combined as needed):

- Screw osteosynthesis (e.g., compression with corticalis-traction screw, **a**)
- Plate osteosynthesis (e.g., compression plate, **b**)
- Intramedullary nail, rod, or fixation (e.g., in diaphyseal fracture, **c**)
- Tension-band wiring (e.g., using a wire loop, **d**)
- External fixation (e.g., three-dimensional frame construction, **e**)

5.1 Skeletal Muscles: Overview

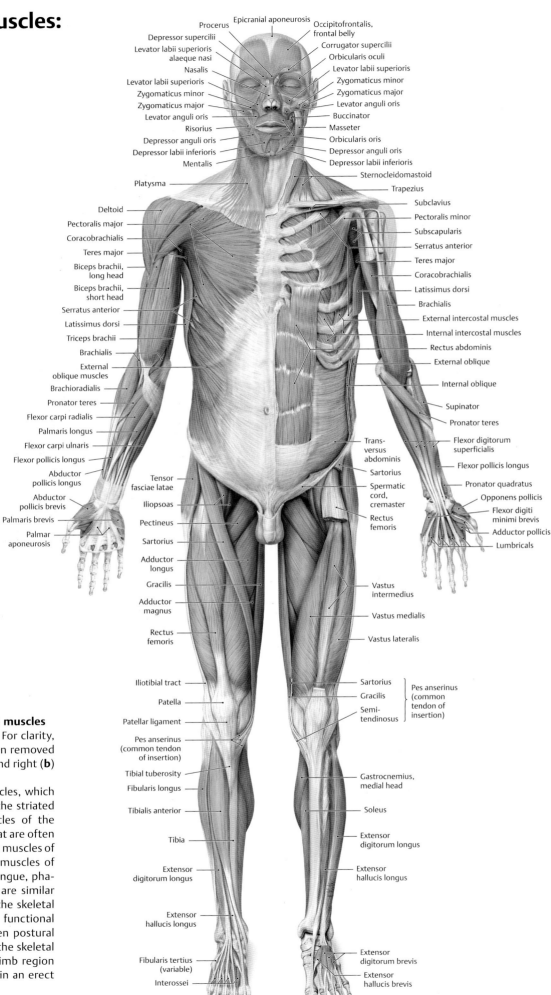

Procerus — Epicranial aponeurosis — Occipitofrontalis, frontal belly
Depressor supercilii — Corrugator supercilii
Levator labii superioris alaeque nasi — Orbicularis oculi
Nasalis — Levator labii superioris
Levator labii superioris — Zygomaticus minor
Zygomaticus minor — Zygomaticus major
Zygomaticus major — Levator anguli oris
Levator anguli oris — Buccinator
Risorius — Masseter
Depressor anguli oris — Orbicularis oris
Depressor labii inferioris — Depressor anguli oris
Mentalis — Depressor labii inferioris
— Sternocleidomastoid
Platysma — Trapezius
— Subclavius
Deltoid — Pectoralis minor
Pectoralis major — Subscapularis
Coracobrachialis — Serratus anterior
Teres major — Teres major
Biceps brachii, long head — Coracobrachialis
Biceps brachii, short head — Latissimus dorsi
Serratus anterior — Brachialis
Latissimus dorsi — External intercostal muscles
Triceps brachii — Internal intercostal muscles
Brachialis — Rectus abdominis
External oblique muscles — External oblique
Brachioradialis — Internal oblique
Pronator teres — Supinator
Flexor carpi radialis — Pronator teres
Palmaris longus — Flexor digitorum superficialis
Flexor carpi ulnaris — Flexor pollicis longus
Flexor pollicis longus — Pronator quadratus
Abductor pollicis longus — Tensor fasciae latae — Opponens pollicis
Abductor pollicis brevis — Iliopsoas — Spermatic cord, cremaster — Flexor digiti minimi brevis
Palmaris brevis — Pectineus — Adductor pollicis
Palmar aponeurosis — Sartorius — Rectus femoris — Lumbricals
Trans-versus abdominis — Sartorius
Adductor longus — Vastus intermedius
Gracilis — Vastus medialis
Adductor magnus — Vastus lateralis
Rectus femoris
Iliotibial tract — Sartorius — Pes anserinus (common tendon of insertion)
Patella — Gracilis
Patellar ligament — Semi-tendinosus
Pes anserinus (common tendon of insertion)
Tibial tuberosity — Gastrocnemius, medial head
Fibularis longus — Soleus
Tibialis anterior — Extensor digitorum longus
Tibia — Extensor hallucis longus
Extensor digitorum longus
Extensor hallucis longus — Extensor digitorum brevis
Fibularis tertius (variable) — Extensor hallucis brevis
Interossei

A Overview of skeletal (striated) muscles
a Anterior view, **b** posterior view. For clarity, some superficial muscles have been removed or windowed on both the left (**a**) and right (**b**) side of the body.
Approximately 220 individual muscles, which differ in shape and size, make up the striated muscles. Overall, these are muscles of the active musculoskeletal system (what are often referred to as skeletal muscles). The muscles of facial expression and masticatory muscles of the face and the muscles of the tongue, pharynx, larynx, eye, and tympanum are similar in form to these muscles. Within the skeletal muscles (extrafusal muscles), for functional reasons, one differentiates between postural and phasic muscles. Two thirds of the skeletal muscles are located in the lower limb region and mainly help to hold the body in an erect

a

Sternocleidomastoid

Thoracolumbar fascia (= deep layer of nuchal fascia)

Trapezius, descending part

Trapezius, transverse part

Scapular spine

Deltoid

Trapezius, ascending part

Teres major

Triceps brachii

Latissimus dorsi

Thoracolumbar fascia, superficial layer

Aponeurosis of origin of latissimus dorsi

Brachioradialis

Extensor carpi radialis brevis

Extensor carpi radialis longus

Anconeus

Extensor digitorum

Extensor carpi ulnaris

Flexor carpi ulnaris

Abductor pollicis longus

Extensor pollicis brevis

Extensor retinaculum

First dorsal interosseus

Second dorsal interosseus

Third dorsal interosseus

Iliac crest

Gluteus medius

Extensor digiti minimi

Tensor fasciae latae

Abductor digiti minimi

Fourth dorsal interosseus

Gluteus maximus

Adductor magnus

Gracilis

Semitendinosus

Biceps femoris, long head

Semimembranosus

Popliteal fossa

Plantaris

Gastrocnemius, lateral head

Gastrocnemius, medial head

Calcaneal (Achilles') tendon

Semispinalis capitis

Splenius capitis

Splenius cervicis

Rhomboid minor

Levator scapulae

Clavicle

Acromion

Supraspinatus

Rhomboid major

Infraspinatus

Teres minor

Scapula, medial border

Teres major

Serratus anterior

Latissimus dorsi

Serratus posterior inferior

External oblique muscles

Extensor carpi radialis longus

Extensor carpi radialis brevis

Supinator

Internal oblique muscles

Flexor digitorum profundus

Brachioradialis

Abductor pollicis longus

Extensor pollicis longus

Extensor pollicis brevis

Extensor indicis

Abductor digiti minimi

Dorsal interossei

Gluteus minimus

Tensor fasciae latae

Piriformis

Gemellus superior

Gemellus inferior

Obturator internus

Quadratus femoris

Adductor magnus

Iliotibial tract

Semitendinosus

Biceps femoris, long head

Semimembranosus

Plantaris

Gastrocnemius

Popliteus

Soleus

Tibialis posterior

Flexor digitorum longus

Flexor hallucis longus

Fibularis brevis

Fibularis longus

b

position in the field of gravity (= antigravity = postural = muscles) and in movement (= locomotion = phasic muscles).

Depending on gender, age, and physical condition, the skeletal muscles account on average for 40% of the total weight of a person and are thus the heaviest organ. They consist of up to 75% water, 20% proteins (mainly contractile proteins of muscles: myosin, actin, troponin, and tropomyosin), 2% low molecular weight organic components (e.g., triglycerides), and 3% inorganic components (e.g., calcium ions). As people age, their percentage of muscle mass decreases, and their percentage of fat increases (due to physical inactivity and the influence of hormonal factors, see p. 56).

5.2 Skeletal Muscles: Muscle Fiber Types and Pennate and Nonpennate Skeletal Muscles

A Muscle fiber types for postural muscles and muscles of movement: a comparison

All striated skeleton muscles basically consist of two different muscle fiber types (type I and type II fibers), which differ in their metabolic, physiological, histochemical, and biochemical characteristics (see **B**). The type II muscle fibers can be further divided into type IIA and type IIB fibers based on weight of isoforms in their myosin chains. Since the type I and type II fibers respond to a single action potential from the innervated axon with a single twitch in an all-or-none response, they are also known as twitch fibers. In contrast, tonic fibers, which are only found in muscle spindles and external eye muscles, gradually depolarize, leading to gradual fiber shortening.

The twitch duration of type I and II fibers differs. Type I fibers twitch more slowly (slow-twitch, or ST, fibers) than type II fibers (fast-twitch, or FT, fibers). The basic distribution pattern of type I and type II fibers in individual skeletal muscles is apparently genetically determined. In each case, the muscle fiber type of a motor unit is determined by the innervating neuron, so that all fibers of a motor unit belong to the same fiber type. Muscles with small motor units (< 100) have mostly fast-twitch (type II) fibers; muscles with large motor units (several thousand muscle fibers) have mostly slow-twitch (type I) fibers (see p. 59). The fiber type and its twitch duration are linked to a specific form of capacity and thus a particular type of twitch duration. Due to their high oxidative metabolism, type I fibers have endurance capacity and are thus mainly found in the postural muscles. Due to their high glycolytic metabolism, type II fibers can perform short, forceful contractions and are thus mainly found in phasic or elastic muscles. However, as skeletal muscles are highly adaptable, the genetically programmed distribution of type I and type II fibers can be influenced through neuromuscular activity (exercise). Accordingly, muscles that predominantly consist of type I fibers are found in endurance athletes, such as long-distance runners, cyclists, rowers, and cross-country skiers. Muscles that predominantly consist of type II fibers are found in explosive athletes, such as sprinters, high or long jumpers, and weight lifters (Pette and Saron, 2001). This phenotypic plasticity of the muscle is based on qualitative and quantitative changes in gene expression and mainly involves contractile and regulatory proteins of the myofibril apparatus, as well as the enzymes in metabolism (Pette, 1999).

	Postural muscles (red muscles)	Muscles of movement (white muscles)
Characteristics:	• Phylogenetically older • Predominantly slow-twitch fibers (type I fibers, approximately 100 ms) • Function best in endurance • Fatigue slowly • Large motor units • Rich in myoglobin • Abundant mitochondria • Energy derived from oxidative (aerobic) metabolism • Little glycogen (PAS-negative) • Relatively highly vascularized • Prone to shortening (increased resting tonus) and require regular stretching	• Phylogenetically more recent • Predominantly fast-twitch fibers (type II fibers, approximately 30 ms) • Brief periods of intense activity • Fatigue more rapidly • Small motor units • Scant myoglobin • Few mitochondria • Energy derived mainly from anaerobic glycolysis • Abundant glycogen (PAS-positive) • Much smaller capillary supply • Prone to atrophy and require regular strengthening
Examples:	Intercostal muscles, masticatory muscles, trapezius (descending part), hamstrings, iliopsoas, adductors, rectus femoris, soleus, intrinsic back muscles (mainly the cervical and lumbar part)	Biceps brachii, vastus lateralis and medialis, tibialis anterior, serratus anterior, gluteus maximus, gastrocnemius *Abbreviation:* PAS, periodic acid–Schiff.

Note: The loss of muscle mass (sarcopenia) in old age and the associated loss of muscular force and endurance are the most important causes for impaired physical mobility and, as a result, impaired ability to live independently. Sarcopenia is prevalent among the old and is a heavy financial burden on the health care system. Between the ages of 25 and 75, a person loses almost 40% of muscle mass (mainly type II muscle fibers). Especially dramatic is the loss of muscle mass after the age of 50 (15% per decade). Taking into account that muscle weakness is the most common factor in the risk of falling, exercises that target a specific muscle group (especially for elasticity) can efficiently counteract the loss of strength and in combination with balance exercises significantly reduce the risk of falling.

B Histochemical differences between type I and type II skeletal muscle fibers

Microscopic cross section of a skeletal muscle (tibialis anterior, rat, 200X magnification, 8-μm-thick frozen section). Succinated dehydrogenase (SDH), a mitochondrial enzyme of muscle metabolism, catalyzes the transformation of succinate into fumarate (reduction of fumarate leads to a brownish black reaction product, histochemical proof for the presence of SDH). The activity of mitochondrial SDH makes the varying percentage of mitochondria in the individual muscle fibers visible: heavily colored type I fibers with numerous mitochondria between the myofibrils and underneath the sarcolemma, and pale-colored type II fibers with few mitochondria.

Type I fibers

Type II fibers

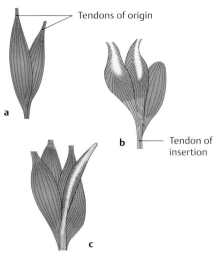

Tendons of origin

Tendon of insertion

Inter-mediate tendons

Muscle bellies

Cut surface of the sphincter muscle

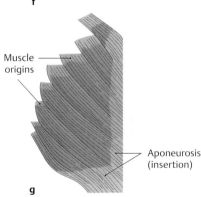

Muscle origins

Aponeurosis (insertion)

C Morphological forms of muscles

a Two heads = bicipital
(e.g., the biceps brachii).

b Three heads = tricipital
(e.g., the triceps surae).

c Four heads = quadricipital
(e.g., the quadriceps femoris).

d Two bellies = digastric
(e.g., the digastric muscle).

e Multiple bellies = multigastric
(e.g., the rectus abdominis).

f Radial (e.g., the external anal sphincter).

g Flat (e.g., the external oblique).

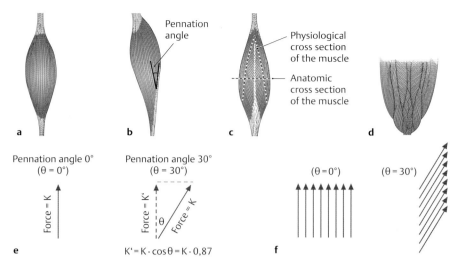

Pennation angle

Physiological cross section of the muscle

Anatomic cross section of the muscle

Pennation angle 0° (θ = 0°)

Pennation angle 30° (θ = 30°)

(θ = 0°)   (θ = 30°)

Force = K

Force = K'

Force = K

θ

$K' = K \cdot \cos \theta = K \cdot 0{,}87$

D Pennate and nonpennate skeletal muscles

Muscle fibers may have a parallel arrangement or may show varying degrees of convergence, or pennation, at their attachment.

a Nonpennate muscle (with parallel fibers); **b** unipennate muscle; **c** bipennate muscle; **d** multipennate muscle; **e** effect of pennation angle on force (at a 30° pennation angle, the tendon force F' amounts to 87% of the force generated in the muscle fibers); **f** effect of fiber arrangement on the number of fibers in a given cross section of muscle.

Whereas almost all fibers of skeletal muscles are of the same thickness (average diameter approximately 60 μm, see p. 58), their length varies considerably (ranging from a few millimeters to up to 20 cm), as does their ratio of fiber length to muscle length (between 0.2 and 0.6, meaning the fiber length amounts to between 20 and 60% of the length of the muscle) and their pennation angle.

All three factors play a significant role in lifting force and lifting height and thus in muscle "power output" (power = force x velocity or lifting force x lifting height):

- The longer the fibers, the greater the maximum shortening and thus the maximum lifting height of the muscle.
- The longer the fibers relative to the length of the muscle, the smaller the physiological cross-sectional area of the muscle and thus the lifting force of the muscle.
- The greater the pennation angle, the greater the physiological cross-sectional area and thus the lifting force.

Note: The physiological cross section is perpendicular to the cross sections of the muscle fibers, whereas the anatomic cross section is measured at the thickest part of the muscle.

E Nonpennate and pennate muscles: a comparison

Nonpennate (parallel-fibered) muscle	Pennate muscle
• Fibers run roughly along the longitudinal direction of the tendon (= muscle line of action) and are thus able to transmit almost all of their force to the tendon, see **f** • Maximum fiber shortening (= lifting height) and extent of actual fiber shortening during muscle activity are almost identical • Anatomic cross section (perpendicular to the longitudinal axis of the muscle, at its thickest part) and physiological cross section (perpendicular to the longitudinal axis of the fibers, see **c**) are roughly the same size	• The fibers form a (pennation) angle (up to 30°) with the longitudinal axis of the tendon and thus can transmit only a portion of their force to the tendon • Due to pennation angle, maximum fiber shortening (= lifting height) is greater than actual fiber shortening during muscle activity (= path gain) • Physiological cross section is larger than anatomic cross section, meaning (due to the angle) more muscle fibers can insert into the tendon in a given cross section as compared to a parallel-fibered muscle, thus increasing the lifting height, which depends on the size of the physiological cross section

Note: In nonpennate (parallel-fibered) muscles, force production is greater (direct force transmission from muscle to tendon, as there is no pennation angle); in pennate muscles, force development is greater (there are more fibers in a given cross section, since fibers are arranged obliquely to a tendon, resulting in greater lifting height, see above). The lesser force production of pennate muscles is compensated for by the greater force development. A huge advantage of pennate muscles compared to nonpennate muscles is their smaller size for similar size power output. If there were only nonpennate muscles, the body, in a lot of places, would not have space for a sufficient number of strong muscles.

5.3 Skeletal Muscles: Structure and Function

A Structure of a skeletal muscle

a Cross section of a skeletal muscle; **b** detail from **a** (cross section); **c** detail from **a** (longitudinal section); **d** structure of a muscle fiber (= muscle cell); **e** structure of a myofibril.

In striated skeletal muscle, muscle fibers and connective tissue are tightly interwoven and collaborate to carry out particular functions. The connective tissue is arranged in sheaths, which perform the following functions:

- Endomysium: most interior connective tissue sheaths (important for the tensile strength of the muscles); surrounds and condenses 200 to 250 muscle fibers (= muscle cells) into primary bundles. Each primary bundle, or muscle cell, contains the end branches of the motor axons to the motor end plates, as well as numerous (300–400 per mm²) heavily gyrose capillaries, see **c** (important for the supply of the muscles).
- Perimysium (important for the transmission of muscle tensile force to tendons): surrounds and condenses numerous primary bundles into secondary bundles (see **a**), which are several millimeters thick and thus are clearly visible to the naked eye (meat fibers); in contrast, the primary bundles (see above) have an average medial cross-sectional area of 1 mm².
- Epimysium: loose connective tissue layer directly beneath the muscle fascia (see **b**); establishes the connection to the muscle.

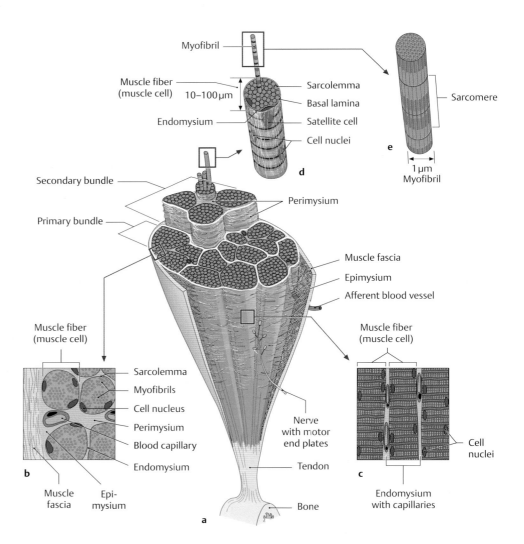

B Structure of a skeletal muscle fiber

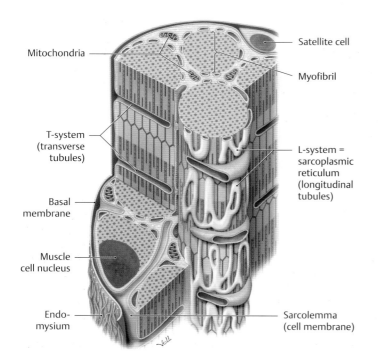

Skeletal muscle fibers are especially large cells, with average diameters of roughly 60 µm (10–100 µm) and lengths up to 20 cm. The dominant structures in the cytoplasm are myofibrils, mitochondria, and the L- and T-systems. The L-, or longitudinal, system is a cavity system (sarcoplasmic reticulum, longitudinal tubules), which is arranged lengthwise to the myofibrils and offers a pool for calcium ions. The T-, or transverse, system is created when a cell membrane periodically invaginates deeply into the interior of the muscle cell and as a result develops transverse tubules. It enlarges the membrane surface of a muscle fiber by 5 to 10 times, and the extracellular space can extend over the entire muscle fiber cross section. It guarantees the fast spread of an action potential deep into the muscle fiber.

Characteristic for the skeletal muscle cell are the numerous cell nuclei (approximately 50 nuclei/mm length), which are located directly underneath the cell membrane (sarcolemma). This very large number of cell nuclei arises during embryonic development, when the progenitor cells (myoblasts), arranged in a chainlike pattern, fuse with each other. Scattered between the sarcolemma and basal membrane are satellite cells (approximately 800/mm³ muscle tissue), which as dormant myoblasts (stem cells) represent some sort of cell pool.

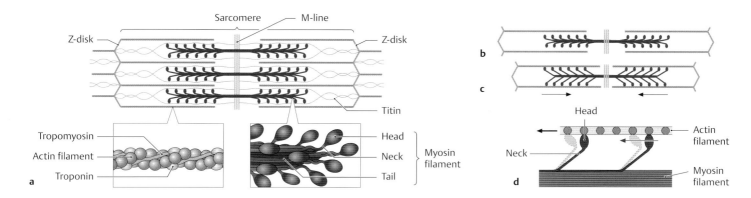

C Structure of a sarcomere

a Schematic representation of a sarcomere (= structural unit of a striated muscle cell); **b** myosin heads at rest; **c** myosin heads during contraction; **d** interaction between myosin heads and actin.

The arrangement of myofibrils in skeletal muscle fibers (see **B**) shows a cross-striation under the light microscope. It arises as the result of an alternating arrangement of thin actin (diameter: 7 nm) and thick myosin filaments (diameter: 15 nm). While actin filaments and their accompanying proteins (tropomyosin and troponin) of two adjacent sarcomeres are connected with each other at the Z-disks, the myosin filaments in the M-line among others are cross-linked by the myosin protein and in addition are kept in place by the elastic protein titin.

With the bipolar structure of the myosin filaments, a distinction is made between three parts: the head, neck, and tail. During muscle contraction, the myosin heads migrate along the actin filaments (so-called filament sliding) toward the Z-disks. Thereby, when at rest, each sarcomere shortens maximally to 70% of their optimal length of 2.2 μm; however, the individual filaments maintain their original length. This sliding mechanism is based on a quick succession of reaction cycles, during which cross-bridges between myosin heads and actin filaments are developed and detached again. It is associated with a tilting and rowing movement of the myosin head toward the middle of the sarcomere, with the myosin heads snapping off in an articulated manner (red arrow), and the actin filaments shoving on (black arrow). A single tilting movement shifts the actin filaments by about 10 to 20 mm, meaning the sarcomere shortens by about 1% of its original length. Greater changes in length are enabled by numerous repetitions of the interaction between actin and myosin. The basis for these cyclical processes is the fission of adenosine triphosphate (ATP) through the myosin head ATPase and the increase in cytosolic Ca+ concentration (electromechanical coupling; for more details, see books about physiology).

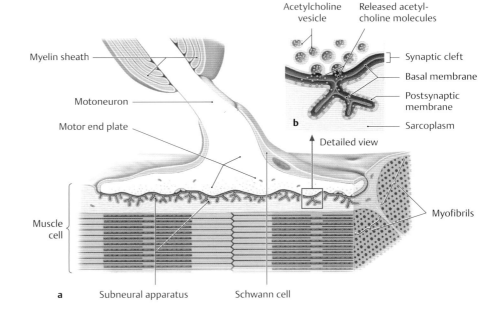

D Motor Unit

A motor unit is the sum of all muscle fibers that are innervated by a motor nerve fiber (the axon of a motor nerve cell of the spinal cord = α-motoneuron). There are small motor units (< 100 fibers) with mostly fast-twitching muscle fibers and large motor units (several thousand muscle fibers) with mostly slow-twitching muscle fibers. The fewer the muscle fibers combined in a motor unit, the more precise and finely tuned the movements of the muscle (e.g., finger muscles and external eye muscles). However, in muscles whose main function is to maintain posture or to produce movement (e.g., gluteal and back muscles), several thousand muscle fibers are innervated by one motor nerve cell.

E Motor end plate

a Schematic representation of a motor end plate; components of the synaptic contact (detailed view of **a**).

The motor axon divides at its end into several branches (one branch per muscle fiber), loses its myelin sheath, and develops on each of the branches a motor end plate (neuromuscular synapse), where the synaptic transmission of action potentials of the motoneuron occurs. Acetylcholine serves as a neurotransmitter and is stored in synaptic vesicles in the axoplasm of the end plate. As a result of folds in the sarcolemma (see **B**), the postsynaptic membrane with its acetylcholine receptors is greatly enlarged (subneural folding apparatus). In the entire 100-nm-wide system, there is one basal lamina, to which the acetylcholinesterase (an enzyme responsible for breaking down acetylcholine) is attached. The functional sequence at the motor end plate is generally identical to that at other synapses.

5.4 The Tendons and Mechanisms That Assist Muscle Function

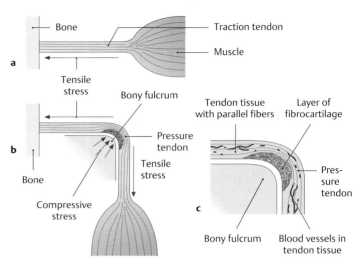

A Structure of a tendon (after Kristic)

a The tendon is connected to its surroundings by the loose, richly vascularized paratenon.

b Detail from **a**: The individual primary bundles are surrounded by peritendineum and are grouped into the actual tendon by the epitendineum. The function of a tendon is to transmit force from the muscle to the bone.

B Pressure tendons and traction tendons

a Traction tendons are subject to tensile stresses and consist of strong connective tissue with parallel fibers.

b Pressure tendons are strained by pressure and change their direction by running around the bone (unlike traction tendons). They consist of fibrocartilage on the side in contact with the bone, which acts as a fulcrum.

c Detail from **b**: The fibrocartilage layer in the compressed area, unlike the strong connective tissue in a traction tendon, is not vascularized.

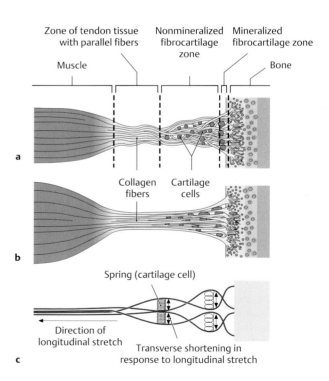

C Structure and function of a periosteal diaphyseal tendon insertion

a Tendon in the lax condition.

b Tendon on stretch.

D Structure and function of a chondral apophyseal tendon insertion

a Tendon in the lax condition (muscle relaxed).

b Tendon on stretch (muscle contracted).

c The principle of stretch protection: cartilage cells in the nonmineralized fibrocartilage zone act like taut springs to resist transverse shortening.

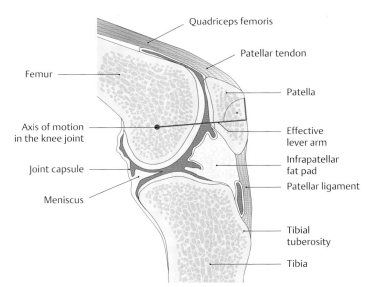

E Muscle fasciae

Proximal view. Cross section through the middle third of the right arm. Muscle fasciae (fibrous sheaths enclosing muscle) are composed of tough collagenous connective tissue. They help to maintain the shape and position of muscles and permit adjacent muscles or muscle groups to glide past each other with relatively little friction (less friction means less loss of force).

F Structure of a tendon sheath (synovial sheath)

Tendon sheaths serve to protect and facilitate the gliding of tendons that run directly on bone. The wall structure of the sheath, consisting of an outer fibrous membrane and an inner synovial membrane, resembles that of a joint capsule. The inner layer of the synovial membrane is firmly attached to the tendon, while its outer layer is attached to the fibrous membrane of the tendon sheath. The space between the two layers is filled with synovial fluid. The mesotendineum (sometimes referred to as *vincula brevia* and *longa* in different locations) transmits blood vessels to the tendon.

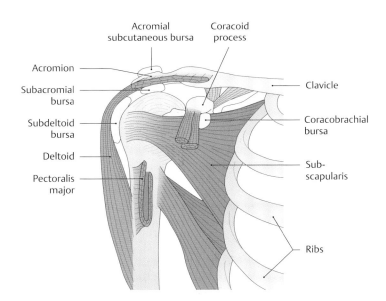

G Synovial bursae in the shoulder region

Right shoulder viewed from the anterior aspect, with some of the muscles removed. Bursae are pouchlike structures of varying size, usually flattened, that contain synovial fluid. Their wall structure is similar to that of a joint capsule. The bursae may become inflamed (*bursitis*), causing severe pain.

H Functional significance of sesamoid bones

Sagittal section through a knee joint. Sesamoid bones are bones that are embedded in tendons and protect the tendons from excessive friction. Their occurrence is variable, so everyone does not have an equal number of sesamoid bones. Their main functional role is to *lengthen the effective lever arm of a muscle*, increasing its mechanical efficiency. The diagram illustrates this principle for the patella, which is the largest sesamoid bone in the body. The patella significantly lengthens the effective lever arm, represented by a perpendicular line from the joint axis to the tendon of insertion of the quadriceps femoris.

6.1 Overview of the Human Cardiovascular System

A Schematic representation of the circulatory system

Special circulatory organs are needed to transport and distribute the blood, ensuring that it is made accessible to all the cells in the body. These organs consist of the heart and vascular system (blood vessels and lymphatics). The **system of blood vessels** consists of arteries, capillaries, and veins. The *arteries* carry the blood from the heart and distribute it throughout the body. The *veins* return the blood to the heart. The exchange of gases, nutrients, and waste products takes place in the *capillary* region. All blood vessels leading away from the heart are called arteries, and all vessels leading toward the heart are called veins, regardless of their oxygen content (the umbilical vein, for example, carries oxygen-rich blood). The blood flow in this closed vascular system is maintained by the **pumping action of the heart**. The **lymphatic system** runs parallel to the venous system. It originates with blind-ended vessels in the capillary region, collects the *extracellular* fluid that is deposited there, and returns it to the venous blood through *lymphatic vessels*. *Lymph nodes* are interposed along these pathways to filter the lymph. Functionally, the circulatory system is divided into two main circuits:

- **The pulmonary circulation:** *Deoxygenated venous blood* from the upper and lower body regions is returned through the superior and inferior vena cava to the *right* atrium. It then enters the *right* ventricle, which pumps it through the pulmonary arteries to the lungs.
- **The systemic circulation:** *Oxygen-enriched blood* from the lungs returns through the pulmonary veins to the *left* atrium. From the left atrium it enters the *left* ventricle, which pumps the blood through the aorta into the systemic circulation. A special part of the systemic circuit is the **portal circulation,** which includes two successive capillary beds. *Before* venous blood returns to the inferior vena cava from the capillary beds of the unpaired abdominal organs (stomach, bowel, pancreas, and spleen), it is carried by the portal vein to the capillary bed of the liver. This ensures that nutrient-rich blood from the digestive organs undergoes numerous filtering and metabolic processes in the liver before it is returned to the inferior vena cava via the hepatic veins.

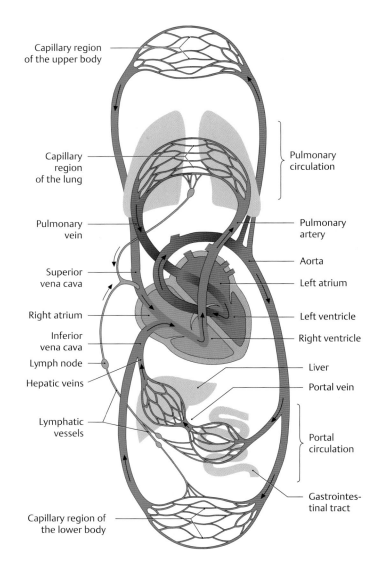

B Basic functional diagram of the circulatory system
(no distinction is made between the systemic and pulmonary systems in the diagram; after Klinke, Silbernagl)

Blood is transported through the circulatory system along a *pressure gradient* created by the different pressure levels in the arterial and venous systems. While the average blood pressure in the *arterial high-pressure system* is approximately 100 mmHg (13.3 N), the pressure in the *venous low-pressure system* generally does not exceed 20 mmHg (2.6 N). The two systems meet in the capillary region of the terminal vascular bed, where metabolic exchange takes place. When the heart expels blood during systole, the *arteries surrounding the heart (elastic-*type arteries) can temporarily expand to accommodate the ejected blood volume. During the diastole that follows, the vessel lumen undergoes an *elastic recoil* that transforms the intermittently ejected blood volumes into continuous flow. *Arteries distant from the heart (muscular-*type arteries) can actively expand (*vasodilation*) and contract (*vasoconstriction*), providing a very effective means of controlling vascular resistance and regulating local blood flow. The veins are also called *capacitance vessels* because of the high volume of blood contained within the veins. They can accommodate 80% of the total blood volume and thus serve an important reservoir function.

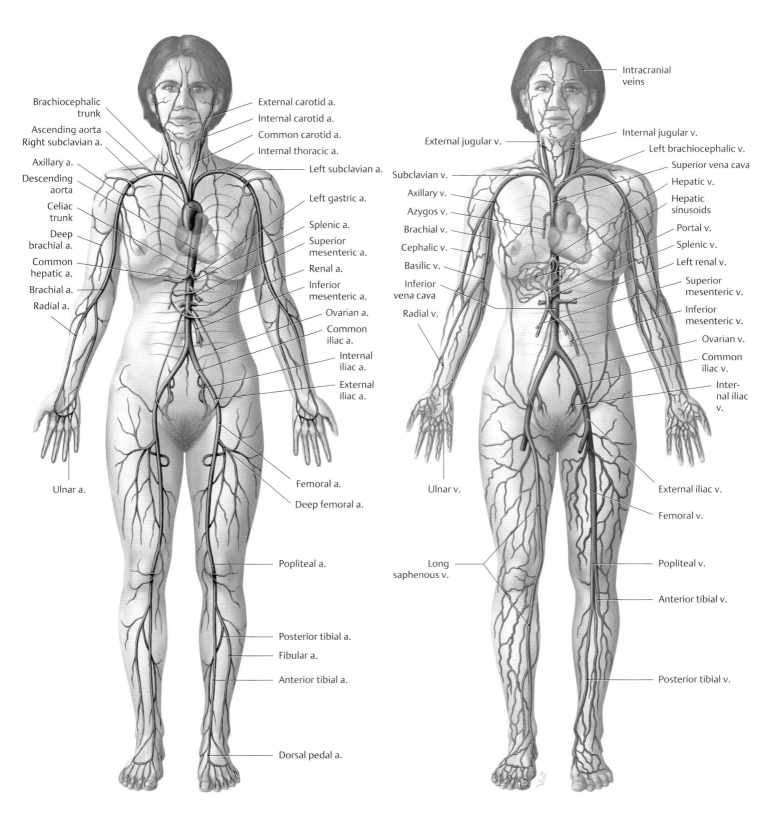

Brachiocephalic trunk

Ascending aorta
Right subclavian a.

Axillary a.

Descending aorta

Celiac trunk

Deep brachial a.

Common hepatic a.

Brachial a.

Radial a.

External carotid a.

Internal carotid a.

Common carotid a.

Internal thoracic a.

Left subclavian a.

Left gastric a.

Splenic a.

Superior mesenteric a.

Renal a.

Inferior mesenteric a.

Ovarian a.

Common iliac a.

Internal iliac a.

External iliac a.

Ulnar a.

Femoral a.

Deep femoral a.

Popliteal a.

Posterior tibial a.

Fibular a.

Anterior tibial a.

Dorsal pedal a.

External jugular v.

Subclavian v.

Axillary v.

Azygos v.

Brachial v.

Cephalic v.

Basilic v.

Inferior vena cava

Radial v.

Intracranial veins

Internal jugular v.

Left brachiocephalic v.

Superior vena cava

Hepatic v.

Hepatic sinusoids

Portal v.

Splenic v.

Left renal v.

Superior mesenteric v.

Inferior mesenteric v.

Ovarian v.

Common iliac v.

Internal iliac v.

Ulnar v.

External iliac v.

Femoral v.

Long saphenous v.

Popliteal v.

Anterior tibial v.

Posterior tibial v.

C Overview of the principal arteries in the systemic circulation

D Overview of the principal veins in the systemic circulation

The venous system is comprised of superficial veins, deep veins, and perforator veins, which interconnect the superficial and deep venous systems.

Note the portal circulation (portal vein), which carries nutrient-rich blood (shown here in purple) from the digestive organs directly to the liver (compare to the left side of **A**).

6.2   The Structure of Arteries and Veins

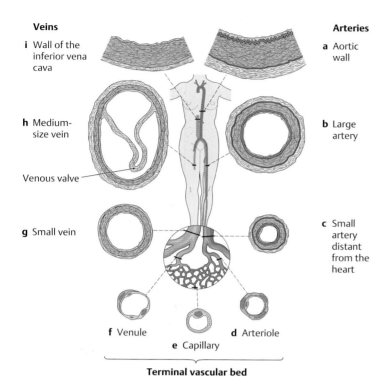

Veins

i Wall of the inferior vena cava

h Medium-size vein

Venous valve

g Small vein

f Venule

e Capillary

d Arteriole

Terminal vascular bed

Arteries

a Aortic wall

b Large artery

c Small artery distant from the heart

B Organization of the blood vessel system

Arteries (high-pressure system = supply function)

- Elastic-type arteries
- Muscular-type arteries

Terminal vascular bed (microcirculation = exchange function)

- Arterioles
- Capillaries
- Venules

Veins (low-pressure system = reservoir function)

- Small and medium-size veins (with valves)
- Large venous trunks

	Arteries		Terminal vascular bed		Veins	
	Aorta	Small artery	Arteriole	Venule	Vein	Vena cava
Wall thick-ness (w)	2.5 mm	1 mm	20 µm	5 µm	0.5 mm	1.5 mm
Luminal radius (ri)	12.5 mm	2 mm	20 µm	20 µm	2.5 mm	15 mm

A Structure of the blood vessels in different regions of the systemic circulation

Consistent with changing demands, the vessels in different regions of the systemic circulation (high- and low-pressure systems, microcirculation) show significant local structural differences despite a basic similarity in the arrangement of their wall layers. Whereas a relatively high internal pressure prevails throughout the *arterial system*, and the arterial vessels have correspondingly thick walls, the *veins* have a considerably lower intravascular pressure, resulting in thinner walls and larger luminal diameters than in the arteries. In the terminal vascular bed, on the other hand, the vessel wall layers are reduced to permit the exchange of gases, fluids, and other substances.

a–c Arteries, **d–f** terminal vascular bed, **g–i** veins. **a** Close-up view of the aortic wall (elastic-type artery). **b,c** Large and small arteries distant from the heart (muscular-type arteries). **d** Arteriole. **e** Capillary. **f** Venule. **g,h** Small and medium-size veins (some with venous valves). **i** Close-up view of the wall of the inferior vena cava.

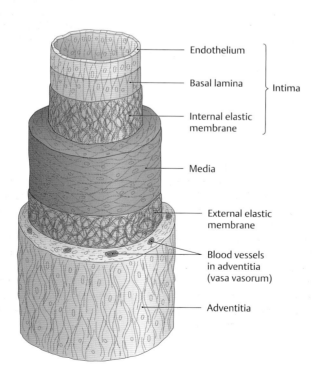

Endothelium

Basal lamina

Internal elastic membrane

} Intima

Media

External elastic membrane

Blood vessels in adventitia (vasa vasorum)

Adventitia

C Wall structure of a blood vessel, illustrated for a muscular-type artery

The wall of a blood vessel basically consists of *three layers*: the *intima*, *media*, and *adventitia*. The three-layered structure is clearly apparent in the walls of arteries and is less conspicuous in veins (see **D**).

- The **intima** consists of a layer of spindle-shaped endothelial cells that are aligned along the vessel axis and rest upon a basement membrane and a thin layer of subendothelial connective tissue. In muscular-type arteries, the intima is consistently separated from the media by an internal elastic membrane.
- The **media** consists of an approximately circular arrangement of smooth muscle cells, elastic and collagenous fibers, and proteoglycans. Muscular-type arteries may have an external elastic membrane that separates the media from the adventitia.
- The **adventitia**, like the intima, is composed of longitudinally aligned elements, mostly connective tissue. The adventitia of veins may additionally contain smooth muscle. The adventitia transmits autonomic nerves to the muscle of the vessel wall, and, especially in larger vessels, it also transmits the vasa vasorum, which supply blood to the outer third of the vessel wall.

Specific functions can be assigned to all three layers. The intima is concerned with the exchange of gases, fluids, and other substances through the vessel wall; the media regulates blood flow, and the adventitia integrates the blood vessel into its surroundings.

Vein — Artery

- Adventitia
- Media
- Intima

a

- Intraluminal clotted blood
- Perivascular connective tissue

- Adventitia
- Media
- Intima
- Vessel lumen

- Media of vein
- Media of artery
- Elastic fibers
- Internal elastic membrane
- External elastic membrane

b

D Differences in the wall structure of arteries and veins

Wall sections from a muscular-type artery and an accompanying vein. Comparison of tissue cross sections treated with different stains.
a H & E-resorcin-fuchsin stain of the posterior tibial artery and vein.
b Resorcin-fuchsin stain of the femoral artery and vein.
Note the characteristic structural differences in the media. While the arterial media consists of densely packed layers of smooth muscle cells, the venous media contains a far greater amount of connective tissue elements (collagenous and elastic fibers), giving it a much looser structure. The veins also lack a conspicuous layered structure and an internal elastic membrane (from Lüllmann-Rauch: *Histologie*, 2nd ed. Stuttgart: Thieme; 2006).

Veins Pressure (mmHg) — **Arteries** Pressure (mmHg)

- –30 / +35
- –15 / +50
- –3 / +100
- Hydrostatic indifference level (0)
- +20
- +90 / +180

E Arterial and venous pressure changes in the standing position

Changing from a recumbent to a standing position radically alters the pressure relationships in the circulatory system. The hydrostatic effects of this change cause the pressure to rise sharply in the lower parts of the body, while the pressures in the upper body decrease (the pressures remain unchanged at the "hydrostatic indifference level" just below the diaphragm). Along with the hydrostatic pressure changes, approximately 500 mL of blood volume is shifted into the lower limb veins. This rise of venous pressure greatly increases the transmural pressure in the lower limb veins, while the pressure in the head and neck veins may fall so low that the veins collapse. This explains why analogous veins in the lower and upper body regions have wall layers of different thickness; i.e., the veins on the dorsum of the foot are much more muscular than on the dorsum of the hand. The wall of the inferior vena cava, however, is paper-thin due to the low venous pressures at that level.

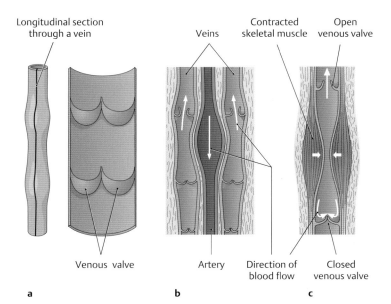

- Longitudinal section through a vein
- Veins
- Contracted skeletal muscle
- Open venous valve
- Venous valve
- Artery
- Direction of blood flow
- Closed venous valve

a   **b**   **c**

F Venous return to the heart

The following factors promote the return of venous blood to the heart:
a opening and closing of the venous valves, **b** arteriovenous coupling (the pulse wave in the artery is transmitted to the accompanying vein), and **c** the muscle pump.
Venous return is also aided by the "suction effect" of the heart, i. e., the negative pressure produced when the valve plane moves toward the cardiac apex during systole. A lack of muscular movement due to prolonged standing or sitting, for example, can cause the damming back of venous blood, leading to a raised intravascular pressure and incompetence of the venous valves. This can result in edema, varicose veins, and circulatory impairment.

65

6.3 The Terminal Vascular Bed

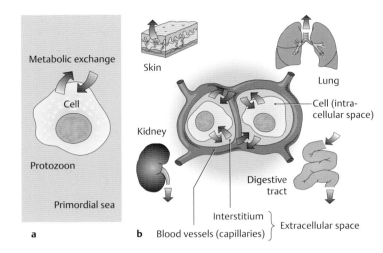

a   **b**   Blood vessels (capillaries)

A The milieu in which a cell lives (after Silbernagl, Despopoulos)

a Protozoan: The first single-cell organisms lived in an environment, the primordial sea, that provided a milieu of constant composition. The internal and external milieus were the same, and so neither of them changed during metabolism.

b Human: The cells of a multicellular organism are bathed by extracellular fluid, whose volume is substantially smaller than the intracellular volume. The extra- and intracellular fluids also have a different composition. In this situation the internal milieu would change very quickly if the intercellular space (interstitium) were not linked via the bloodstream to organs such as the lungs, kidneys, and digestive tract, which absorb nutrients and excrete metabolic products. Nutrients absorbed from the bowel are distributed to the cells of the various organs (interstitium of the capillary beds) via the bloodstream. The blood also transports the metabolic products of the cells to the organs that are responsible for their excretion (e.g., the lungs and kidneys).

B Characteristics of different vascular regions (after Silbernagl, Despopoulos)

The terminal vascular bed is the site of the microcirculation and therefore is the site where gases, fluids, and other substances are exchanged. It consists of

- an *afferent arterial limb* (precapillary arterioles),
- the *capillary bed* itself, and
- an *efferent venous limb* (postcapillary venules).

The smallest vessels, the capillaries, consist only of an endothelial layer and a basal lamina to which pericytes may be externally attached (contrast with the more complex structure of large vessels, p. 46). Owing to the extensive branching of the vessels in the capillary bed, the total vascular cross section is greatly increased (approximately 800 times), while the flow velocity is correspondingly reduced (from 50 cm/s in the aorta to 0.05 cm/s in the capillaries). With an average capillary length of 0.5 mm, a time of approximately 1 second is available for metabolic exchange. The increased vascular resistance in the arterioles and capillaries caused by contact of the blood with the large endothelial surface area (increased friction) lowers the blood pressure and eliminates pressure spikes. Thus, the capillaries provide ideal conditions for exchange processes to occur between the blood and the interstitial fluid that bathes the body's cells.

Number of vessels

Diameter of the individual vessel (cm)

Total cross-sectional area (cm²)

Flow velocity (cm/s)

Intravascular pressure (mmHg)

Percentage of total resistance

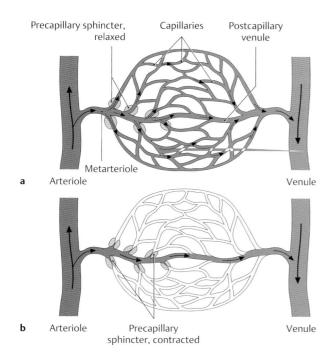

a Arteriole — Venule

b Arteriole — Precapillary sphincter, contracted — Venule

C Blood flow in the capillary bed
a Sphincter relaxed, **b** sphincter contracted.
Precapillary sphincters, with their circular array of muscle cells, are located at the junction of the metarterioles and capillaries and regulate blood flow within the capillary network. When the sphincters contract, the branching capillaries are closed, and the capillary bed is unperfused except for the metarterioles (e.g., only about 25 to 35% of all capillaries are perfused under resting conditions). The arterioles and venules may also be interconnected by shunts called *arteriovenous anastomoses*.

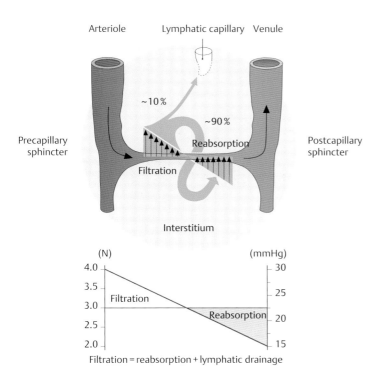

E Mechanism of fluid exchange in a capillary (after Silbernagl, Despopoulos)
Fluid exchange between capillaries and the surrounding tissue (interstitium) is regulated by a changing pressure gradient between the blood pressure in the capillaries (hydrostatic pressure) and the intra-

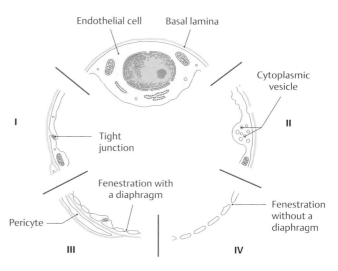

D Different forms of capillary endothelial cells (scheme of ultrastructural features)
Capillaries range from 5 to 15 μm in diameter and consist of endothelial cells, basal lamina, and external pericytes. Pericytes have various properties and functions, including a role in vascular development and angiogenesis. The individual endothelial cells are connected to one another by adhesion contacts, tight junctions, and gap junctions, largely preventing any metabolic exchange between individual endothelial cells. The endothelia of different capillaries have varying degrees of permeability, and several types of endothelium are distinguished on that basis:

I Closed endothelium without fenestrations and with a continuous basal lamina (e.g., nervous system)
II Closed endothelium with pinocytotic activity (e.g., cardiac and skeletal muscle)
III Endothelial cells fenestrated by a diaphragm (e.g., gastrointestinal tract)
IV Endothelial cells with intercellular gaps (large fenestrations) and without a continuous basal lamina (e.g., liver)

vascular colloid osmotic pressure. The driving force behind the fluid exchange is the hydrostatic blood pressure. The pressure at the arterial end of the capillary is 35 mmHg (= 4.6 N), which is 10 mmHg *higher* than the colloid osmotic pressure of approximately 25 mmHg (= 3.3 N). This positive pressure differential makes it possible for fluid as well as dissolved particles to filter out of the capillaries and into the surrounding tissue. These relationships are reversed at the venous end of the capillary—there, the hydrostatic blood pressure falls to approximately 15 mmHg (2.0 N), while the colloid osmotic pressure remains essentially unchanged at about 25 mmHg. As a result of this, the hydrostatic pressure on the *venous side of the capillary* is 10 mmHg *lower* than the colloid osmotic pressure (15–25 = –10 mmHg), causing fluid with its solute particles to flow back into the vessel (*reabsorption*).
Of the 20 L of fluid that leave the capillaries each day, only about 18 L (90%) are reabsorbed. Approximately 2 L (10%) of the filtered volume is removed by lymphatic vessels in the form of lymph. If this fluid exchange does not occur in the manner described, edema may develop (i. e., a persistent accumulation of fluids in the interstitium). The reason for this may be an *elevated hydrostatic pressure* (due to blood pooling on the venous side of the capillaries) or a *decreased colloid osmotic pressure* (due to a decrease in plasma proteins). In both cases there is an imbalance of fluid exchange, allowing fluid to accumulate in the tissue, known as edema.

7.1 The Human Lymphatic System

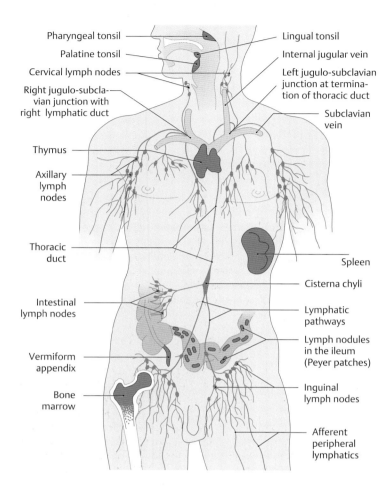

Pharyngeal tonsil
Palatine tonsil
Cervical lymph nodes
Right jugulo-subclavian junction with right lymphatic duct
Thymus
Axillary lymph nodes
Thoracic duct
Intestinal lymph nodes
Vermiform appendix
Bone marrow

Lingual tonsil
Internal jugular vein
Left jugulo-subclavian junction at termination of thoracic duct
Subclavian vein
Spleen
Cisterna chyli
Lymphatic pathways
Lymph nodes in the ileum (Peyer patches)
Inguinal lymph nodes
Afferent peripheral lymphatics

A The human lymphatic system

This system includes the lymphatic vessels and the lymphatic organs (immune organs, see **B**). The **lymphatic vascular system** runs parallel to the venous system and performs several functions:

- Its primary function is to clear the interstitial spaces of tissue fluid and substances that cannot be reabsorbed in the venous capillary bed. The composition of the lymph varies in different regions and is similar to that of the surrounding interstitial fluid.
- It carries away food lipids (chylomicrons) that are absorbed in the bowel.
- It returns lymphocytes from the lymphatic organs to the blood.

The lymphatic vascular system consists of

- *lymphatic capillaries*, which begin peripherally as blind-ended vessels;
- the *lymphatic vessels* and interposed *lymph nodes*; and
- the *major lymphatic trunks* (thoracic duct and right lymphatic duct).

The lymphatic capillaries collect fluid from the interstitium and transport it via the lymphatic vessels and lymph nodes to the major lymphatic trunks. The fluid reenters the venous system from these trunks at the junctions of the left and right subclavian and internal jugular veins. The lymph drained from three body quadrants enters the left jugulo-subclavian venous junction, while only lymph from the right upper quadrant enters the right jugulo-subclavian venous junction.

The **lymphatic organs** are part of the specific immune system and, as such, are situated at likely portals of entry for infectious microorganisms. The spleen is the only immune organ that is directly integrated into the bloodstream.

B Primary and secondary lymphatic organs

The functions of the lymphatic organs include mounting a specific immune response. A distinction is drawn between primary and secondary lymphatic organs. The primary lymphatic organs are concerned with the production, maturation, and selection of immune cells. The secondary lymphatic organs are subsequently populated by the immunocompetent lymphocytes and are sites for various processes, such as antigen presentation, lymphocyte proliferation, and antibody formation.

- **Primary lymphatic organs:**
  - Thymus (selection of T-lymphocytes)
  - Bone marrow (selection of B-lymphocytes)
- **Secondary lymphatic organs:**
  - Spleen
  - Lymph nodes
  - Mucosa-associated lymphatic tissue (MALT) and the pharyngeal lymphatic (Waldeyer's) ring—the pharyngeal, palatine, and lingual tonsils.
  - Bronchus-associated lymphatic tissue (BALT)
  - Gut-associated lymphatic tissue (GALT), such as Peyer patches and the vermiform appendix

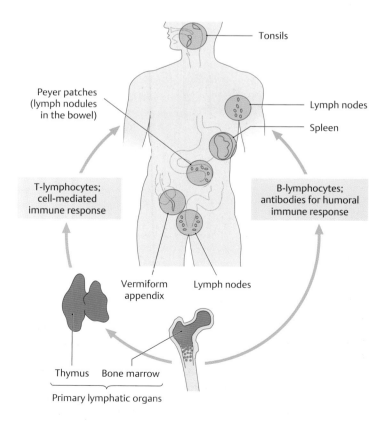

Tonsils
Peyer patches (lymph nodes in the bowel)
Lymph nodes
Spleen
T-lymphocytes; cell-mediated immune response
B-lymphocytes; antibodies for humoral immune response
Vermiform appendix
Lymph nodes
Thymus   Bone marrow
Primary lymphatic organs

C Organization of the lymphatic vascular system (after Kubik)

Three compartments can be distinguished in the lymphatic vascular system based on **topographical** and **functional** criteria:

1. A superficial system → drains the skin and subcutaneous tissue.
2. A deep system → drains lymph from the muscles, joints, tendon sheaths, and nerves.
3. An organ-specific system → drains the organs and shows organ-specific differences.

A system of **perforator vessels** interconnects the superficial and deep systems, conveying lymphatic fluid toward the surface from deeper tissues.

The lymphatic vascular system can be subdivided into *four different regions* based on the **histologic structure of the vessel walls**:

1. Lymphatic capillaries
2. Precollectors
3. Collectors
4. Lymphatic trunks

Lymphatic capillaries and precollectors are also known as *initial lymphatics*.

D Organization and structure of the different lymphatic regions
(after Kubik)
a Lymphatics in the skin and muscles.
b Detail from **a**, showing the structure and function of a collector segment.

Both the superficial and deep lymphatics originate with the extremely thin-walled **lymphatic capillaries**, which are approximately 50 μm in diameter. Their endothelium is bounded by an incomplete basal lamina, and they are attached by collagenous "anchoring filaments" to elastic fibers and collagen fibers in their surroundings. The network of lymphatic capillaries opens into larger **precollectors** approximately 100

μm in diameter. Unlike the lymphatic capillaries, these vessels contain valve cusps, and their walls are reinforced by a layer of connective tissue. They open into **collectors**, which also contain valves and have a transverse diameter of 150 to 600 μm. Like the larger lymphatic vessels and the lymphatic trunks, the collectors have a venous-type wall structure divided indistinctly into an intima (endothelium and basement membrane), a smooth-muscle media, and a fibrous adventitia. *Lymph transport* is effected by a series of rhythmic contractile waves (10–12/min) that are generated in the smooth-muscle, valveless collector segments. The *direction* of lymph flow is controlled by closing the distal valves and opening the proximal valves of the precollectors and collectors.

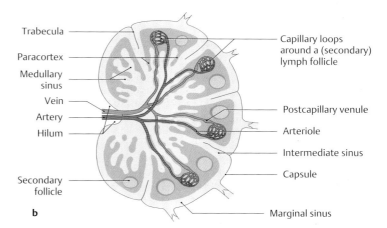

E Structure of a lymph node
a Lymph circulation, b blood supply to the lymph node.

Lymph nodes are small filtering stations located in the course of lymphatic vessels and are components of the specific immune response (they contain T- and B-lymphocytes). *Regional lymph nodes* are distinguished from the *collecting lymph nodes* that receive lymph from multiple regional nodes. The lymph enters the lymph node through multiple afferent vessels. As the fluid passes along the various lymph sinuses to the efferent vessels, it comes into contact with the lymph node tissue

over a broad surface area. From outside to inside, a lymph node consists of the cortex, paracortex, and medulla. The numerous secondary follicles in the *cortex* form the *B-lymphocyte region*, and the lymphocyte-rich areas between and below the secondary follicles are the *T-lymphocyte regions (paracortex)*. Lymphocytes leave the bloodstream in the high-endothelial postcapillary venules of the T-lymphocyte region; then, after differentiating, they leave the lymph node with the draining lymph via efferent lymph vessels, which often become the afferent vessel of another lymph node of a lymph node group.

7.2 Exocrine and Endocrine Glands

A Development and classification of glands

Glands are epithelial aggregations of highly specialized single cells (goblet cells, multicellular intraepithelial glands) or of larger cell groups that have migrated to deeper levels. Their function is to synthesize and release secretions. Glands fall into two main categories:

- **Exocrine glands** (e.g., salivary glands, sweat glands): These glands release their secretion *externally* to the skin or mucosa, either directly or through excretory ducts.
- **Endocrine glands:** Their secretions (in this case hormonal messengers) are released *internally*, i.e., into the bloodstream, lymphatics, or intercellular spaces. Endocrine glands do not have excretory ducts (see **F** for mechanisms of hormone release). Once released into the bloodstream, the hormones are distributed throughout the body and are transported to their target cells, where they bind to specific receptors and exert their effect.

B Mechanisms by which exocrine glands release their secretions
(light-microscopic scale)

a Exocytosis: In this mechanism, the secretion is released *without an enclosing membrane* (merocrine or eccrine secretion). The membrane-bound vesicles containing the secretion fuse with the apical cell membrane and discharge their contents to the outside with no loss of membranous material (the secretory mechanism of most glands, see also **C**).

b Apocytosis: The membrane-bound vesicles form a bulge in the apical cell membrane and are finally *pinched off* by it (apocrine secretion). The pinched-off secretory products are enclosed within a membrane. This mechanism is necessary in the secretion of fats. The membrane encloses the fats and keeps them emulsified (e.g., scent glands, mammary glands).

c Holocytosis: In this mechanism the *entire glandular cell disintegrates and becomes the secretory product* (holocrine secretion). As a result, the glandular cells must be constantly replaced by a basal regenerative cell layer (e.g., sebaceous glands in the skin).

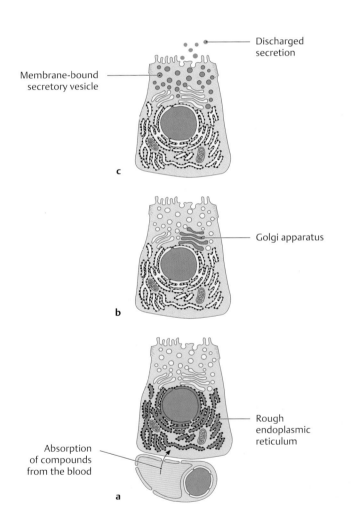

C Production and release of secretions by exocytosis (electron-microscopic scale)

After the glandular cell has absorbed essential compounds from the blood and synthesized necessary materials such as secretory proteins in the rough endoplasmic reticulum (**a**), the secretions are transported by the Golgi apparatus (**b**) to the apical part of the cell, where they are discharged by exocytosis (**c**).

D Principal sites where hormones and hormonelike substances are formed

Hormones are vitally important chemical messengers that enable cells to communicate with one another. Usually, very small amounts of these messengers act on metabolic processes in their target cells. Different hormones can be classified on the basis of their

- site of formation,
- site of action,
- mechanism of action, or
- chemical structure.

Examples are steroid hormones (e.g., testosterone, aldosterone), amino acid derivatives (e.g., epinephrine, norepinephrine, dopamine, serotonin), peptide hormones (e.g., insulin, glucagon), and fatty acid derivatives (e.g., prostaglandins).

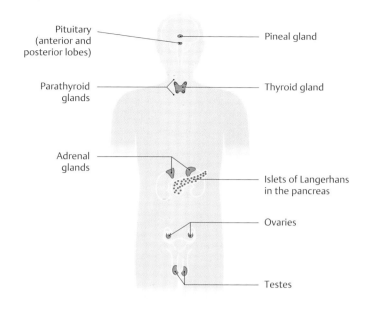

Principal sites of formation	Hormones and hormonelike substances
Classic endocrine hormonal glands	
Pituitary gland (anterior and posterior lobes)	ACTH (adrenocorticotropic hormone, corticotropin)
	TSH (thyroid-stimulating hormone, thyrotropin)
	FSH (follicle-stimulating hormone, follitropin)
	LH (luteinizing hormone, lutropin)
	STH (somatotropic hormone, somatotropin)
	MSH (melanocyte-stimulating hormone, melanotropin)
	PRL (prolactin)
	ADH (antidiuretic hormone or vasopressin)
	Oxytocin (formed in the hypothalamus and secreted by the posterior pituitary)
Pineal gland	Melatonin
Thyroid gland	Thyroxine (T_4) and triiodothyronine (T_3)
C cells of the thyroid gland	Calcitonin
Parathyroid glands	Parathyroid hormone
Adrenal glands	Mineralocorticoids and glucocorticoids
	Androgens
	Epinephrine and norepinephrine
Pancreatic islet cells (Langerhans cells)	Insulin, glucagon, somatostatin, and pancreatic polypeptide
Ovary	Estrogens and progestins
Testis	Androgens (mainly testosterone)
Placenta	Chorionic gonadotropin, progesterone
Hormone-producing tissues and single cells	
Central and autonomic nervous system	Neuronal transmitters
Parts of the diencephalon (e.g., the hypothalamus)	Releasing and inhibitory hormones (liberins and statins)
System of gastrointestinal cells in the GI tract	Gastrin, cholecystokinin, secretin
Cardiac atria	Atrial natriuretic peptide
Kidney	Erythropoietin, renin
Liver	Angiotensinogen, somatomedins
Immune organs	Thymus hormones, cytokins, lymphokines
Tissue hormones	Eicosanoids, prostaglandins, histamine, bradykinin

E Overview of the human endocrine glands

The diffuse or disseminated endocrine cell system (individual endocrine cells dispersed among the cells of the surface epithelium) in the gastrointestinal tract is not shown.

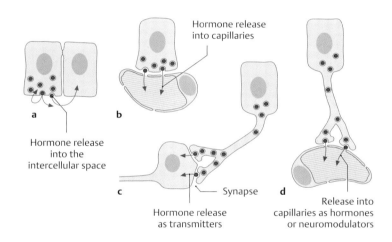

F Types of hormone-mediated information transmission

The endocrine system is closely linked to the autonomic nervous system and immune system in terms of its biological tasks. It functions as a kind of wireless communication system that coordinates the functions of target tissues and target organs, which may be located at distant sites.

a **Paracrine and autocrine secretion:** The hormones are not released into the bloodstream but into the intercellular space. Hence they act only in close proximity to their site of synthesis.

b **Endocrine secretion:** The hormones are synthesized and released into the bloodstream (fenestrated capillaries).

c **Neurocrine secretion:** Hormones of the neurocrine system (neurotransmitters) act in the form of synaptic transmitter substances and are concerned with local information transmission.

d **Neurosecretion:** Hormones or neuromodulators (neurohormones) are produced in specialized nerve cells and released to blood vessels in neurohemal regions (e.g., the pituitary). This enables them to act on distant organs.

8.1 Development of the Central Nervous System (CNS)

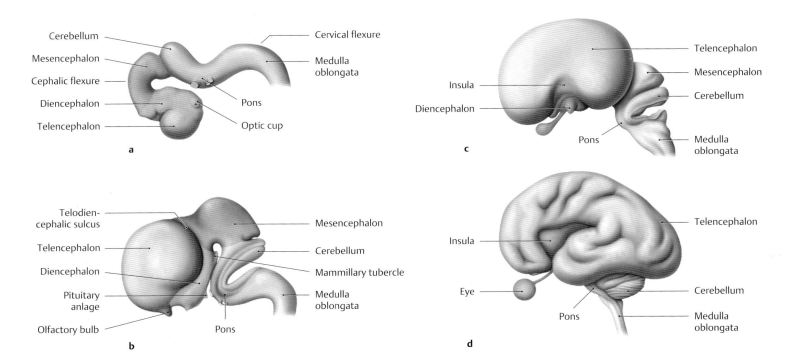

A Development of the brain

a Embryo with a greatest length (GL, see p. 4) of 10 mm, *at the beginning of the 2nd month of development.* Even at this stage we can see the differentiation of the neural tube into segments that will generate various brain regions (see **C**):

- Medulla oblongata (gray)
- Pons (gray)
- Cerebellum (light blue)
- Midbrain (mesencephalon, dark blue)
- Interbrain (diencephalon, yellow)
- Forebrain (telencephalon, red)

Note: The telencephalon grows over all the other brain structures as development proceeds.

b Embryo with a GL of 27 mm, *near the end of the 2nd month of development* (end of the embryonic period). The olfactory bulb is developing from the telencephalon, part of the pituitary anlage (*neurohypophysis*) from the diencephalon.

c Fetus with a GL of 53 mm, in approximately the *3rd month of development.* By this time the telencephalon has begun to overgrow the other brain areas. The insula is still on the surface but will subsequently be covered by the cerebral hemispheres (compare with **d**).

d Fetus with a crown–rump length (CRL, see p. 4) of 27 cm (270 mm), in approximately the *7th month of development.* The brain has begun to develop conspicuous gyri and sulci.

B Brain vesicles and their derivatives

The cranial end of the neural tube expands to form three primary brain vesicles: the forebrain (prosencephalon), the midbrain (mesencephalon), and the hindbrain (rhombencephalon). The forebrain (telencephalon) and interbrain (diencephalon) develop from the prosencephalon. The mesencephalon gives rise to the superior and inferior colliculi and related structures. The rhombencephalon differentiates into the pons, cerebellum, and medulla oblongata. The pons and cerebellum are also known collectively as the metencephalon. Some important structures of the adult brain are listed at far right to illustrate the derivatives of the brain vesicles. They can be traced back in the diagram to their developmental precursors.

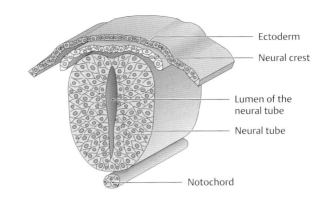

Ectoderm

Neural crest

Lumen of the neural tube

Neural tube

Notochord

C Development of the nervous system: cross section through the neural tube, neural crest, and dorsal ectoderm
During development, the neural groove folds away from the overlying dorsal ectoderm and closes to form the *neural tube*. Cells migrate from the lateral portions of the neural groove to form the *neural crest* on each side. The *central* nervous system (brain and spinal cord) develops from the neural *tube,* while the *peripheral* nervous system develops from derivatives of the neural *crest* (see p. 74).

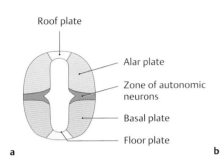

Roof plate

Alar plate

Zone of autonomic neurons

Basal plate

Floor plate

a

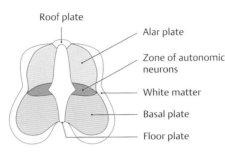

Roof plate

Alar plate

Zone of autonomic neurons

White matter

Basal plate

Floor plate

b

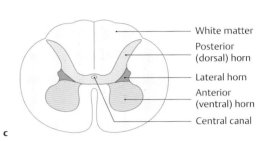

White matter

Posterior (dorsal) horn

Lateral horn

Anterior (ventral) horn

Central canal

c

D Differentiation of the neural tube in the spinal cord region during development
Cross section, cranial view.
a Early neural tube, **b** intermediate stage, **c** adult spinal cord.
The neurons that form in the *basal plate* are *efferent* (motor) neurons, while those that form in the *alar plate* are *afferent* (sensory) neurons.

The area between them—the future thoracic, lumbar, and sacral cord—is another zone that gives rise to preganglionic autonomic neurons. The roof plate and floor plate do not form neurons. A knowledge of how these neuron populations are distributed is helpful in understanding the structure of the hindbrain (rhombencephalon, see **E**).

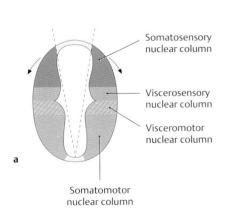

Somatosensory nuclear column

Viscerosensory nuclear column

Visceromotor nuclear column

a

Somatomotor nuclear column

b

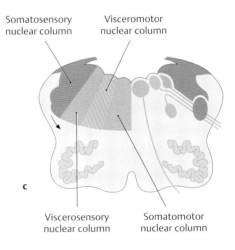

Somatosensory nuclear column

Visceromotor nuclear column

Viscerosensory nuclear column

Somatomotor nuclear column

c

E Embryonic migratory movements of neuron populations and their effect on the location of the cranial nerve nuclei
Cross section, cranial view. (Visual aid: If we compare the spinal cord to a book, it would be closed in **a** and open in **b** and **c**.)

a In the **initial stage,** the motor neurons are ventral (anterior), and the sensory neurons are dorsal (posterior). The arrows indicate the directions of migration.
b In the **early embryonic stage,** the neurons of the alar plate migrate laterally and ventrally (anteriorly).

c In the adult brain (medulla oblongata and pons, derivatives of the rhombencephalon), we can distinguish **four nuclear columns** (after His and Herrick) that contain functionally distinct cranial nerve nuclei (from medial to lateral):

1. Somatomotor column (lilac)
2. Visceromotor column (orange and green stripes)
3. Viscerosensory column (light blue)
4. Somatosensory column (dark blue)

73

8.2 Neural Crest Derivatives and the Development of the Peripheral Nervous System (PNS)

A Development of the neural crest cells

At 3 weeks' development, the notochord induces surface ectoderm in the medial embryonic disc to thicken and form the neural plate (neuro-ectoderm). The neural plate differentiates to form the primordia of the nervous system. Neural folds are raised on each side of the neural plate, and a median groove develops between them—the neural groove. This groove subsequently deepens and closes to form the neural tube, which sinks below the ectoderm. Portions of the folds that do not contribute to neural tube formation differentiate to form the neural crest. While neural crest cells in the future head region start to migrate even before the neural tube is closed, crest migration in the trunk is delayed until tube closure. Cells destined to form the neural crest detach from the ectoderm at the fusing margins of the neural tube and undergo an *epithelio-mesenchymal transition*, diving into underlying mesoderm, where they begin a long and tortuous migration. As the neural tube differentiates into the central nervous system, migrating neural crest cells settle in different locations and develop into sensory and autonomic ganglia, endocrine glands, melanocytes, cartilage, and other structures (see **B** and **C**) (after Wolpert).

B Main migratory pathways and derivatives of the neural crest

(after Christ and Wachtler)

Neural crest cells originated in different regions have different migration paths and fates. Those from cranial levels contribute to cartilage and bone in the head and neck, and to cranial parasympathetic ganglia (see **C**). Those from thoracolumbar levels do not become skeletal cells, but generate peripheral neurons, endocrine cells, melanocytes, and Schwann cells. This diagram shows the migration of the neural crest cells *in the trunk of the early embryo* (4 weeks' development, see p. 7). They follow three **main migratory pathways**:

① Dorsolateral pathway (melanoblasts, which differentiate into melanocytes)
② Ventrolateral pathway (ganglioblasts, which differentiate into sensory nerve cells in the dorsal (posterior) root [spinal] ganglia)
③ Ventral pathway (cells differentiate into neurons and associated cells of the paravertebral sympathetic ganglia, into chromaffin cells of the adrenal medulla, and into autonomic plexuses in the gastrointestinal tract)

Thus, the neural crest can develop into a variety of seemingly unrelated *nonneuronal* cells as well as peripheral ganglion cells. These unusual characteristics of the neural crest— its pluripotential capacity and wide-ranging migration—have consequences when its differentiation or migration is defective. Disruption of neural crest development may deprive organs of their autonomic innervation (Hirschsprung disease). Tumors derived from neural crest cells tend to be highly malignant and difficult to treat. (See **D**.)

a   **b**

C Neural crest derivatives in the head and neck region

Besides the equivalents of the structures named in **B** (e.g., melano-cytes), other structures in the head and neck region that originate from the cranial neural crest are skeletal and cartilaginous muscles and muscles of facial expression.

a Cranial neural crest derivatives in the adult skeleton: facial bones, hyoid bone, portions of the thyroid cartilage.

b Most of the facial skin is derived from the neural crest.

D Diseases of neural crest derivatives (selected examples)

Neural crest	Disease
Parasympathetic visceral ganglia	Neuroblastoma (malignant childhood tumor)
Enteric nervous system	Hirschsprung disease (aganglionic colon)
Glial cells (Schwann cells, satellite cells)	Neurofibromatosis (Recklinghausen disease)
Melanocytes	Malignant melanoma, albinism
Adrenal medulla	Pheochromocytoma (adrenal gland tumor)
Endocrine cells of the lung and heart	Carcinoids (malignant tumors with endocrine activity)
Parafollicular cells (C cells) of the thyroid gland	Medullary thyroid carcinoma

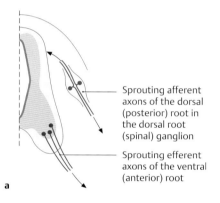

Sprouting afferent axons of the dorsal (posterior) root in the dorsal root (spinal) ganglion

Sprouting efferent axons of the ventral (anterior) root

a

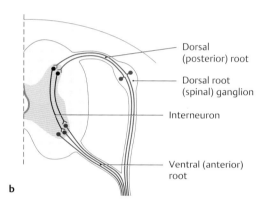

Dorsal (posterior) root

Dorsal root (spinal) ganglion

Interneuron

Ventral (anterior) root

b

E Development of a peripheral nerve

Afferent (blue) and efferent (red) axons sprout *separately* from the neuron cell bodies during early development (**a**). Primary afferent (sensory) neurons develop in the dorsal (posterior) root (spinal) ganglia, and primary motor neurons develop from the basal plate of the spinal cord (**b**). *Interneurons* (black), which connect sensory ganglia and motor neurons, develop later.

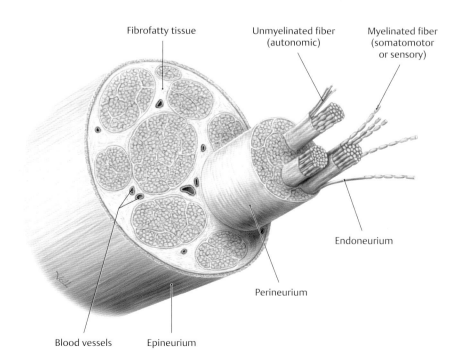

Fibrofatty tissue

Unmyelinated fiber (autonomic)

Myelinated fiber (somatomotor or sensory)

Endoneurium

Perineurium

Blood vessels   Epineurium

F Structure of a peripheral nerve

A peripheral nerve consists entirely of axons (also called neurites) and sheath tissue (Schwann cells, fibroblasts, blood vessels). The axons transmit information either from the periphery to the CNS (*afferents*) or in the opposite direction from the CNS to the periphery (*efferents*). Axons may be myelinated or unmyelinated. The latter have a much slower conduction velocity and are usually fibers of the autonomic nervous system (see p. 95). Among the investing layers of the nerve, the *perineurium* ensheaths the nerve fascicles and provides an important tissue barrier (see p. 93).

8.3   Topography and Structure of the Nervous System

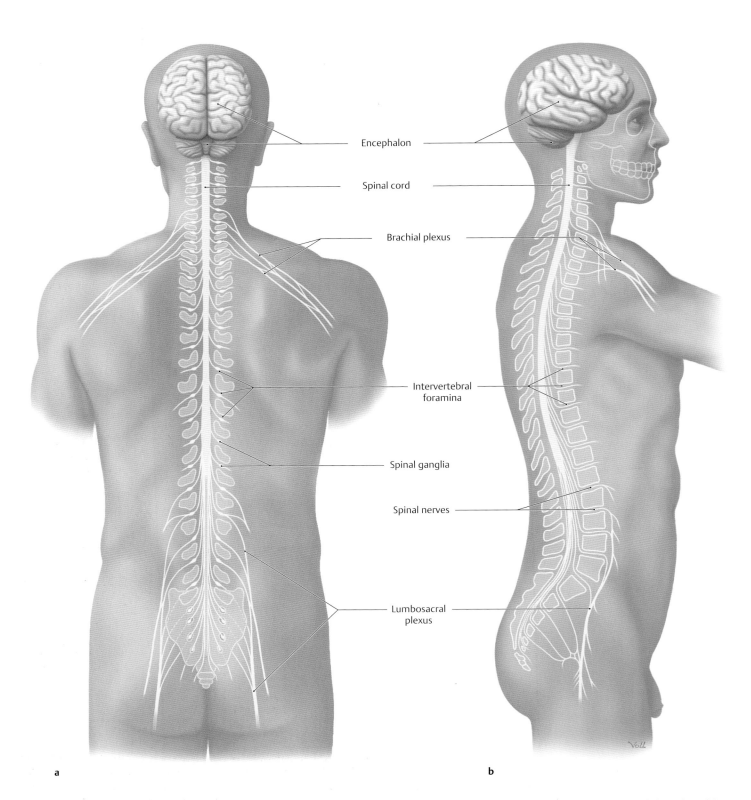

Encephalon

Spinal cord

Brachial plexus

Intervertebral foramina

Spinal ganglia

Spinal nerves

Lumbosacral plexus

a   b

A Topography of the nervous system
a Posterior view, **b** right lateral view.
The *central nervous system* (CNS), consisting of the brain (encephalon) and spinal cord, is shown in pink. The *peripheral nervous system* (PNS), consisting of nerves and ganglia, is shown in yellow. The nerves arising from the spinal cord leave their bony canal through the *intervertebral foramina* and are distributed to their target organs. The *spinal nerves* are formed in the foramina by the union of their dorsal (posterior) roots and ventral (anterior) roots (see p. 81). The small *spinal ganglion* in the intervertebral foramen appears as a slight swelling of the dorsal root (visible only in the posterior view; its function is described on p. 81).
In the limbs, the ventral rami of the spinal nerves come together to form plexuses. These plexuses then give rise to the peripheral nerves that supply the limbs.

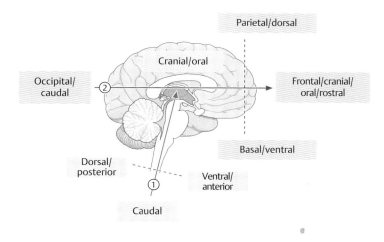

C Terms of location and direction in the CNS
Midsagittal section, right lateral view.
Note two important axes:

① The almost vertical brainstem axis (corresponds approximately to the body axis).
② The horizontal axis through the diencephalon and telencephalon.
Keep these reference axes in mind when using directional terms in the CNS.

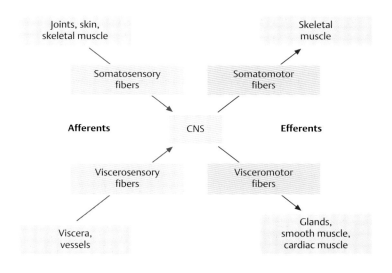

B Spinal nerves and cranial nerves
Anterior view. *Thirty-one pairs of spinal nerves* arise from the spinal cord in the peripheral nervous system, compared to *12 pairs of cranial nerves* that arise from the brain. The cranial nerve pairs are traditionally designated by roman numerals.
Note: The first two cranial nerves, the olfactory (II) and optic (I) nerves, are not peripheral nerves in the strict sense, but outpouchings from the brain, which means they are pathways of the central nervous system. They are enclosed within the meninges and contain cells that are exclusively found in the central nervous system, oligondendrocytes and microglial cells.

D Schematic representation of information flow in the nervous system
The information encoded in nerve fibers is transmitted either *to the CNS* (brain and spinal cord) or *from the CNS* to the periphery (PNS, including the peripheral parts of the autonomic nervous system, see p. 72). Fibers that carry information to the CNS are called afferent fibers or *afferents* for short; fibers that carry signals away from the CNS are called efferent fibers or *efferents*.

8.4 Cells of the Nervous System

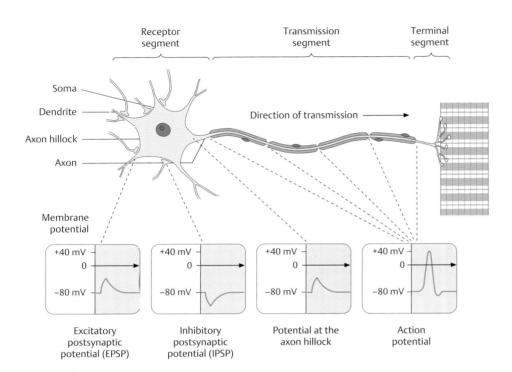

Receptor segment | Transmission segment | Terminal segment

Soma
Dendrite
Axon hillock
Axon

Direction of transmission

Membrane potential

+40 mV
0
−80 mV

Excitatory postsynaptic potential (EPSP)

+40 mV
0
−80 mV

Inhibitory postsynaptic potential (IPSP)

+40 mV
0
−80 mV

Potential at the axon hillock

+40 mV
0
−80 mV

Action potential

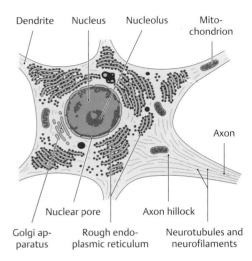

Dendrite   Nucleus   Nucleolus   Mito-chondrion

Axon

Nuclear pore   Axon hillock

Golgi apparatus | Rough endoplasmic reticulum | Neurotubules and neurofilaments

A The nerve cell (neuron)

The neuron is the smallest functional unit of the nervous system. Neurons communicate with other nerve cells through synapses. The *synapses that end at nerve cells* usually do so at dendrites (as seen here). The transmitter substance that is released at the synapses to act on the dendrite membrane may have an *excitatory* or *inhibitory* action, meaning that the transmitter either increases or decreases the local action potential at the nerve cell membrane. All of the excitatory and inhibitory potentials of a nerve cell are integrated in the axon hillock. If the excitatory potentials predominate, the stimulus exceeds the excitation threshold of the neuron, causing the axon to fire (transmit an impulse) according to the all-or-nothing rule.

B Electron microscopy of the neuron

Neurons are rich in *rough endoplasmic reticulum* (protein synthesis, active metabolism). This endoplasmic reticulum (known also as *Nissl substance*) is easily demonstrated by light microscopy using cationic dyes, which bind to the phosphodiester backbone of the ribosomal RNAs. The distribution pattern of the Nissl substance is used in neuropathology to evaluate the functional integrity of neurons. Neurotubules and neurofilaments are referred to collectively as *neurofibrils* in light microscopy, as they are too fine to be identified as separate structures under a light microscope. Neurofibrils can be demonstrated in light microscopy by impregnating the nerve tissue with silver salts. This is of interest in neuropathology because the clumping of neurofibrils is an important histologic feature of Alzheimer disease.

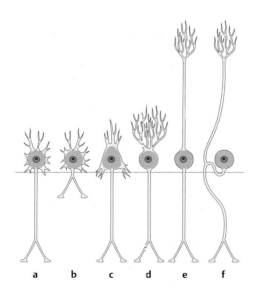

a   b   c   d   e   f

C Basic forms of the neuron and its functionally adapted variants

The horizontal line marks the region of the axon hillock, which represents the initial segment of the axon. (The structure of a peripheral nerve, consisting only of axons and sheath tissue, is shown on p. 75.)

a Multipolar neuron (multiple dendrites) with a *long* axon (= long transmission path). Examples are projection neurons such as α-motoneurons in the spinal cord.

b Multipolar neuron with a short axon (= short transmission path). Examples are interneurons like those in the gray matter of the brain and spinal cord.

c Pyramidal cell: Dendrites are present only at the apex and base of the *tridentate* cell body, and the axon is long. Examples are efferent neurons of the cerebral motor cortex.

d Purkinje cell: An elaborately branched dendritic tree arises from a circumscribed site on the cell body. The Purkinje cell receives many synaptic contacts from afferents to the cerebellum and is also the efferent cell of the cerebellar cortex.

e Bipolar neuron: The dendrite branches in the periphery. Examples are bipolar cells of the retina.

f Pseudounipolar neuron: The dendrite and axon are not separated by a cell body. An example is the primary afferent (= first sensory) neuron in the spinal ganglion (see p. 89).

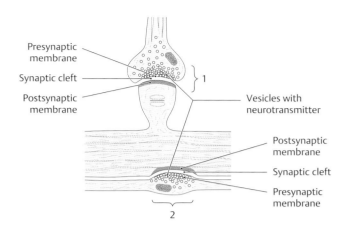

D Synaptic patterns in a small group of neurons

Axons can terminate at various sites on the target neuron and form synapses there. The synaptic patterns are described as axodendritic, axosomatic, or axoaxonal. Axodendritic synapses are the most common (see also **A**).

E Electron microscopy of synapses in the CNS

Synapses are the functional connection between two neurons. They consist of a presynaptic membrane, a synaptic cleft, and a postsynaptic membrane. In a *spine synapse* (1), the presynaptic knob (bouton) is in contact with a specialized protuberance (spine) of the target neuron. The side-by-side synapse of an axon with the flat surface of a target neuron is called a parallel contact or *bouton en passage* (2). The vesicles in the presynaptic expansion contain the neurotransmitters that are released into the synaptic cleft by exocytosis when the axon fires. From there the neurotransmitters diffuse to the postsynaptic membrane, where their receptors are located. A variety of drugs and toxins act upon synaptic transmission (antidepressants, muscle relaxants, toxic gases, botulinum toxin).

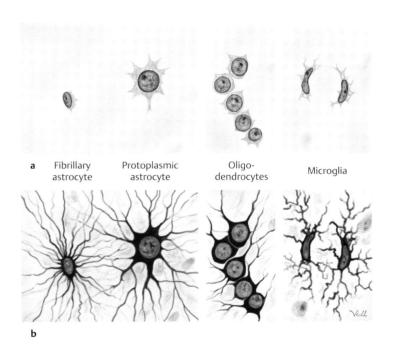

a Fibrillary astrocyte   Protoplasmic astrocyte   Oligo-dendrocytes   Microglia

b

F Cells of the neuroglia in the CNS

Neuroglial cells surround the neurons, providing them with structural and functional support (see **G**). Various staining methods are available in light microscopy for selectively demonstrating different portions of the neuroglial cells:

a Cell nuclei demonstrated with a basic stain.
b Cell body demonstrated by silver impregnation.

G Summary: cells of the CNS and PNS and their functional importance

Type of cell	Function
Neurons (CNS and PNS)	1. Impulse formation 2. Impulse conduction 3. Information processing
Glial cells	
Astrocytes (CNS only)	1. Maintain a constant internal milieu in the CNS 2. Contribute to the structure of the blood–brain barrier (see p. 93) 3. Phagocytize dead synapses 4. Form scar tissue in the CNS (e.g., in multiple sclerosis or following a stroke)
Microglial cells (CNS only)	Phagocytosis ("macrophages of the brain")
Oligodendrocytes (CNS only)	Myelin sheath formation in the CNS
Schwann cells (PNS only)	Myelin sheath formation in the PNS
Satellite cells (PNS only)	Modified Schwann cells; surround the cell body of neurons in PNS ganglia

8.5 Structure of a Spinal Cord Segment

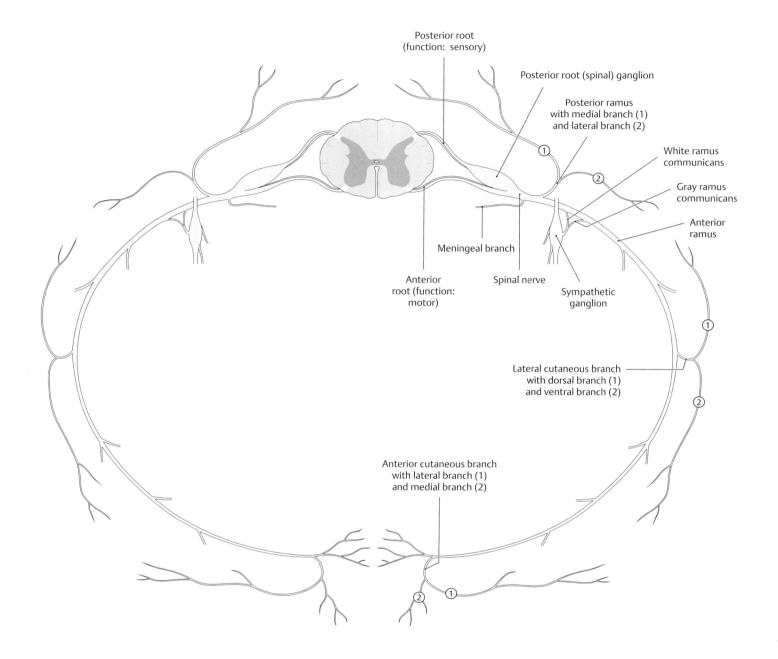

Posterior root
(function: sensory)

Posterior root (spinal) ganglion

Posterior ramus
with medial branch (1)
and lateral branch (2)

White ramus
communicans

Gray ramus
communicans

Anterior
ramus

Meningeal branch

Anterior
root (function:
motor)

Spinal nerve

Sympathetic
ganglion

Lateral cutaneous branch
with dorsal branch (1)
and ventral branch (2)

Anterior cutaneous branch
with lateral branch (1)
and medial branch (2)

A Structure of a spinal cord segment with its spinal nerve
Superior view. The spinal cord is made up of 31 consecutive segments arranged one above the other (see **B**). An *anterior root* and a *posterior root* emerge from the sides of each segment. The *anterior* root consists of *efferent* (motor) fibers, while the *posterior* root consists of *afferent* (sensory) fibers. Both roots from one segment unite in the intervertebral foramen to form the *spinal nerve*. The afferent (sensory) fibers and efferent (motor) fibers intermingle at this junction, so that the branches into which the spinal nerve divides (see below) contain motor *and* sensory elements (except for the meningeal branch, which is purely sensory). This division into branches (rami) occurs shortly after the anterior and posterior roots unite to form the spinal nerve. Consequently, the spinal nerve itself is only about 1 cm long.

The principal branches of the spinal nerve have the following functions:

- The anterior ramus innervates the anterior and lateral body wall and the limbs.
- The posterior ramus innervates the skin of the back and the intrinsic back muscles.
- The meningeal branch reenters the spinal canal, providing sensory innervation to the spinal membranes and other structures.
- The white ramus communicans carries white (= myelinated) fibers *to* the ganglion of the sympathetic trunk.
- The gray ramus communicans carries gray (= unmyelinated) fibers *from* the sympathetic ganglion back to the spinal nerve (the functional significance of this is described on p. 95). The anterior and posterior rami of the spinal nerves subdivide into further branches.

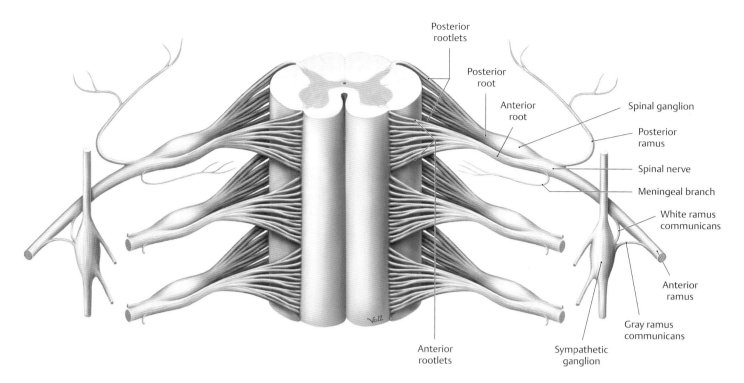

B Spinal cord segments

Anterior view. The spinal cord is composed of many segments, each of which gives rise to one pair of spinal nerves (for clarity, only the upper segment of the spinal cord is shown). Several rootlets unite to form the anterior and the posterior roots of a spinal nerve, which then divides into five branches (see **A**). The segmental structure of the spinal cord is visible externally only at the rootlets; the spinal cord itself does not show any external segmentation.

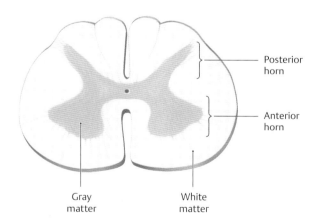

C Embryological origins of the topographical and functional anatomy of a spinal cord segment

The afferent fibers (e.g., from cutaneous receptors) pass through the *posterior root* into the posterior horn of the spinal cord, which is derived embryologically from the alar plate. The efferent fibers arise from neurons located in the anterior horn of the spinal cord, which is a derivative of the basal plate. They leave the spinal cord by the *anterior root* and are distributed to their target organ, such as a skeletal muscle.

D Cross section of a spinal cord segment

Superior view. A cross section of the spinal cord shows the centrally located gray matter arranged in a butterfly-shaped pattern and the white matter surrounding it. Cell bodies of neurons are located in the gray matter; axons move up and down in the white matter. The gray matter is divided into anterior and posterior horns. The cell bodies of efferent neurons are located in the anterior horns, and those of afferent neurons in the posterior horns. Thus, the spinal cord is functionally arranged from anterior (motor) to posterior (sensory) (horizontal arrangement). For the relationship between spinal cord segments and dermatomes (vertical arrangement of the spinal cord), see p. 82.

8.6 Sensory Innervation: An Overview

A Location and designation of spinal cord segments in relation to the vertebral canal

Right lateral view. The spinal cord consists of 31 segments that are arranged from top to bottom:

- 8 cervical segments,
- 12 thoracic segments,
- 5 lumbar segments,
- 5 sacral segments, and
- 1 coccygeal segment (no clinical significance)

The growth of the spinal cord lags behind that of the spinal column, so in an adult it extends only to the first lumbar vertebra, as shown here (compare p. 128). The spinal cord segments are equivalent to the dermatomes on the body surface (see **C**). In other words, a dermatome is an area on the body surface, the sensory receptors of which (e.g., for pressure, temperature, pain, vibration) pull with their afferents into a spinal cord segment, thus enabling a 1:1 relationship between body surface and spinal cord segment. In clinical terms, it means that in the case of sensory disorder (dermatome malfunction), it is possible to determine at which level of the spinal cord the malfunction is located. A myotome (see p. 7) is the equivalent of a dermatome, as regards motor function.

Note: There are seven cervical vertebrae (C1–C7) but eight pairs of cervical nerves (C1–C8). The highest pair of cervical nerves exit the vertebral canal superior to the first cervical vertebra. The remaining pairs of cervical nerves, like all the other spinal nerve pairs, exit inferior to the cervical vertebral body. The pair of coccygeal nerves (gray) has no clinical importance.

B Dermatomes and limb buds (after Sadler)

From the somites, which give rise to limbs, cells migrate, and limb buds form. These migrating cells drag their original segmental innervation along behind them. Thus, dermatomes reflect the segmental arrangement, which is based on the somites (see p. 7).

a In a 5-week-old embryo, the dermatomes are still segmentally arranged.

b In a 6-week-old embryo, migrations have already taken place: the preaxial segments are positioned cranially, the postaxial seg-

ments caudally. The segments lying in between have shifted in a distal direction toward the hand.

c In a 7-week-old embryo, the proportions are similar to those postbirth.

This dermatome diagram, similar to the diagram in **C**, is simplified, because the cells, which form the dermatomes, migrate (for details, see p. 14).

C Simplified scheme for learning the dermatomes (after Mumenthaler)

The distribution of dermatomes on the human limbs results from the sprouting of the limb buds that occurs during embryonic development. When the limbs are positioned at right angles to the body as in a quadruped, it is easier to appreciate the pattern of innervation. Compare the location of the dermatomes to those of the spinal cord sections in **A**. The more complex pattern of dermatomes resulting from cell migration is shown on p. 86.

Note: The C1 segment contains only motor fibers; thus, there is not a C1 dermatome.

8.7 Sensory Innervation: Principles of Dermatome and Plexus Formation

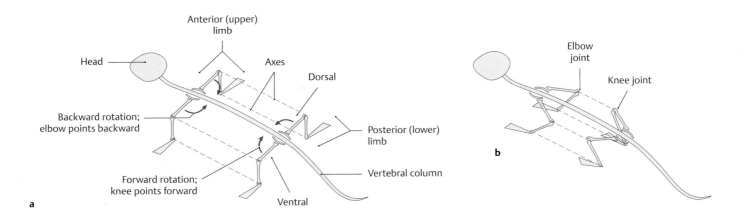

A Phylogenetic development of dermatomes
In lower tetrapods, the trunk is located between the limbs (**a**). In mammals, the limbs are also rotated (**b**). The posterior (= lower) limbs are rotated forward, and the original posterior position of the limb muscles shifts anteriorly when picturing the mammal walking erect (for details,

see p. 20). This is not the case for the anterior (= upper) limbs, which are rotated backward. That is why the cells that form dermatomes in the lower limb region migrate more than similar cells in the upper limb region. That leads to a screwlike distribution of dermatomes in the lower limbs, unlike that in the upper limbs (see p. 86).

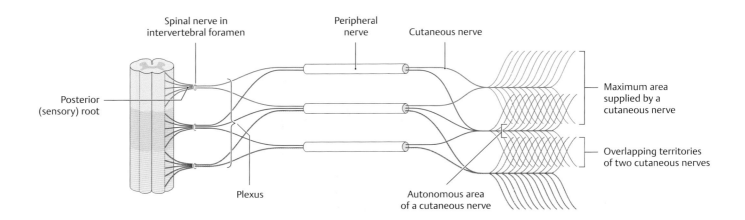

B Course of sensory fibers from the posterior root to the dermatome
Sensory fibers pass from the posterior root to the intervertebral foramen, where they unite with motor fibers to form the spinal nerve. The sensory fibers are then distributed to the anterior and posterior rami of the spinal nerve. The simple segmental arrangement of the sensory territories that occurs on the trunk is not found in the limbs (see **D**). This results from the migratory movements of various muscular and cutaneous primordia, or precursors, during the development of the limbs. Because these primordia carry their segmental innervation with them, the sensory fibers from different segments become intermingled in the limbs (plexus formation, see **C**). After fibers have been distributed in the plexus, the fibers in peripheral nerves travel to their destinations, their terminal portions often consisting entirely of sensory cutaneous nerves. The area of skin that is innervated by one spinal cord segment is called a *dermatome*. The dermatomes of adjacent spinal cord segments are often located so close together that their territories broadly overlap. This explains why the clinically detectable

area of sensory loss caused by a segmental nerve lesion may be considerably smaller than the dermatome itself. The area that receives all of its sensory supply from one cutaneous nerve is called the autonomous area of that nerve. When a segmental nerve lesion occurs, the cutaneous nerves from the two adjacent spinal cord segments are still available to supply at least the peripheral part of the affected skin area. This helps in understanding the difference between radicular (= segmental) and peripheral sensory innervation. When a nerve root becomes damaged (e.g., due to a herniated intervertebral disk), the resulting sensory loss will follow a radicular innervation pattern (see p. 86). But when a peripheral nerve is damaged (e.g., due to a limb injury), the sensory loss will conform to a peripheral innervation pattern (see p. 87).

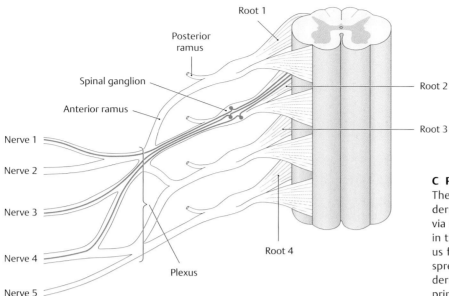

- Root 1
- Posterior ramus
- Spinal ganglion
- Anterior ramus
- Nerve 1
- Nerve 2
- Nerve 3
- Nerve 4
- Plexus
- Nerve 5
- Root 2
- Root 3
- Root 4

C Principles of plexus formation

The axons, which form the afferents from a dermatome, extend from that dermatome via several peripheral nerves to a single root in the spinal cord. As part of embryonic plexus formation, afferent axons of that one root spread via several peripheral nerves to the dermatome, in response to signals from the primordia of the dermatome.

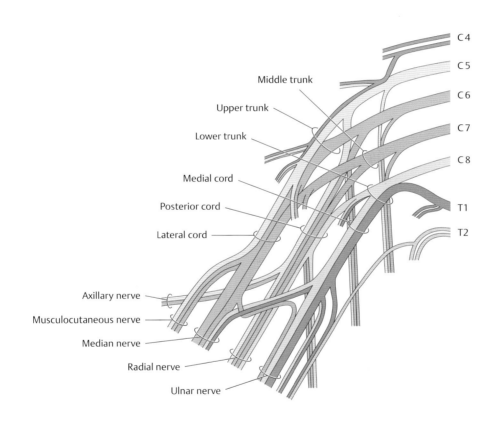

- Middle trunk
- Upper trunk
- Lower trunk
- Medial cord
- Posterior cord
- Lateral cord
- Axillary nerve
- Musculocutaneous nerve
- Median nerve
- Radial nerve
- Ulnar nerve
- C 4
- C 5
- C 6
- C 7
- C 8
- T 1
- T 2

D Plexus formation as illustrated by the brachial plexus

During embryonic development, migration and, associated with it, mixing of dermatome and myotome primordia occur with the primordia dragging their innervation along behind them. Dermatomes and myotomes have an identical developmental pattern. In the following, we will discuss only dermatomes (for more on myotomes, see p. 88). During their development, the primordia of dermatomes transmit signals to the budding sensory axons (see p. 75). This leads to every dermatome receiving its axons from its spinal cord segment. (To exhibit features more clearly, every spinal cord segment is individually colored). In order for the axons to leave their spinal cord segment and reach "their" dermatome, they have to be paired with the various peripheral nerves. The place where the shifting and mixing of axons (= fibers) occurs is called a plexus. With the brachial plexus, a distinction is made between different parts of the plexus. Prior to plexus formation, axons from one spinal cord segment combine to form roots. The axons from the roots of C5 and C6 merge to form the upper trunk, the axons from the root of C7 form the middle trunk, and those of C8 and T1 form the lower trunk. The anterior branches of the upper and middle trunks form the lateral and medial cords, and the posterior branches of all three trunks form the posterior cord. Finally, from the cords arise the large nerves of the arm and shoulder, where the axons travel on their way to the dermatomes.

8.8 Sensory Innervation: Dermatomes and Cutaneous Nerve Territories

A Pattern of radicular (segmental) sensory innervation (dermatomes)

The skin area supplied by a posterior spinal nerve root is called a *dermatome*. Because the C1 segment consists entirely of motor fibers, it lacks a corresponding sensory field. A knowledge of radicular innervation is very important clinically. For example, when a herniated intervertebral disk is impinging on a sensory root, it will cause sensory losses in the affected dermatome. The area of sensory loss can then be used to locate the level of the lesion: Which intervertebral disk is affected? In a patient with shingles (herpes zoster inflammation of a spinal ganglion), the dermatome supplied by that ganglion will be affected (after Mumenthaler).

B Pattern of nuclear sensory innervation in the head region

The head receives its sensory innervation from the trigeminal nerve (cranial nerve V). A lesion of the sensory nucleus of the trigeminal nerve within the brain (= central lesion) causes an onion-skin pattern of sensory alteration along the concentric *Sölder lines* that encircle the mouth and nostrils. The pattern of these lines corresponds to the distribution of the neurons in the sensory nucleus of the trigeminal nerve (somatotopic organization, i.e., certain groups of neurons in the CNS are linked to certain territories in the periphery). Territory 1 is supplied by the cranial nuclear column, territory 2 by the middle column, and territory 3 by the caudal column. This pattern of sensory loss is like that associated with radicular neuropathy affecting a peripheral nerve.

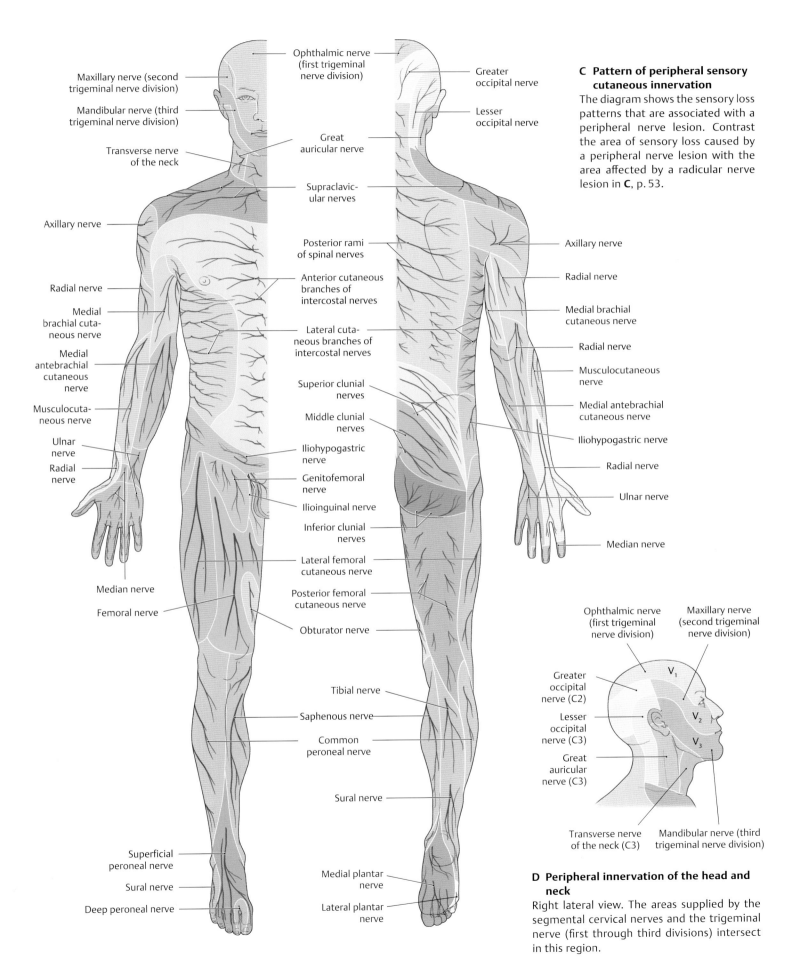

Maxillary nerve (second trigeminal nerve division)

Mandibular nerve (third trigeminal nerve division)

Transverse nerve of the neck

Axillary nerve

Radial nerve

Medial brachial cutaneous nerve

Medial antebrachial cutaneous nerve

Musculocutaneous nerve

Ulnar nerve

Radial nerve

Median nerve

Femoral nerve

Superficial peroneal nerve

Sural nerve

Deep peroneal nerve

Ophthalmic nerve (first trigeminal nerve division)

Great auricular nerve

Supraclavicular nerves

Posterior rami of spinal nerves

Anterior cutaneous branches of intercostal nerves

Lateral cutaneous branches of intercostal nerves

Superior clunial nerves

Middle clunial nerves

Iliohypogastric nerve

Genitofemoral nerve

Ilioinguinal nerve

Inferior clunial nerves

Lateral femoral cutaneous nerve

Posterior femoral cutaneous nerve

Obturator nerve

Tibial nerve

Saphenous nerve

Common peroneal nerve

Sural nerve

Medial plantar nerve

Lateral plantar nerve

Greater occipital nerve

Lesser occipital nerve

Axillary nerve

Radial nerve

Medial brachial cutaneous nerve

Radial nerve

Musculocutaneous nerve

Medial antebrachial cutaneous nerve

Iliohypogastric nerve

Radial nerve

Ulnar nerve

Median nerve

C Pattern of peripheral sensory cutaneous innervation

The diagram shows the sensory loss patterns that are associated with a peripheral nerve lesion. Contrast the area of sensory loss caused by a peripheral nerve lesion with the area affected by a radicular nerve lesion in **C**, p. 53.

Ophthalmic nerve (first trigeminal nerve division)

Maxillary nerve (second trigeminal nerve division)

Greater occipital nerve (C2)

Lesser occipital nerve (C3)

Great auricular nerve (C3)

V_1

V_2

V_3

Transverse nerve of the neck (C3)

Mandibular nerve (third trigeminal nerve division)

D Peripheral innervation of the head and neck

Right lateral view. The areas supplied by the segmental cervical nerves and the trigeminal nerve (first through third divisions) intersect in this region.

87

8.9 Motor Innervation: Organization of the Spinal Cord and Reflexes

A Organization of anterior horns in the spinal cord

Whereas the dermatomes are areas of sensory innervation (= afferents), myotomes are areas of motor innervation of the skeletal muscles (= efferents). Just as in the posterior horn, in the anterior horn, too, the spinal cord segments are stacked on top of each other. With regard to innervation, a distinction is generally made between two types of skeletal muscles:

- Those with monosegmental innervation
- Those with polysegmental innervation

In monosegmentally innervated muscles (green muscle), the cell bodies of the motoneurons innervating these muscles are located at the level of a single spinal cord segment. In polysegmentally innervated muscles (blue and orange muscle), the cell bodies of the motoneurons reside inside a column that extends over several spinal cord segments. Muscles that are exclusively or predominantly innervated by one spinal cord segment are called segment-indicating muscles. They can be clinically evaluated by testing a corresponding reflex.

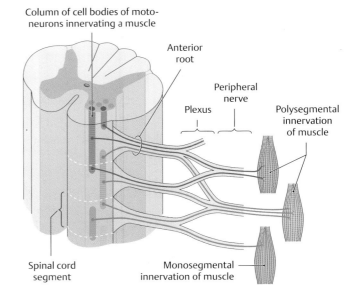

B Principles of plexus formation

In the plexus region, efferent axons from various spinal cord roots that innervate a polysegmentally innervated muscle combine into one peripheral nerve, which then extends to the muscle.

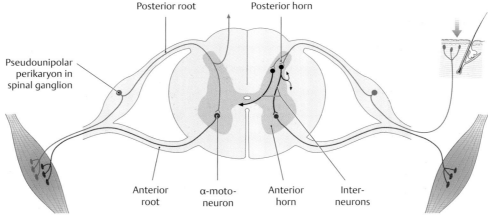

C Reflexes

The gray matter in the spinal cord, among other things, helps to coordinate muscle action on the spinal cord level (without involvement of the cortex), that is, reflexes. Broadly speaking, a distinction is made between a monosynaptic proprioceptive reflex (shown on the left) and a polysynaptic exteroceptive reflex (shown on the right).

Monosynaptic proprioceptive reflex: Receptors in a muscle transmit information about the condition of the muscle (length, muscle tension) via neurons in the spinal ganglia, the synapses of which end on the motor neuron of the muscle in the spinal cord, thereby influencing its activity.

Polysynaptic exteroceptive reflex: Receptors in the skin, rather than a muscle, transmit information to an interneuron; the interneuron synapses with the motoneuron of the muscle in the spinal cord. Since there is more than one neuron involved in the transmission of sensory information, the reflex is referred to as polysynaptic.

C5/C6

C6/C7

a

b

L3/L4

S1/S2

c

d

D Clinically important reflexes

a Biceps reflex; **b** triceps reflex; **c** patellar tendon reflex (quadriceps reflex); **d** calcaneal (Achilles') tendon reflex.

For each reflex, the muscles, reflex trigger points, involved nerves (afferents in blue, efferents in red), and corresponding spinal cord segments are shown. The most important proprioceptive reflexes should be tested during every clinical examination. The reflex is triggered by a brief blow with the reflex hammer, in most cases hitting the tendon of the muscle. As a result, the muscle stretches. If the muscle then contracts in reaction to the expansion, the reflex arc is intact. Although the reflex involves one muscle and the nerve supplying it, several spinal cord segments are involved in the innervation (multisegmental muscles, see **A**). As part of reflex testing, it is important to compare each reflex to its contralateral counterpart in order to detect one-sided augmentation, impairment, or pathologic deviations.

E Topographical and functional organization of a spinal cord segment

The **afferent fibers** from the skin, muscles, and joints (somatosensory, blue) and from the viscera (viscerosensory, green) pass through the posterior root into the spinal cord and terminate in the posterior horn. Both fibers arise from pseudounipolar cells in the posterior root (spinal) ganglion.

The **efferent fibers** for the skeletal musculature (somatomotor, red) and for the viscera (visceromotor, brown) pass through the anterior root to their respective target organs, i.e., the skeletal muscles, the vascular smooth muscles, and the smooth muscles of the internal organs. The fibers differ in their origin. Fibers for the skeletal muscles originate in the anterior horn of the spinal cord, and fibers for the viscera originate in the lateral horn. The axons of somatic motoneurons in the anterior horn synapse directly on skeletal muscle fibers (p. 90). Visceral motoneurons in the lateral horn, however, provide indirect innervation to most of their target organs. Their axons form synapses with autonomic neurons in larger discrete sympathetic ganglia or in scattered clusters embedded in the visceral organs (p. 95).

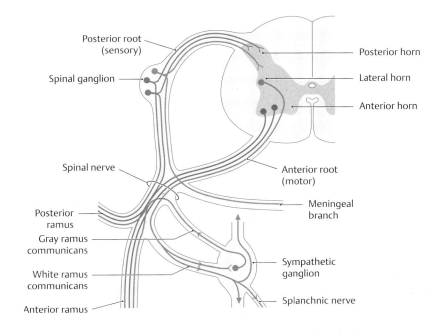

Posterior root (sensory)

Spinal ganglion

Posterior horn

Lateral horn

Anterior horn

Spinal nerve

Anterior root (motor)

Posterior ramus

Meningeal branch

Gray ramus communicans

White ramus communicans

Sympathetic ganglion

Anterior ramus

Splanchnic nerve

8.10 Motor Innervation: Upper (First) and Lower (Second) Motor Neurons

A Simplified scheme of motor innervation

The simplest common path of motor innervation originates in the primary cerebral motor cortex. Large neurons (dark red) contribute axons to bundles collected into massive *corticospinal* tracts. Many axons pass uninterrupted to the spinal cord, where they synapse upon motor neurons in the anterior horn (orange). In the brainstem the bundles of corticospinal axons are designated *pyramids* or *pyramidal tracts*. In the medulla oblongata, most corticospinal axons cross the midline in the *pyramidal decussation* and continue on the opposite side. Axons from motor neurons in the anterior horn of the spinal cord exit in *anterior roots* (p. 62) and reach their targets, skeletal muscles, via peripheral nerves, where they synapse directly at *neuromuscular junctions*.

The typical spinal motor neuron receives inputs from multiple sources. The simplest local circuit involves afferent (sensory) synapses from fibers from posterior root (spinal) ganglion cells (blue). Although most afferent information is relayed to spinal motor neurons through multiple intermediate *interneurons*, some sensory input—particularly from tendon stretch receptors—is transmitted directly via a single synapse, as depicted. This chain of connections is called a *reflex arc*. One such arc produces the knee-jerk or patellar tendon reflex.

This pattern of motor connections is responsible for two fundamental principles in the diagnosis of neurologic disorders. Because of their positions in the pathway, the cerebral cortical cells are referred to as *upper motor neurons*, those in the spinal cord as *lower motor neurons*. Damage to lower motor neurons or their axons leads to denervation of muscles, with *flaccid paralysis* and eventual muscle atrophy. In contrast, interruption of corticospinal axons or destruction of the upper motor neurons themselves, resulting, for instance, from a cerebral infarction (stroke), leads to a loss of voluntary control over the lower motor neurons. With such an upper motor neuron lesion, the lower motor neuron is controlled solely by local spinal circuits. Local reflexes remain or are enhanced, but muscles show sustained contractions and increased tone, with *spastic paralysis*.

The second fundamental correlation between the anatomy of the motor pathway and neurologic diagnosis involves the crossing of corticospinal axons in the pyramidal decussation. Upper motor lesions that occur above (cranial to) this decussation will produce spastic paralysis on the *contralateral* side of the body; lesions in corticospinal axons below (caudal to) this point will cause spastic paralysis on the same side as (*ipsilateral* to) the lesion.

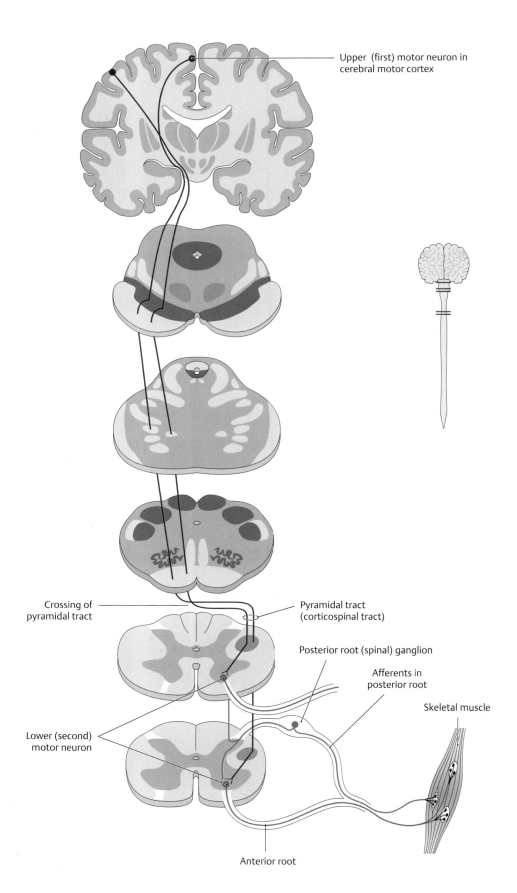

Upper (first) motor neuron in cerebral motor cortex

Crossing of pyramidal tract

Pyramidal tract (corticospinal tract)

Posterior root (spinal) ganglion

Afferents in posterior root

Skeletal muscle

Lower (second) motor neuron

Anterior root

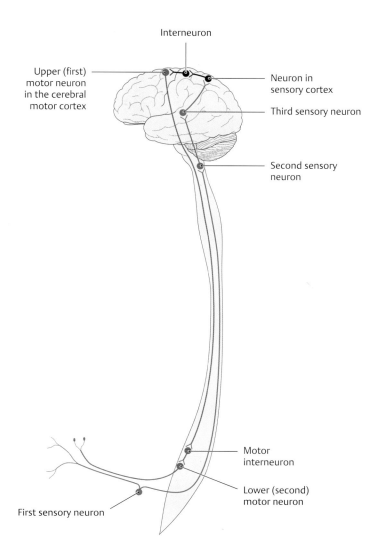

Interneuron

Upper (first)
motor neuron
in the cerebral
motor cortex

Neuron in
sensory cortex

Third sensory neuron

Second sensory
neuron

Motor
interneuron

Lower (second)
motor neuron

First sensory neuron

B Neural circuit for sensory and motor innervation
Left lateral view. Information processing in the CNS is actually more complex than shown in **A** because motor innervation is influenced by afferents of a kind not illustrated here (= sensorimotor circuit). Although a great many neurons are active at each step in the circuit, the diagram shows only one at each level. Sensory information, encoded as electrical impulses, enters the spinal cord through a primary afferent neuron (first sensory neuron) whose cell body is in the spinal ganglion (afferent neurons shown in blue). The information is relayed synaptically to the second and third afferent (sensory) neurons, which transfer it to the sensory cortex (black). Associative neurons (interneurons, black) transmit the information to the upper motor neuron in the cerebral motor cortex, where the information is modified by many associated inputs. The cortical motor neuron (upper motor neuron) redirects the information to the spinal cord, where it reaches the spinal (lower) motor neuron, either directly or via interneurons and additional synaptic relays. Finally, the lower motor neuron in the spinal cord transmits the impulses to the voluntary skeletal muscle. Corticospinal projections are most direct and numerous for lower motor neurons that innervate muscles, like those in the human hand, which are often under fine control and coordinated cognitive direction. Other motor pathways, not depicted here, are more important for controlling posture and balance. Because the axons in some of these other pathways are not in the corticospinal and pyramidal tracts, they are sometimes referred to as *extrapyramidal*.

C Obersteiner–Redlich zone in a posterior root
The Obersteiner–Redlich zone marks the morphological junction between the CNS and PNS (arrows). Oligodendrocytes in the CNS form a myelin sheath around the axons only as far as this zone, which is located just past the emergence of the posterior root from the spinal cord. The myelin sheaths in the PNS are formed by Schwann cells (see p. 92 for details). The myelin is so thin at these sites that the fibers appear almost unmyelinated. This creates a site of predilection for immunologic diseases such as the immune reactions that occur in the late stages of syphilis.

8.11 Differences between the Central and Peripheral Nervous Systems

A Myelination differences in the PNS and CNS

The purpose of myelination is to provide the axons with electrical insulation, which significantly increases the nerve conduction velocity. The very lipid-rich membranes of myelinating cells are wrapped around the axons to produce this insulation. Schwann cells (left) myelinate the axons in the *PNS*, while oligodendrocytes (right) form the myelin in the *CNS*.

Note: In the *CNS*, *one* oligodendrocyte *always* wraps around *multiple* axons. In the *PNS*, *one* Schwann cell *may* ensheath *multiple* axons if the peripheral nerve is *unmyelinated*. If the peripheral nerve is *myelinated*, *one* Schwann cell *always* wraps around *one* axon.

Owing to this improved insulation, the nerve conduction velocity is higher in myelinated nerves than in unmyelinated nerves. Myelinated fibers occur in areas where fast reaction speeds are needed (muscular contractions), while unmyelinated fibers occur in areas that do not require rapid information transfer, as in the transmission of visceral pain. Because of the different cell types, myelin has a different composition in the CNS and PNS. This difference in myelination is also important clinically. An example is multiple sclerosis, in which the oligodendrocytes are damaged, but the Schwann cells are not, so that the central myelin sheaths are disrupted, while the peripheral myelin sheaths remain intact.

B Myelination

Principles
• Myelinated axons are generally thicker than unmyelinated axons.
• Myelinated axons transmit impulses faster than unmyelinated axons.
• Unmyelinated axons reside only in the PNS.

CNS
• Oligodendrocytes myelinate axons, with the oligodendrocyte enveloping from several up to 50 axons.

PNS
• With myelinated axons, Schwann cells wrap many layers around a single axon.
• Somatomotor and somatosensory axons are usually myelinated (exception: small pain fibers).
• Axons of the autonomic nervous system are often unmyelinated (exception: e.g., white rami communicantes of preganglionic fibers).
• With unmyelinated axons, Schwann cells wrap one layer around several axons.
• The transition from Schwann cell to oligodendrocyte occurs in the Obersteiner–Redlich zone (see **C**, p. 91).

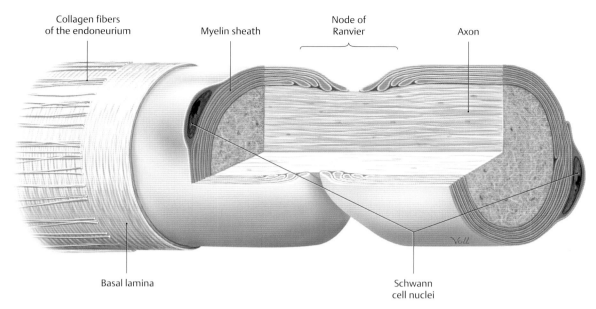

Collagen fibers of the endoneurium — Myelin sheath — Node of Ranvier — Axon

Basal lamina — Schwann cell nuclei

C Structure of a node of Ranvier in the PNS

In the PNS, the *node of Ranvier* is the site where two Schwann cells come together. That site is marked by a small gap in the myelin sheath, which forms the morphological basis for *saltatory nerve conduction*, allowing impulses to be transmitted at a higher velocity.

Astro-cytes — Endothelial cell — Endothelial cell — Basal lamina — Brain milieu

Brain capillary — Capillary lumen — Tight junction — Astrocytic processes

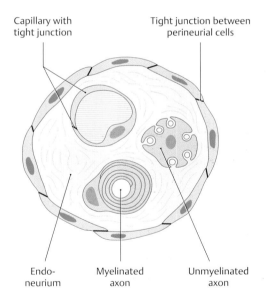

Capillary with tight junction — Tight junction between perineurial cells

Endo-neurium — Myelinated axon — Unmyelinated axon

D Structure of the blood–brain barrier in the CNS

Besides the type of myelination, there is also a difference in tissue barriers between the CNS and PNS. The CNS is isolated from surrounding tissues by the blood–brain barrier. The components of the blood–brain barrier include (1) most importantly, a continuous capillary endothelial cell layer, sealed by tight junctions; (2) a continuous basal lamina surrounding the endothelial cells; and (3) enveloping astrocytic processes surrounding the brain capillary. This barrier serves to exclude macromolecules, as well as many small molecules that are not actively transported by the endothelial cells, thus protecting the delicate environment of the CNS. The barrier is vulnerable, however, to lipid-soluble molecules that can traverse the endothelial cell membranes. The perineurial sheath creates a similar barrier in the PNS (see **E**).

E Structure of the perineurial sheath in the PNS

The perineurial sheath, like the blood–brain barrier, is formed by tight junctions between the epithelium-like fibroblasts (perineurial cells; the perineurium is described on p. 75). It isolates the milieu of the axon from that of the surrounding endoneural space (endoneurium), thereby preventing harmful substances from invading the axon. This tissue barrier must be surmounted by drugs that are designed to act on the axon, such as local anesthetic agents.

8.12   The Autonomic Nervous System

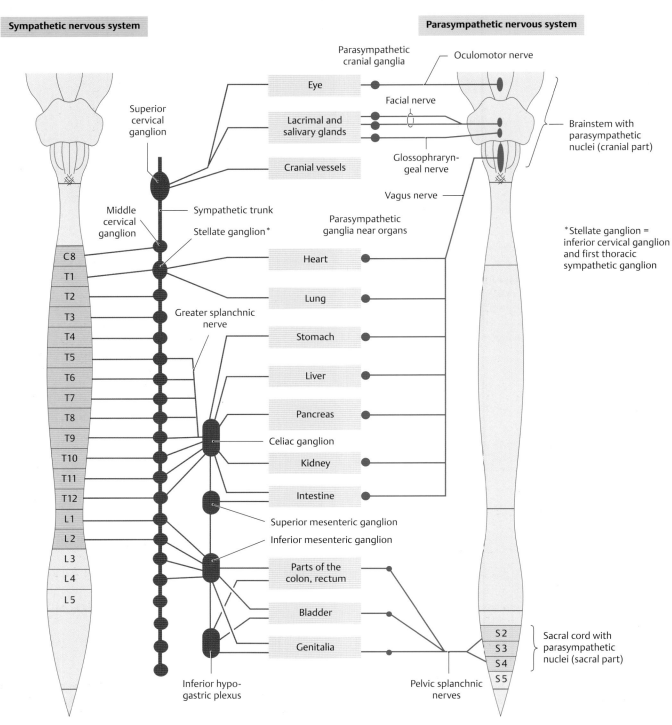

Sympathetic nervous system

Parasympathetic nervous system

Parasympathetic cranial ganglia

Oculomotor nerve

Eye

Superior cervical ganglion

Facial nerve

Lacrimal and salivary glands

Cranial vessels

Glossophraryn-geal nerve

Brainstem with parasympathetic nuclei (cranial part)

Middle cervical ganglion

Sympathetic trunk

Stellate ganglion*

Vagus nerve

Parasympathetic ganglia near organs

*Stellate ganglion = inferior cervical ganglion and first thoracic sympathetic ganglion

Heart

Lung

Greater splanchnic nerve

Stomach

Liver

Pancreas

Celiac ganglion

Kidney

Intestine

Superior mesenteric ganglion

Inferior mesenteric ganglion

Parts of the colon, rectum

Bladder

Genitalia

Sacral cord with parasympathetic nuclei (sacral part)

Inferior hypo-gastric plexus

Pelvic splanchnic nerves

A Structure of the autonomic nervous system

The system of motor innervation of skeletal muscle is complemented by the *autonomic nervous system*, with two divisions: sympathetic (red) and parasympathetic (blue). Both divisions have a two-neuron path between the CNS and their targets: a *preganglionic* CNS neuron and a ganglion cell in the PNS that is close to the target. The preganglionic neurons of the sympathetic system are in the lateral horns of the cervical, thoracic, and lumbar spinal cord. Their axons exit the CNS via the anterior roots and synapse in sympathetic ganglia in bilateral *paravertebral* chains (*sympathetic trunks*), or as single midline *prevertebral ganglia* (see **E**). Axons from these ganglion cells course in unmyelinated bundles on blood vessels or in peripheral nerves to their targets. The preganglionic neurons of the parasympathetic system are located in the brainstem and sacral spinal cord. Their axons exit the CNS via

cranial and pelvic splanchnic nerves to synapse with parasympathetic ganglion cells. In the head, these cells are in discrete ganglia associated with the cranial nerves. In other locations the parasympathetic ganglion cells are in tiny clusters embedded in their target tissues. The sympathetic and parasympathetic systems regulate blood flow, secretions, and organ function; the two divisions often act in antagonistic ways on the same target (see **B**). Although this basic dichotomy of visceral motor activity was identified early, by Langley (1905) and others, it has been shown more recently that autonomic control of various organs, particularly in the gastrointestinal and urogenital tracts, is highly sophisticated, dependent upon feedback from local visceral afferents that relay pain and stretch information, etc., through complex local circuits.

B Synopsis of the sympathetic and parasympathetic nervous systems

1. The sympathetic nervous system can be considered the excitatory part of the autonomic nervous system that prepares the body for a "fight or flight" response.
2. The parasympathetic nervous system is the part of the autonomic nervous system that coordinates the "rest and digest" responses of the body.
3. Although there are separate control centers for the two divisions in the brainstem and spinal cord, they have close anatomic and functional ties in the periphery.
4. The principal transmitter at the target organ is *acetylcholine* in the parasympathetic nervous system and *norepinephrine* in the sympathetic nervous organ.
5. Stimulation of the sympathetic and parasympathetic nervous systems produces the following different effects on specific organs:

Organ	Sympathetic nervous system	Parasympathetic nervous system
Eye	Pupillary dilation	Pupillary constriction and increased curvature of the lens
Salivary glands	Decreased salivation (scant, viscous)	Increased salivation (copious, watery)
Heart	Elevation of the heart rate	Slowing of the heart rate
Lungs	Decreased bronchial secretions and bronchial dilation	Increased bronchial secretions and bronchial constriction
Gastrointestinal tract	Decreased secretions and motor activity	Increased secretions and motor activity
Pancreas	Decreased secretion from the endocrine part of the gland	Increased secretion
Male sex organs	Ejaculation	Erection
Skin	Vasoconstriction, sweat secretion, piloerection	No effect

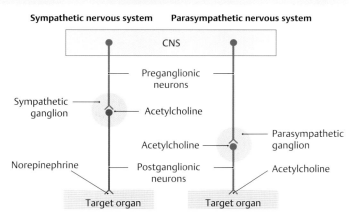

Sympathetic nervous system   Parasympathetic nervous system

CNS

Preganglionic neurons

Sympathetic ganglion — Acetylcholine

Acetylcholine — Parasympathetic ganglion

Norepinephrine   Postganglionic neurons — Acetylcholine

Target organ   Target organ

C Circuit diagram of the autonomic nervous system
The synapse of the central, preganglionic neuron uses *acetylcholine* as a transmitter in both the sympathetic *and* parasympathetic nervous systems (cholinergic neuron, shown in blue). In the sympathetic nervous system, the transmitter changes to *norepinephrine* at the synapse of the postganglionic neuron with the target organ (adrenergic neuron, shown in red), while the parasympathetic system continues to use acetylcholine at that level.
Note: Various types of receptors for acetylcholine (= neurotransmitter sensors) are located in the membrane of the target cells. As a result, acetylcholine can produce a range of effects depending on the receptor type.

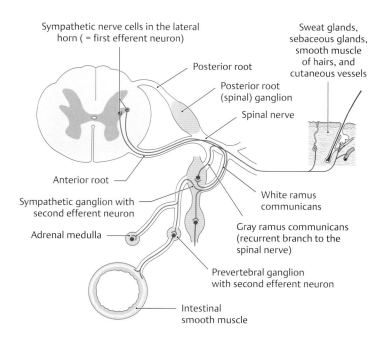

Sympathetic nerve cells in the lateral horn (= first efferent neuron)

Sweat glands, sebaceous glands, smooth muscle of hairs, and cutaneous vessels

Posterior root

Posterior root (spinal) ganglion

Spinal nerve

Anterior root

White ramus communicans

Sympathetic ganglion with second efferent neuron

Gray ramus communicans (recurrent branch to the spinal nerve)

Adrenal medulla

Prevertebral ganglion with second efferent neuron

Intestinal smooth muscle

D Distribution of sympathetic fibers in the periphery
Skin (blood vessels, cutaneous glands, and smooth muscle cells attached to hair follicles) and blood vessels of skeletal muscles are only innervated sympathetically. For these, synapses between the first and second neurons occur in the ganglia of the sympathetic trunk. For the sympathetic fibers to the organs, the synapses occur in the prevertebral ganglia or in the organ itself (see **E**).
Note: Skin and skeletal muscles are not parasympathetically innervated.

E Location of synapses in the sympathetic nervous system
Acetylcholine is the neurotransmitter released by both the first and second neurons in the parasympathetic system, but in the sympathetic system the second neuron releases norepinephrine. Synapses of the first (preganglionic cholinergic) neuron (blue) with the second neuron (red) may be located

① In the paravertebral ganglia on either side of the vertebral column, which are linked to one another as the sympathetic trunk. The synapses for the blood vessels of the skin and skeletal muscles mainly reside in these ganglia (see **D**).
② In prevertebral ganglia located in front of the spinal column. The synapses for visceral fibers of the abdomen and pelvis reside here.
③ In the target organ, or effector, itself, i.e., the adrenal medulla.

8.13 Lesions of Peripheral Nerves

Myelinated fiber (somatomotor or sensory)

Unmyelinated fiber (vegetative)

A Damage to a peripheral nerve

A peripheral nerve is a cluster of afferent (pain, temperature, pressure, vibration, sense of position) and efferent (somatomotor and visceromotor) axons. Pressure (left) or cuts (right) can damage the occasionally long course of the nerve.

Damage through pressure: It only takes slight pressure for the peripheral nerves to respond sensitively, with the afferent system being the first to be affected. Already a mild stimulus leads to paresthesia (e.g., tingling when the ulnar nerve is stimulated due to a slight tap on the medial elbow); longer and heavier pressure leads to loss of sensation in the area innervated by the receptive field. Finally, the efferent system is damaged, causing motor loss. There are numerous anatomic bottlenecks

(e.g., tunnel or slit-shaped [osteo] fibrous canals), which can occasionally lead to compression syndromes. They are first perceived as pain and later as loss of function in the affected muscles. Some of the important syndromes are listed under **B**.

Damage through cutting: As a result of a cut (a mixed nerve has been completely severed), the afferent and efferent systems fail at the same time. The muscles innervated by this nerve can no longer be moved, resulting in flaccid paralysis (for more about the difference between flaccid and spastic paralysis, see p. 90). In addition, the loss of afferents leads to a loss of sensation, and the loss of sympathetic fibers leads to vegetative symptoms (increased sweat secretion and increased cutaneous perfusion) in the skin area innervated by the nerve.

B Selected nerve compression (bottleneck) syndromes

This provides an overview of the syndromes or symptoms that can be caused by the compression of individual nerves (for more details about the syndromes, see textbooks of neurology).

Affected nerve	Anatomic region	Syndrome/symptoms
Shoulder girdle and upper limb		
Brachial plexus	Upper thoracic aperture	Thoracic outlet syndrome (e.g., scalene syndrome, cervical rib syndrome, costoclavicular syndrome)
Suprascapular nerve	Scapular notch	Scapular notch syndrome
Axillary nerve	Lateral axillary hiatus	Lateral axillary hiatus syndrome
Ulnar nerve	Ulnar sulcus Flexor carpi ulnaris tendon of origin, ulnar palmar branches	Ulnar nerve entrapment (ulnar sulcus syndrome) Cubital tunnel syndrome Ulnar tunnel syndrome (Guyon–Logen syndrome)
Radial nerve	Groove for radial nerve	Park bench paralysis
– Deep branch	Supinator (arcade of Frohse)	Supinator syndrome (distal radial compression syndrome)
– Superficial branch	Distal radial forearm	Wartenberg disease
Median nerve	Passage through pronator teres Carpal tunnel	Pronator teres syndrome Carpal tunnel syndrome
Pelvic girdle and lower limb		
Sciatic nerve	Gluteal region	Piriformis syndrome
Femoral nerve	Inguinal region	Pain/weakness of the front upper leg
Obturator nerve	Anterior pubic bone area	Howship–Romberg syndrome
Saphenous nerve	Adductor canal	Dysesthesia at the interior lower leg
Lateral femoral cutaneous nerve	Lateral inguinal/upper leg region	Meralgia paresthetica (inguinal ligament syndrome)
Common fibular nerve	Head and neck of the fibula	Fibular tunnel syndrome
Deep fibular nerve	Anterior upper ankle joint	Anterior tarsal tunnel syndrome
Tibial nerve/plantar nerves	Inner malleolus region	Posterior tarsal tunnel syndrome
Plantar digital nerves	Toe ball area 3/4	Interdigital Morton neuralgia

C Damage to a peripheral nerve exemplified by loss of sensitivity

Functionally speaking, in the innervated area of an afferent nerve, the nerve is only a part of a conduit cable for stimuli, which ends in the sensory area of the cerebral cortex, where conscious perception of the respective sensory stimulus occurs (see p. 91). The brain always locates damage to an afferent nerve in the area innervated by that cutaneous nerve, regardless of whether the damage occurs close to the spinal cord or not. In case of sensitivity loss, the damage is not necessarily located where sensation is lost.

a Skeletal muscle fiber

b Denervated skeletal muscle fiber

c Reinnervated skeletal muscle fiber

d

D Regeneration of a peripheral nerve after having been cut

In the peripheral nervous system (PNS), a nerve can usually regenerate after its axon has been severed.

a A few days after the axon has been severed, it first degenerates distally to the lesion (so-called Waller degeneration). Its myelin sheath disintegrates, and the axon dissipates, as it is no longer nourished through the perikaryon (the so-called trophic function of the perikaryon is no longer required). In the affected perikarya, the cell nucleus shifts to the margin, and the Nissl substance partially dissolves (tigrolysis). At the same time, the Schwann cells divide, forming a cluster of cells from which the so-called Büngner ligaments arise.

b Weeks later, the severed axons begin to sprout again proximally (axonal sprouting) and extend by 1 mm/day into the areas they originally innervated. From adjacent axons, which have not been affected by the lesions, axon collaterals can also extend into the affected area. The process of axonal sprouting can be tested with the help of the Hoffmann–Tinel sign. When percussing over the course of the nerve, patients experience a tingling around the area where the axons sprout.

c Months later, the regeneration is complete. The axons have reached the skeletal muscles again and innervate them. Axons that have not made it to their relevant skeletal muscles and axons that have sprouted from the axon collaterals perish. As the Schwann cells divide distally along the lesion, the same segment of axons is now being myelinated by more Schwann cells than previously. This leads to an increased number of nodes of Ranvier, thus slowing down the saltatory conduction. This process can be measured by determining the nerve conduction velocity. The position of the nuclei and the texture of the Nissl substance in the perikarya have normalized.

After the peripheral nerve has been severed, its ends are sutured back together end-to-end. The goal of the nerve suture is to maintain the continuity of the connective tissue tube with its Schwann cell tubes as the anatomic landmark for the sprouting axons. In case of an injury to a large segment of the nerve, a nerve transplant may be performed. This transplant bridges the gap; it, too, only provides a conduction for the spouting axons. Such a conduction is crucial for sprouting axons because axons cannot penetrate into the scar tissue. If, because of such a scar, axons cannot find their way back to their muscle, it can lead to amputation or scar neuroma (see **d**), which is a conglomerate of Schwann cells and axonal sprouts.

Trunk Wall

9.1 The Skeleton of the Trunk

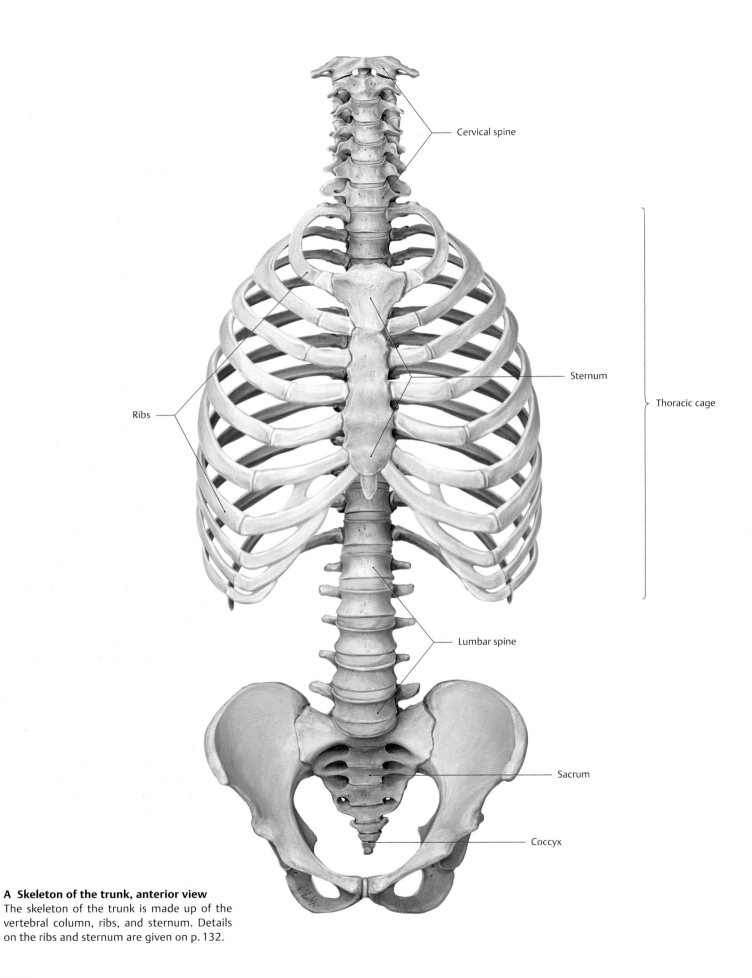

A Skeleton of the trunk, anterior view
The skeleton of the trunk is made up of the vertebral column, ribs, and sternum. Details on the ribs and sternum are given on p. 132.

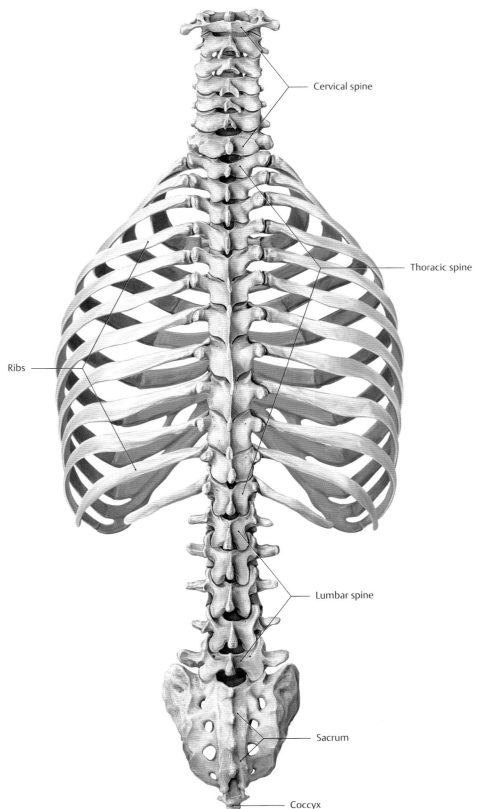

B **Skeleton of the trunk, posterior view**

C The spinous processes as anatomical landmarks

Posterior view. The spinous processes of the vertebrae appear as variable prominences beneath the skin and provide important landmarks during the physical examination. With few exceptions, they are easily palpated.

- The spinous process of the seventh cervical vertebra, located at the junction of the cervical and thoracic spine. Usually it is the most prominent of the spinous processes, causing the seventh cervical vertebra to be known also as the *vertebra prominens*.
- The spinous process of the third thoracic vertebra, located on a horizontal line connecting the scapular spines
- The spinous process of the seventh thoracic vertebra, located at the level of the inferior angles of the scapulae
- The spinous process of the twelfth thoracic vertebra, located slightly below the attachment of the last rib
- The spinous process of the fourth lumbar vertebra, located on a horizontal line connecting the highest points of the iliac crests

Note: The spinous processes of the thoracic vertebrae are angled downward (see p. 110), so the spinous process of the fifth thoracic vertebra, for example, is at the level of the sixth thoracic vertebral body.

9.2 The Bony Spinal Column

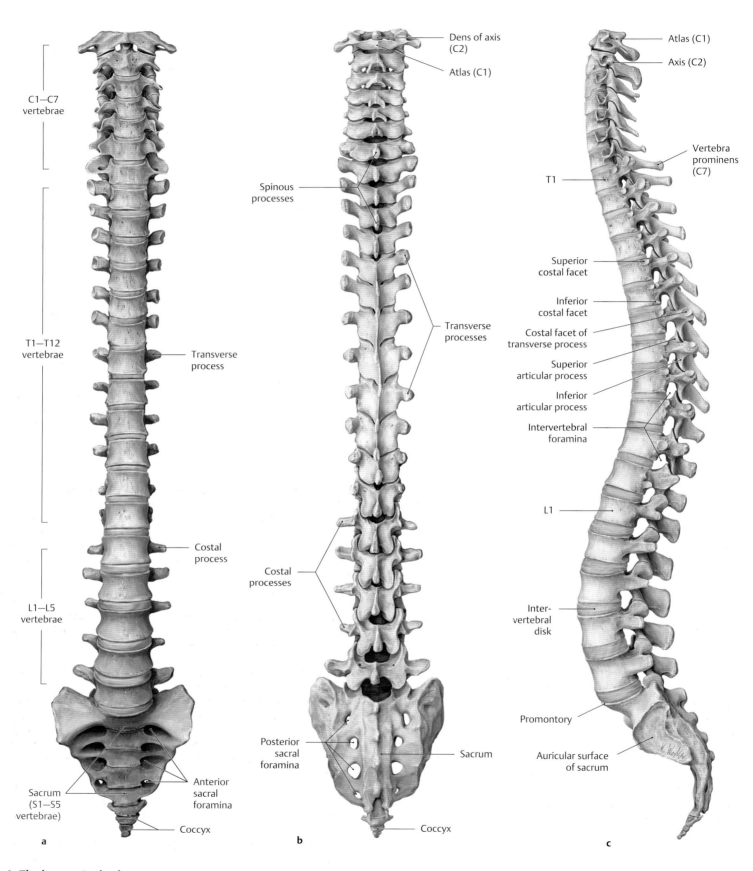

C1—C7
vertebrae

T1—T12
vertebrae

Transverse
process

L1—L5
vertebrae

Costal
process

Sacrum
(S1—S5
vertebrae)

Anterior
sacral
foramina

Coccyx

a

Dens of axis
(C2)

Atlas (C1)

Spinous
processes

Transverse
processes

Costal
processes

Posterior
sacral
foramina

Sacrum

Coccyx

b

Atlas (C1)

Axis (C2)

Vertebra
prominens
(C7)

T1

Superior
costal facet

Inferior
costal facet

Costal facet of
transverse process

Superior
articular process

Inferior
articular process

Intervertebral
foramina

L1

Inter-
vertebral
disk

Promontory

Auricular surface
of sacrum

c

A The bony spinal column
a Anterior view, **b** posterior view, **c** left lateral view.

Note: Phylogenetically, the transverse processes of the lumbar vertebrae are rudimentary ribs. They therefore are known as costal processes (see also p. 106).

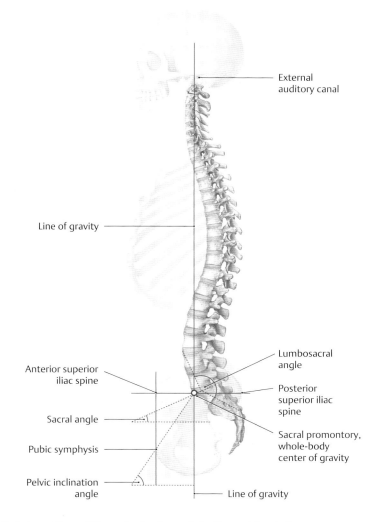

B Regions and curvatures of the spinal column

Left lateral view. The spinal column of an adult is divided into four regions and presents four characteristic curvatures in the sagittal plane. These curves are the result of human adaptation to upright bipedal locomotion, acting as springs to cushion axial loads. The following regions and curvatures are distinguished in the craniocaudal direction:

- Cervical spine – cervical lordosis
- Thoracic spine – thoracic kyphosis
- Lumbar spine – lumbar lordosis
- Sacral spine – sacral kyphosis

The cervical, thoracic, and lumbar regions of the spinal column are also known collectively as the *presacral spine*. The transitional areas between the different regions are of clinical importance because they are potential sites for spinal disorders (e.g., herniated disks). Occasionally, the vertebrae in these transitional areas have an atypical morphology that identifies them as *transitional vertebrae*. This is particularly common at the lumbosacral junction, where *sacralization* or *lumbarization* may be seen, depending on the appearance of the atypical vertebra. With lumbarization, the first sacral vertebra is not fused to the sacrum and constitutes an extra lumbar vertebra. With sacralization, there are only four lumbar vertebrae, the fifth being "sacralized" by fusion to the sacrum. These *assimilation disorders* are often unilateral (hemilumbarization, hemisacralization).

C Integration of the spinal column into the pelvic girdle

Skeleton of the trunk with the skull and pelvic girdle, left lateral view. Normally, the spinal column is curved and integrated into the pelvic girdle in such a way that characteristic angles are formed between certain imaginary lines and axes. These angles and lines are useful in the radiographic evaluation of positional abnormalities and deformities of the spine and trunk.

Lumbosacral angle: angle formed by the axes of the L 5 and S 1 vertebrae, averaging 143°. It results from the fact that the sacrum is a fixed component of the pelvic ring (see p. 138) and thus contributes little to straightening the vertebral column. The result is a characteristic sharp angle at the junction of the presacral part of the spinal column with the sacrum.

Sacral angle: angle between the horizontal plane and the superior surface of the sacrum, averaging approximately 30°

Pelvic inclination angle: angle formed by the pelvic inlet plane (connecting the sacral promontory to the upper border of the symphysis) with the horizontal. It measures approximately 60° in upright stance. The pelvic inclination angle increases or decreases as the pelvis is tilted forward or backward (see p. 157). With an ideal pelvic position in upright stance, the anterior and posterior superior iliac spines are at the same horizontal level, and the anterior superior iliac spine is directly above the pubic symphysis. By knowing this, the examiner can easily evaluate the position of the pelvis by using palpable bony landmarks.

Line of gravity: the line of gravity passes through landmarks that include the external auditory canal, the dens of the axis (C 2), the functional-anatomical transition points in the spinal column (between lordosis and kyphosis), and the whole-body center of gravity just anterior to the sacral promontory

103

9.3 Development of the Spinal Column

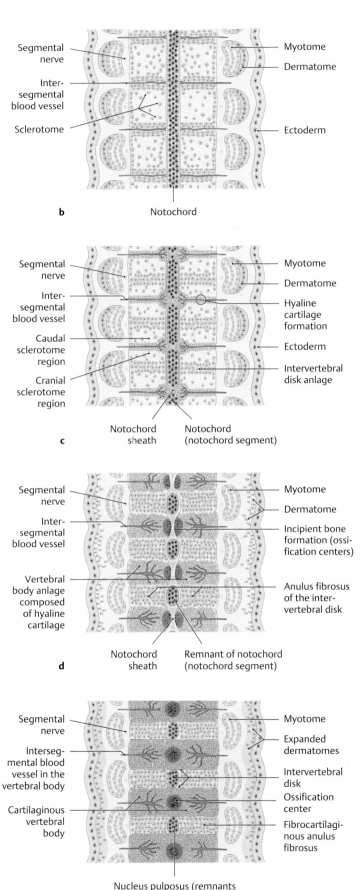

A Development of the spinal column (weeks 4–10)

a Schematic cross section, **b–e** schematic coronal sections (the plane of section in **b–e** is indicated in **a**).

a, b The former somites have differentiated into the myotome, dermatome, and sclerotome. The sclerotome cells separate from the other cells at 4 weeks, migrate toward the notochord, and form a cluster of mesenchymal cells around the notochord (anlage of the future spinal column).

c Adjacent cranial and caudal sclerotome segments above and below the intersegmental vessels join together and begin to chondrify in the sixth week, displacing the notochord material superiorly and inferiorly (notochord segments).

d The intervertebral disks with their nucleus pulposus and anulus fibrosus develop between the rudimentary vertebral bodies. Ossification begins at the center of the vertebral bodies in the eighth week of development.

e By fusion of the caudal and cranial sclerotome segments, the segmentally arranged myotomes interconnect the processes of two adjacent vertebral anlages, bridging the gap across the intervertebral disks. This is how the *motion segments* are formed (see p. 124). The segmental spinal nerve courses at the level of the future intervertebral foramen, and the intersegmental vessels become the *nutrient vessels* of the vertebral bodies (week 10).

Clinical aspects: If the neural tube or the dorsal portions of the vertebral arches fail to close normally during embryonic development, the result is *spina bifida*—a cleft spine. In this anomaly, the spinal column is open posteriorly, and the spinous processes are absent (the various forms and manifestations are described in textbooks of embryology). Usually there is a bilateral defect in the vertebral arches (generally affecting the L 4 and L 5 region), known as *spondylolysis*. This defect may be congenital or acquired (e.g., due to trauma). Acquired cases are common in sports that pose a risk of vertebral arch fractures (javelin throwing, gymnastics, high jumping). If the associated intervertebral disk is also damaged, the vertebral body will begin to slip forward (*spondylolisthesis*). In cases of *congenital spondylolysis* (which are associated with varying degrees of spondylolisthesis), the slippage progresses slowly during growth, and the condition tends to stabilize after 20 years of age.

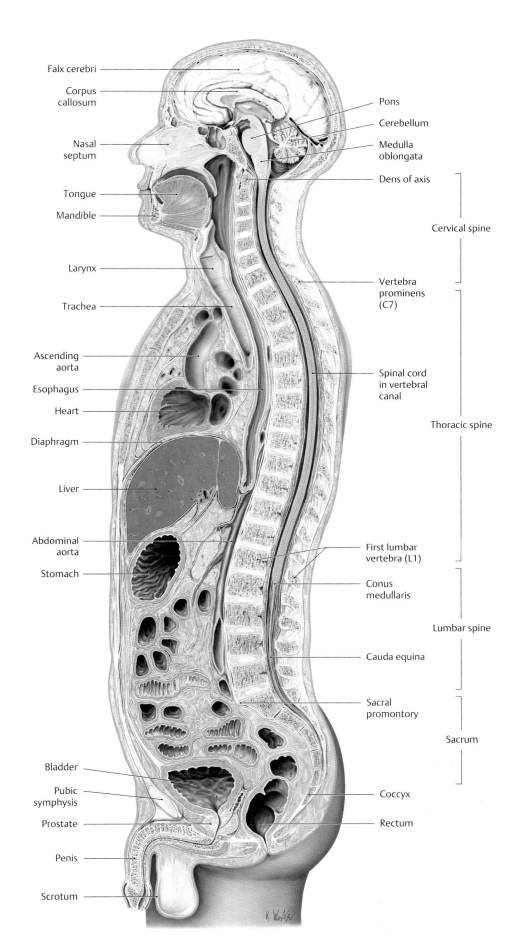

Falx cerebri
Corpus callosum
Nasal septum
Tongue
Mandible
Larynx
Trachea
Ascending aorta
Esophagus
Heart
Diaphragm
Liver
Abdominal aorta
Stomach
Bladder
Pubic symphysis
Prostate
Penis
Scrotum

Pons
Cerebellum
Medulla oblongata
Dens of axis
Cervical spine
Vertebra prominens (C7)
Spinal cord in vertebral canal
Thoracic spine
First lumbar vertebra (L1)
Conus medullaris
Lumbar spine
Cauda equina
Sacral promontory
Sacrum
Coccyx
Rectum

D Physiological curvatures of the adult spinal column

Midsagittal section through an adult male, left lateral view.

B Neonatal kyphosis
Midsagittal section through a newborn, left lateral view. Owing to the curved intrauterine position of the fetus, the newborn has a "kyphotic" spinal curvature with no lordotic straightening of the cervical and lumbar spine (after Rohen, Yokochi, Lütjen-Drecoll).

Kyphotic curvature

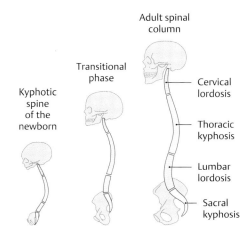

Adult spinal column
Transitional phase
Kyphotic spine of the newborn
Cervical lordosis
Thoracic kyphosis
Lumbar lordosis
Sacral kyphosis

C Straightening of the spine during normal development (after Debrunner)
The characteristic curvatures of the adult spine are only partially present in the newborn (compare with **B**) and appear only during the course of postnatal development. First cervical lordosis develops to balance the head in response to the growing strength of the posterior neck muscles. Lumbar lordosis develops later as the child learns to sit, stand, and walk. The degree of lordosis increases until the legs can be fully extended at the hips, and it finally becomes stable during puberty. A similar transformation of the spinal column is observed in the phylogenetic transition from quadrupedal to bipedal locomotion.

9.4 The Structure of a Vertebra

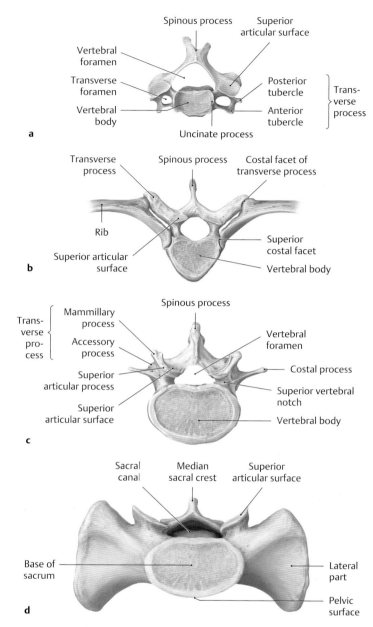

A Structural elements of a vertebra

Left posterosuperior view. All vertebrae except the atlas and axis (see p. 109) consist of the same basic structural elements:

- A vertebral body
- A vertebral arch
- A spinous process
- Two transverse processes (called costal processes in the lumbar vertebrae)
- Four articular processes

The processes give attachment to muscles and ligaments, and the bodies of the thoracic vertebrae have costovertebral joints. The vertebral bodies and arches enclose the vertebral foramen, and all of the vertebral foramina together constitute the vertebral (spinal) canal.

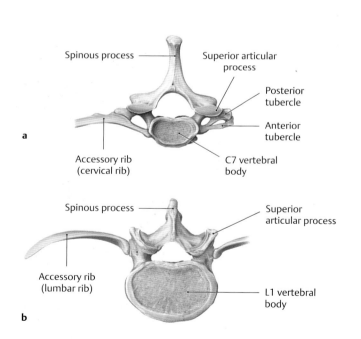

B Accessory ribs

Superior view. **a** Cervical rib, **b** lumbar rib.

The presence of anomalous cervical ribs can narrow the scalene interval, causing compression of the brachial plexus and subclavian artery (scalenus syndrome or cervical rib syndrome, see also p. 362). An accessory lumbar rib, on the other hand, has no adverse clinical effects.

C Costal elements in different regions of the spinal column

Superior view. The shape and configuration of the vertebrae are closely related to the development of the ribs and their rudiments (indicated here by color shading).

a Cervical vertebrae: Here the rudimentary rib forms a process called the anterior tubercle. It unites with the posterior tubercle to form the transverse foramen.

b Thoracic vertebrae: Because these vertebrae give attachment to the ribs, their bodies and transverse processes bear corresponding cartilage-covered articular surfaces (costal facets on the transverse processes, also superior and inferior costal facets).

c Lumbar vertebrae: The costal elements in the lumbar spine take the form of "transverse processes," which are much larger than in the cervical spine. Because of their size, they are also known as costal processes.

d Sacrum: Here the rudimentary rib forms the anterior portion of the lateral part of the sacral vertebra. It is fused to the transverse processes.

D Typical vertebrae from different regions of the spinal column

Superior and left lateral view.

a, b First cervical vertebra (atlas).
c, d Second cervical vertebra (axis).
e, f Fourth cervical vertebra.
g, h Sixth thoracic vertebra.
i, j Fourth lumbar vertebra.
k, l Sacrum.

The vertebrae in different regions of the spinal column differ not only in their size but also in their special features. While the vertebral *bodies* gradually become larger from superior to inferior to accommodate the increasing stresses imposed by the gravity and body weight, the vertebral *foramina* gradually become smaller to match the decreasing diameter of the spinal cord. The arrangement of the vertebral arches and adjacent processes also varies at different levels in the spine (for details see pp. 109, 111, and 113).

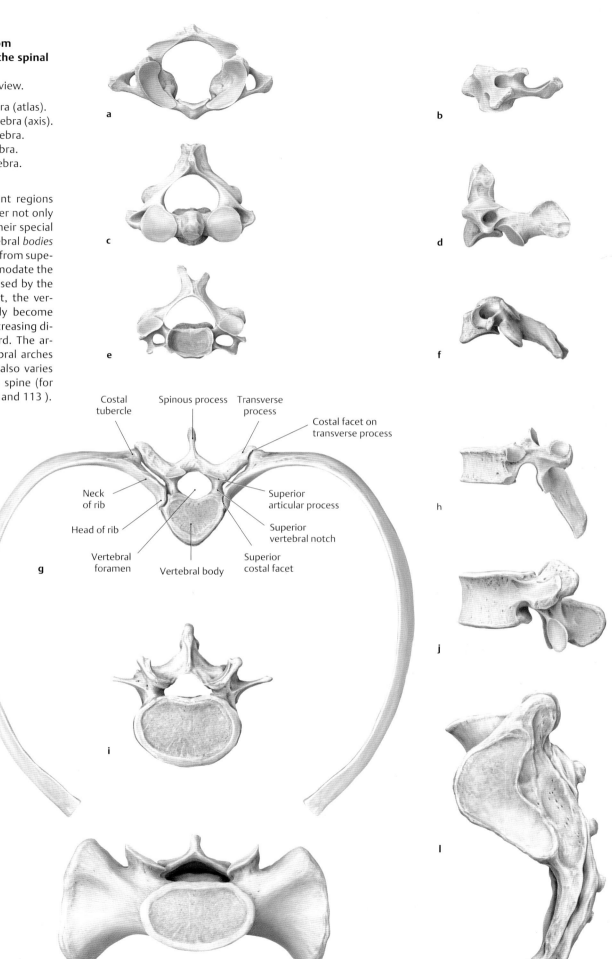

Costal tubercle

Spinous process

Transverse process

Costal facet on transverse process

Neck of rib

Superior articular process

Head of rib

Superior vertebral notch

Vertebral foramen

Vertebral body

Superior costal facet

Shaft of rib

107

9.5 The Cervical Spine

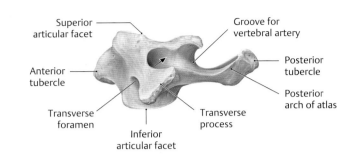

a First cervical vertebra (C1, atlas)

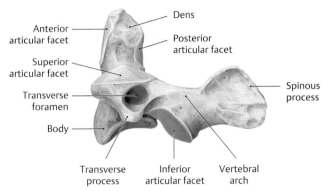

b Second cervical vertebra (C2, axis)

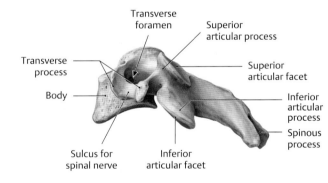

c Fourth cervical vertebra (C4)

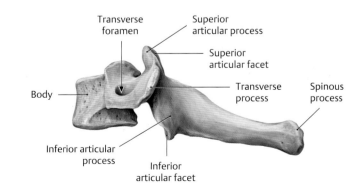

d Seventh cervical vertebra (C7, vertebra prominens)

B Cervical vertebrae, left lateral view

A Cervical spine, left lateral view

Of the cervical vertebrae, which number seven in all, the **first and second cervical vertebrae** (C1 and C2, atlas and axis) differ most conspicuously from the common vertebral morphology. They are specialized for bearing the weight of the head and allowing the head to move in all directions, similar to a ball-and-socket joint. Each of the **remaining five cervical vertebrae** (C3–C7) has a relatively small body, which presents a more or less square shape when viewed from above, and a large, triangular vertebral foramen (see **Cc**). The superior and inferior surfaces of the vertebral bodies are saddle-shaped, the superior surfaces bearing lateral uncinate processes that do not appear until about the tenth year of life (see p.126). The transverse process consists of an anterior and a posterior bar, which terminate laterally in two small tubercles (anterior and posterior tubercles). These bars enclose the transverse foramen, through which the vertebral artery ascends from the C6 to the C1 level. The superior surface of the transverse process of the first three cervical vertebrae bears a broad, deep notch (spinal nerve sulcus), in which lies the emerging spinal nerve at that level. The superior and inferior articular processes are broad and flat. Their articular surfaces are flat and are inclined approximately 45° from the horizontal plane. The spinous processes of the third through sixth cervical vertebrae are short and bifid. The spinous process of the seventh cervical vertebra is longer and thicker than the others and is the first of the spinous processes that is distinctly palpable through the skin (vertebra prominens).

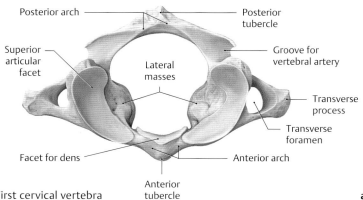

Posterior arch — Posterior tubercle

Superior articular facet

Lateral masses

Groove for vertebral artery

Transverse process

Transverse foramen

Facet for dens — Anterior arch

Anterior tubercle

a First cervical vertebra (atlas)

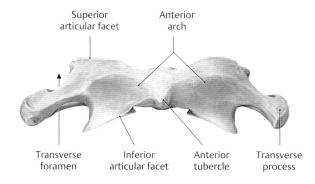

Superior articular facet — Anterior arch

Transverse foramen — Inferior articular facet — Anterior tubercle — Transverse process

a First cervical vertebra (atlas)

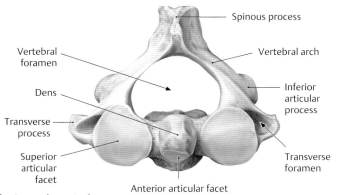

Spinous process

Vertebral foramen — Vertebral arch

Dens — Inferior articular process

Transverse process — Transverse foramen

Superior articular facet

Anterior articular facet

b Second cervical vertebra (axis)

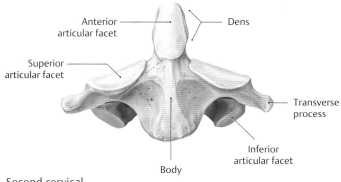

Anterior articular facet — Dens

Superior articular facet

Transverse process

Inferior articular facet

Body

b Second cervical vertebra (axis)

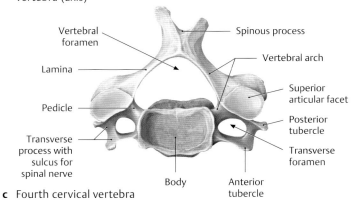

Vertebral foramen — Spinous process

Lamina — Vertebral arch

Pedicle — Superior articular facet

Transverse process with sulcus for spinal nerve

Posterior tubercle

Transverse foramen

Body — Anterior tubercle

c Fourth cervical vertebra

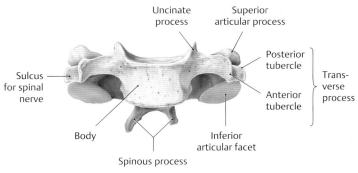

Uncinate process — Superior articular process

Sulcus for spinal nerve

Posterior tubercle

Anterior tubercle

Trans- verse process

Body — Inferior articular facet

Spinous process

c Fourth cervical vertebra

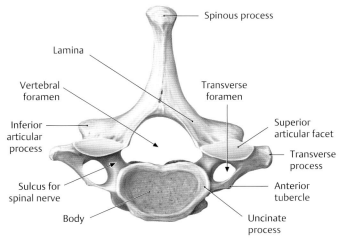

Spinous process

Lamina

Vertebral foramen — Transverse foramen

Inferior articular process

Superior articular facet

Transverse process

Sulcus for spinal nerve

Anterior tubercle

Body — Uncinate process

d Seventh cervical vertebra (vertebra prominens)

C Cervical vertebrae, superior view

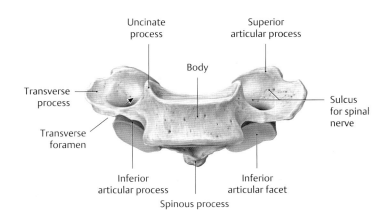

Uncinate process — Superior articular process

Body

Transverse process — Sulcus for spinal nerve

Transverse foramen

Inferior articular process — Inferior articular facet

Spinous process

d Seventh cervical vertebra (vertebra prominens)

D Cervical vertebrae, anterior view

9.6 The Thoracic Spine

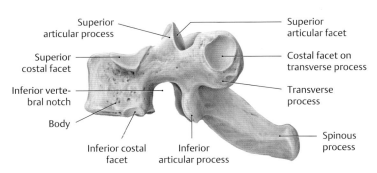

a Second thoracic vertebra (T2)

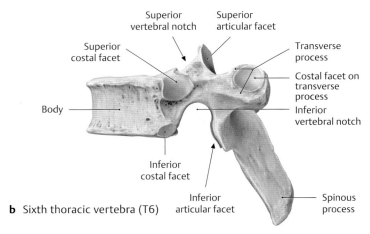

b Sixth thoracic vertebra (T6)

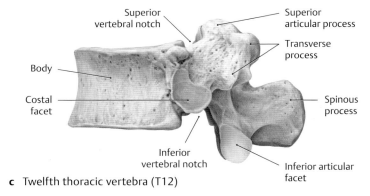

c Twelfth thoracic vertebra (T12)

A Thoracic spine, left lateral view
The thoracic vertebral bodies gradually become taller and broader from superior to inferior, the lower vertebral bodies assuming a transverse oval shape like that of the lumbar vertebrae. The vertebral foramen is roughly circular and is smaller than in the cervical and lumbar vertebrae. The end plates are rounded and triangular. The spinous processes are long and angled sharply inferiorly, creating an overlapping arrangement that interlinks the thoracic vertebrae. The facets of the *inferior* articular processes are directed anteriorly, while the facets of the *superior* articular processes face posterior so that they can articulate with the inferior facets to form the zygapophyseal or facet joints (p.124). Another feature of the thoracic vertebrae is that their transverse processes are angled backward to allow for articulations with the ribs.

B Thoracic vertebrae, left lateral view
The costal facets are cartilage-covered surfaces that articulate with the corresponding ribs (see p. 137). The bodies of the second through ninth thoracic vertebrae (T1–T9) bear two articular facets on each side —a superior costal facet and an inferior costal facet—such that two adjacent vertebrae combine to articulate with the head of a rib. Thus, a given numbered rib articulates with its own numbered vertebra and the vertebra above. Exceptions to this scheme are ribs 1 and 10 to 12, which articulate only with the vertebral body of the same number. The body of the tenth thoracic vertebra has only superior articular facets, and the tenth rib usually articulates only with the tenth thoracic vertebrae. As mentioned, the transverse processes of the thoracic vertebrae (except for T11 and T12) also bear articular facets for the ribs.

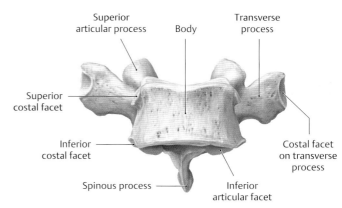

a Second thoracic vertebra (T2)

a Second thoracic vertebra (T2)

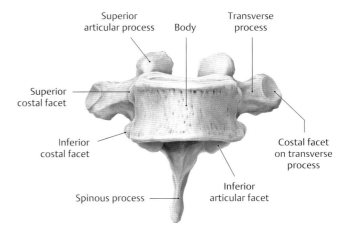

b Sixth thoracic vertebra (T6)

b Sixth thoracic vertebra (T6)

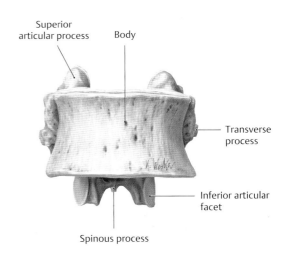

c Twelfth thoracic vertebra (T12)

c Twelfth thoracic vertebra (T12)

C Thoracic vertebrae, superior view
The laminae and pedicles make up the vertebral arch.

D Thoracic vertebrae, anterior view

9.7　The Lumbar Spine

a Second lumbar vertebra

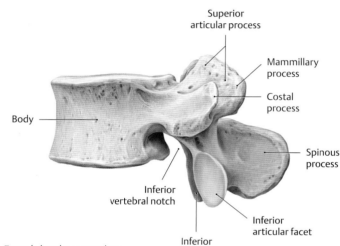

b Fourth lumbar vertebra

A Lumbar spine, left lateral view

The bodies of the lumbar vertebrae are large and have a transverse oval shape when viewed from above (see **C**). The massive vertebral arches enclose an almost triangular vertebral foramen, and they unite posteriorly to form a thick spinous process that is flattened on each side. The "transverse processes" of the lumbar vertebrae correspond phylogenetically to rudimentary ribs (see p. 106). Thus, they are more accurately termed costal processes and are not homologous with the transverse processes of the other vertebrae. The thick costal process is fused with the actual transverse process, which is a small, pointed eminence located at the root of each costal process (accessory process, see **Cb**). The relatively massive superior and inferior articular processes bear slightly inclined articular facets that have a vertical, almost sagittal orientation. The articular facets of the superior articular processes are slightly concave and face medially, while those of the inferior articular processes are slightly convex and face laterally. The mammillary processes on the lateral surfaces of the superior articular processes serve as origins and insertions for the intrinsic back muscles (see **Bb** and **Ca**).

c　Fifth lumbar vertebra

B Lumbar vertebrae, left lateral view

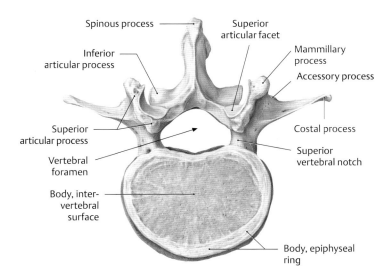

Spinous process

Superior articular facet

Inferior articular process

Mammillary process

Accessory process

Superior articular process

Costal process

Vertebral foramen

Superior vertebral notch

Body, intervertebral surface

Body, epiphyseal ring

a Second lumbar vertebra

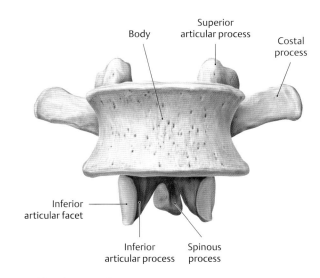

Body

Superior articular process

Costal process

Inferior articular facet

Inferior articular process

Spinous process

a Second lumbar vertebra

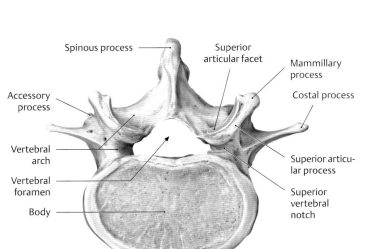

Spinous process

Superior articular facet

Mammillary process

Accessory process

Costal process

Vertebral arch

Superior articular process

Vertebral foramen

Superior vertebral notch

Body

b Fourth lumbar vertebra

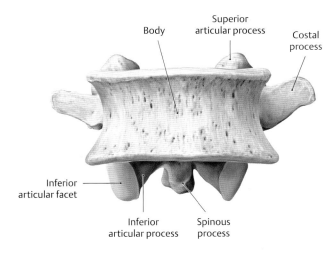

Body

Superior articular process

Costal process

Inferior articular facet

Inferior articular process

Spinous process

b Fourth lumbar vertebra

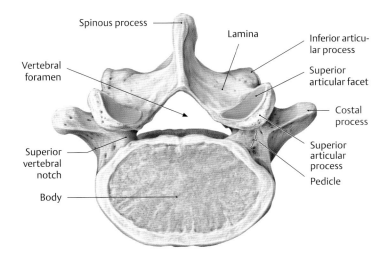

Spinous process

Lamina

Inferior articular process

Superior articular facet

Vertebral foramen

Costal process

Superior articular process

Pedicle

Superior vertebral notch

Body

c Fifth lumbar vertebra

C Lumbar vertebrae, superior view

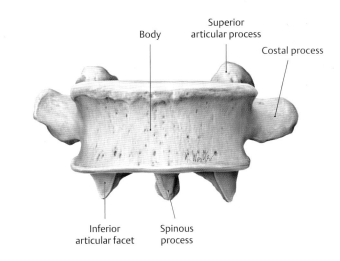

Body

Superior articular process

Costal process

Inferior articular facet

Spinous process

c Fifth lumbar vertebra

D Lumbar vertebrae, anterior view

113

9.8 The Sacrum and Coccyx

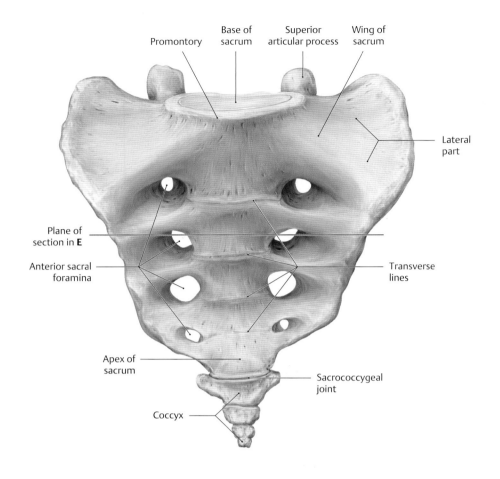

Promontory — Base of sacrum — Superior articular process — Wing of sacrum

Lateral part

Plane of section in **E**

Anterior sacral foramina

Transverse lines

Apex of sacrum

Sacrococcygeal joint

Coccyx

A Sacrum and coccyx, anterior (pelvic) view

The sacrum at birth is composed of five separate sacral vertebrae. Postnatally, they fuse to form a single bone that is flattened anteroposteriorly and has a triangular shape when viewed from the front. The *base of the sacrum,* located at the superior end of the bone, articulates with the body of the fifth lumbar vertebra by a wedge-shaped intervertebral disk. The *apex of the sacrum* is at the inferior end of the bone and articulates with the coccyx. The anterior or *pelvic surface* of the sacrum is concave in both the sagittal and transverse planes (see **C**). Between the anterior sacral foramina are four transverse ridges (transverse lines), which mark the sites of fusion between the five sacral vertebrae. The coccyx consists of three or four rudimentary vertebrae. Only the first coccygeal vertebra exhibits some of the typical structural elements of a fully formed vertebra. A cartilaginous disk usually connects the base of the coccyx to the apex of the sacrum (sacrococcygeal joint). This joint allows passive forward and backward motion of the coccyx, increasing the anteroposterior diameter of the pelvic outlet during childbirth (see p. 139).

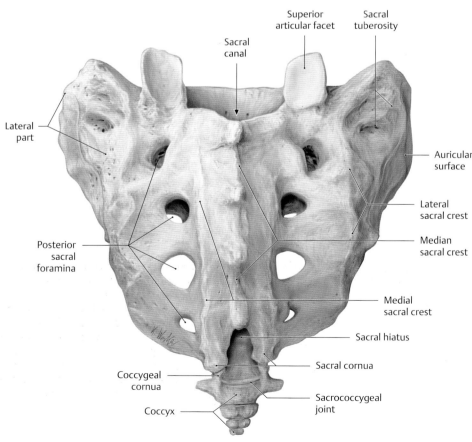

Superior articular facet — Sacral tuberosity

Sacral canal

Lateral part

Auricular surface

Lateral sacral crest

Median sacral crest

Posterior sacral foramina

Medial sacral crest

Sacral hiatus

Sacral cornua

Coccygeal cornua

Sacrococcygeal joint

Coccyx

B Sacrum and coccyx, posterior view

The fused spinous processes form a jagged bony ridge on the convex dorsal surface of the sacrum, the *median sacral crest.* This ridge is flanked on each side by the paired *medial sacral crests,* formed by fusion of the articular processes. The medial crests are continuous below with the rudimentary inferior articular processes of the fifth sacral vertebra (the sacral cornua); they are continuous above with the two superior articular processes that face posteriorly. Between the sacral cornua is an aperture, the sacral hiatus, which is formed by the incomplete vertebral arch of the fifth sacral vertebrae and provides access to the sacral canal (e.g., for anesthesia). Lateral to the posterior sacral foramina are another pair of longitudinal ridges, the *lateral sacral crests,* formed by the fused transverse processes. The bony union of the transverse processes with the rudimentary ribs forms the thick *lateral* parts of the sacral wing that flank the body of the sacrum. Each lateral part bears an ear-shaped ("auricular") surface that articulates with the ilium (see **C**). In this view, the two small coccygeal cornua representing the superior articular processes and the two rudimentary transverse processes of the coccyx are visible.

C Sacrum, left lateral view

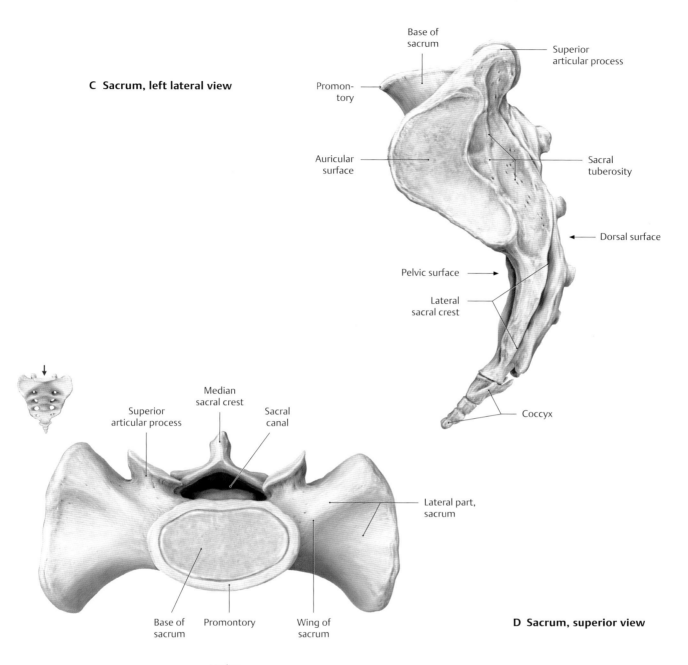

Base of sacrum

Superior articular process

Promontory

Auricular surface

Sacral tuberosity

Dorsal surface

Pelvic surface

Lateral sacral crest

Coccyx

Median sacral crest

Superior articular process

Sacral canal

Lateral part, sacrum

Base of sacrum

Promontory

Wing of sacrum

D Sacrum, superior view

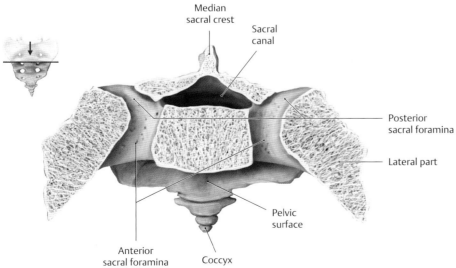

Median sacral crest

Sacral canal

Posterior sacral foramina

Lateral part

Pelvic surface

Anterior sacral foramina

Coccyx

E Transverse section through the sacrum
Superior view (the level of the section is shown in **A**). Fusion of the upper four sacral vertebrae creates four T-shaped bony canals at the level of the intervertebral foramina on each side, providing sites of emergence for the first through fourth sacral nerves. The corresponding ventral and dorsal rami of the spinal nerves exit the bony canals through the anterior and posterior sacral foramina (see p. 237).

9.9 The Intervertebral Disk: Structure and Function

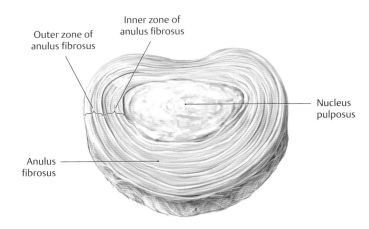

A Structure of an intervertebral disk

Isolated lumbar intervertebral disk, anterosuperior view.

The intervertebral disk consists of an external fibrous ring, the *anulus fibrosus,* and a gelatinous core, the *nucleus pulposus.* The anulus fibrosus consists of an outer zone and an inner zone. The outer zone is a fibrous sheath that possesses high tensile strength and is made up of concentric laminae of type I collagen fibers. Its fiber systems crisscross due to their varying obliquity and interconnect the marginal ridges of two adjacent vertebrae (see **B**), to which they are attached. At the junction with the inner zone of the anulus fibrosus, the tough fibrous tissue of the outer zone blends with a fibrocartilaginous tissue whose type II collagen fibers are attached to the hyaline cartilage end plates of the vertebral bodies (see **Da** and **Ea**).

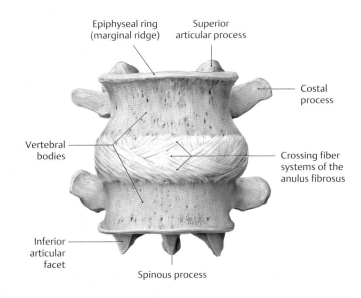

B Outer zone of the anulus fibrosus

Intervertebral disk between the third and fourth lumbar vertebrae, anterior view.

The connective-tissue fiber bundles in the outer zone of the anulus fibrosus cross one another at various angles, interconnecting the bony marginal ridges of two adjacent vertebral bodies.

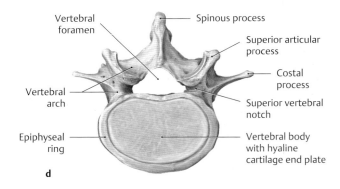

C Main structural components of an intervertebral disk

Fourth lumbar vertebra with its associated upper disk, superior view.

a Intervertebral disk with the anulus fibrosus and nucleus pulposus.
b Anulus fibrosus (with the nucleus pulposus removed).
c Outer zone of the anulus fibrosus (with the inner zone removed).
d Hyaline cartilage end plate within the bony marginal ridge (entire intervertebral disk removed).

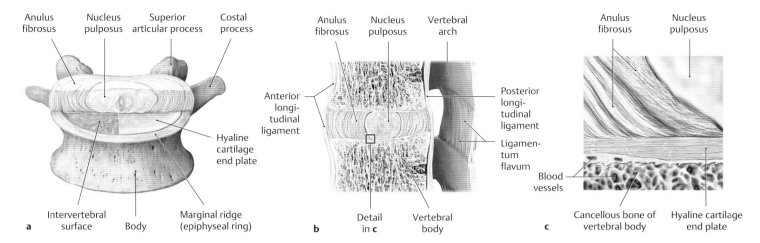

a — Anulus fibrosus, Nucleus pulposus, Superior articular process, Costal process, Anterior longitudinal ligament, Hyaline cartilage end plate, Intervertebral surface, Body, Marginal ridge (epiphyseal ring)

b — Anulus fibrosus, Nucleus pulposus, Vertebral arch, Posterior longitudinal ligament, Ligamentum flavum, Blood vessels, Detail in c, Vertebral body

c — Anulus fibrosus, Nucleus pulposus, Cancellous bone of vertebral body, Hyaline cartilage end plate

D Position of the intervertebral disk in the motion segment

a Hyaline cartilage end plate, anterosuperior view (the anterior half of the disk and right half of the end plate have been removed).

b Sagittal section through a motion segment (see p.124), left lateral view.

c Detail from **b.**

Except for the outer zone of the anulus fibrosus, the entire disk is in contact superiorly and inferiorly with the hyaline cartilage layer of the adjacent vertebral endplates. The subchondral, bony portion of the end plate consists of compact bone (intervertebral surface) permeated by myriad pores (see **c**) through which the vessels in the bone marrow spaces of the vertebral bodies can supply nutrients to the disk tissue.

a — Vertebral body, Vertebral arch, Superior articular process, Spinous process, Anulus fibrosus, Nucleus pulposus, Inferior articular process

b — **Pressure applied** — Vertebral body, Intervertebral foramen, Spinous process, Costal process, Intervertebral disk, Vertebral body

c — **Pressure released** — Vertebral end plate, Vertebral end plate

E Load-dependent fluid shifts in the intervertebral disk

a The nucleus pulposus functions as a "water cushion" to absorb transient axial loads on the intervertebral disk. Mechanically, the disk represents a hydrostatic system that is resilient under pressure. It is composed of a tension-resistant sheath (the anulus fibrosus) and a watery, incompressible core, the nucleus pulposus. This core consists of 80 to 85% water, which it can reversibly bind in its paucicellular, gelatinous, mucoviscous tissue (owing to its high content of glycosaminoglycans). The nucleus pulposus is under a very high hydrostatic pressure, particularly when acted upon by gravity and other forces. This pressure can be absorbed by the adjacent cartilaginous end plates and also by the anulus fibrosus (which transforms compressive forces into tensile forces). In this way the nucleus pulposus functions as a "water cushion" or hydraulic press between two adjacent vertebral bodies. Combined with the anulus fibrosus, it acts as an effective shock absorber that can distribute pressures uniformly over the adjacent vertebral end plates.

b Fluid outflow from the intervertebral disk (green arrows) in response to a sustained pressure load (thick red arrows). While transient loads are cushioned by the shock-absorber function of the nucleus pulposus and anulus fibrosus (see **a**), sustained loads cause a gradual but permanent outflow of fluid from the disk. The turgor and height of the disk are reduced, while the end plates and eventually the bony vertebral elements move closer together (see p.131 for further details on disk degeneration).

c Fluid uptake by the intervertebral disk (green arrows) when pressure is released (thin red arrows). The process described in **b** is reversed when the pressure on the disk is released, and the height of the disk increases. This increase is caused by fluid uptake from the subchondral blood vessels in the bone marrow spaces, which are instrumental in disk nutrition (see **Dc**). As a result of pressure-dependent fluid shifts (convection) in the intervertebral disks, the overall body height decreases temporarily by approximately 1% (1.5–2.0 cm) relative to the initial body height during the course of the day.

9.10 The Ligaments of the Spinal Column: Overview and Thoracolumbar Region

A The ligaments of the spinal column at the level of the thoracolumbar junction (T11–L3)

Left lateral view. The two uppermost thoracic vertebrae have been sectioned in the midsagittal plane.

B The ligaments of the spinal column

The ligaments of the spinal column bind the vertebrae securely to one another and enable the spine to withstand high mechanical loads and shearing stresses. The ligaments are subdivided into vertebral *body* ligaments and vertebral *arch* ligaments.

Vertebral body ligaments
• Anterior longitudinal ligament
• Posterior longitudinal ligament

Vertebral arch ligaments
• Ligamenta flava
• Interspinous ligaments
• Supraspinous ligament
• Nuchal ligament*
• Intertransverse ligaments

* The sagittally oriented nuchal ligament runs between the external occipital protuberance and the seventh cervical vertebra; it corresponds to a supraspinal ligament that is broadened superiorly (see p. 121).

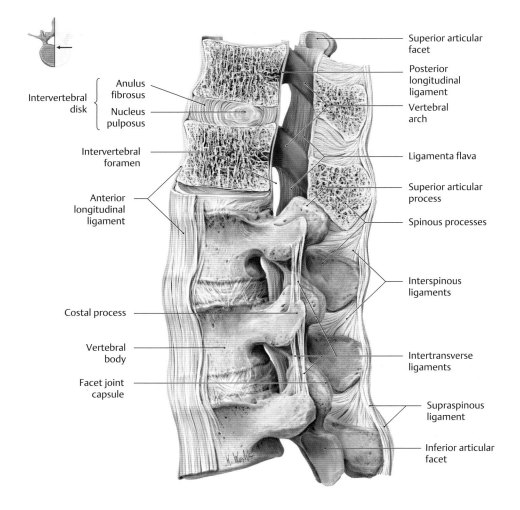

C Schematic representation of the vertebral body and vertebral arch ligaments

Viewed obliquely from the left posterior view.

a Vertebral body ligaments.
b–d Vertebral arch ligaments.

Intervertebral disk

Costal process

Vertebral body

Anterior longitudinal ligament

a

Nutrient foramina

Posterior longitudinal ligament

Intervertebral disk

Gap in ligamentous reinforcement of the disk

Vertebral arch, pedicle

Intervertebral foramen

Vertebral body

Superior articular facet

Costal process

Inferior articular process

Spinous process

b

D The ligaments surrounding the lumbar spine

a Anterior longitudinal ligament, anterior view.

b Posterior longitudinal ligament, posterior view after removal of the vertebral arches at the pedicular level.

c Ligamenta flava and intertransverse ligaments, anterior view (after removal of the L2–L4 vertebral bodies). (The other vertebral arch ligaments are not visible in this view.)

The **anterior longitudinal ligament** runs broadly on the anterior side of the vertebral bodies, extending from the skull base to the sacrum. Its deep fibers bind adjacent vertebral bodies together, while its superficial fibers span multiple segments. Its collagenous fibers are attached firmly to the vertebral bodies but have only a loose attachment to the intervertebral disks. The thinner **posterior longitudinal ligament** descends from the clivus along the posterior surface of the vertebral bodies, passing into the sacral canal. The portion over the vertebral bodies is narrow and is attached to their superior and inferior margins. The ligament broadens at the levels of the intervertebral disks, to which it is firmly attached by tapered lateral extensions. Despite the attachment of the ligament to the anulus fibrosus of the intervertebral disks (not seen clearly here, being hidden by the posterior longitudinal ligament), a large portion of the intervertebral disk has no ligamentous reinforcement, especially laterally (predisposing to lateral disk herniation, see p.131). Both longitudinal ligaments contribute to maintaining the normal curvature of the spinal column. The **ligamenta flava** consist mainly of elastic fibers, which give these ligaments their characteristic yellow color. They are thick, powerful ligaments that connect the laminae of adjacent vertebral arches and reinforce the wall of the vertebral canal posterior to the intervertebral foramina (see **A**). When the spinal column is erect, the ligamenta flava are under tension and help the back muscles to stabilize the spine in the sagittal plane. They also act as reins to limit forward flexion of the spinal column, thereby helping to maintain the position of the flexed spine. The tips of the transverse processes are connected on each side by the **intertransverse ligaments**, which serve to limit rocking movements of one vertebra upon another.

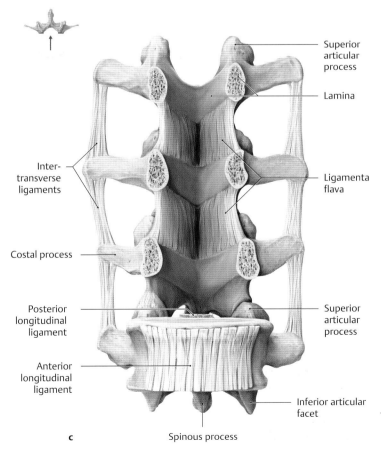

Superior articular process

Lamina

Ligamenta flava

Inter-transverse ligaments

Costal process

Posterior longitudinal ligament

Anterior longitudinal ligament

Superior articular process

Inferior articular facet

Spinous process

c

9.11 Overview of the Ligaments of the Cervical Spine

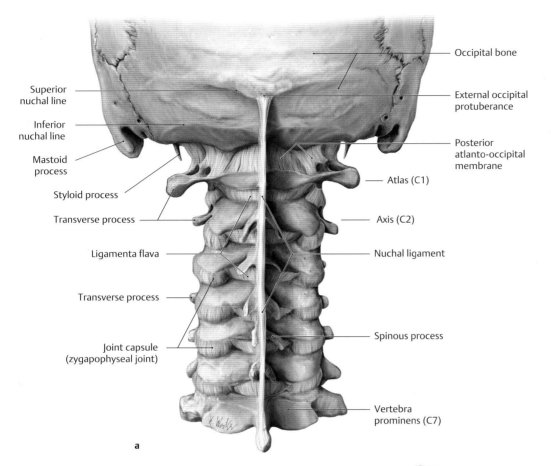

Superior
nuchal line

Inferior
nuchal line

Mastoid
process

Styloid process

Transverse process

Ligamenta flava

Transverse process

Joint capsule
(zygapophyseal joint)

Occipital bone

External occipital
protuberance

Posterior
atlanto-occipital
membrane

Atlas (C1)

Axis (C2)

Nuchal ligament

Spinous process

Vertebra
prominens (C7)

a

A The ligaments of the cervical spine
a Posterior view.
b Anterior view after removal of the anterior skull base (see p. 122 for the ligaments of the upper cervical spine, especially the craniovertebral joints).

b → ← a

B The craniovertebral joints

The craniovertebral joints are the articulations between the atlas (C1) and occipital bone (atlanto-occipital joints) and between the atlas and axis (C2, atlantoaxial joints). While these joints, which number six in all, are anatomically distinct, they are mechanically interlinked and comprise a functional unit (see p. 125).

Atlanto-occipital joints

Paired joints where the oval, slightly concave superior articular facets of the atlas articulate with the convex occipital condyles.

Atlantoaxial joints

- *Lateral atlantoaxial joint* = paired articulation between the inferior articular facets of the atlas and the superior articular facets of the axis
- *Median atlantoaxial joint* = unpaired articulation (comprising an anterior and posterior compartment) between the dens of the axis, the fovea of the atlas, and the cartilage-covered anterior surface of the transverse ligament of the atlas (see p. 123)

Internal occipital
protuberance

Internal
occipital crest

Atlanto-occipital
joint (capsule)

Atlas (C1)

Transverse
foramina

Axis (C2)

Anterior
longitudinal
ligament

Sulcus for
spinal nerve

Intervertebral
disk

Occipital bone,
basilar part

Anterior
atlanto-occipital
membrane

Transverse process

Lateral atlantoaxial
joint (capsule)

Zygapophyseal
joint (capsule)

Posterior
tubercle

Anterior
tubercle

Vertebra
prominens (C7)

b

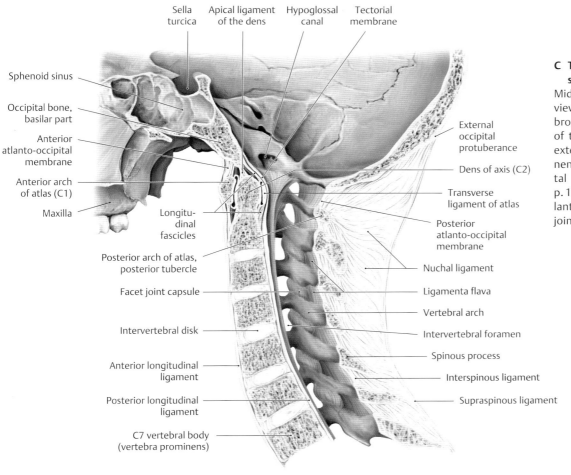

Sella turcica

Apical ligament of the dens

Hypoglossal canal

Tectorial membrane

Sphenoid sinus

Occipital bone, basilar part

Anterior atlanto-occipital membrane

Anterior arch of atlas (C1)

Maxilla

Longitudinal fascicles

Posterior arch of atlas, posterior tubercle

Facet joint capsule

Intervertebral disk

Anterior longitudinal ligament

Posterior longitudinal ligament

C7 vertebral body (vertebra prominens)

External occipital protuberance

Dens of axis (C2)

Transverse ligament of atlas

Posterior atlanto-occipital membrane

Nuchal ligament

Ligamenta flava

Vertebral arch

Intervertebral foramen

Spinous process

Interspinous ligament

Supraspinous ligament

C The ligaments of the cervical spine: nuchal ligament
Midsagittal section, left lateral view. The nuchal ligament is the broadened, sagittally oriented part of the supraspinous ligament that extends from the vertebra prominens (C1) to the external occipital protuberance (see **A**; see also p. 122 for the ligaments of the atlanto-occipital and atlantoaxial joints).

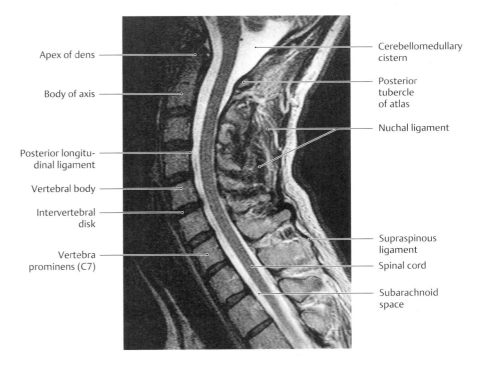

Apex of dens

Body of axis

Posterior longitudinal ligament

Vertebral body

Intervertebral disk

Vertebra prominens (C7)

Cerebellomedullary cistern

Posterior tubercle of atlas

Nuchal ligament

Supraspinous ligament

Spinal cord

Subarachnoid space

D Plain lateral radiograph of the cervical spine

E Magnetic resonance image of the cervical spine
Midsagittal section, left lateral view T2-weighted TSE sequence (from Vahlensieck M, Reiser M. MRT des Bewegungsapparates. 2nd ed. Stuttgart: Thieme; 2001).

121

9.12 The Ligaments of the Upper Cervical Spine (Atlanto-occipital and Atlantoaxial Joints)

a

b

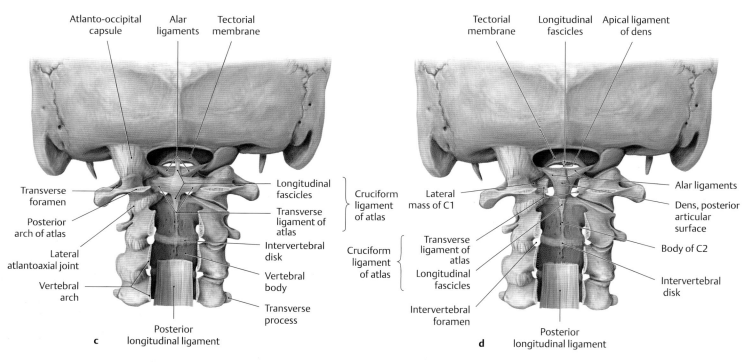

c

d

A The ligaments of the craniovertebral joints

Skull and upper cervical spine, posterior view.

a The posterior atlanto-occipital membrane—the "ligamentum flavum" between the atlas and occipital bone (see p. 120)—stretches from the posterior arch of the atlas to the posterior rim of the foramen magnum. This membrane has been removed on the right side.

b With the vertebral canal opened and the spinal cord removed, the tectorial membrane, a broadened expansion of the posterior longitudinal ligament, is seen to form the anterior boundary of the vertebral canal at the level of the craniovertebral joints.

c With the tectorial membrane removed, the cruciform ligament of the atlas can be seen. The transverse ligament of the atlas forms the thick horizontal bar of the cross, and the longitudinal fascicles form the thinner vertical bar.

d The transverse ligament of the atlas and longitudinal fascicles have been partially removed to demonstrate the paired alar ligaments, which extend from the lateral surfaces of the dens to the corresponding inner surfaces of the occipital condyles, and the unpaired apical ligament of the dens, which passes from the tip of the dens to the anterior rim of the foramen magnum.

B The ligaments of the median atlantoaxial joint
Atlas and axis, superior view. (The fovea, while part of the median atlantoaxial joint, is hidden by the joint capsule.)

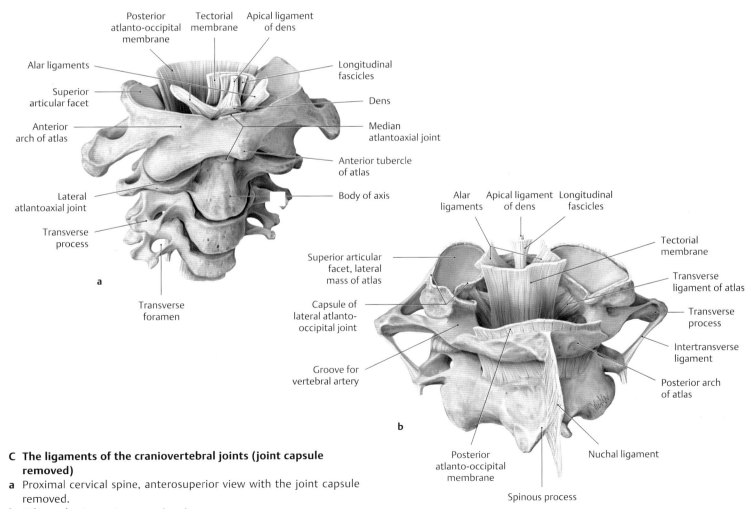

C The ligaments of the craniovertebral joints (joint capsule removed)

a Proximal cervical spine, anterosuperior view with the joint capsule removed.

b Atlas and axis, posterosuperior view.

9.13 The Intervertebral Facet Joints, Motion Segments, and Range of Motion in Different Spinal Regions

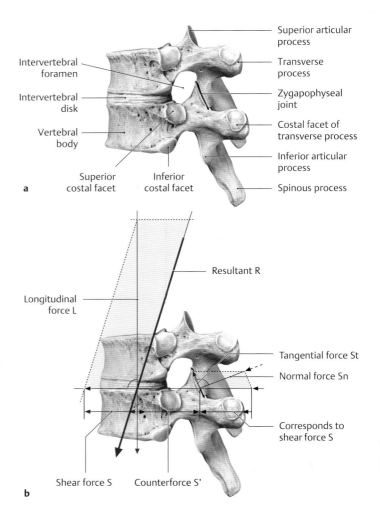

A The intervertebral facet joints (zygapophyseal joints)

The diagrams show the position of the articular surfaces of the intervertebral facet joints in different regions of the spinal column, shown from the left posterosuperior view: **a** cervical spine, **b** thoracic spine, **c** lumbar spine. Panel **d** is a sagittal section through the facet joints at the level of the third, fourth, and fifth cervical vertebrae, shown from the lateral view (drawing based on a specimen from the Anatomical Collection at Kiel University).

The paired facet joints are true synovial joints formed by the articular processes of the vertebral arches (see p. 106). Their articular surfaces, called **facets,** show varying degrees of inclination from the horizontal (and vertical) in different spinal regions and are therefore specialized for certain directions and ranges of motion (the movements that can occur in different spinal regions are shown in **D**). The **joint capsule** of the facet joint is inserted into the margins of the articular facets and is often firmly attached to the ligamentum flavum (see **d**). The joint capsule tends to be broad and lax in the cervical spine but is narrower in the thoracic and lumbar regions. Almost all the intervertebral joints contain *meniscoid synovial folds,* which form a crescent-shaped projection into the joint space. The folds consist of some loose but mostly firm connective tissue that has a rich vascular supply. The function of these folds is to fill the spaces around the articular surfaces (**d**).

B Structure and loading of a motion segment, illustrated for two thoracic vertebrae

Lateral view. "Motion segment" is the term applied to the articular and muscular connection between two adjacent vertebrae (**a**). It consists of the intervertebral disk, the paired intervertebral facet joints (zygapophyseal joints), and the associated ligaments and muscles (not depicted here). For clinical purposes, the motion segment is also considered to include the contents of the intervertebral foramina (nerves and blood vessels, see pp. 190 and 196) and the contents of the vertebral canal. In all, the spinal column contains 25 of these motion segments, which constitute distinct functional and morphological units. However, because of the interdependence of these units, abnormalities in a circumscribed portion of the spinal column tend to affect the other spinal segments as well. Each of these motion segments is subjected to certain loads that can be represented as applied forces (**b**): a forward-directed *shear force* and a downward-directed *longitudinal force,* which combine to give the resultant force R. The longitudinal force acts on the vertebral body and intervertebral disk, while the shear force is absorbed mainly by the ligaments and facet joints (counterforce S'). The shear force can be subdivided into a normal force (Sn) and a tangential force (St). Because the shearing forces are not perpendicular to the articular surfaces of the facet joints, these surfaces are loaded by the axially directed *normal force* (Sn), which is weaker than the original shear force. Displacement of the vertebrae by the upward-directed *tangential force* (St) is prevented by the ligaments and intrinsic back muscles (after Kummer).

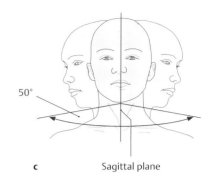

| a | Clavicular line | Eyeline | b | Occlusal plane | c | Sagittal plane |

C Total range of motion of the cervical spine
a Lateral flexion, **b** flexion/extension, **c** rotation.

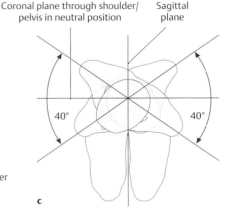

D Total range of motion of the thoracic and lumbar spine
a Lateral flexion, **b** flexion/extension, **c** rotation.

The clinical examination, particularly function testing, is of key importance in examinations of the spine. Because the total range of spinal motion is comprised of the movements of a total of 25 motion segments, generally the examiner can detect only movement disorders that affect individual regions. For example, clinical testing can show clear evidence of ankylosis affecting particular spinal segments. The examiner makes use of standard reference lines (e.g., the clavicular line or occlusal plane) in determining whether the range of spinal motion is normal or decreased.

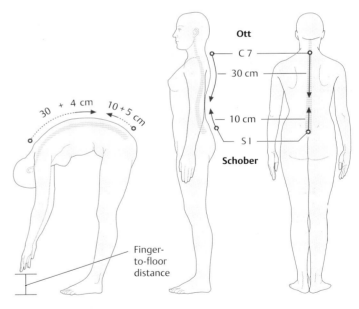

E Average ranges of motion in different spinal regions (degrees)

	Cervical spine			Thoracic spine	Lumbar spine	Cervical + thoracic + lumbar
	A-o joint	A-a joint	Entire cervical spine			
Flexion	20	—	65	35	50	150
Extension	10	—	40	25	35	100
Lateral flexion*	5	—	35	20	20	75
Rotation*	—	35	50	35	5	90

A-o joint = Atlanto-occipital joint
A-a joint = Atlantoaxial joint

* To each side

F Measurement of the range of thoracic and lumbar spinal flexion by the method of Schober and Ott

In the method of Schober and Ott, the patient stands erect while the examiner marks the S1 spinous process and a second point 10 cm higher. When the patient bends as far forward as possible, the distance between the two skin markings will increase to approximately 15 (10 + 5) cm (range of motion of the lumbar spine). The thoracic range of motion is determined by measuring 30 cm down from the spinous process of the C7 vertebra (vertebra prominens) and marking that point on the skin. When the patient bends forward, the distance between the markings may increase by up to 4 cm. An alternative method is to measure the smallest finger-to-floor distance (FFD) with the knees extended.

125

9.14 The Uncovertebral Joints of the Cervical Spine

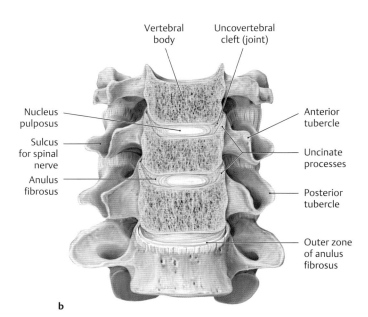

A The uncovertebral joints in a young adult
Cervical spine of an 18-year-old man, anterior view.

a The upper end plates of the C3 through C7 vertebral bodies have lateral projections (uncinate processes) that develop during childhood. Starting at about 10 years of age, the uncinate processes gradually come into contact with the oblique, crescent-shaped margin on the undersurface of the next higher vertebral body. This results in the formation of lateral clefts (uncovertebral clefts or joints, see **b**) in the outer portions of the intervertebral disks.

b C4 through C7 vertebrae. The bodies of the C4–C6 vertebrae have been sectioned in the coronal plane to demonstrate more clearly the uncovertebral joints or clefts. These clefts are bounded laterally by a connective tissue structure, a kind of joint capsule, which causes them to resemble true joint spaces. These clefts or fissures in the intervertebral disk were first described by the anatomist Hubert von Luschka in 1858, who called them *lateral hemiarthroses*. He interpreted them as primary mechanisms designed to enhance the flexibility of the cervical spine and confer a functional advantage (drawings based on specimens from the Anatomical Collection at Kiel University).

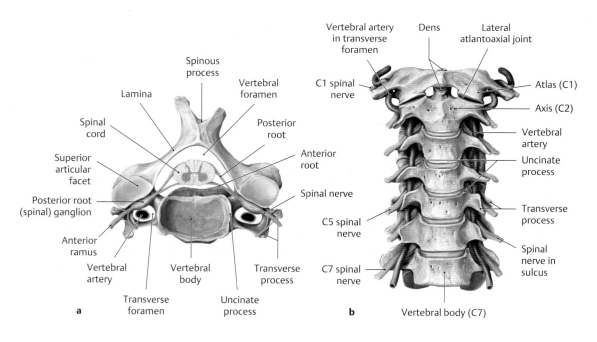

B Topographical relationship of the spinal nerve and vertebral artery to the uncinate process

a Fourth cervical vertebra with spinal cord, spinal roots, spinal nerves, and vertebral arteries, superior view.

b Cervical spine with both vertebral arteries and the emerging spinal nerves, anterior view.

Note the course of the vertebral artery through the transverse foramina and the course of the spinal nerve at the level of the intervertebral foramina. Given their close proximity, both the artery and nerve may be compressed by osteophytes (bony outgrowths) caused by uncovertebral arthrosis (see **D**).

Atlas (C1)

Dens

Lateral atlantoaxial joint

Transverse foramen

C2 vertebral body

Vertebral artery

Uncovertebral joint

Uncinate processes

Intervertebral disks with horizontal clefts

C7 vertebral body

C Degenerative changes in the cervical spine (uncovertebral arthrosis)

Coronal section through the cervical spine of a 35-year-old man, anterior view. *Note* the course of the vertebral arteries on both sides of the vertebral bodies.

The development of the uncovertebral joints at approximately 10 years of age initiates a process of cleft formation in the intervertebral disks. This process spreads toward the center of the disk with aging, eventually resulting in the formation of complete transverse clefts that subdivide the intervertebral disks into two slabs of roughly equal thickness. The result is a progressive degenerative process marked by flattening of the disks and consequent instability of the motion segments (drawing based on specimens from the Anatomical Collection at Kiel University).

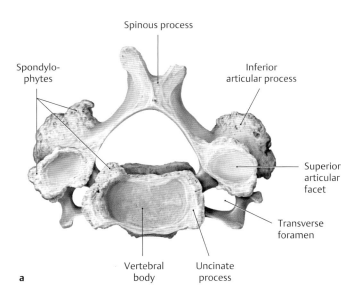

Spinous process

Spondylophytes

Inferior articular process

Vertebral body

Superior vertebral notch

Superior articular process

Zygapophyseal joint (facet joint)

Spondylophytes

Superior articular facet

Intervertebral foramen

Transverse foramen

Vertebral body

Uncinate process

Uncovertebral joint

Sulcus for spinal nerve

Spinous process

a

b

D Advanced uncovertebral arthrosis of the cervical spine

a Fourth cervical vertebra, superior view.
b Fourth and fifth cervical vertebrae, lateral view (drawings based on specimens from the Anatomical Collection at Kiel University).

The uncovertebral joints undergo degenerative changes comparable to those seen in other joints, including the formation of osteophytes (called spondylophytes when they occur on vertebral bodies). These sites of new bone formation serve to distribute the imposed forces over a larger area, thereby reducing the pressure on the joint. With progres-

sive destabilization of the corresponding motion segment, the facet joints undergo osteoarthritic changes leading to osteophyte formation. Osteophytes of the uncovertebral joints have major clinical importance because of their relation to the intervertebral foramen and vertebral artery (uncovertebral arthrosis). They cause a progressive narrowing of the intervertebral foramen, with increasing compression of the spinal nerve and often of the vertebral artery as well (see **C**). Meanwhile, the spinal canal itself may become significantly narrowed (spinal stenosis) by the same process.

9.15 Cross-sectional Anatomy of the Lumbar Spine

A Midsagittal section through the lower part of the spinal column

Left lateral view.

Note: The caudal end of the spinal cord, the conus medullaris, terminates in most people at the level of the first lumbar vertebra but in a few at the level of the second lumbar vertebra. The spinal cord and spinal canal are approximately the same length until the 12th week of prenatal development, so that each spinal cord segment and its pair of spinal nerves lie adjacent to the vertebra of the same number. With further growth, however, the vertebral column lengthens more rapidly than the spinal cord, resulting in an increasing cephalad displacement of the conus medullaris. At birth the conus medullaris has already reached the level of the third lumbar vertebra, and it continues its gradual upward shift until about the 10th year of life. Because of these disparate growth rates, the spinal roots run obliquely downward from their segment of origin in the cord to reach their corresponding intervertebral foramen. The spinal roots that descend from the lower end of the cord are collectively termed the *cauda equina* ("horse's tail"). Because the membranes that enclose the spinal cord (the meninges) extend into the sacral canal (lumbar cistern), a needle can be safely introduced into the subarachnoid space below the conus medullaris to sample cerebrospinal fluid without injuring the cord *(lumbar puncture)*. This site is also used for *lumbar spinal anesthesia* to block both the afferent nerve roots (for analgesia) and the efferent nerve roots (for muscular paralysis) that supply the pelvic region and lower limbs.

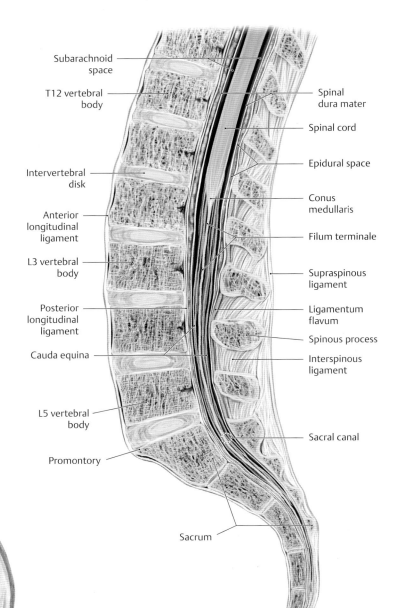

Labels (top figure): Subarachnoid space · T12 vertebral body · Intervertebral disk · Anterior longitudinal ligament · L3 vertebral body · Posterior longitudinal ligament · Cauda equina · L5 vertebral body · Promontory · Sacrum · Spinal dura mater · Spinal cord · Epidural space · Conus medullaris · Filum terminale · Supraspinous ligament · Ligamentum flavum · Spinous process · Interspinous ligament · Sacral canal · Coccyx

Labels (bottom figure): Posterior longitudinal ligament · Spinal dura mater · Cauda equina · Epidural space with fat tissue and venous plexus · Ligamentum flavum · Posterior internal vertebral venous plexus · Anterior internal vertebral venous plexus · Dural sleeve with spinal nerve · Dural sac

B Cauda equina at the level of the second lumbar vertebra

Transverse section, superior view. Because the spinal cord ends at the level of the first lumbar vertebra in most people, at the level of the second lumbar vertebra, the dural sac, which ends at the level of the second sacral vertebrae, consists only of the cauda equina and the filum terminale (see **A**). Here the epidural space is enlarged and filled with extended venous plexus and fatty tissue.

Cauda equina
Ligamentum flavum
Posterior longitudinal ligament
Basivertebral veins
Anterior longitudinal ligament
Epidural adipose tissue

a

Spinal (sensory) ganglion
Zygapophyseal joint
Intraforaminal fat
Intraforaminal veins
Ligamentum flavum

b

Anterior longitudinal ligament
Conus medullaris
Cauda equina
Basivertebral veins
Epidural fat
Nucleus pulposus
Ligamentum flavum

c

Vertebral arch
Intervertebral foramen
Intraforaminal fat
Zygapophyseal joint
Intraforaminal vessels
Spinal (sensory) ganglion

d

C MRI of the normal lumbar spine: Sagittal and transverse sections (photos from Vahlensieck M, Reiser M. MRT des Bewgungsapparates. 3rd ed. Stuttgart: Thieme; 2006)

a, **b** structures visible in the median and para-sagittal section.

c, **d** T1-weighted SE sequence of the lumbar spine in median and parasagittal section.

Sectional plane of
— **F** and **I**
— **G** and **J**
— **H** and **K**

e

e motion segment L4–L5 after removal of vertebral arch, dorsal view; position of the transverse planes:

f supradisk level.
g disk level L4–L5.
h infradisk level.

In **f** and **g**, the intervertebral foramen is shown; in **h**, the pedicle is shown.

i–k T1-weighted SE sequences of the motion segment L4–L5 in the corresponding axial (transverse) planes.

Note the position of the spinal roots in relation to the dural sac. The spinal roots extend in so-called dural bags, which reach into the intervertebral foramen, so the roots and the spinal ganglion are completely bathed in fluid (see Fig. **B**).

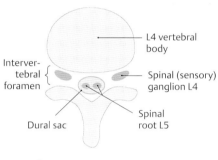

L4 vertebral body
Intervertebral foramen
Spinal (sensory) ganglion L4
Dural sac
Spinal root L5

f

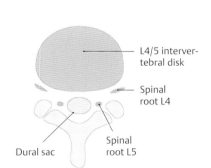

L4/5 intervertebral disk
Spinal root L4
Dural sac
Spinal root L5

g

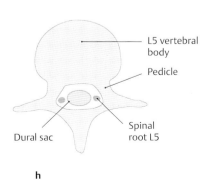

L5 vertebral body
Pedicle
Dural sac
Spinal root L5

h

i Spinal (sensory) ganglion L4   Spinal root L5

j Spinal root L4   Spinal root L5

k Spinal root L5   Dural sac

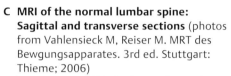

129

9.16 Degenerative Changes in the Lumbar Spine

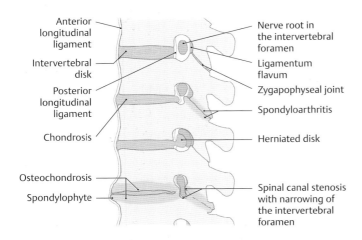

Labels (clockwise):
Anterior longitudinal ligament — Nerve root in the intervertebral foramen — Ligamentum flavum — Zygapophyseal joint — Spondyloarthritis — Herniated disk — Spinal canal stenosis with narrowing of the intervertebral foramen
Intervertebral disk — Posterior longitudinal ligament — Chondrosis — Osteochondrosis — Spondylophyte

A Degenerative spine changes at a glance

Degenerative spine changes are among the most common disorders. They are age-dependent and increase dramatically after the age of 30. The intervertebral disk, the adjacent osseous end plates, the vertebrae, and the ligaments of the participating motion segment are most often affected.

Degeneration of the intervertebral disks and disk herniation: As a result of fluid depletion in the nucleus pulposus (decreased water-binding capacity — a typical symptom of old age), the intervertebral disk space increasingly narrows, and the affected motion segment be-

comes increasingly unstable. The resulting locally increased mechanical loading of the disk causes fraying and cracking in the anulus fibrosus (chondrosis) and eventually leads to a herniated disk (protrusion or prolapse, see **D**).

Lumbar spinal stenosis: The body tries to withstand disk degeneration through reactive bone changes, similar to what happens with osteoarthritis in the limb joints (see p. 46). At the vertebral bodies, marginal spikes (osteophytes = spondylophytes) form, which are supposed to enlarge the force-transmitting surface, thereby relieving the relevant vertebral joint and stabilizing the motion segment, causing end plate sclerosis (osteochondrosis). Similar processes occur at the small vertebral joints (spondylarthrosis). The increasing narrowing of the vertebral canal and the intervertebral foramina leads to degenerative lumbar spinal stenosis (see **B**). Later, the marginal spikes grow toward each other until they finally touch and as a result bridge and ossify the motion segment ("formation of bone bridges," see **Cc**). This increasingly impairs spine movement, often decreasing discomfort. A herniated disk is no longer possible, which is why herniated disks do not occur in old age.

Vertebral body fractures and deformities: In old age, the vertebral body is often the weakest link. Advanced osteoporosis or osteolytic bone metastasis accompanied by loss of stability in the bone can lead to vertebral body fractures and deformities. The symptoms include initially localized pain, which can spread if, at the same time, nerve roots are compressed.

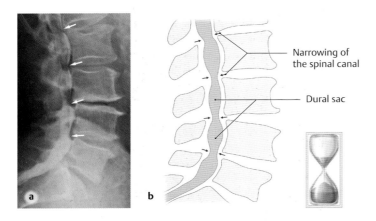

Labels: Narrowing of the spinal canal — Dural sac

B Degenerative lumbar spinal stenosis

Symptoms of this disorder include the concentric narrowing of the vertebral canal at the level of the relevant motion segment. It develops based on a congenital narrowing and/or acquired degenerative changes, such as dorsal spondylophytes and arthrotically transformed vertebral joints (spondylarthrosis). Although rare, ligamentous hypertrophy, too, particularly of the posterior longitudinal ligament and the ligamenta flava, can contribute to narrowing of the vertebral canal. Typical symptoms include load-dependent neurogenic pain in the lumbar region and legs. It is caused by walking for long periods of time but also by standing, and subsides only by supporting the body (e.g., by propping oneself up) and by kyphosis of the lumbar spine (sitting with the upper body bent forward). Pain, sensory disturbance, and paralysis lead to drastically impaired walking distance (spinal claudication). The diagnosis is made using MRI and/or with the help of lumbar myelography with the spine positioned in lateral projection (**a**).

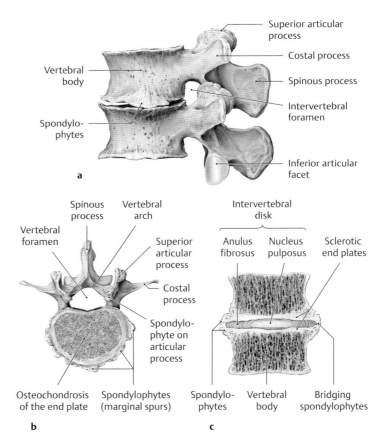

Labels (a): Superior articular process — Costal process — Spinous process — Intervertebral foramen — Inferior articular facet — Vertebral body — Spondylophytes
Labels (b): Spinous process — Vertebral arch — Intervertebral disk — Vertebral foramen — Superior articular process — Anulus fibrosus — Nucleus pulposus — Sclerotic end plates — Costal process — Spondylophyte on articular process — Osteochondrosis of the end plate — Spondylophytes (marginal spurs)
Labels (c): Spondylophytes — Vertebral body — Bridging spondylophytes

C Lumbar disk herniation

a Posterolateral herniation, superior view
b Posterior herniation, superior view
c Posterolateral herniation, posterior view (the vertebral arches have been removed to demonstrate the lumbar dural sac and corresponding nerve roots)

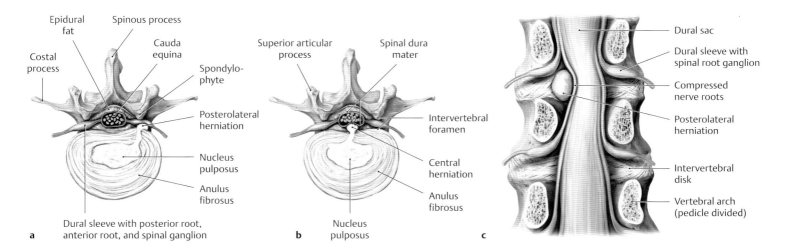

a Dural sleeve with posterior root, anterior root, and spinal ganglion

b Nucleus pulposus

c

D Lumbar disk herniation

a Posterolateral herniation, superior view.
b Posterior herniation, superior view.
c Posterolateral herniation, posterior view (the vertebral arches have been removed at the level of the pedicle to demonstrate the lumbar dural sac and corresponding nerve roots).

In old age, not only does the intervertebral disk get thinner (due to loss of water in the nucleus pulposus, see **A**), it also shifts more easily, as a result of a decrease in resistance in the intervertebral disk sleeve, the anulus fibrosus, which begins to tear and fray. The tissue of the jelly-like nucleus pulposus shifts initially toward the weak spots of the anu-

lus fibrosus (intervertebral disk protrusion). If it tears as a result of continuous strain, it protrudes (disk prolapse) and compresses the content of the intervertebral foramen. Sequestration occurs when a part of the intervertebral disk that has shifted forward no longer shows any connection to the rest of the intervertebral disk. A posterolateral herniation generally compresses the subjacent lying nerve root (**c**), causing pain and paralysis that affect inferiorly adjacent dermatomes and corresponding muscles (see **E**).

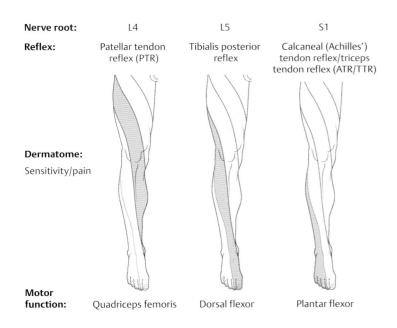

Nerve root:	L4	L5	S1
Reflex:	Patellar tendon reflex (PTR)	Tibialis posterior reflex	Calcaneal (Achilles') tendon reflex/triceps tendon reflex (ATR/TTR)
Dermatome: Sensitivity/pain			
Motor function:	Quadriceps femoris	Dorsal flexor	Plantar flexor

E Schematic representation of neurologic disorders in lumbar root compression syndromes as a result of herniated disks (L4, L5, and S1)

In over 90% of all cases, herniated lumbar disks affect the L5 and S1 roots. Patients complain about pain and sensitivity loss in the affected dermatomes, as well as weakness or paralysis in the muscles innervated by these nerve roots. Patients experience the symptoms of root compression syndrome in the following order with increasing severity: pain, sensitivity loss, and paralysis. Often the cause is a weakening or abnormal proprioceptive reflex associated with the affected root.

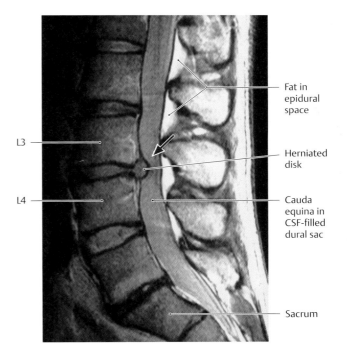

F Posterior disk herniation in the lumbar spine

Midsagittal T2-weighted magnetic resonance image of the lumbar spine, left lateral view (from Vahlensieck M, Reiser M. MRT des Bewegungsaparates. 2nd ed. Stuttgart: Thieme; 2001). The image shows a conspicuous herniated disk at the L3–L4 level (red arrow), which protrudes posteriorly (transligamentous herniation). The dural sac at that level is deeply indented (see **Db**).

9.17 The Thoracic Skeleton

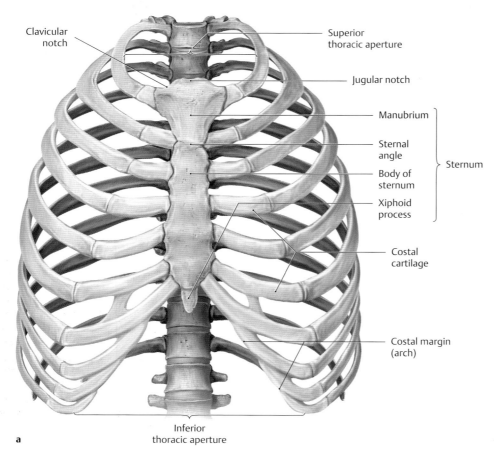

Clavicular notch
Superior thoracic aperture
Jugular notch
Manubrium
Sternal angle
Body of sternum
Xiphoid process
Sternum
Costal cartilage
Costal margin (arch)
Inferior thoracic aperture

a

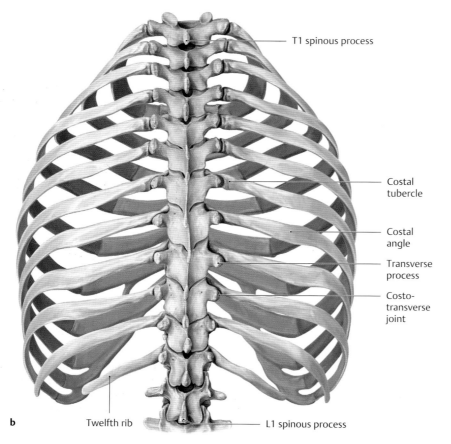

T1 spinous process
Costal tubercle
Costal angle
Transverse process
Costotransverse joint
Twelfth rib
L1 spinous process

b

A Thoracic skeleton
a Anterior view, **b** posterior view.
The thoracic skeleton (thoracic cage, thorax) consists of the vertebral column, the 12 pairs of ribs, and the sternum. These structures are movably interconnected by ligaments, true joints, and synchondroses. Tension is imparted to the thorax by the intercostal muscles. The thoracic cage encloses the chest cavity and has a superior aperture (the thoracic inlet) and an inferior aperture (the thoracic outlet). Its shape is subject to marked variations relating to age and gender. The ribs of an infant have very little obliquity and are approximately horizontal. With increasing age, the ribs incline downward, while the thoracic cage becomes flattened anteroposteriorly. This is associated with a relative decrease in the size of the thoracic outlet. Generally, the female thorax is narrower and shorter than in the male. From a functional standpoint, the thoracic skeleton and its muscular wall structures form a rugged, stable enclosure that permits the respiratory excursions that are necessary for normal breathing. This is apparent in patients with severe chest injuries such as multiple rib fractures due to blunt trauma, where instability of the chest wall leads to paradoxical respiration: the affected side of the rib cage moves inward during inspiration and outward during expiration. This results in a *pendelluft* effect (from the German *Pendel*, pendulum, and *Luft*, air): air streams back and forth between the lungs, leading to increased dead space ventilation, decreased alveolar gas exchange, and respiratory failure. Patients thus affected generally require intubation.

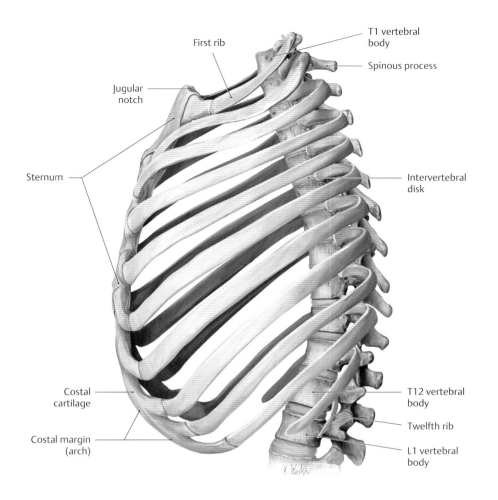

B Thoracic skeleton, lateral view

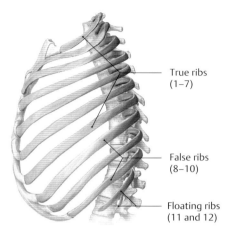

C True, false, and floating ribs

Lateral view. Each of the 12 pairs of ribs is bilaterally symmetrical, but the shapes of the ribs vary at different levels. The first seven pairs of ribs, called the *true ribs,* are normally connected anteriorly to the sternum. Of the remaining five, called the *false ribs,* the eighth, ninth, and tenth ribs are joined by their costal cartilage to the cartilage of the rib directly above, contributing to the structure of the costal margin (arch) (see **Aa**). The last two pairs of "false" ribs, called the *floating ribs,* usually terminate freely between the muscles of the lateral abdominal wall.

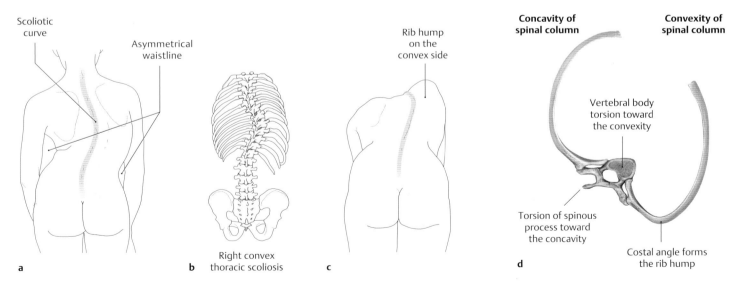

D Lateral curvature of the spinal column (scoliosis)

a, b Posterior view. Scoliosis commonly presents as a *right convex* curve of the spinal column at the level of the T8–T9 vertebrae (**b**). It is manifested by a typical postural deformity in upright stance (**a**).

c, d When a patient with right convex scoliosis bends forward, a typical rib hump appears on the convex side of the curve (**c**). This happens because the adjacent ribs also occupy an abnormal position due to torsion of the vertebral bodies (**d**, superior view).

133

9.18 The Sternum and Ribs

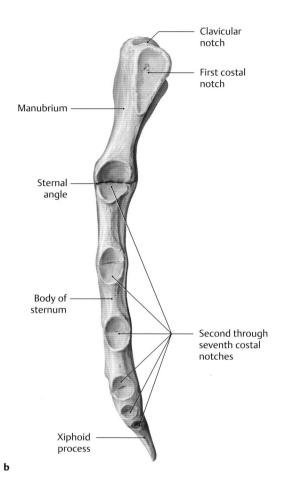

a

b

A The sternum
a Anterior view.
b Lateral view.

The sternum is a flattened bone, slightly convex anteriorly, with multiple indentations along its lateral borders (costal notches). The adult sternum consists of three bony parts:

- The manubrium
- The body of the sternum
- The xiphoid process

The manubrium, body, and xiphoid process in adolescents and young adults are connected to one another by cartilaginous plates (manubriosternal synchondrosis and xiphosternal synchondrosis), which gradually ossify with increasing age. The fully ossified, mature adult form is depicted here. The depression in the superior border of the manubrium (jugular notch) is clearly palpable through the skin and marks the inferior margin of the jugular fossa. On each side of the jugular notch is a depression for articulation with the clavicle on that side (clavicular notch), and just below that is a shallow concavity (first costal notch) for the synchondrosis with the first rib. At the junction of the sternal manubrium and body is an articular facet for the second rib (second costal notch). At that site the manubrium is usually angled slightly backward in relation to the body of the sternum (sternal angle). The lateral borders of the sternal body bear additional costal notches that articulate with the third through seventh costal cartilages, the notches for the sixth and seventh costal cartilages being placed very close together. The sometimes bifid and perforated xiphoid process itself is devoid of costal attachments and is highly variable in its form. Frequently, the xiphoid process is still cartilaginous in adults.

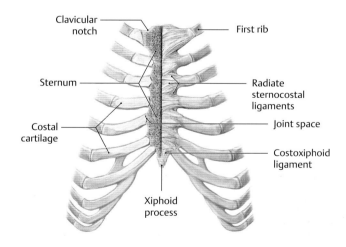

B The sternocostal joints
Anterior view (the right half of the sternum has been sectioned frontally to show the sternocostal joints). The connections between the costal cartilages for the first through seventh ribs and the costal notches of the sternum consist partly of synchondroses and partly of true joints. Generally, a joint space is found only at the second through fifth ribs, while the first, sixth, and seventh ribs are attached to the sternum by synchondroses. In the true joints as well as the synchondroses, ligaments (radiate sternocostal ligaments) radiate from the perichondrium of the costal cartilage to the anterior surface of the sternum, where they blend with the periosteum to form a dense fibrous membrane (the sternal membrane). The second rib is typically the most superior palpable rib.

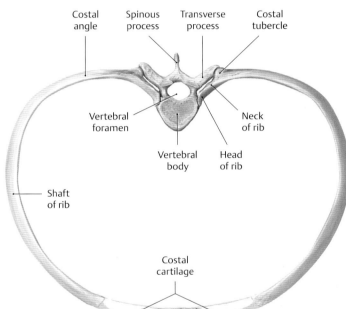

C Variable size and shape of the ribs

a First rib, **b** second rib, **c** fifth rib, **d** eleventh rib (all are right ribs, viewed from above).

The neck of the rib extends from the head of the rib to the costal tubercle. Except on the first rib, the neck bears a sharp superior ridge (crest of the neck of the rib). Lateral to the costal tubercle is the shaft (body) of the rib, which curves forward to form the costal angle. The shafts of the second through twelfth ribs in particular show irregular curvatures (on the flat and on the edges) and are also twisted about their long axis. Because of this torsion, the external surfaces of the ribs face slightly downward at their vertebral end and slightly upward at their anterior end. Normally, the first and twelfth ribs are the shortest, while the seventh rib is the longest. The costal cartilage increases in length from the first to the seventh rib and shortens again past the eighth rib. Every rib except the first, eleventh, and twelfth has a groove along its inferior border (costal groove) that affords some protection for the intercostal vessels and nerves (see pp. 173 and 205).

D Segments of the rib and structure of a thoracic segment

Sixth pair of ribs, superior view. Each rib consists of a bony part (costal bone) and a cartilaginous part (costal cartilage). The bony part consists of the following segments, starting from its vertebral end:

- Head
- Neck
- Costal tubercle
- Shaft (body), which includes the costal angle

9.19 The Costovertebral Joints and Thoracic Movements

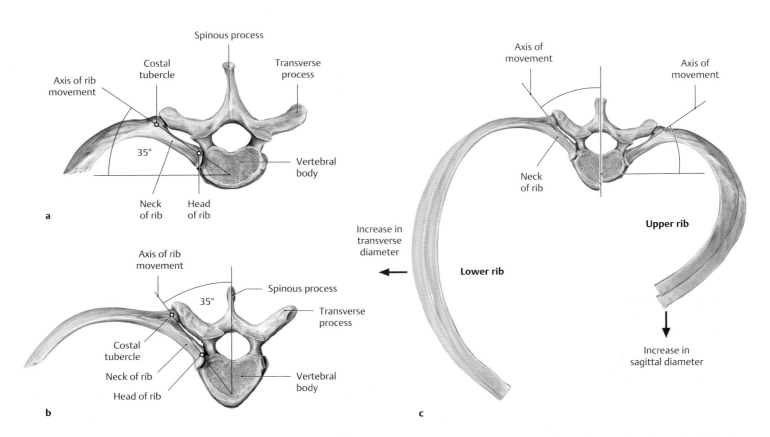

A Axes for movements of the costovertebral joints and ribs
(after Kapandji)
Superior view.

a Axis of upper rib movements.
b Axis of lower rib movements.
c Direction of rib movements (see **C** for the costovertebral joints).

The axes of rib movements are directed parallel to the necks of the ribs. The axes for the upper ribs are closer to the coronal plane (**a**), while those for the lower ribs are closer to the sagittal plane (**b**). For this reason, a rib excursion in the upper part of the rib cage mainly increases the sagittal thoracic diameter, while a lower rib excursion increases the transverse diameter (see **B**).

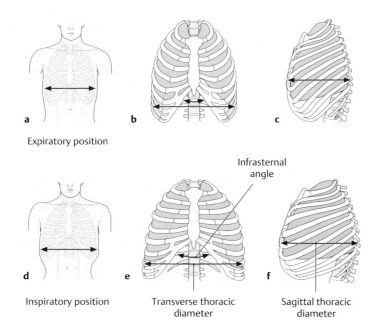

B Movements of the rib cage during costal or chest breathing (sternocostal breathing)
Respiration (ventilation) is effected through changes in the thoracic volume. The increase in thoracic volume that is necessary for inspiration can be accomplished in two ways:

1. By lowering the diaphragm (costodiaphragmatic breathing or abdominal breathing, see p.160)
2. By elevating the ribs (sternocostal breathing, also known as costal or chest breathing)

While breathing at rest is almost entirely abdominal, respiration during physical effort is augmented by chest breathing with the intercostal muscles and the auxiliary muscles of respiration. The drawings illustrate the thoracic volume changes that occur during *chest or costal breathing,* in which the thoracic volume decreases and increases in both the coronal and sagittal planes. Panels **a–c** show the *decrease* in the transverse and sagittal chest diameters at end-expiration, and **d–f** show the *increase* at end-inspiration.

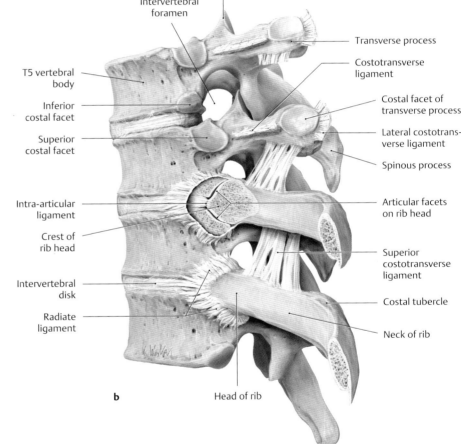

C Ligaments of the costovertebral joints

The costovertebral joints are the joints by which the ribs articulate with the vertebrae. They consist of two types: the joints of the heads of the ribs and the costotransverse joints. Though morphologically distinct, these different joint types are functionally interrelated.

a Articulation of the eighth rib with the eighth thoracic vertebra, superior view (the joint of the head of the rib and costotransverse joint on the left side have been transversely sectioned).

b The fifth through eighth thoracic vertebrae and associated ribs (seventh and eighth ribs), left lateral view (the joint of the head of the seventh rib has been transversely sectioned).

Joint of the head of the rib: This joint consists of two articular surfaces:

1. An articular facet on the head of the rib
2. A costal facet on the vertebral body

The articular facets on the head of the second through tenth ribs (defined by the crest of the rib head) articulate with the fossa formed by the superior and inferior costal facets on two adjacent vertebral bodies and the intervertebral disk between them. The intra-articular ligament, which extends from the crest of the rib head to the intervertebral disk, separates the joint cavity of the second through tenth rib heads into two compartments. By contrast, the heads of the first, eleventh, and twelfth ribs each articulate with only one thoracic vertebral body (see **A**, p. 110). In all the joints of the heads of the ribs, the joint capsule is reinforced by the *radiate ligament.*

Costotransverse joint: In the costotransverse joints of the first through tenth ribs, the articular surface of the costal tubercle articulates with the costal facet on the transverse process of the corresponding thoracic vertebra. The eleventh and twelfth ribs do not have a costotransverse joint because their transverse processes do not have articular facets (see **A**, p. 110). Three ligaments stabilize the costotransverse joint and also strengthen the joint capsule:

1. The lateral costotransverse ligament (from the tip of the transverse process to the costal tubercle)
2. The costotransverse ligament (between the neck of the rib and the transverse process)
3. The superior costotransverse ligament (between the neck of the rib and the transverse process of the vertebra above it)

137

9.20 The Bony Pelvis

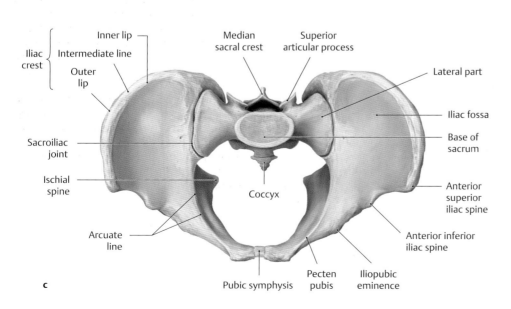

A The male pelvis
a Anterior view.
b Posterior view.
c Superior view.

B The pelvic girdle and pelvic ring
Anterosuperior view. The pelvic girdle consists of the two hip bones (coxal bones). The sacroiliac joints and the cartilaginous pubic symphysis unite the bony parts of the pelvic girdle with the sacrum to form a stable ring called the pelvic ring (indicated by color shading). It allows very little mobility, because stability throughout the pelvic ring is an important prerequisite for transmitting the trunk load to the lower limbs.

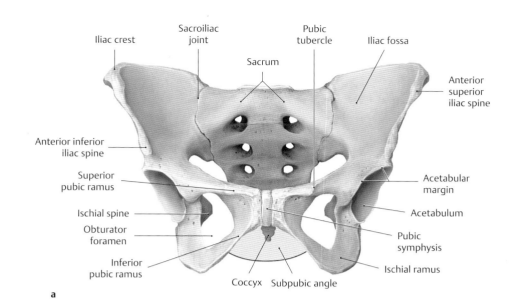

C The female pelvis
a Anterior view.
b Posterior view.
c Superior view.

a

b

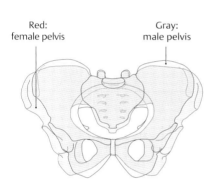

Red:
female pelvis

Gray:
male pelvis

D Gender-specific features of the pelvis
Anterosuperior view. A male and female pelvis have been superimposed to illustrate the gender-specific differences. Comparison reveals that the female pelvis is larger and broader than the male pelvis, while the latter is taller, narrower, and more massive than the female pelvis. The inlet of the female pelvis is larger and has an almost oval shape, while the sacral promontory shows a greater projection in the male pelvis (**Cc**). Sex differences are also noted in the angle of the pubic arch formed by the inferior pubic rami, which is acute in men (70°) but significantly larger in women (almost 90–100°). Accordingly, this angle is called the subpubic angle (see **D**, p.141). The sacrum also exhibits differences between the sexes. In women the sacrum is angled at the level of the third and fourth vertebrae (see p.114), while in men it presents a uniform curvature.

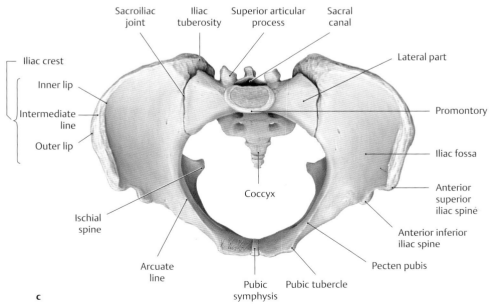

c

9.21 The Pelvic Ligaments and Pelvic Measurements

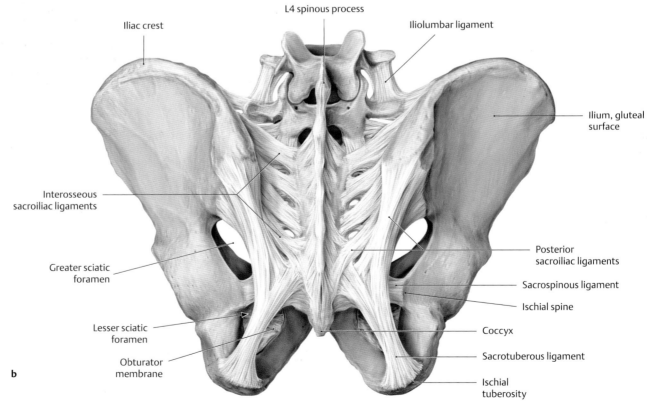

A Ligaments of the male pelvis

a Anterosuperior view.

b Posterior view.

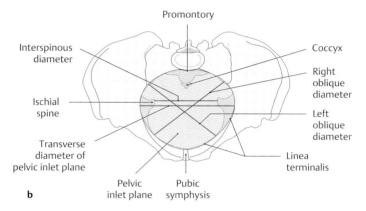

Promontory
Diagonal conjugate
True conjugate
Pelvic inlet plane
Pubic tubercle
Symphyseal surface
Linea terminalis
Coccyx
AP diameter of pelvic outlet

a   ~60°   ~15°

Promontory
Interspinous diameter
Ischial spine
Transverse diameter of pelvic inlet plane
Coccyx
Right oblique diameter
Left oblique diameter
Linea terminalis
Pelvic inlet plane   Pubic symphysis

b

Sacroiliac joint
Intertubercular distance
Interspinous distance
Pelvic inlet plane

c

B Internal and external pelvic measurements
a Right half of a female pelvis, medial view.
b Female pelvis, superior view.
c Male pelvis, superior view.

The linea terminalis is marked in red in **a**. The pelvic inlet plane is color-shaded in **b** and **c**.

C Internal and external pelvic measurements, linea terminalis, and pelvic inlet plane

The internal and external pelvic measurements provide direct or indirect information on the size and shape of the bony boundaries of the lesser pelvis. Because the lesser pelvis functions as the birth canal, the internal and external pelvic dimensions have special practical significance in obstetrics, determining whether the pelvic cavity is broad enough to allow for a vaginal delivery. A particularly important measurement is the true conjugate of the pelvic inlet (the obstetric conjugate), which is the smallest anteroposterior dimension of the lesser pelvis. With *pelvimetry,* a method of measuring pelvic dimensions, potential obstructions to labor can be identified prior to the delivery. Generally, the measurements are performed by transvaginal sonography. Some pelvic dimensions, such as the diagonal conjugate, can be accurately determined by bimanual examination.

Internal pelvic measurements in women (see **Ba** and **Bb**)

- True conjugate = 11 cm (distance from the sacral promontory to the posterior border of the symphysis)
- Diagonal conjugate = 12.5–13 cm (distance from the sacral promontory to the lower border of the symphysis)
- Anteroposterior (AP) diameter of the pelvic outlet = 9 (+2) cm (distance from the lower border of the symphysis to the tip of the coccyx)
- Transverse diameter of the pelvic inlet plane = 13 cm (greatest distance between the lineae terminales)
- Interspinous diameter = 11 cm (distance between the ischial spines)
- Right and left oblique diameter = 12 cm (distance from the sacroiliac joint at the level of the linea terminalis to the iliopectineal eminence on the opposite side)

External pelvic measurements in men (see **Bc**)

- Intertubercular distance = 25–26 cm (distance between the anterior superior iliac spines)
- Intercristal distance = 28–29 cm (greatest distance between the left and right iliac crests in the coronal plane)
- External conjugate = 20–21 cm (distance from the upper border of the symphysis to the spinous process of the L5 vertebra)

Linea terminalis (see **B**)

Boundary line between the greater and lesser pelvis, consists of the pubic symphysis and crest + pecten pubis + the arcuate line and sacral promontory.

Pelvic inlet plane (see **Bb** and **Bc**)

Plane through the pelvic inlet at the level of the linea terminalis, below which is the lesser pelvis

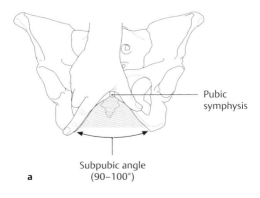

Pubic symphysis
Subpubic angle (90–100°)

a

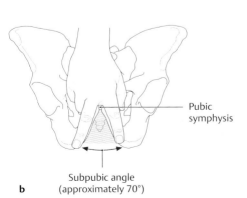

Pubic symphysis
Subpubic angle (approximately 70°)

b

D Subpubic angle
Anterior view.

a Female pelvis.
b Male pelvis.

9.22 The Sacroiliac Joint

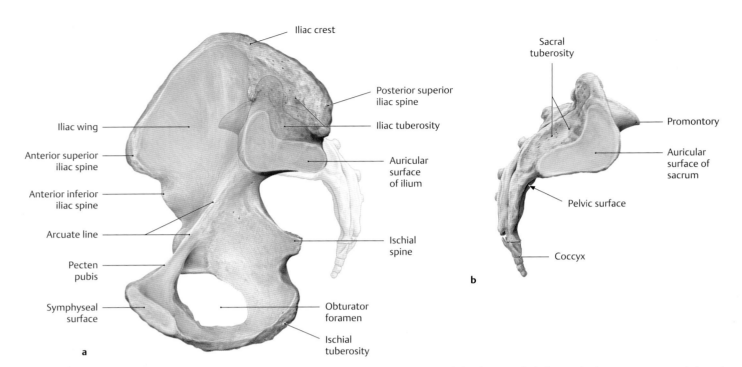

A Articular surfaces of the sacroiliac joint
a Auricular surface of the ilium, right hip bone, medial view (the sacrum is transparent in this view).
b Auricular surface of the sacrum, right lateral view.

The two ear-shaped articular surfaces of the ilium and sacrum (auricular surfaces) are brought together at the sacroiliac joint. The auricular surface of the ilium is slightly notched at its center, and there is a reciprocal ridge on the articular surface of the ilium. The shape and size of both articular surfaces show considerable individual variation—more so than in other joints. Their cartilaginous covering is generally irregular, the articular cartilage on the sacral side being approximately twice as thick as on the iliac side.

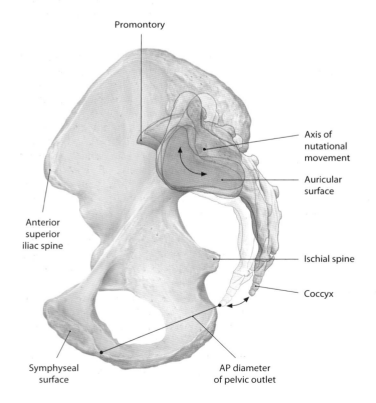

B Nutation in the sacroiliac joint
Right half of pelvis, medial view. Movements in the sacroiliac joints alter the width of the pelvic ring and thus have practical importance in obstetrics. The amplitude of the movements is greatly limited by tight ligaments and varies considerably in different individuals and between the sexes. Basically, very slight rotational and translational movements can be distinguished in the joints. Nutation, as shown here, is a rotational or "tilting" movement of the sacrum about an axis located at the attachments of the interosseous sacroiliac ligaments. With *anterior rotation of the sacrum*, the promontory moves forward and downward, while the coccyx moves upward and backward, thereby increasing the AP diameter of the pelvic outlet. With *posterior rotation of the sacrum*, the AP diameter of the pelvic inlet plane increases, while the AP diameter of the pelvic outlet is decreased.

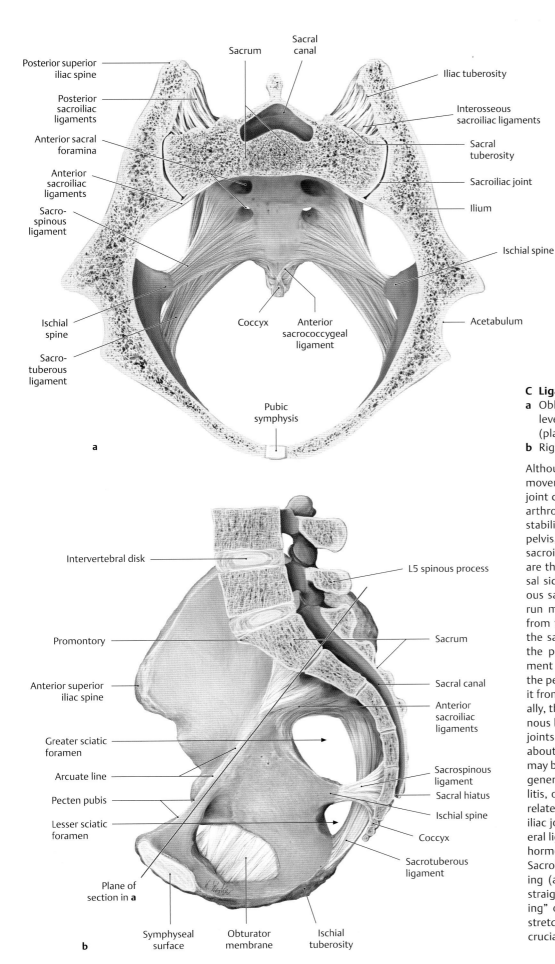

a

Posterior superior iliac spine

Posterior sacroiliac ligaments

Anterior sacral foramina

Anterior sacroiliac ligaments

Sacro-spinous ligament

Ischial spine

Sacro-tuberous ligament

Sacrum

Sacral canal

Iliac tuberosity

Interosseous sacroiliac ligaments

Sacral tuberosity

Sacroiliac joint

Ilium

Ischial spine

Acetabulum

Coccyx

Anterior sacrococcygeal ligament

Pubic symphysis

b

Intervertebral disk

Promontory

Anterior superior iliac spine

Greater sciatic foramen

Arcuate line

Pecten pubis

Lesser sciatic foramen

Plane of section in **a**

Symphyseal surface

Obturator membrane

Ischial tuberosity

L5 spinous process

Sacrum

Sacral canal

Anterior sacroiliac ligaments

Sacrospinous ligament

Sacral hiatus

Ischial spine

Coccyx

Sacrotuberous ligament

C Ligaments of the sacroiliac joint
a Oblique section through the pelvis at the level of the pelvic inlet plane, superior view (plane of section indicated in **b**).
b Right half of pelvis, medial view.

Although the sacroiliac joint is a true joint, its movements are greatly restricted by a tight joint capsule and powerful ligaments (amphiarthrosis). The anterior sacroiliac ligaments stabilize the joint on the anterior side of the pelvis, while the interosseous and posterior sacroiliac ligaments and iliolumbar ligaments are the main stabilizing elements on the dorsal side (see p.140). The powerful interosseous sacroiliac ligaments are deep bands that run medially just behind the sacroiliac joint from the iliac tuberosity to the tuberosity of the sacrum. They are completely covered by the posterior sacroiliac ligaments. The ligament complex helps to anchor the sacrum in the pelvic ring during upright stance and keep it from sliding into the pelvic cavity. Additionally, the sacrotuberous ligament and sacrospinous ligament (see **b**) stabilize both sacroiliac joints and prevent posterior tilting of the pelvis about the transverse axis. *Sacroiliac joint pain* may be caused by chronic inflammatory or degenerative changes (e.g., ankylosing spondylitis, osteoarthritis) or by trauma (e.g., sport-related injuries). Hypermobility of the sacroiliac joint may also develop as a result of general ligamentous weakness or a pregnancy- or hormone-related laxity of the ligaments. Sacroiliac dysfunction may include joint locking (a sudden force like that occurring in a straight-legged jump may cause a "wedging" of the sacrum with joint locking). This stretches the joint capsule and can cause excruciating pain during most body movements.

143

10.1 The Muscles of the Trunk Wall: Their Origin and Function

Overview of the Trunk Wall Muscles

The muscles of the trunk wall in the strict sense consist of the intrinsic back muscles and the muscles of the chest and abdominal wall. In the broad sense, they include the muscles of the pelvic floor (which form the inferior boundary of the abdominopelvic cavity) and the diaphragm (which separates the thoracic and abdominal cavities). Besides the muscles of the trunk wall, the back and thorax also contain muscles of the shoulder girdle and upper limb that migrated to the trunk dur-

ing the course of development *(nonintrinsic back and thoracic muscles)*. Examples are the *thoracohumeral muscles* anteriorly, the *spinohumeral* muscles laterally and posteriorly, and the *spinocostal* muscles. Other muscles that have migrated to the trunk, such as the trapezius, are derived from the mesenchyme of the branchial arches (branchial musculature). They are innervated by cranial nerves (the trapezius by the accessory nerve) and were incorporated secondarily into the trunk wall (see p. 298 ff).

A Trunk wall muscles in the strict sense

Intrinsic back muscles

Lateral tract
- Sacrospinal system
  - Iliocostalis
  - Longissimus
- Spinotransverse system
  - Splenius
- Intertransverse system
  - Intertransversarii
  - Levatores costarum

Medial tract
- Spinal system
  - Interspinales
  - Spinalis
- Transversospinal system
  - Rotatores breves and longi
  - Multifidus
  - Semispinalis

Short nuchal and craniovertebral joint muscles (suboccipital muscles)
- Rectus capitis posterior major
- Rectus capitis posterior minor
- Obliquus capitis superior
- Obliquus capitis inferior

Prevertebral neck muscles (belong topographically to the group of deep neck muscles but act mainly on the cervical spine)

- Longus capitis
- Longus colli
- Rectus capitis lateralis
- Rectus capitis anterior

Muscles of the thoracic cage and wall

- Intercostal muscles
- Transversus thoracis
- Subcostal muscles
- Scalene muscles (belong topographically to the group of deep neck muscles but are functionally related to thoracic breathing)

Muscles of the abdominal wall

Anterolateral abdominal muscles
- External oblique
- Internal oblique
- Transversus abdominis

Anterior (straight or strap) abdominal muscles
- Rectus abdominis
- Pyramidalis

Posterior (deep) abdominal muscles
- Quadratus lumborum
- Psoas major (belongs functionally to the hip muscles, see p. 476)

B Trunk wall muscles in the broad sense

Muscles of the pelvic floor and perineum

Pelvic diaphragm
- Levator ani muscle
  - Puborectalis
  - Pubococcygeus
  - Iliococcygeus
  - Coccygeus
Deep perineal muscles
- Deep transverse prineal (in male)
- External urethral sphincter
- Compressor urethra (in female)
- Urethrovaginal sphincter (in female)
Superficial perineal muscles
- Superficial transverse perineal
- Bulbospongiosus
- Ischiocavernosus
- External anal sphincter

Diaphragm

- Costal part
- Lumbar part (crura)
- Sternal part

C Muscles that migrated secondarily to the trunk wall
(described in the Upper Limb unit, p. 238)

Spinocostal muscles (see also p. 164)

- Serratus posterior superior
- Serratus posterior inferior

Spinohumeral muscles between the trunk and shoulder girdle

- Rhomboid major and minor
- Levator scapulae
- Serratus anterior
- Subclavius
- Pectoralis minor
- Trapezius

Spinohumeral muscles between the trunk and arm

- Latissimus dorsi

Thoracohumeral muscles

- Pectoralis major

* The suboccipital muscles in the strict sense are the short or deep nuchal muscles that are counted among the intrinsic back muscles (because they are innervated by a posterior ramus). The rectus capitis anterior and lateralis muscles are *not* classified as intrinsic back muscles because they are innervated by anterior rami, even though they are also suboccipital in their location.

Origin of the Trunk Wall Muscles

The striated muscles of the trunk wall (including the muscles of the diaphragm and pelvic floor), like the limb muscles, develop embryologically from the myotomes of the somites (see p. 6) and are therefore called the *somatic muscles*. In all, approximately 42 to 44 pairs of segmental somites are formed in the paraxial mesoderm between the 20th and 30th day of development. Five occipital, 7 cervical, 12 thoracic, 5 lumbar, 5 sacral, and 8 to 10 coccygeal somites are formed in a craniocaudal sequence (see **D**). Some of these somites regress with further development, particularly the first occipital somites and most of the coccygeal somites, so that the number of original somites is greater than the number of subsequent vertebral segments. The boundary between the head and neck runs through the fifth pair of occipital somites. At the end of the sixth week of development, the somite myotomes migrate in the dorsoventral direction and become separated into a dorsal part

(epimere or epaxial muscles) and a ventral part (hypomere or hypaxial muscles) (**E**). While the epaxial muscles develop into intrinsic (local) back muscles and retain their original location, the hypomere develops into the anterolateral muscles of the chest and abdominal wall and the limb musculature (**F**). As the myotomes become segregated, the spinal nerves undergo a corresponding division into a *dorsal (posterior) ramus* for the epaxial muscles and a *ventral (anterior) ramus* for the hypaxial muscles (see **Ea**). The original segmental (metameric) arrangement of the trunk muscles mostly disappears with further development. It persists only in the deep layers of the intrinsic back muscles (e.g., the rotator, interspinal, and intertransverse muscles) and the thoracic muscles (e.g., the internal and external intercostal muscles), while the superficial portions of the myotomes fuse together to form long, continuous muscles ("polymerization") in which only the neurovascular supply still exhibits the original segmental arrangement (see **F**).

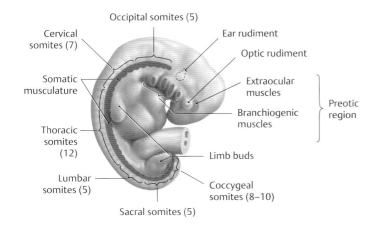

D Somites in a 5-week-old human embryo

Right lateral view. The somites formed from the paraxial mesoderm are classified as *preotic* (shown in blue and green) or *postotic* (shown in red), meaning that they are located cranial or caudal to the ear rudiment. The somatic muscles develop from postotic somites. Segmentation into different somites is not observed in the preotic region, which contains the rudiments for the branchiogenic pharyngeal arch muscles and the extraocular muscles. The structures in this region are innervated by cranial nerves (after Boyd, Hamilton, and Mossmann, quoted in Starck).

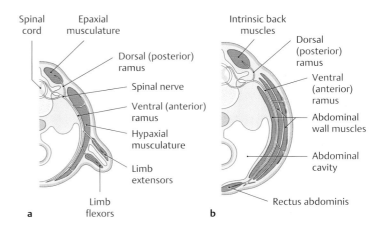

E Transverse sections through a 6-week-old human embryo

a Transverse section at the level of a limb bud.
b Transverse section through the abdominal wall.

Muscle precursor cells with replicative capacity located at the level of the limb buds migrate from the myotomes into the limb buds, and the myotome that remains in these regions develops into intrinsic back muscles. With further growth of the limb bud, the muscle tissue differentiates into a dorsal rudiment (blastema) for the extensor muscles and a ventral rudiment for the flexor muscles of the upper and lower limbs (see p. 20). As in the hypomere, the limb muscles are innervated by ventral (anterior) spinal nerve rami (brachial plexus and lumbosacral plexus, see pp. 360 and 530).
Note the different innervation of the epaxial muscles (dorsal [posterior] ramus) and hypaxial muscles (ventral [anterior] ramus).

F Diagram of the principal muscle groups in an 8-week-old human embryo

Right lateral view. Red = somatic muscles, blue = branchiogenic (branchial arch) muscles, green = extraocular muscles (after Boyd, Hamilton, and Mossmann, quoted in Starck).

10.2 The Intrinsic Back Muscles: Lateral Tract

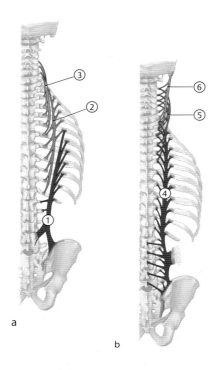

A Lateral tract: schematic of the sacrospinal system
a Iliocostalis muscles.
b Longissimus muscles.

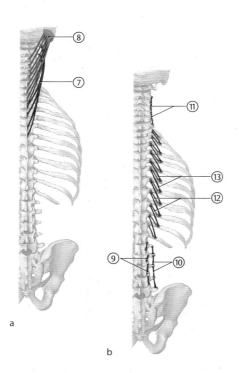

B Lateral tract: schematic of the spinotransverse and intertransverse systems
a Splenius muscles.
b Intertransversarii and levatores costarum muscles.

Iliocostalis muscles (*see p. 147, opposite, lower right)

Origin:	① Iliocostalis lumborum: sacrum, iliac crest, superficial layer of the thoracolumbar fascia
	② Iliocostalis thoracis: seventh to twelfth ribs
	③ Iliocostalis cervicis: third to seventh ribs
Insertion:	• Iliocostalis lumborum: sixth to twelfth ribs, deep layer of thoracolumbar fascia, transverse processes of upper lumbar vertebrae
	• Iliocostalis thoracis: first to sixth ribs
	• Iliocostalis cervicis: transverse processes of C4–C6 vertebrae
Action:	Entire muscle: bilateral contraction extends the spine, unilateral contraction bends the spine laterally to the same side.
Innervation:	Lateral branches of posterior rami of spinal nerves C8–L1

Longissimus muscles

Origin:	④ Longissimus thoracis: sacrum, iliac crest (common tendon of origin with iliocostalis), spinous processes of lumbar vertebrae, transverse processes of lower thoracic vertebrae
	⑤ Longissimus cervicis: transverse processes of T1–T6 vertebrae
	⑥ Longissimus capitis: transverse processes of T1–T3 vertebrae and transverse and articular processes of C4–C7 vertebrae
Insertion:	• Longissimus thoracis: second to twelfth ribs, costal processes of lumbar vertebrae, transverse processes of thoracic vertebrae
	• Longissimus cervicis: transverse processes of C2–C5 vertebrae
	• Longissimus capitis: mastoid process of temporal bone
Action:	• Entire muscle: bilateral contraction extends the spine, unilateral contraction bends the spine laterally to the same side.
	• Longissimus capitis: bilateral contraction extends the head, unilateral contraction flexes and rotates the head to the same side.
Innervation:	Lateral branches of posterior rami of spinal nerves C1–L5

Splenius muscles

Origin:	⑦ Splenius cervicis: spinous processes of the T3–T6 vertebrae
	⑧ Splenius capitis: nuchal ligament, spinous processes of the C7–T3 vertebrae
Insertion:	• Splenius cervicis: transverse processes of C1 and C2
	• Splenius capitis: lateral superior nuchal line, mastoid process
Action:	Entire muscle: bilateral contraction extends the cervical spine and head, unilateral contraction flexes and rotates the head to the same side.
Innervation:	Lateral branches of dorsal rami of spinal nerves C1–C6

Intertransversarii

Origin and insertion:	⑨ Intertransversarii mediales lumborum: course between adjacent mammillary processes of all lumbar vertebrae
	⑩ Intertransversarii laterales lumborum: course between adjacent costal processes of all lumbar vertebrae
	⑪ Intertransversarii posteriores cervicis: course between adjacent posterior tubercles of the C2–C7 vertebrae
	• Intertransversarii anteriores cervicis: course between adjacent anterior tubercles of the C2–C7 vertebrae
Action:	• Bilateral contraction stabilizes and extends the cervical and lumbar spine.
	• Unilateral contraction bends the cervical and lumbar spine laterally to the same side.
Innervation:	Posterior rami of the spinal nerves for intertransversarii mediales lumborum, intertransversarii laterales lumborum, and intertransversarii posteriores cervicis; anterior rami of the spinal nerves for intertransversarii anteriores cervicis

Levatores costarum

Origin:	⑫ Levatores costarum breves: transverse processes of the C7 and T1–T11 vertebrae
	⑬ Levatores costarum longi: transverse processes of the C7 and T1–T11 vertebrae
Insertion:	• Levatores costarum breves: costal angle of the next lower rib
	• Levatores costarum longi: costal angle of second lower rib
Action:	• Bilateral contraction extends the thoracic spine.
	• Unilateral contraction bends the thoracic spine to the same side, rotates it to the opposite side.
Innervation:	Posterior rami of the spinal nerves

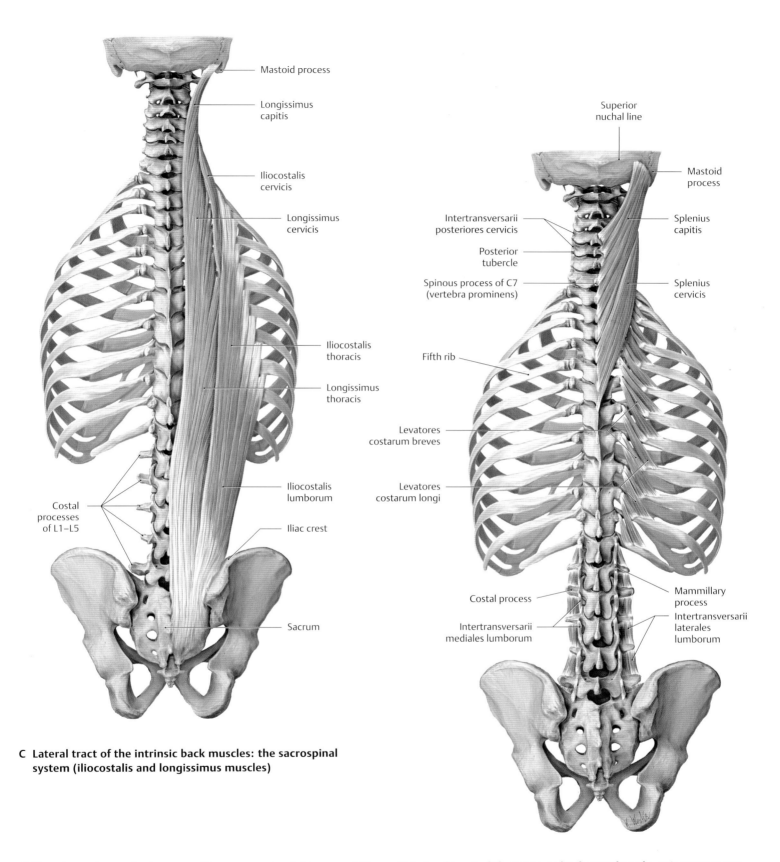

C Lateral tract of the intrinsic back muscles: the sacrospinal system (iliocostalis and longissimus muscles)

Mastoid process

Longissimus capitis

Iliocostalis cervicis

Longissimus cervicis

Iliocostalis thoracis

Longissimus thoracis

Iliocostalis lumborum

Costal processes of L1–L5

Iliac crest

Sacrum

Superior nuchal line

Mastoid process

Intertransversarii posteriores cervicis

Splenius capitis

Posterior tubercle

Spinous process of C7 (vertebra prominens)

Splenius cervicis

Fifth rib

Levatores costarum breves

Levatores costarum longi

Costal process

Mammillary process

Intertransversarii mediales lumborum

Intertransversarii laterales lumborum

D Lateral tract of the intrinsic back muscles: the spinotransverse system (splenius muscles) and intertransverse system (intertransversarii and levatores costarum muscles)

* The schematic muscle diagrams with accompanying tables on p. 146 are intended to give a systematic overview of the muscles and their actions. The drawings on the right-hand page are intended to display the muscles as they would appear in a dissection. Not all the structures listed in the tables on p. 146 are labeled in the drawings above, as they are not all visible in the views shown.

147

10.3 The Intrinsic Back Muscles: Medial Tract

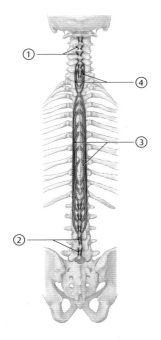

A Medial tract of the intrinsic back muscles: schematic of the spinal system

The interspinales and spinalis muscles.

a
b
c

B Medial tract of the intrinsic back muscles: schematic of the transversospinal system

a Rotatores breves and longi.
b Multifidus.
c Semispinalis.

Interspinales muscles

Origin and insertion:
① Interspinales cervicis: course between the spinous processes of adjacent cervical vertebrae
② Interspinales lumborum: course between the spinous processes of adjacent lumbar vertebrae

Action: Extends the cervical and lumbar spine
Innervation: Posterior rami of the spinal nerves

Spinalis muscles

Origin:
③ Spinalis thoracis: lateral surface of the spinous processes of the T10–T12 and L1–L3 vertebrae
④ Spinalis cervicis: spinous processes of the C5–C7 and T1–T2 vertebrae

Insertion:
• Spinalis thoracis: lateral surface of the spinous processes of the T2–T8 vertebrae
• Spinalis cervicis: spinous processes of the C2–C5 vertebrae

Action:
• Bilateral contraction extends the cervical and thoracic spine.
• Unilateral contraction bends the cervical and thoracic spine to the same side.

Innervation: Posterior rami of the spinal nerves

Rotatores breves and longi

Origin and insertion:
⑤ Rotatores breves: from transverse process of thoracic vertebrae to spinous process of the next higher vertebra
⑥ Rotatores longi: from transverse process of thoracic vertebrae to spinious process of the vertebra two levels higher

Action:
• Bilateral contraction extends the thoracic spine.
• Unilateral contraction rotates it to the opposite side.

Innervation: Posterior rami of the spinal nerves

⑦ Multifidus (most fully developed in lumbar spine)

Origin: Sacrum, ilium, mammillary processes of L1–L5, transverse and articular processes of T1–T4, C4–C7

Insertion: Superomedially to spinous process of vertebra two to four levels higher

Action:
• Bilateral contraction extends the spine.
• Unilateral contraction flexes the spine to the same side and rotates it to the opposite side.

Innervation: Posterior rami of the spinal nerves

Semispinalis muscles

Origin:
⑧ Semispinalis thoracis: transverse processes of the T6–T12 vertebrae
⑨ Semispinalis cervicis: transverse processes of the T1–T6 vertebrae
⑩ Semispinalis capitis: transverse processes of the C3–T6 vertebrae

Insertion:
• Semispinalis thoracis: spinous processes of the C6–T4 vertebrae
• Semispinalis cervicis: spinous processes of the C2–C5 vertebrae
• Semispinalis capitis: occipital bone between the superior and inferior nuchal lines

Action:
• Bilateral contraction extends the thoracic spine, cervical spine, and head (stabilizes the craniovertebral joints).
• Unilateral contraction bends the head, cervical spine, and thoracic spine to the same side and rotates them to the opposite side.

Innervation: Posterior rami of the spinal nerves

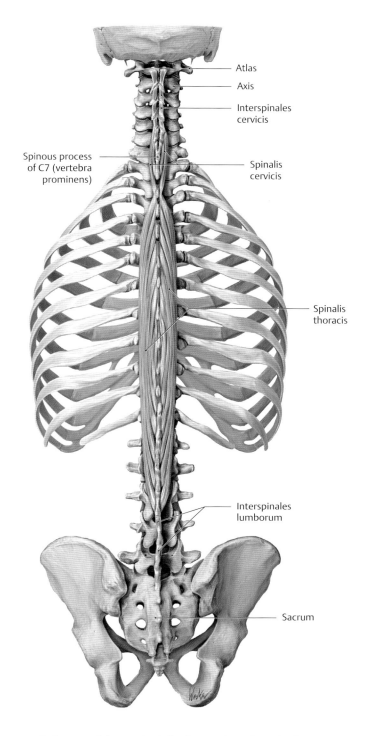

Atlas

Axis

Interspinales cervicis

Spinous process of C7 (vertebra prominens)

Spinalis cervicis

Spinalis thoracis

Interspinales lumborum

Sacrum

C Medial tract of the intrinsic back muscles: the spinal system (interspinales and spinalis muscles)

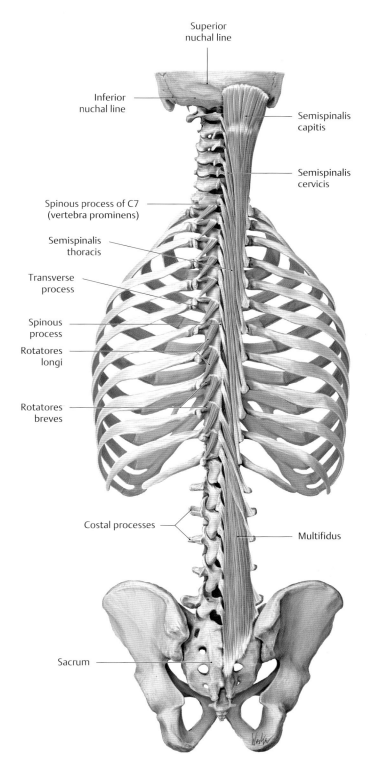

Superior nuchal line

Inferior nuchal line

Semispinalis capitis

Semispinalis cervicis

Spinous process of C7 (vertebra prominens)

Semispinalis thoracis

Transverse process

Spinous process

Rotatores longi

Rotatores breves

Costal processes

Multifidus

Sacrum

D Medial tract of the intrinsic back muscles: the transversospinal system (rotatores breves and longi, multifidus, and semispinalis muscles)

10.4 The Intrinsic Back Muscles (Short Nuchal and Craniovertebral Joint Muscles) and the Prevertebral Muscles

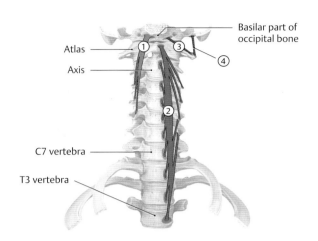

A Schematic of the short nuchal and craniovertebral joint muscles (suboccipital muscles): recti capitis posterior major and minor and obliquii capitis superior and inferior
Posterior view.

① Rectus capitis posterior major

Origin:	Spinous process of the axis
Insertion:	Middle third of the inferior nuchal line
Action:	• Bilateral: extends the head
	• Unilateral: rotates the head to the same side
Innervation:	Posterior ramus of C1 (suboccipital nerve)

② Rectus capitis posterior minor

Origin:	Posterior tubercle of the atlas
Insertion:	Inner third of the inferior nuchal line
Action:	• Bilateral: extends the head
	• Unilateral: rotates the head to the same side
Innervation:	Posterior ramus of C1 (suboccipital nerve)

③ Obliquus capitis superior

Origin:	Transverse process of the atlas
Insertion:	Above the insertion of the rectus capitis posterior major or middle third of nuchal line
Action:	• Bilateral: extends the head
	• Unilateral: tilts the head to the same side and rotates it to the opposite side
Innervation:	Posterior ramus of C1 (suboccipital nerve)

④ Obliquus capitis inferior

Origin:	Spinous process of the axis
Insertion:	Transverse process of the atlas
Action:	• Bilateral: extends the head
	• Unilateral: rotates the head to the same side
Innervation:	Posterior ramus of C1 (suboccipital nerve)

Note: The prevertebral muscles are not included among the intrinsic back muscles as they are innervated by the anterior rami of the spinal nerves.

B Schematic of the prevertebral neck muscles (colli and cervicis muscles): longi capitis and colli and recti capitis anterior and lateralis
Anterior view.

① Longus capitis

Origin:	Anterior tubercle of the transverse processes of the C3–C6 vertebrae
Insertion:	Basilar part of the occipital bone
Action:	• Unilateral: tilts and slightly rotates the head to the same side
	• Bilateral: flexes the head
Innervation:	Direct branches from the cervical plexus (C1–C3)

② Longus colli (cervicis)

Origin:	• Vertical (medial) part: anterior sides of the C5–C7 and T1–T3 vertebral bodies
	• Superior oblique part: anterior tubercle of the transverse processes of the C3–C5 vertebrae
	• Inferior oblique part: anterior sides of the T1–T3 vertebral bodies
Insertion:	• Vertical part: anterior sides of the C2–C4 vertebrae
	• Superior oblique part: anterior tubercle of the atlas
	• Inferior oblique part: anterior tubercle of the transverse processes of the C5 and C6 vertebrae
Action:	• Unilateral: tilts and rotates the cervical spine to the same side
	• Bilateral: flexes the cervical spine
Innervation:	Anterior rami of C2–C6

③ Rectus capitis anterior

Origin:	Lateral mass of the atlas
Insertion:	Basilar part of the occipital bone
Action:	• Unilateral: lateral flexion at the atlanto-occipital joint
	• Bilateral: flexion at the atlanto-occipital joint
Innervation:	Anterior ramus of the C1 nerve

④ Rectus capitis lateralis

Origin:	Transverse process of the atlas
Insertion:	Basilar part of the occipital bone (lateral to the occipital condyles)
Action:	• Unilateral: lateral flexion at the atlanto-occipital joint
	• Bilateral: flexion at the atlanto-occipital joint
Innervation:	Anterior ramus of the C1 nerve

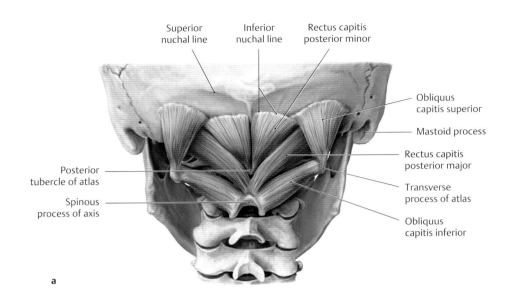

Superior nuchal line

Inferior nuchal line

Rectus capitis posterior minor

Obliquus capitis superior

Mastoid process

Rectus capitis posterior major

Transverse process of atlas

Obliquus capitis inferior

Posterior tubercle of atlas

Spinous process of axis

a

C The short nuchal and craniovertebral joint muscles: rectus capitis posterior and obliquus capitis

a Posterior view, **b** lateral view.

In a strict sense, the short nuchal muscles consist only of the muscles innervated by the posterior ramus of the first spinal nerve (suboccipital nerve). They include representatives of the lateral tract (obliquus capitis inferior) and the medial tract (obliquus capitis superior and recti capitis posterior major and minor). The anterior group of short nuchal muscles (recti capitis lateralis and anterior) is innervated by the anterior rami, placing them among the prevertebral neck muscles (see **D**).

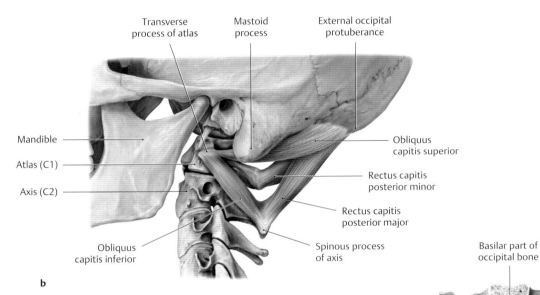

Transverse process of atlas

Mastoid process

External occipital protuberance

Mandible

Atlas (C1)

Axis (C2)

Obliquus capitis superior

Rectus capitis posterior minor

Rectus capitis posterior major

Obliquus capitis inferior

Spinous process of axis

b

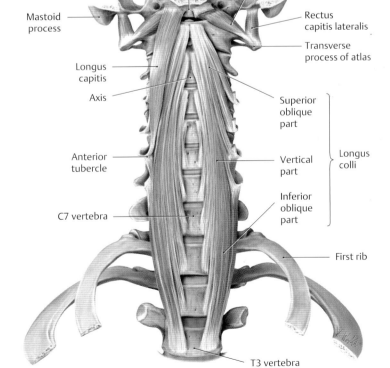

Basilar part of occipital bone

Rectus capitis anterior

Mastoid process

Rectus capitis lateralis

Transverse process of atlas

Longus capitis

Axis

Superior oblique part

Anterior tubercle

Vertical part

Longus colli

Inferior oblique part

C7 vertebra

First rib

T3 vertebra

D The prevertebral neck muscles: longi capitis and colli and recti capitis anterior and lateralis

Anterior view after removal of the cervical viscera. The longus capitis muscle has been partially removed on the left side.

10.5 The Muscles of the Abdominal Wall: Anterolateral Muscles

A Schematic of the external oblique

External oblique

Origin:	Outer surface of the fifth to twelfth ribs
Insertion:	• Outer lip of the iliac crest
	• Anterior layer of the rectus sheath, linea alba
Action:	• Unilateral: bends the trunk to the same side, rotates the trunk to the opposite side
	• Bilateral: flexes the trunk, stabilizes the pelvis, active in expiration, compresses the abdomen
Innervation:	Intercostal nerves (T5–T11), subcostal nerve (T12), iliohypogastric nerve

B Schematic of the internal oblique

Internal oblique

Origin:	Deep layer of the thoracolumbar fascia, intermediate line of the iliac crest, anterior superior iliac spine, iliopsoas fascia
Insertion:	• Lower borders of the tenth to twelfth ribs
	• Anterior and posterior layers of the rectus sheath, linea alba
Action:	• Junction with the cremaster muscle
	• Unilateral: bends the trunk to the same side, rotates the trunk to the same side
	• Bilateral: flexes the trunk, stabilizes the pelvis, active in expiration, compresses the abdomen
Innervation:	• Intercostal nerves (T8–T11), subcostal nerve (T12), iliohypogastric nerve, ilioinguinal nerve
	• Cremaster muscle (genital branch of genitofemoral nerve)

Transversus abdominis

Origin:	• Inner surfaces of the seventh to twelfth costal cartilages
	• Deep layer of the thoracolumbar fascia
	• Inner lip of the iliac crest, anterior superior iliac spine
	• Lateral part of the inguinal ligament
Insertion:	• Posterior layer of the rectus sheath, linea alba
	• Pubic crest
Action:	• Unilateral: rotates the trunk to the same side
	• Bilateral: active in expiration, compresses the abdomen
Innervation:	Intercostal nerves (T5–T11), subcostal nerve (T12), iliohypogastric nerve, ilioinguinal and genitofemoral nerves

C Schematic of the transversus abdominis

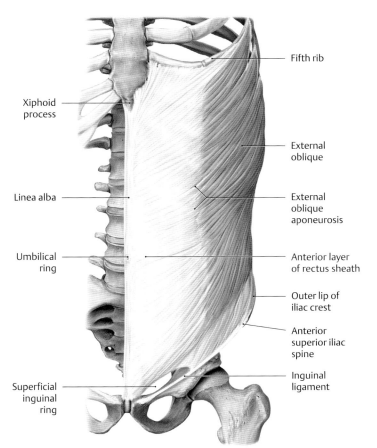

D External oblique
Left side, anterior view.

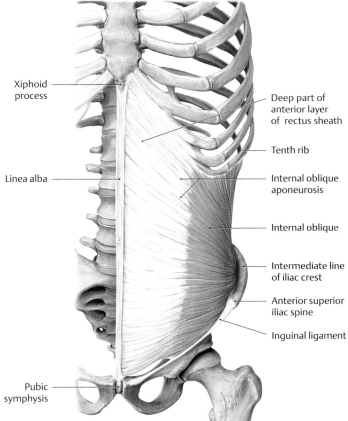

E Internal oblique
Left side, anterior view.

F Transversus abdominis
Left side, anterior view.
(For structure of the rectus sheath, see p.179.)

10.6 The Muscles of the Abdominal Wall: Anterior and Posterior Muscles

Linea alba

A Schematic of the anterior (straight, or strap) muscles of the abdominal wall: rectus abdominis and pyramidalis

① **Rectus abdominis**

Origin: Cartilages of the fifth to seventh ribs, xiphoid process of the sternum
Insertion: Pubis (between the pubic tubercle and symphysis)
Action: Flexes the lumbar spine, stabilizes the pelvis, active in expiration, compresses abdomen
Innervation: Intercostal nerves (T5–T11) and subcostal nerve (T12)

② **Pyramidalis**

Origin: Pubis (anterior to insertion of the rectus abdominis)
Insertion: Linea alba (runs within the rectus sheath)
Action: Tenses the linea alba
Innervation: Subcostal nerve (T12)

B Schematic of the posterior (deep) muscles of the abdominal wall: quadratus lumborum and psoas major

Quadratus lumborum

Origin: Iliac crest
Insertion: Twelfth rib, costal processes of the L1–L4 vertebrae
Action: • Unilateral: bends the trunk to the same side
• Bilateral: bearing down and expiration
Innervation: Subcostal nerve (T12)

Iliopsoas (① psoas major and ② iliacus)*

Origin: • Psoas major (superficial layer): lateral surfaces of the T12 vertebral body, the L1–L4 vertebral bodies, and the associated intervertebral disks
• Psoas major (deep layer): costal processes of the L1–L5 vertebrae
• Iliacus: iliac fossa
Insertion: Insert jointly as the iliopsoas muscle on the lesser trochanter of the femur
Action: • Hip joint: flexion and external rotation
• Lumbar spine: unilateral contraction (with the femur fixed) bends the trunk laterally, bilateral contraction raises the trunk from the supine position
Innervation: Direct branches from spinal nerves (L1–L4) and femoral nerve (L2–L4)

* Of these two muscles, only the psoas major belongs topographically to the posterior abdominal muscles. It is classified functionally as a hip muscle (see p. 476).

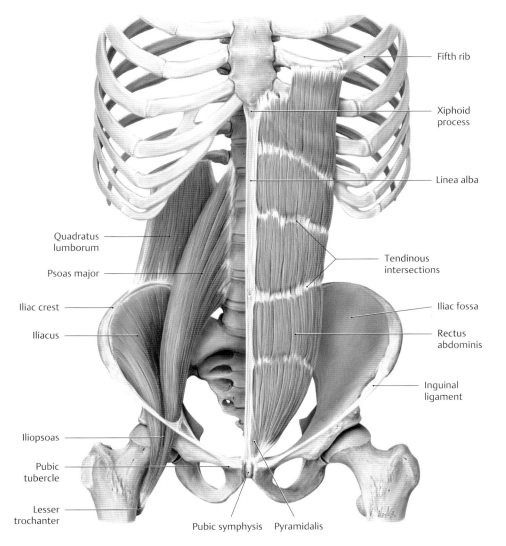

Fifth rib

Xiphoid process

Linea alba

Quadratus lumborum

Psoas major

Tendinous intersections

Iliac crest

Iliacus

Iliac fossa

Rectus abdominis

Inguinal ligament

Iliopsoas

Pubic tubercle

Lesser trochanter

Pubic symphysis   Pyramidalis

C Anterior muscles (rectus abdominis and pyramidalis) and posterior muscles (quadratus lumborum and iliopsoas) of the abdominal wall
Anterior view. The anterior abdominal wall muscles are shown on the left side and the posterior muscles on the right side.

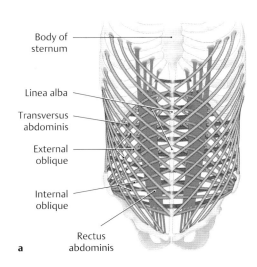

Body of sternum

Linea alba

Transversus abdominis

External oblique

Internal oblique

Rectus abdominis

a

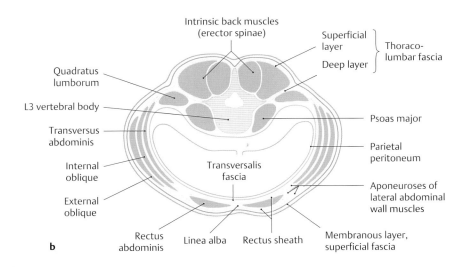

Intrinsic back muscles (erector spinae)

Superficial layer

Deep layer

Thoraco-lumbar fascia

Quadratus lumborum

L3 vertebral body

Transversus abdominis

Internal oblique

External oblique

Psoas major

Parietal peritoneum

Transversalis fascia

Aponeuroses of lateral abdominal wall muscles

Rectus abdominis

Linea alba   Rectus sheath

Membranous layer, superficial fascia

b

D Arrangement of the abdominal wall muscles and rectus sheath
a Anterior view, **b** transverse section at the level of L3.
The rectus abdominis and lateral oblique abdominal wall muscles and their aponeuroses comprise a functional unit. Fusion of the aponeuroses of the oblique muscles creates a sheath enclosing the rectus muscles that in turn meets the aponeurosis from the opposite side to form the linea alba in the abdominal midline. For the upper three fourths of the length of the rectus muscles, the aponeurosis of the internal oblique muscle splits, so portions pass both anterior and posterior to the rectus muscles. Therefore, in the upper region of the rectus, an anterior rec-

tus sheath (external oblique and a portion of the internal oblique aponeuroses) and a posterior rectus sheath (the rest of the internal oblique and transversus abdominis aponeuroses) are formed (see p. 179). Over the lower one fourth of the rectus muscles, the aponeuroses of all three abdominal muscles pass anterior to the rectus muscles. No posterior sheath is present. The inferior edge of the posterior rectus sheath is called the arcuate line.

155

10.7 The Functions of the Abdominal Wall Muscles

a

b

Functions of the Abdominal Wall Muscles
The different abdominal wall muscles perform numerous functions, which very often are carried out in concert with other muscle groups (e.g., the back and gluteal muscles and the diaphragm). The principal actions of the abdominal wall muscles are as follows:

- Maintenance of abdominal tone: tensing the abdominal wall and compressing the abdominal viscera (abdominal press)
- Stabilizing the vertebrae and reducing stresses on the spinal column
- Moving the trunk and pelvis
- Assisting in respiration

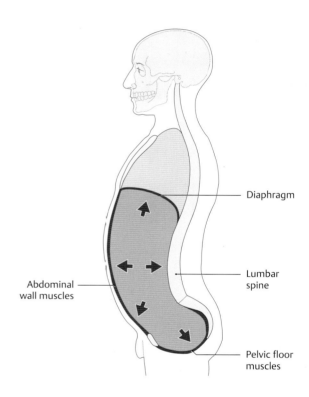

A Abdominal press = raising the intra-abdominal pressure by tensing the abdominal wall and pelvic floor muscles and the diaphragm
Schematic coronal section through the abdominal cavity, anterior view.

a The walls of the abdominal and pelvic cavity are formed by bony structures (spinal column, thoracic cage, pelvis) and also by muscles (diaphragm, muscles of the abdominal wall and pelvic floor).

b When the muscles about the abdomen contract (abdominal press), they reduce the volume of the abdominal cavity, thereby raising the intra-abdominal pressure and actively compressing the abdominal viscera. This action is important, for example, in expelling stool from the rectum (defecation), expelling urine from the bladder (micturition), and emptying the gastric contents (vomiting). The abdominal press is also an essential part of maternal pushing during the expulsive phase of labor.

B Abdominal press = stabilizing the spinal column by raising the intra-abdominal pressure
Schematic midsagittal section through the trunk, left lateral view. Simultaneous contraction of the diaphragm and the muscles of the abdominal wall and pelvic floor raises the pressure in the abdominal cavity (abdominal press). The hydrostatic effect of this maneuver stabilizes the trunk, reduces stresses on the spinal column (especially at the lumbar level), and stiffens the trunk wall like the wall of an inflated ball. This action is performed automatically during the lifting of heavy loads. The "inflatable space" of the trunk can be employed in this way to lighten the pressure load on the intervertebral disks by up to 50% in the upper lumbar spine and by approximately 30% in the lower lumbar spine. Meanwhile, the forces exerted by the intrinsic back muscles are reduced by more than 50%. This explains the importance of well-conditioned abdominal muscles in preventing and treating diseases of the spinal column.

Sternum

Rectus abdominis

External oblique

Transversus abdominis

Internal oblique

Linea alba

Pubic symphysis

C Trunk movements aided by the straight and oblique muscles of the abdominal wall

a Course and arrangement of the straight and oblique abdominal wall muscles.

b Trunk flexion to the right with simultaneous rotation of the trunk to the left side by contraction of the external oblique muscle on the right side and the internal oblique muscle on the left side.

c Trunk flexion to the right by contraction of the right lateral abdominal muscles (aided by the right intrinsic back muscles).

d Rotating the trunk to the right side is effected by the right lateral abdominal muscles and the left intrinsic back muscles.

e Flexion of the trunk is effected by bilateral contraction of the rectus abdominis, lateral abdominal and psoas muscles.

.

Psoas major

Abdominal muscles

Pelvic tilt 12°

Anterior superior iliac spine

Quadriceps femoris

Intrinsic back muscles

Posterior superior iliac spine

Gluteus maximus

Iliopsoas

Hamstrings

D Effect of the abdominal wall muscles on pelvic movements: active and passive posture

a Normal active posture, **b** active rigid posture, **c** passive slumped posture.

An imbalance between the intrinsic back muscles and abdominal muscles is particularly evident in the curvature of the lower spine and in the degree of pelvic tilt. In a normal active posture, the pelvis is tilted forward by approximately 12° (**a**). When a rigid posture is assumed ("stomach in, chest out"), the pelvis is held in a more upright position so that the anterior superior iliac spine and the posterior superior iliac spine are at the same level (**b**). The most active muscles are the abdominal wall muscles, the gluteal muscles, and the hamstrings. When the abdominal muscles are lax and are not well conditioned, the result is a passive slumped posture (**c**) with an excessive degree of anterior pelvic tilt. Also, the lordotic curvature of the lumbar spine is accentuated due to progressive shortening of the intrinsic back muscles. This posture is reinforced by the tendency of the iliopsoas muscles (psoas major and iliacus) to become shortened.

157

10.8 The Muscles of the Thoracic Cage: Scalenes, Intercostals, Subcostals, and Transversus Thoracis

A Overview of the thoracic wall muscles:
(**a**) scalenes and (**b**) intercostals
Anterior view.

B Overview of the thoracic wall muscles: transversus thoracis
Posterior view.

Scalene muscles

Origin:	① Anterior scalene: anterior tubercle of the transverse processes of the C3–C6 vertebrae
	② Middle scalene: posterior tubercle of the transverse processes of the C3–C7 vertebrae
	③ Posterior scalene: posterior tubercle of the transverse processes of the C5–C7 vertebrae
Insertion:	• Anterior scalene: anterior scalene tubercle of first rib
	• Middle scalene: first rib (posterior to the groove for the subclavian artery)
	• Posterior scalene: outer surface of the second rib
Action:	• With the ribs mobile: raises the upper ribs (in inspiration)
	• With the ribs fixed: bends the cervical spine toward the same side (with unilateral contraction) and flexes the neck (with bilateral contraction)
Innervation:	• Anterior scalene: anterior rami of C4–C6
	• Middle scalene: anterior rami of C3–C8
	• Posterior scalene: anterior rami of C6–C8

Intercostal muscles

Origin and insertion:	④ External intercostal muscles (costal tubercle to chondro-osseous junction): arise at the lower margin of a rib and insert on the upper margin of the next lower rib (course obliquely forward and downward)
	⑤ Internal intercostal muscles (costal angle to sternum): arise at the lower margin of a rib and insert on the upper margin of the next lower rib (course obliquely backward and downward)
	• Innermost intercostal muscles: division of the internal intercostals (same course and action)
Action:	• External intercostals: elevate (raise) the ribs (in inspiration), support the intercostal spaces, stabilize the chest wall
	• Internal intercostals: depress (lower) the ribs (in expiration), support the intercostal spaces, stabilize the chest wall
Innervation:	First through eleventh intercostal nerves

Transversus thoracis

Origin:	Inner surface of the sternum and xiphoid process
Insertion:	Inner surface of the costal cartilage of the second through sixth ribs
Action:	Lowers the ribs (in expiration)
Innervation:	Second through seventh intercostal nerves

Atlas

Axis

C Anterior, middle, and posterior scalenes and the internal and external intercostals

Anterior view with anterior thoracic cage partially removed. Topographically, the scalene muscles are included among the deep neck muscles, but functionally they play an important role in thoracic breathing. Subcostal muscles have the same orientation as internal intercostals but skip over one or two ribs to form continuous sheets, especially at the angle of the sixth through eleventh ribs.

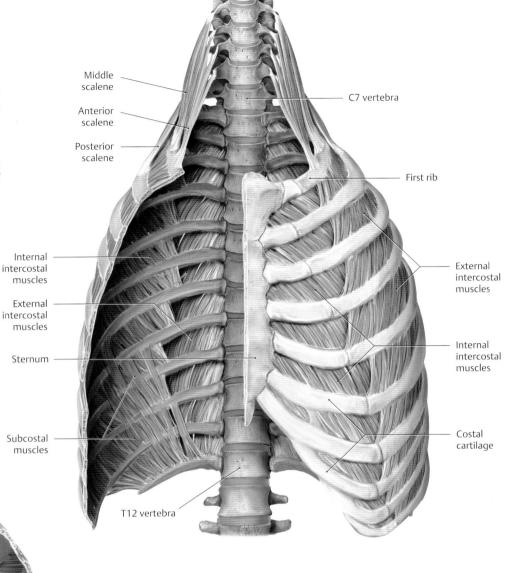

Middle scalene

Anterior scalene

Posterior scalene

C7 vertebra

First rib

Internal intercostal muscles

External intercostal muscles

External intercostal muscles

Sternum

Internal intercostal muscles

Subcostal muscles

Costal cartilage

T12 vertebra

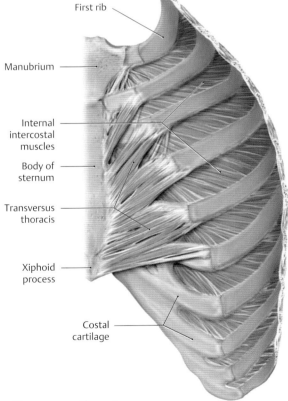

First rib

Manubrium

Internal intercostal muscles

Body of sternum

Transversus thoracis

Xiphoid process

Costal cartilage

D Transversus thoracis

Posterior surface of the anterior thoracic cage removed in **C** (right half of the transversus thoracis muscle).

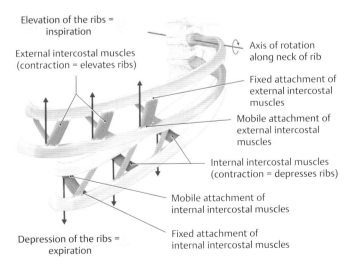

Elevation of the ribs = inspiration

External intercostal muscles (contraction = elevates ribs)

Axis of rotation along neck of rib

Fixed attachment of external intercostal muscles

Mobile attachment of external intercostal muscles

Internal intercostal muscles (contraction = depresses ribs)

Mobile attachment of internal intercostal muscles

Fixed attachment of internal intercostal muscles

Depression of the ribs = expiration

E Action of the external and internal intercostals

Note the position of the axis of motion along the neck of the rib.

10.9 The Muscles of the Thoracic Cage: The Diaphragm

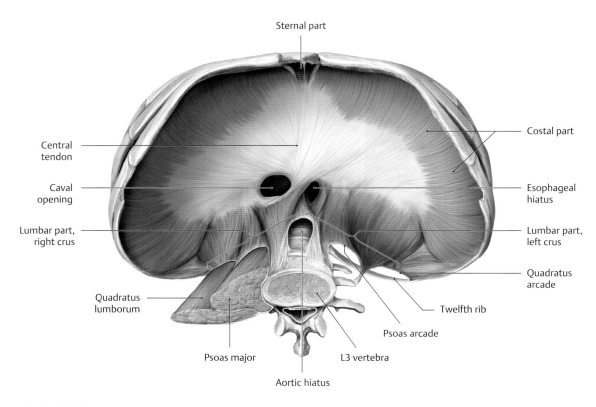

A Overview of the diaphragm

Origin:	• Costal part: lower margin of costal arch (inner surface of seventh through twelfth ribs) • Lumbar part (right and left crura): – Medial parts: L1–L3 vertebral bodies, second and third intervertebral disks, anterior longitudinal ligament – Lateral parts: first tendinous arch of the abdominal aorta (median arcuate ligament) at L1 associated with its anterior surface; second tendinous arch of the psoas arcade (medial arcuate ligament) from L2 vertebral body to associated costal process; third tendinous arch of the quadratus lumborum arcade (lateral arcuate ligament) from the costal process of L2 to the tip of rib 12 • Sternal part: posterior surface of the xiphoid process
Insertion:	Central tendon
Action:	Principal muscle of respiration (diaphragmatic and thoracic breathing), aids in compressing the abdominal viscera (abdominal press)
Innervation:	Phrenic nerve from the cervical plexus (C3–C5)

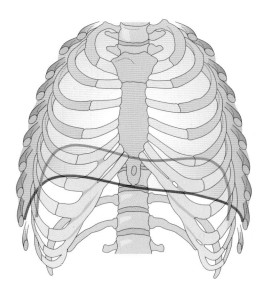

B Position of the diaphragm and ribs at full inspiration and expiration

Thoracic cage, anterior view.

Note the different positions of the diaphragm at full inspiration (red) and full expiration (blue). During a physical examination, the posterior lung boundaries can be identified by percussion (tapping the body surface). The respiratory movement of the diaphragm from end-expiration to end-inspiration should be determined; it is approximately 4 to 6 cm (see p. 174f).

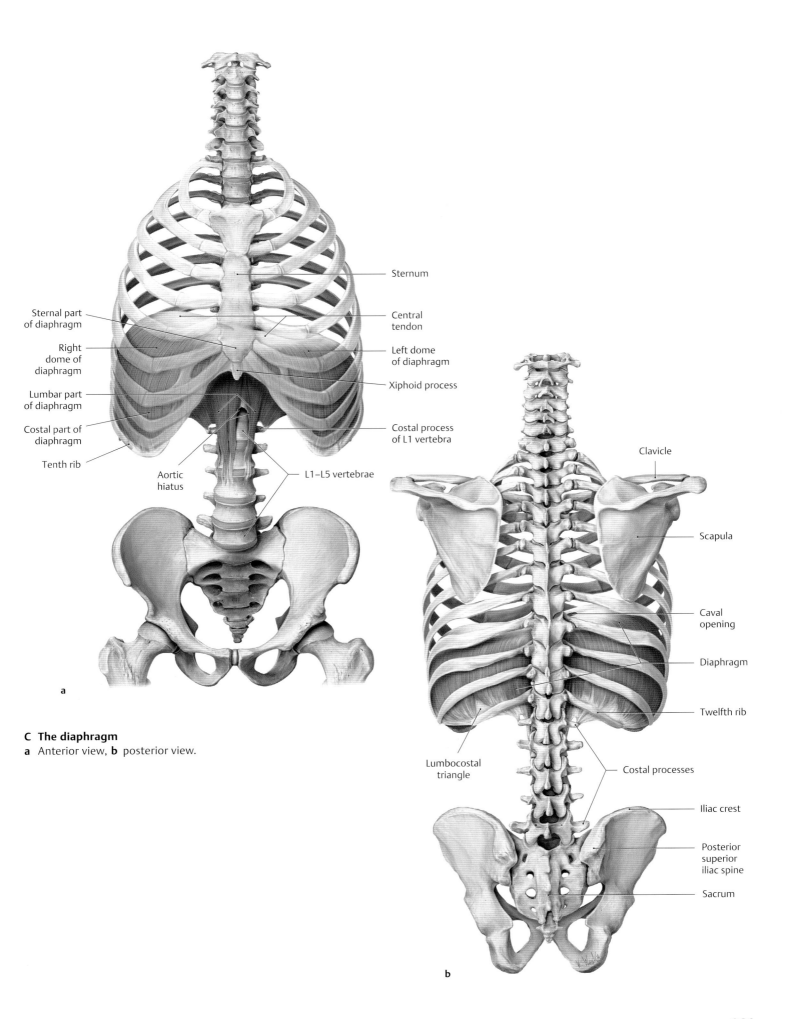

Sternum

Sternal part
of diaphragm

Central
tendon

Right
dome
of
diaphragm

Left dome
of diaphragm

Lumbar part
of diaphragm

Xiphoid process

Costal part of
diaphragm

Costal process
of L1 vertebra

Tenth rib

Aortic
hiatus

L1–L5 vertebrae

a

Clavicle

Scapula

Caval
opening

Diaphragm

Twelfth rib

Lumbocostal
triangle

Costal processes

Iliac crest

Posterior
superior
iliac spine

Sacrum

b

C The diaphragm
a Anterior view, **b** posterior view.

161

10.10 The Muscles of the Pelvic Floor and Perineum: Pelvic Diaphragm and Deep and Superficial Perineal Muscles

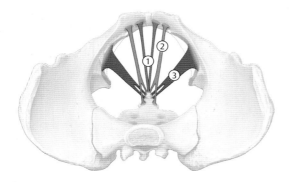

A Schematic of the pelvic diaphragm: the levator ani (puborectalis, pubococcygeus, and iliococcygeus) and coccygeus (not shown)
Superior view.

B Schematic of the deep and superficial transverse perineal
Inferior view.

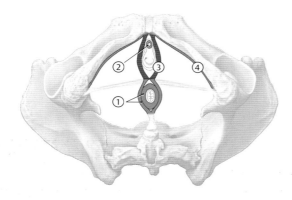

C Schematic of the external anal sphincter, external urethral sphincter, bulbospongiosus, and ischiocavernosus
Inferior view.

③ **Bulbospongiosus**

Runs anteriorly from the perineal body to the clitoris in females or to the penile raphe in males

Action:	Narrows the vaginal introitus in females, surrounds the corpus spongiosum in males
Innervation:	Pudendal nerve (S2–S4)

Levator ani

① **Puborectalis**

Origin:	Superior pubic ramus on both sides of the pubic symphysis
Insertion:	Loop-shaped around the anorectal junction, interwoven with the deep part of the external anal sphincter
Innervation:	Pudendal nerve and direct branches of sacral plexus (S2–S4)

② **Pubococcygeus**

Origin:	Pubis (lateral at origin of the puborectalis)
Insertion:	Anococcygeal ligament, coccyx
Innervation:	Pudendal nerve (S2–S4)

③ **Iliococcygeus**

Origin:	Tendinous arch of the internal obturator fascia (of the levator ani)
Insertion:	Levator (iliococcygeal) raphe, anococcygeal ligament, coccyx
Innervation:	Pudendal nerve (S2–S4)
Function of the pelvic diaphragm:	Holds the pelvic organs in place

Coccygeus (not shown)

Origin:	Inferior end of sacrum
Insertion:	Ischial spine
Innervation:	Direct branches of sacral plexus (S4, S5)
Function:	Holds pelvic organs in place, flexes the coccyx

① **Deep transverse perineal** (in males; smooth muscle, in females–see note p. 163)

Origin:	Inferior pubic ramus, ischial ramus
Insertion:	Wall of vagina or prostate, urethra
Innervation:	Pudendal nerve (S2–S4)

② **Superficial transverse perineal**

Origin:	Ischial ramus
Insertion:	Perineal body
Innervation:	Pudendal nerve (S2–S4)
Function of the transverse perineal muscles:	Holds the pelvic organs in place, closes the urethra

① **External anal sphincter**

The external anal sphincter is a circular muscle that closes the orifice around the anal canal, extends from the perineal body to the anococcygeal ligament, and is divided into subcutaneous, superficial, and deep parts.

Action:	Closes the anus
Innervation:	Pudendal nerve (S2–S4)

② **External urethral sphincter**

Division of the deep transverse perineal (encircles the urethra)

Action:	Closes the urethra
Innervation:	Pudendal nerve (S2–S4)

④ **Ischiocavernosus**

Origin:	Ischial ramus
Insertion:	Crus of penis or clitoris
Action:	Compresses the crura of the clitoris or penis; helps to promote and maintain erection
Innervation:	Pudendal nerve (S2–S4)

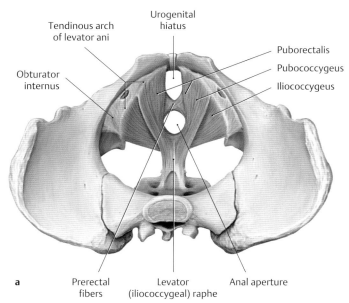

a — Tendinous arch of levator ani, Urogenital hiatus, Puborectalis, Pubococcygeus, Iliococcygeus (Levator ani), Obturator internus, Prerectal fibers, Levator (iliococcygeal) raphe, Anal aperture

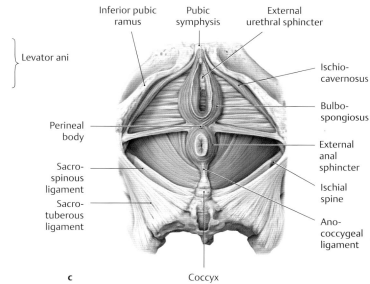

c — Inferior pubic ramus, Pubic symphysis, External urethral sphincter, Perineal body, Ischio-cavernosus, Bulbo-spongiosus, Sacro-spinous ligament, External anal sphincter, Sacro-tuberous ligament, Ischial spine, Ano-coccygeal ligament, Coccyx

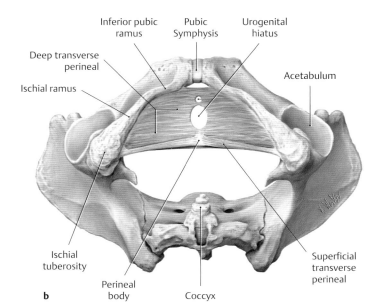

b — Inferior pubic ramus, Pubic Symphysis, Urogenital hiatus, Deep transverse perineal, Acetabulum, Ischial ramus, Ischial tuberosity, Perineal body, Coccyx, Superficial transverse perineal

D The muscles of the female pelvic floor
a Pelvic diaphragm, superior view.
b Transverse perineal muscles, inferior view.
c Sphincter and erectile muscles, inferior view.

Note: The existence of the deep transverse perineal muscle in the female has been called into question. This is because the deep transverse perineal becomes heavily permeated by connective tissue with aging and especially after vaginal deliveries. In older women, the deep perineal space (see p. 183) basically contains connective tissue that completely occupies the urogenital hiatus at the openings of the urethra and vagina (see p. 188). We have noted this replacement by smooth muscle in each illustration of the female pelvis.

Important Functions of the Pelvic Floor Muscles
The pelvic floor performs a dual function:

- It supports the abdominal and pelvic organs by closing the abdominal and pelvic cavities inferiorly, bearing the bulk of the visceral load.
- It controls the openings of the rectum and urogenital passages (sphincter functions), which mechanically weaken the pelvic floor by piercing it.

To accomplish these inherently conflicting functions (sealing off the pelvic cavity while maintaining several apertures), the pelvic floor is lined by overlapping sheets of funnel-shaped muscle and connective tissue. This complex structure, however, also makes the pelvic floor highly susceptible to damage, especially in women.

Repetitive, extreme fluctuations in intra-abdominal pressure and other stresses, particularly at the end of pregnancy, can weaken the connective tissue apparatus and damage the pelvic floor muscles. Stretching and other injuries of the pelvic floor or the nerves supplying it, as during labor and delivery (in multiparous women), can eventually lead to pelvic floor insufficiency and its various clinical sequelae:

- Descent of the pelvic floor and thus the pelvic organs (e.g., *uterine descent*)
- In extreme cases, prolapse of the uterus with eversion of the vagina (*uterine prolapse*)

Visceral descent is generally associated with urinary or fecal incontinence in response to coughing or other acts (*stress incontinence*). Mild degrees of descent often respond well to regular pelvic floor exercises, but more serious cases may require surgical treatment with *pelvic floor repair* (surgical exposure and approximation of the two levator crura = puborectalis muscle) (e.g., approximating the levator muscles by tightening the puborectales) or surgically attaching the pelvic organs (e.g., colpopexy or rectopexy) to the pelvic wall or sacrum.

10.11 Secondarily Incorporated Trunk Muscles: Spinocostal, Spinohumeral, and Thoracohumeral

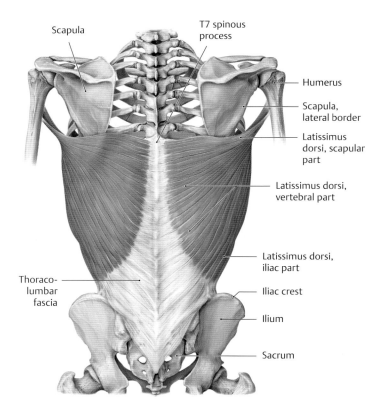

B Latissimus dorsi
Posterior view.

A Overview of spinocostal muscles

Due to their position above the thoracolumbar fascia and their innervation by the anterior rami of the spinal nerves, the two posterior serratus muscles are counted among the secondarily incorporated trunk muscles. These muscles, which are mostly very thin and often markedly segmented, act as auxiliary inspiratory muscles of respiration (see below).

Serratus posterior superior	
Origin:	Nuchal and supraspinous ligaments, spinal processes of C7–T3 vertebrae
Insertion:	Second through fifth ribs lateral to costal angle
Function:	Lifts the ribs, thus supporting inspiration
Innervation:	Intercostal nerves (T2–T5)

Serratus posterior inferior	
Origin:	Spinal processes of the T11–L2 vertebrae and the thoracolumbar fascia
Insertion:	Toward the lower margin of the ninth through twelfth ribs
Function:	Also aids inspiration; by drawing the lower ribs backward and downward, it assists in preventing further narrowing of the thoracic aperture, thus providing a fixed stable base of the diaphragm
Innervation:	Intercostal nerves (T9–T11), subcostal nerve (T12)

C List of secondarily incorporated trunk muscles

(with the exception of the serratus muscles, which are on p. 298 in the Upper Limb unit). All of the intrinsic back muscles are covered by large muscles, which in part extend all the way to the pelvis. In the course of phylogenesis, they have extended their origin to the trunk (incorporated trunk muscles, compare p. 145). These muscles initially migrated from the back as hypaxial muscles (innervation: anterior rami) toward the upper limb (thus shoulder girdle muscles) in order to later relocate again to the back. This probably happened as part of the development of tetrapods, when the pectoral girdle muscles grew and had to carry more weight. A distinction is made between:

Spinocostal or trunk rib muscles
(between spinal column and ribs)

- Serratus posterior superior
- Serratus posterior inferior

Spinohumeral or muscles of the trunk and shoulder girdle or trunk and arm (between spinal column and shoulder girdle or upper arm)

- Muscles of the trunk and shoulder girdle
  - Rhomboid major and rhomboid minor
  - Levator scapulae
  - Serratus anterior
  - Subclavius
  - Pectoralis minor
  - Trapezius

- Muscles of the trunk and arm
  - Latissimus dorsi

- Muscles of the thorax and arm
  - Pectoralis major

Note: All incorporated muscles are innervated by anterior rami of the spinal nerves.

D Trapezius
Posterior view.

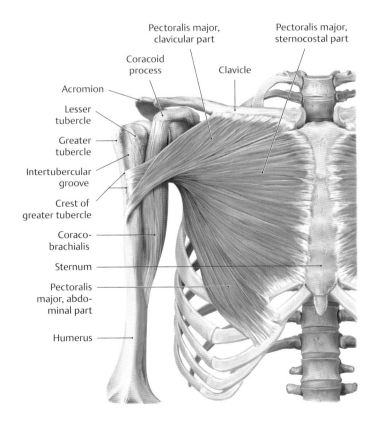

E Pectoralis major and coracobrachialis
Right side, anterior view.

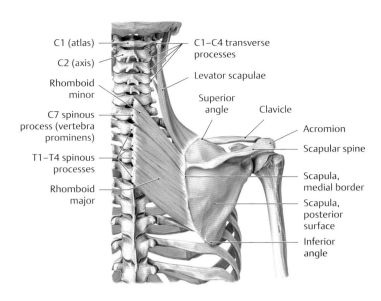

F Levator scapulae, rhomboid major, and rhomboid minor
Right side, posterior view.

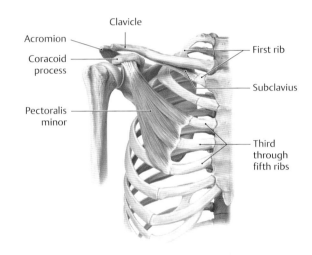

G Pectoralis minor and subclavius
Right side, anterior view.

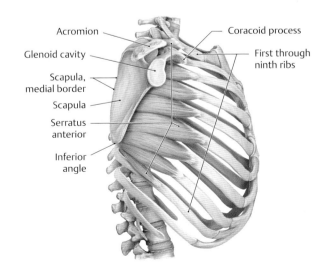

H Serratus anterior
Right side, lateral view.

11.1 The Back Muscles and Thoracolumbar Fascia

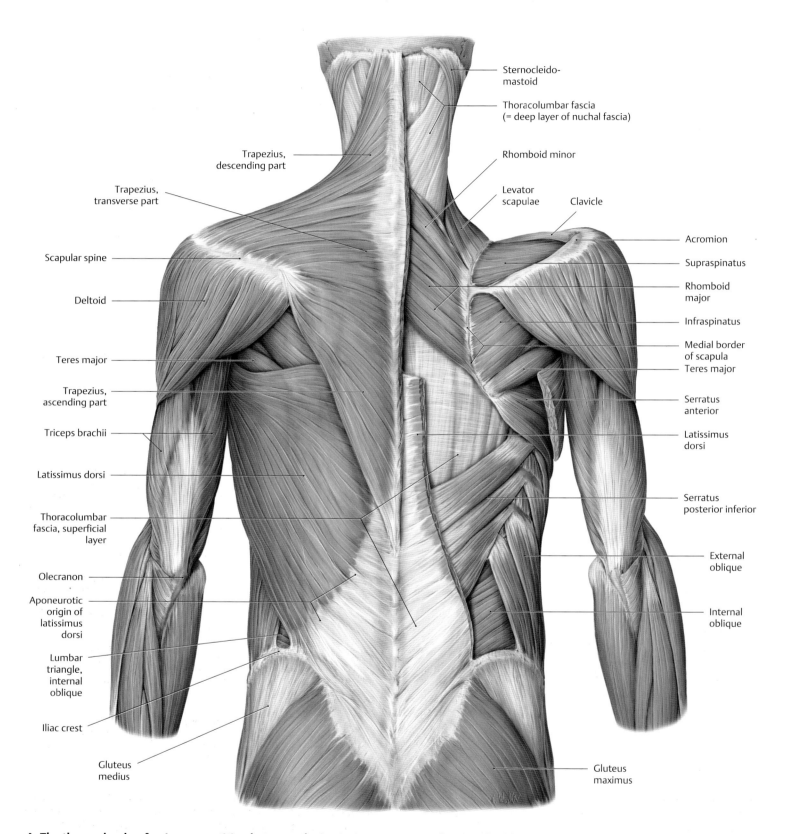

Sternocleido-mastoid

Thoracolumbar fascia (= deep layer of nuchal fascia)

Rhomboid minor

Levator scapulae

Clavicle

Acromion

Supraspinatus

Rhomboid major

Infraspinatus

Medial border of scapula

Teres major

Serratus anterior

Latissimus dorsi

Serratus posterior inferior

External oblique

Internal oblique

Gluteus maximus

Trapezius, descending part

Trapezius, transverse part

Scapular spine

Deltoid

Teres major

Trapezius, ascending part

Triceps brachii

Latissimus dorsi

Thoracolumbar fascia, superficial layer

Olecranon

Aponeurotic origin of latissimus dorsi

Lumbar triangle, internal oblique

Iliac crest

Gluteus medius

A The thoracolumbar fascia as a partition between the intrinsic and nonintrinsic back muscles

The trapezius muscle has been completely removed and the latissimus dorsi has been partially removed on the right side to reveal the thoracolumbar fascia. The superficial layer of the thoracolumbar fascia separates the intrinsic back muscles from the nonintrinsic muscles that have migrated to the back.

Note: The superficial layer of the thoracolumbar fascia is located close to the spinal column just beneath the skin, where it is heavily reinforced and serves as the origin for the extensive tendon of the latissimus dorsi. Lateral to the origin, the superficial layer is pushed beneath both the tendon and the muscle, thereby losing direct contact to the subcutaneous tissue. Along its entire width, medial to lateral, the superficial layer covers the intrinsic back muscles.

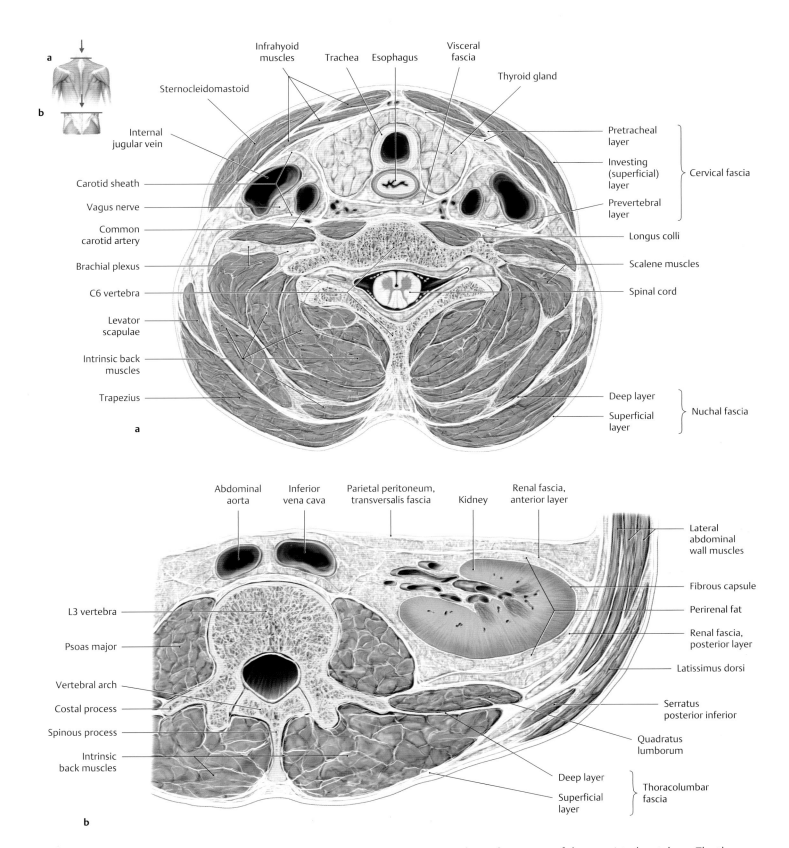

B Thoracolumbar fascia

a Transverse section through the neck at the level of the C6 vertebra, superior view.

b Transverse section through the posterior trunk wall at the level of the L3 vertebra (cauda equina removed), superior view.

The thoracolumbar fascia forms the lateral portion of an osseofibrous canal that encloses all of the *intrinsic back muscles*. In addition to the thoracolumbar fascia, this canal is formed by the vertebral arches and the spinous and costal processes of the associated vertebrae. The thoracolumbar fascia consists of a superficial and a deep layer, especially in the lumbar region; both layers unite at the lateral margin of the intrinsic back muscles. At the back of the neck, the superficial layer of the thoracolumbar fascia blends with the nuchal fascia (deep layer), becoming continuous with the prevertebral layer of the cervical fascia.

11.2 The Intrinsic Back Muscles: Lateral and Medial Tracts

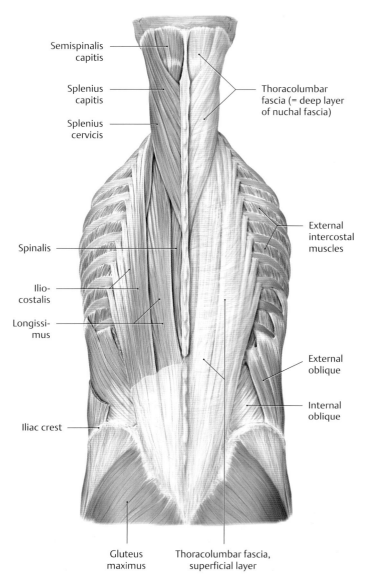

A Course of the thoracolumbar fascia
Posterior view. To reveal the thoracolumbar fascia, both shoulder girdles and the extrinsic back muscles have been removed (except for the serratus posterior superior and inferior and the aponeurotic origin of the latissimus dorsi on the right side).

B Lateral tract of the intrinsic back muscles
Posterior view. Portions of the superficial layer of the thoracolumbar fascia have been removed on the left side of the back to expose the lateral tract muscles (iliocostalis, longissimus, and splenius muscles). The levatores costarum and intertransversarii muscles, also part of the lateral tract, are covered here by the iliocostalis and longissimus muscles (see **C** and **D**).

Note that the thoracolumbar fascia on the back of the neck is continuous with the deep layer of the nuchal fascia.

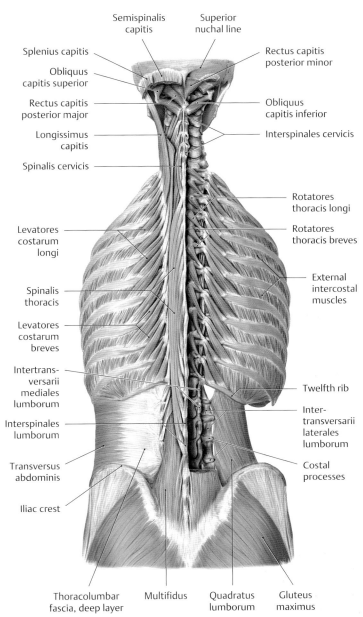

C Medial tract of the intrinsic back muscles (portions of the lateral tract left in place)

Posterior view. The longissimus (except for longissimus capitis) and splenius muscles have been removed on the left side of the back, and the iliocostalis muscles have been removed on the right side (see **D** for the rotatores muscles).

Note the deep layer of the thoracolumbar fascia from which both the internal oblique and the transversus abdominis muscles originate (see **D**).

D Medial tract of the intrinsic back muscles (with the entire lateral tract removed)

Posterior view. The entire lateral tract (except for the intertransversarii and levatores costarum) has been removed, along with portions of the medial tract, to demonstrate the various individual muscles of the medial tract.

Note the origin of the transversus abdominis from the deep layer of the thoracolumbar fascia in the lumbar region (left side).

On the right side, the deep fascial layer and multifidus muscle have been removed to display the intertransversarii (lateral tract) and the quadratus lumborum (posterior [deep] abdominal muscle).

169

11.3 The Intrinsic Back Muscles: Short Nuchal Muscles

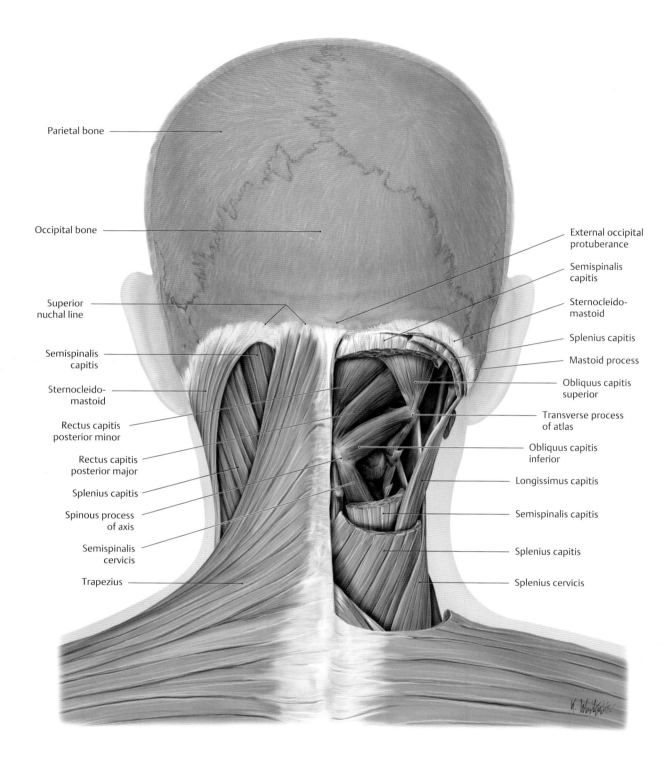

A Location of the short nuchal muscles (suboccipital muscles)
Nuchal region, posterior view. The suboccipital muscles in the strict sense are the short (deep) nuchal muscles that belong to the intrinsic back muscles (recti capitis posterior major and minor and obliquii capitis superior and inferior). They meet the criterion of being innervated by a posterior ramus—in this case the C1 posterior ramus, the suboccipital nerve. The *recti capitis anterior* and *lateralis* are *not* classified as intrinsic back muscles, despite their suboccipital location, because they are innervated by anterior rami. The short nuchal

muscles lie within the thoracolumbar fascia deep at the back of the neck and course between the occiput and the first two cervical vertebrae. They act mainly on the craniovertebral joints (see p. 120) and support differentiated head movements (e.g., for fine adjustments of head position). The following muscles have been partially removed to reveal their location in the right nuchal region: trapezius, sternocleidomastoid, splenius capitis, and semispinalis capitis. An important landmark in the deep nuchal region is the spinous process of the axis.

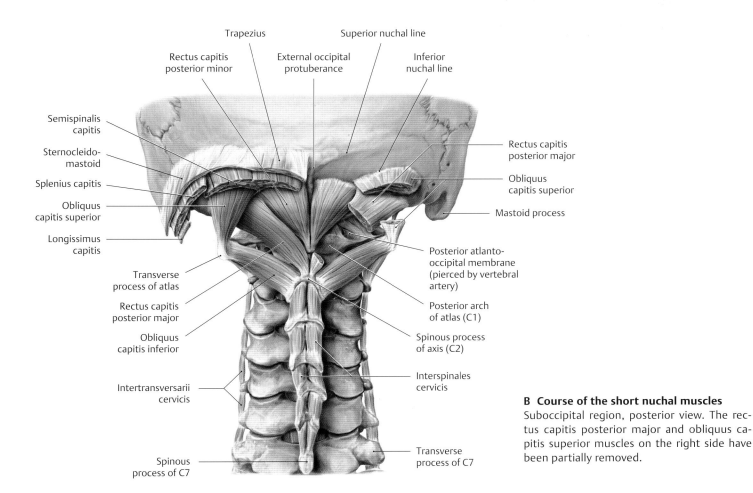

Trapezius

Rectus capitis posterior minor

External occipital protuberance

Superior nuchal line

Inferior nuchal line

Semispinalis capitis

Sternocleido-mastoid

Splenius capitis

Obliquus capitis superior

Longissimus capitis

Transverse process of atlas

Rectus capitis posterior major

Obliquus capitis inferior

Intertransversarii cervicis

Spinous process of C7

Rectus capitis posterior major

Obliquus capitis superior

Mastoid process

Posterior atlanto-occipital membrane (pierced by vertebral artery)

Posterior arch of atlas (C1)

Spinous process of axis (C2)

Interspinales cervicis

Transverse process of C7

B Course of the short nuchal muscles
Suboccipital region, posterior view. The rectus capitis posterior major and obliquus capitis superior muscles on the right side have been partially removed.

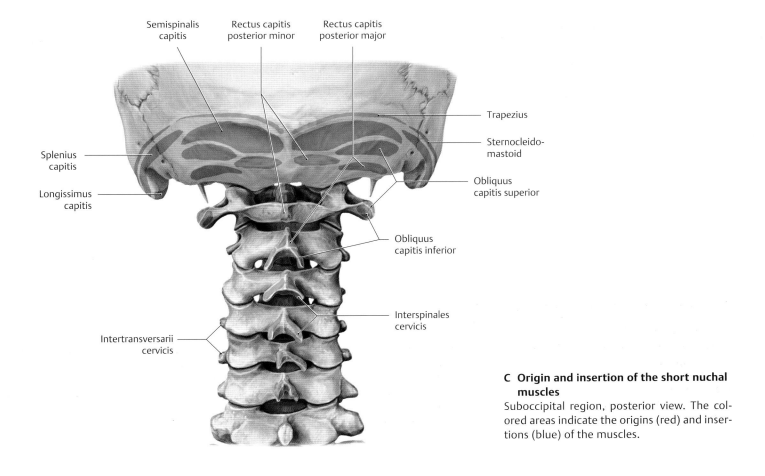

Semispinalis capitis

Rectus capitis posterior minor

Rectus capitis posterior major

Splenius capitis

Longissimus capitis

Intertransversarii cervicis

Trapezius

Sternocleido-mastoid

Obliquus capitis superior

Obliquus capitis inferior

Interspinales cervicis

C Origin and insertion of the short nuchal muscles
Suboccipital region, posterior view. The colored areas indicate the origins (red) and insertions (blue) of the muscles.

171

11.4 The Thoracic Wall Muscles and Endothoracic Fascia

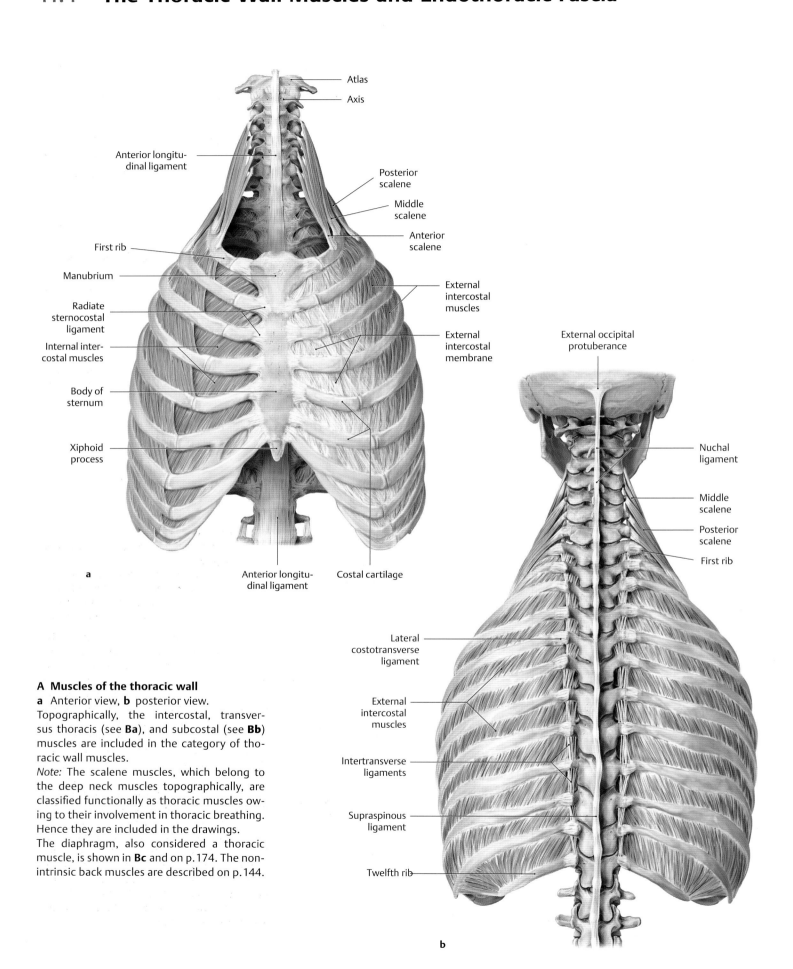

A Muscles of the thoracic wall
a Anterior view, **b** posterior view.
Topographically, the intercostal, transversus thoracis (see **Ba**), and subcostal (see **Bb**) muscles are included in the category of thoracic wall muscles.
Note: The scalene muscles, which belong to the deep neck muscles topographically, are classified functionally as thoracic muscles owing to their involvement in thoracic breathing. Hence they are included in the drawings.
The diaphragm, also considered a thoracic muscle, is shown in **Bc** and on p.174. The non-intrinsic back muscles are described on p.144.

Labels for figure **a**:
Atlas
Axis
Anterior longitudinal ligament
Posterior scalene
Middle scalene
Anterior scalene
First rib
Manubrium
Radiate sternocostal ligament
Internal intercostal muscles
External intercostal muscles
External intercostal membrane
Body of sternum
Xiphoid process
Anterior longitudinal ligament
Costal cartilage

Labels for figure **b**:
External occipital protuberance
Nuchal ligament
Middle scalene
Posterior scalene
First rib
Lateral costotransverse ligament
External intercostal muscles
Intertransverse ligaments
Supraspinous ligament
Twelfth rib

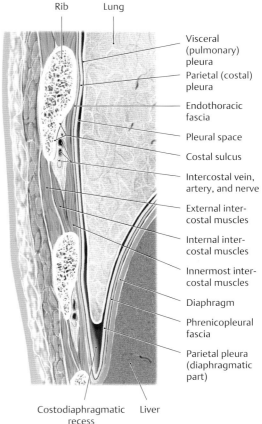

B Endothoracic fascia

a Posterior surface of the anterior thoracic wall segment removed in **b**.

b Posterior thoracic wall, anterior view (endothoracic fascia removed on the left side).

c Coronal section through the lateral thoracic wall and costodiaphragmatic recess.

The thoracic cavity is lined by a fascia-like layer of connective tissue, the *endothoracic fascia.* It lies between the deep muscles of the thoracic wall and the costal portion of the parietal pleura, to which it is firmly attached, and is analogous to the transversalis fascia of the abdominal cavity (**a**). The endothoracic fascia is thickened over the pleural apex to form the *suprapleural membrane (Sibson's fascia).* The *phrenicopleural fascia* is the portion of the endothoracic fascia that connects the diaphragmatic part of the parietal pleura to the upper surface of the diaphragm (**b**). The costodiaphragmatic recess (**c**) between the chest wall and diaphragm is a potential space that enlarges on inspiration (during lowering of the diaphragm) to accommodate the expanding lung. The pleural space is the potential space located between the parietal/costal pleura and the visceral pleura, which directly invests the lung tissue.

173

11.5 The Thoracoabdominal Junction: The Diaphragm

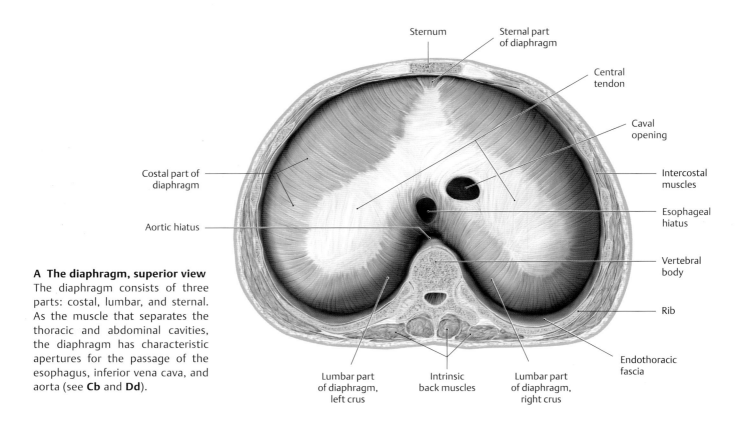

A The diaphragm, superior view
The diaphragm consists of three parts: costal, lumbar, and sternal. As the muscle that separates the thoracic and abdominal cavities, the diaphragm has characteristic apertures for the passage of the esophagus, inferior vena cava, and aorta (see **Cb** and **Dd**).

Labels (clockwise from top): Sternum · Sternal part of diaphragm · Central tendon · Caval opening · Intercostal muscles · Esophageal hiatus · Vertebral body · Rib · Endothoracic fascia · Lumbar part of diaphragm, right crus · Intrinsic back muscles · Lumbar part of diaphragm, left crus · Aortic hiatus · Costal part of diaphragm

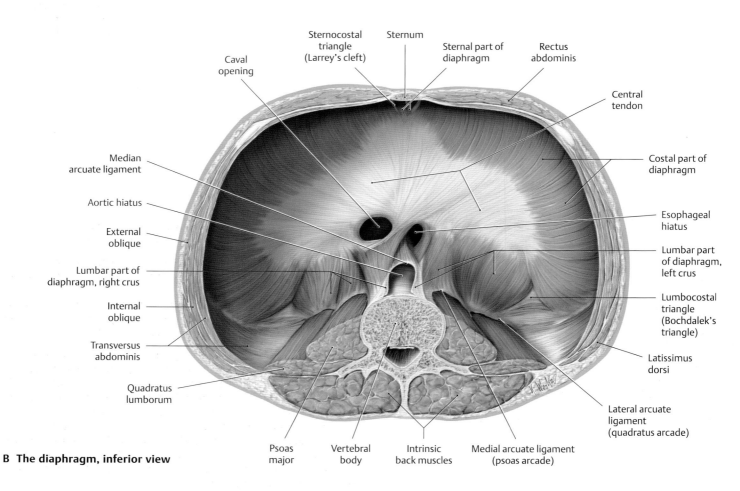

B The diaphragm, inferior view

Labels: Caval opening · Sternocostal triangle (Larrey's cleft) · Sternum · Sternal part of diaphragm · Rectus abdominis · Central tendon · Costal part of diaphragm · Esophageal hiatus · Lumbar part of diaphragm, left crus · Lumbocostal triangle (Bochdalek's triangle) · Latissimus dorsi · Lateral arcuate ligament (quadratus arcade) · Medial arcuate ligament (psoas arcade) · Intrinsic back muscles · Vertebral body · Psoas major · Quadratus lumborum · Transversus abdominis · Internal oblique · Lumbar part of diaphragm, right crus · External oblique · Aortic hiatus · Median arcuate ligament

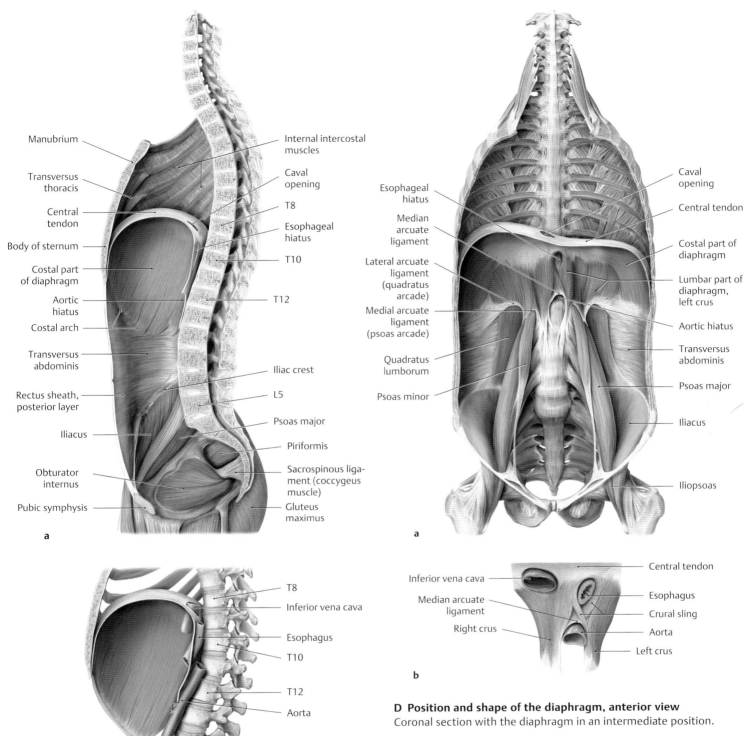

a

Manubrium

Transversus thoracis

Central tendon

Body of sternum

Costal part of diaphragm

Aortic hiatus

Costal arch

Transversus abdominis

Rectus sheath, posterior layer

Iliacus

Obturator internus

Pubic symphysis

Internal intercostal muscles

Caval opening

T 8

Esophageal hiatus

T 10

T 12

Iliac crest

L 5

Psoas major

Piriformis

Sacrospinous ligament (coccygeus muscle)

Gluteus maximus

b

T 8

Inferior vena cava

Esophagus

T 10

T 12

Aorta

Esophageal hiatus

Median arcuate ligament

Lateral arcuate ligament (quadratus arcade)

Medial arcuate ligament (psoas arcade)

Quadratus lumborum

Psoas minor

Caval opening

Central tendon

Costal part of diaphragm

Lumbar part of diaphragm, left crus

Aortic hiatus

Transversus abdominis

Psoas major

Iliacus

Iliopsoas

a

Inferior vena cava

Median arcuate ligament

Right crus

Central tendon

Esophagus

Crural sling

Aorta

Left crus

b

C Position and shape of the diaphragm, viewed from the left side
Midsagittal section demonstrating the right half of the body. The diaphragm is in an intermediate position at end-expiration.

a The apertures in the diaphragm are depicted at vertical positions corresponding to the following landmarks in the lower thoracic spine: caval opening = T 8 vertebral body, esophageal hiatus = T 10 vertebral body, aortic hiatus = T 12 vertebral body.

b The diaphragmatic apertures and the structures that they transmit (see p. 205).

D Position and shape of the diaphragm, anterior view
Coronal section with the diaphragm in an intermediate position.

a The apertures are located in the region of the central tendon (inferior vena cava) and in the lumbar part of the diaphragm (esophageal and aortic hiatus).

b Enlarged view of the diaphragmatic apertures, with vessels transected. The caval opening is located to the right of the midline, the esophageal and aortic hiatus to the left.

In a diaphragmatic hernia (diaphragmatic rupture), abdominal viscera prolapse into the chest cavity through a congenital or acquired area of weakness in the diaphragm. By far the most common herniation site is the esophageal hiatus, accounting for 90% of cases. Typically, the distal end of the esophagus and the gastric cardia (gastric inlet) "slide" upward through the esophageal hiatus into the chest (axial hiatal hernia or sliding hernia; approximately 85% of all hiatal hernias). Typical symptoms are acid reflux, heartburn, and a feeling of retrosternal pressure after meals. More severe cases may present with nausea, vomiting, and functional cardiac complaints.

175

11.6 The Anterolateral and Anterior Abdominal Wall Muscles*

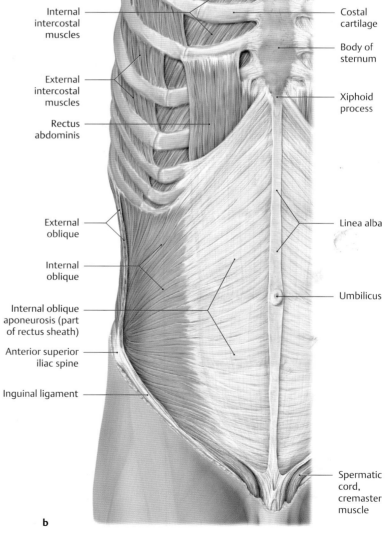

* The posterior (deep) abdominal wall muscles, most notably the psoas major, are actually hip muscles in a functional sense because they act predominantly on the hip joint. For this reason they are described in the Lower Limb unit (see p. 476).

a

b

A Anterolateral abdominal wall muscles in the male

Right side, anterior view. The oblique muscles of the abdominal wall consist of the external and internal oblique and the transversus abdominis.

a The external oblique aponeurosis borders the superficial inguinal ring, its inferior margin forming the inguinal ligament.

b The external oblique, pectoralis major, and serratus anterior muscles have been removed. The inferior border of the internal oblique forms the roof of the inguinal canal (see p. 211) and is continued onto the spermatic cord in the male as the cremaster muscle and cremasteric fascia.

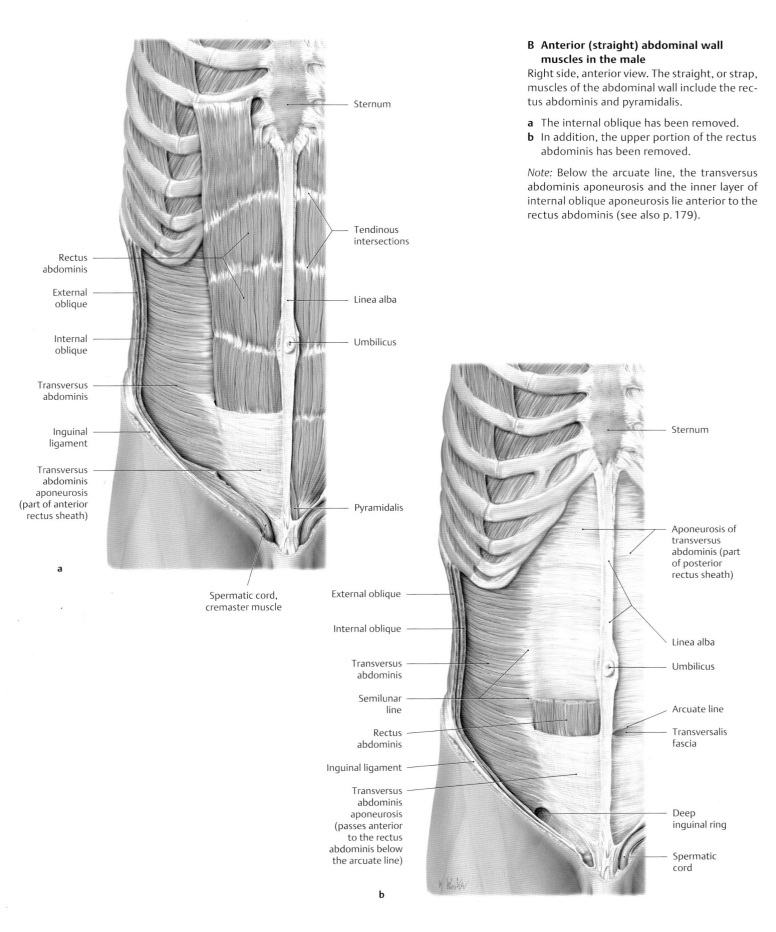

Sternum

Tendinous
intersections

Rectus
abdominis

External
oblique

Linea alba

Internal
oblique

Umbilicus

Transversus
abdominis

Inguinal
ligament

Transversus
abdominis
aponeurosis
(part of anterior
rectus sheath)

Pyramidalis

a

Spermatic cord,
cremaster muscle

**B Anterior (straight) abdominal wall
muscles in the male**

Right side, anterior view. The straight, or strap,
muscles of the abdominal wall include the rectus abdominis and pyramidalis.

a The internal oblique has been removed.
b In addition, the upper portion of the rectus
abdominis has been removed.

Note: Below the arcuate line, the transversus
abdominis aponeurosis and the inner layer of
internal oblique aponeurosis lie anterior to the
rectus abdominis (see also p. 179).

Sternum

Aponeurosis of
transversus
abdominis (part
of posterior
rectus sheath)

Linea alba

External oblique

Internal oblique

Umbilicus

Transversus
abdominis

Semilunar
line

Arcuate line

Transversalis
fascia

Rectus
abdominis

Inguinal ligament

Transversus
abdominis
aponeurosis
(passes anterior
to the rectus
abdominis below
the arcuate line)

Deep
inguinal ring

Spermatic
cord

b

177

11.7 Structure of the Abdominal Wall and Rectus Sheath

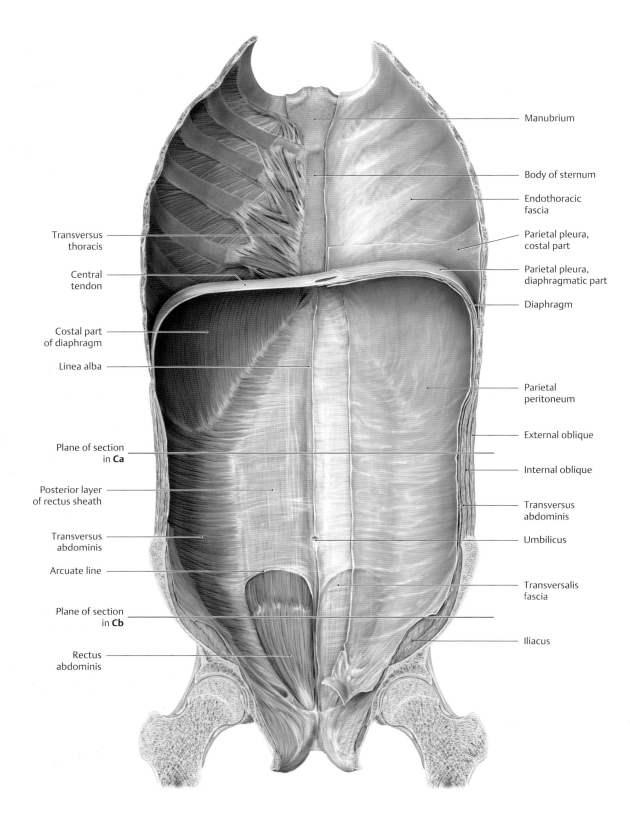

Manubrium

Body of sternum

Endothoracic fascia

Parietal pleura, costal part

Parietal pleura, diaphragmatic part

Diaphragm

Parietal peritoneum

External oblique

Internal oblique

Transversus abdominis

Umbilicus

Transversalis fascia

Iliacus

Transversus thoracis

Central tendon

Costal part of diaphragm

Linea alba

Plane of section in **Ca**

Posterior layer of rectus sheath

Transversus abdominis

Arcuate line

Plane of section in **Cb**

Rectus abdominis

A Overview of the abdominal wall and rectus sheath
Posterior view with the viscera removed. To show how the diaphragm separates the thoracic cavity from the abdominal cavity, the transversalis fascia and parietal peritoneum have been removed from the left abdominal wall, while the endothoracic fascia and Aparietal pleura have been removed from the left chest wall. The rectus sheath (enclosing the rectus abdominis muscle) plays a special role in the abdominal wall, because its structure changes below the arcuate line to accommodate the increasing pressure of the viscera against the body wall (see **C**). The rectus sheath is formed by the aponeuroses of the lateral abdominal muscles (of which only the transversus is visible here; the others are hidden) and is divided into an anterior and a posterior layer.

B Structure of the abdominal wall

Cross section through the abdominal wall above the umbilicus, superior view. The following layers are distinguished in the lateral abdominal wall, from inside to outside:

- Parietal peritoneum
- Transversalis fascia
- Transversus abdominis muscle
- Internal oblique muscle
- External oblique muscle
- Membranous layer, superficial fascia
- Fatty layer, superficial fascia
- Skin

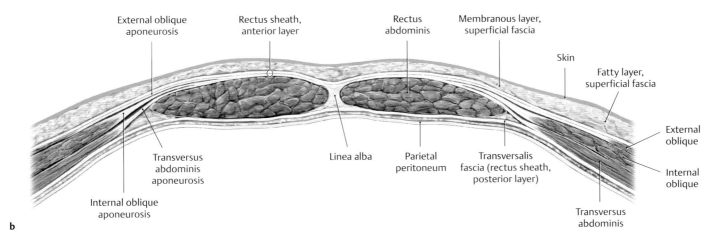

C Structure of the rectus sheath

Cross sections through the rectus sheath superior (**a**) and inferior (**b**) to the arcuate line, superior view. The aponeuroses of the lateral abdominal wall muscles ensheath the anterior strap muscles to form the rectus sheath. This creates a muscular compartment consisting of an anterior layer and a posterior layer. While the aponeuroses of the three lateral abdominal muscles contribute equally to the anterior and posterior layers of the sheath above the umbilicus, the two layers blend together approximately 3 to 5 cm below the umbilicus (at the level of the arcuate line) to form a single (and consequently more stable) sheet that passes in front of the rectus abdominis muscle. Below the arcuate line, the posterior layer of the rectus sheath is absent. The preperitoneal space, a fine layer of loose connective tissue and fat (see also p. 216), is located between transversalis fascia and parietal peritoneum.

179

11.8 The Pelvic Floor Muscles: Overview of the Perineal Region and Superficial Fasciae

a

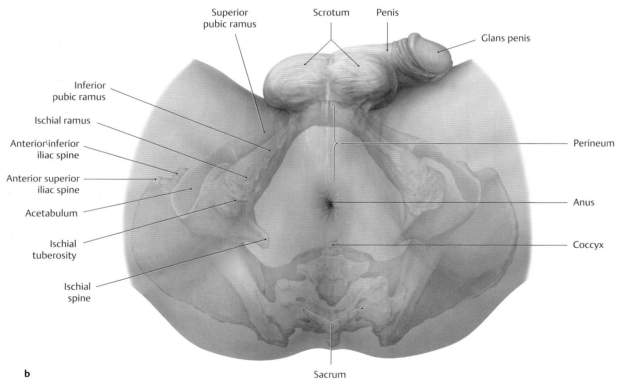

b

A Perineal region in the female (a) and male (b)

Lithotomy position, inferior view. The perineal region in both sexes consists of the urogenital region anteriorly and the adjacent anal region posteriorly. The two regions are separated by a line that runs between the ischial tuberosities. The perineum denotes the soft-tissue area between the thighs and the buttocks. In the female, obstetricians refer to the perineum as the region from the anterior margin of the anus to the posterior commissure of the vagina. It is considerably longer in the male, extending from the anal margin to the root of the scrotum. The perineum is a region containing fibrous and fatty tissue, and the perineal body (see **Ba**) is a fibromuscular mass, also referred to as the central tendon of the perineum. A more detailed structural description of the perineum is given on p. 184.

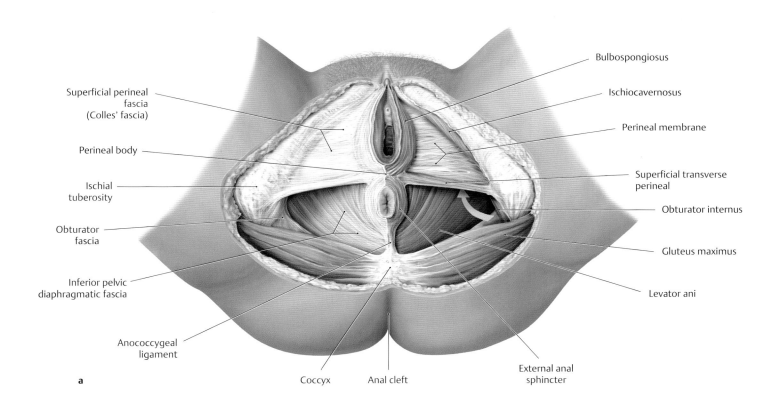

Superficial perineal fascia (Colles' fascia)

Perineal body

Ischial tuberosity

Obturator fascia

Inferior pelvic diaphragmatic fascia

Anococcygeal ligament

Bulbospongiosus

Ischiocavernosus

Perineal membrane

Superficial transverse perineal

Obturator internus

Gluteus maximus

Levator ani

External anal sphincter

Coccyx   Anal cleft

a

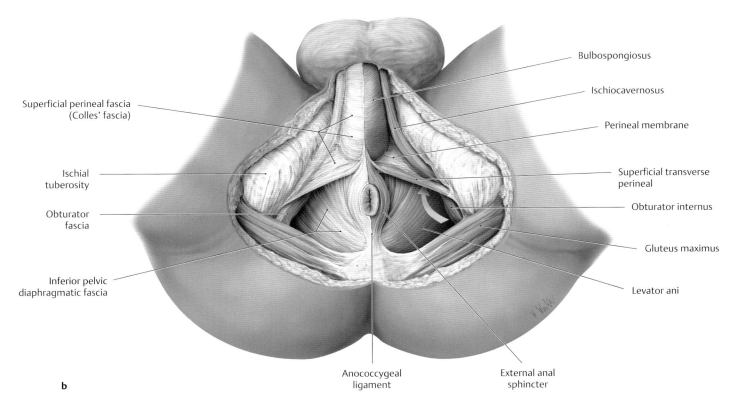

Superficial perineal fascia (Colles' fascia)

Ischial tuberosity

Obturator fascia

Inferior pelvic diaphragmatic fascia

Bulbospongiosus

Ischiocavernosus

Perineal membrane

Superficial transverse perineal

Obturator internus

Gluteus maximus

Levator ani

Anococcygeal ligament

External anal sphincter

b

B Superficial fasciae of the female (a) and male pelvic floor (b)
Lithotomy position, inferior view. The superficial perineal fascia (urogenital region) and the inferior pelvic diaphragmatic fascia (anal region) are intact on the right side but have been removed on the left side. In this way the superficial perineal space has been opened in the urogenital region on the left side of each dissection, and the levator ani muscle has been exposed in the anal region. The superficial perineal space is bounded posteriorly by the superficial transverse perineal muscle and superiorly by the perineal membrane. The bulbospongiosus muscle is located in the medial part of this superficial perineal space; the ischiocavernosusis muscle is located laterally. The green arrow in each figure points to the anterior recess of the left ischioanal fossa (see also p. 556).

11.9 Structure of the Pelvic Floor and Pelvic Spaces: Female versus Male

Plane of section in **A** and **B**

A Coronal section through the female pelvis
Anterior view.

Labels (clockwise from top): Suspensory ligament of the ovary · Rectum · Uterine fundus · External iliac artery and vein · Iliacus · Ovary · Fallopian tube · Cardinal ligament (transverse cervical) · Obturator internus · Ischioanal fossa · Levator ani · Smooth muscle · Superficial perineal fascia · Vestibule of vagina · Vestibular bulb, bulbospongiosus muscle · Crus of clitoris, ischiocavernosus muscle · Inferior pubic ramus · Pudendal (Alcock's) canal · Vagina · Paravaginal tissue (fascia) · Cervix of uterus · Round ligament of uterus

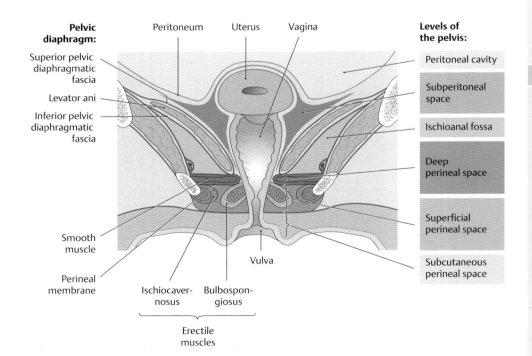

Labels: Pelvic diaphragm: · Superior pelvic diaphragmatic fascia · Levator ani · Inferior pelvic diaphragmatic fascia · Smooth muscle · Perineal membrane · Ischiocavernosus · Bulbospongiosus · Erectile muscles · Peritoneum · Uterus · Vagina · Vulva · Levels of the pelvis: · Peritoneal cavity · Subperitoneal space · Ischioanal fossa · Deep perineal space · Superficial perineal space · Subcutaneous perineal space

B Pelvic spaces, fasciae, and arrangement of the pelvic floor muscles in a female pelvis
Coronal section at the level of the vagina (see small diagram above for the exact location of the plane). The levels of the pelvis are shown in different colors.

C Subdivisions of the pelvis and structure of the pelvic floor (in both sexes)

Subdivisions of the pelvis

The pelvis is the portion of the abdominal cavity located in the lesser pelvis. It is surrounded by the skeleton of the lesser pelvis, which meets the greater pelvis at the *linea terminalis* (see p. 141). The pelvic cavity lies above the pelvic floor (supralevator) and is subdivided into upper and lower levels by the peritoneum:

- **Upper level:** peritoneal cavity of the lesser pelvis
- **Lower level:** subperitoneal space

The perineum lies below the pelvic floor (infralevator) and is separated into

- Deep perineal space with ischioanal fossa
- Superficial perineal space
- Subcutaneous perineal space

Subjacent to the pelvis are three more spaces that are considered to be separate from the pelvis itself: the *deep perineal space*, the *superficial perineal space*, and the *subcutaneous perineal space* (see **B** and **F**).

Structure of the pelvic floor

The three muscular and connective-tissue sheets that contribute to the structure of the pelvic floor are arranged in three levels:

- **Upper level:** pelvic diaphragm
- **Middle level:** deep urogenital muscles
- **Lower level:** sphincters and erectile muscles of the urogenital and intestinal tract

The funnel-shaped pelvic diaphragm is formed by the levator ani and coccygeus muscles and the superior and inferior fasciae of the pelvic diaphragm. The deep urogenital muscles (see p. 184) lie in the **deep perineal pouch**. They include the deep transverse perineal muscle in the male, a sheet of smooth muscle in the female, and the inferior portion of the external urethral sphincter. The perineal membrane separates the deep from the **superficial perineal pouch**, the muscles of which are the superficial transverse perineal, bulbospongiosus, ischiocavernosus, and the external anal sphincter more posteriorly.

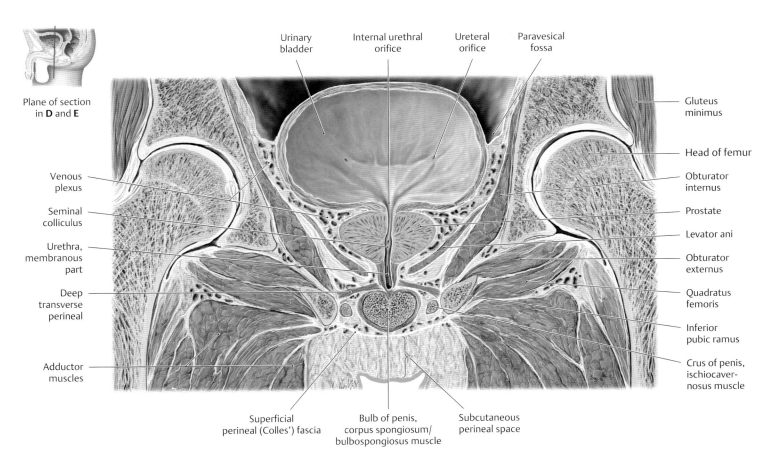

Plane of section in **D** and **E**

D Coronal section through the male pelvis
Anterior view.

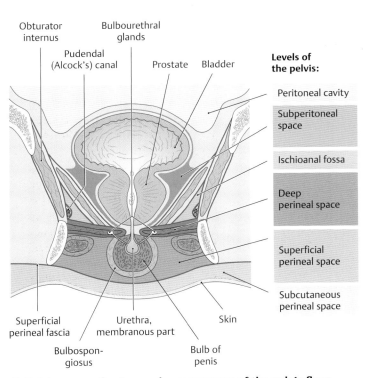

Levels of the pelvis:

- Peritoneal cavity
- Subperitoneal space
- Ischioanal fossa
- Deep perineal space
- Superficial perineal space
- Subcutaneous perineal space

E Pelvic spaces, fasciae, and arrangement of the pelvic floor muscles in a male pelvis

Coronal section at the level of the prostate (see small diagram above for the exact location of the plane). Different colors indicate the various levels of the pelvis and the perineal spaces.

F Boundaries and contents of the deep perineal space and superficial perineal space (Colles' space) in the male [and female]

Deep perineal space

- Boundaries:
  - Perineal membrane
  - Inferior fascia of pelvic diaphragm
  - Inferior portion of inner fascia of obturator internus
- Contents:
  - Deep transverse perineal muscle
  - Inferior portion of external urethral sphincter
  - Compressor urethra muscles (in female)
  - Anterior extension of ischioanal fat pad
  - Intermediate (membranous) portion of urethra (in male)
  - Bulbourethral glands (in male)
  - Branches of related neurovascular structures

Superficial perineal space

- Boundaries:
  - Superficial perineal (Colles') fascia
  - Perineal membrane
  - Ischiopubic rami
- Contents:
  - Superficial transverse perineal muscle
  - Bulbospongiosus muscles
  - Ischiocavernosus muscles
  - Root of penis and proximal portion Tof spongy urethra (in males)
  - Clitoris, bulb of vestibule, and greater vestibular glands (in females)
  - Branches of related neurovascular structures

The **subcutaneous perineal space** is located between the superficial perineal fascia and skin and contains mostly fatty tissue.

11.10 The Muscles of the Female Pelvic Floor and Wall

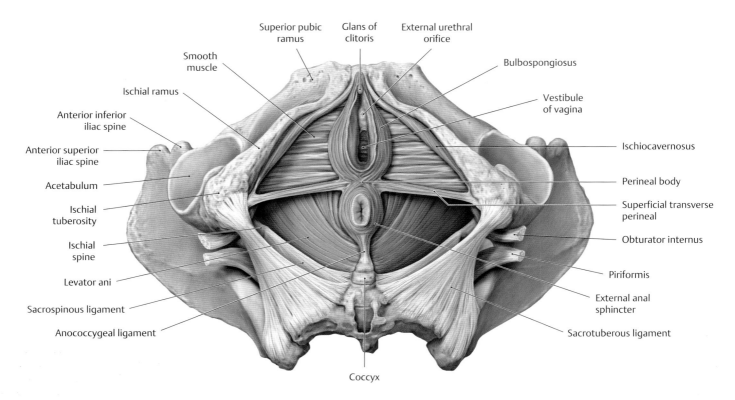

A Muscles of the pelvic floor with the fasciae removed
Female pelvis, inferior view. The muscular layers are progressively removed from **B** through **D** to demonstrate the underlying muscles from a consistent perspective. The levator ani muscle is described more fully on pp. 186–187.

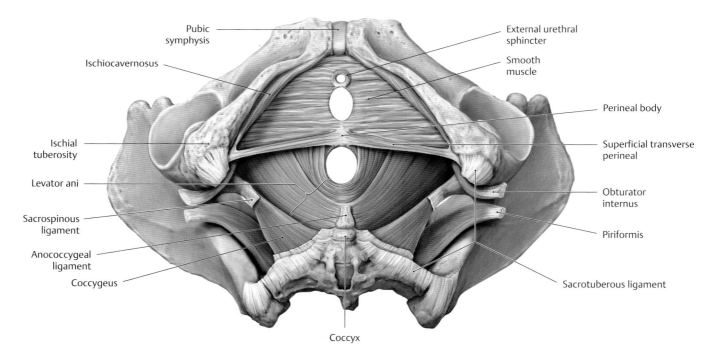

B Muscles of the pelvic floor with the sphincters removed
Female pelvis, inferior view. The sphincter muscles have been removed from the urogenital and intestinal tracts (= bulbospongiosus and external anal sphincter), leaving the external urethral sphincter intact.

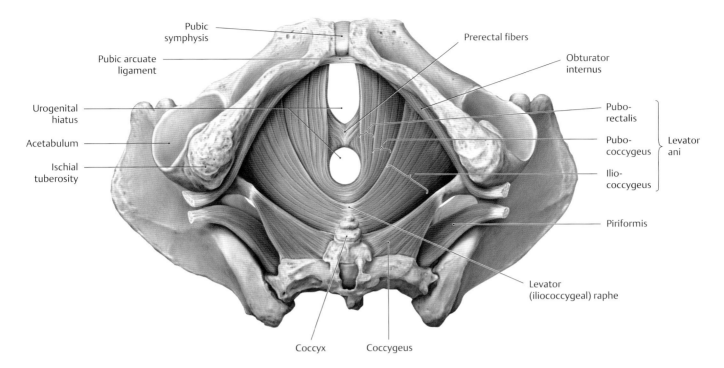

C Muscles of the pelvic floor with the urogenital muscles removed

Female pelvis, inferior view. The urogenital muscles (= superficial and deep transverse perineal and the ischiocavernosi) have been removed. *Note* the opening of the urogenital hiatus, which is bounded by the two crura of the puborectalis muscle (the levator crura). *Note* also the prerectal fibers that have split off from the puborectalis muscle. The prerectal fibers are interwoven with connective-tissue fibers and smooth muscle to form the fibromuscular framework of the perineum (see also p. 180).

D Muscles of the pelvic wall (parietal muscles of the lesser pelvis)

Female pelvis, inferior view. All of the pelvic floor muscles have been removed, leaving the parietal muscles intact (obturator internus, coccygeus, and piriformis). Along with the skeleton of the lesser pelvis, these muscles contribute structurally to the pelvic wall and assist in closing the posterior pelvic outlet. The obturator internus and its fascia provide a tendon of origin for the iliococcygeus, which is part of the levator ani complex (tendinous arch of the levator ani, see p. 187).

11.11 Pelvic Floor Muscles: The Levator Ani

a

b

A Parts of the levator ani and the parietal muscles of the pelvic wall

Female pelvis, superior view.

a The levator ani muscle consists of three parts: the puborectalis, pubococcygeus, and iliococcygeus. It arises from the anterior and lateral pelvic wall on a line running from the center of the pubic symphysis to the ischial spine (= tendinous arch of the levator ani). As a contributor to continence, the puborectalis muscle assists the external anal sphincter (not visible here) in keeping the anus closed. It arises from the superior pubic ramus on both sides of the pubic symphysis and

runs in the shape of a loop around the rectum, where the fibers are connected to the deep part of the external anal sphincter. It has the shape of an arched gateway, with its two crura (the levator crura) forming the boundaries of the urogenital hiatus. In contraction of the puborectal sling, the rectal wall is pulled forward toward the pubic bone, which increases the so-called anorectal angle (angle between rectum and anal canal) and tightens the anal canal by squeezing it.

b The puborectalis and pubococcygeus muscles have been removed. The coccygeus (muscle fibers on the sacrospinous ligament) and the piriformis complete the pelvic outlet posteriorly on both sides of the sacrum.

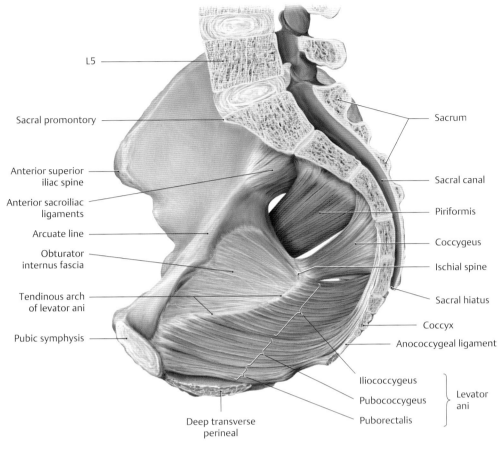

L5

Sacral promontory

Anterior superior iliac spine

Anterior sacroiliac ligaments

Arcuate line

Obturator internus fascia

Tendinous arch of levator ani

Pubic symphysis

Sacrum

Sacral canal

Piriformis

Coccygeus

Ischial spine

Sacral hiatus

Coccyx

Anococcygeal ligament

Iliococcygeus

Pubococcygeus

Puborectalis

} Levator ani

Deep transverse perineal

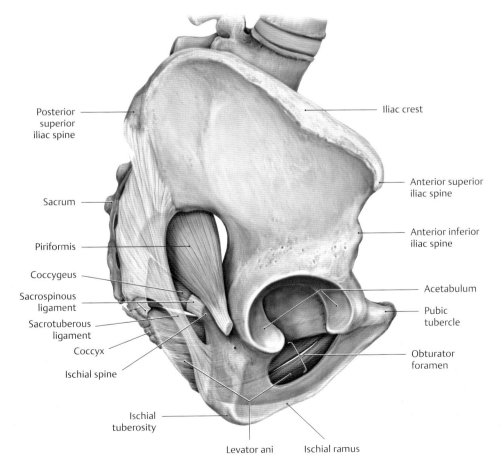

Posterior superior iliac spine

Sacrum

Piriformis

Coccygeus

Sacrospinous ligament

Sacrotuberous ligament

Coccyx

Ischial spine

Ischial tuberosity

Levator ani

Ischial ramus

Iliac crest

Anterior superior iliac spine

Anterior inferior iliac spine

Acetabulum

Pubic tubercle

Obturator foramen

B Tendinous arch of the levator ani

Right hemipelvis, medial view. The tendinous arch of the levator ani is a thickening of the obturator internus fascia that serves as the origin of the iliococcygeus muscle.

a

Anococcygeal ligament

Levator ani

b

External anal sphincter

Gaps in connective tissue

D Gender-related differences in structure of the levator ani (**a** male, **b** female)

Posterior view.

Note the gaps in the connective tissue between the muscular parts of the levator ani in female (**b**).

C Funnel shape of the levator ani

Pelvis viewed from the right side. A portion of the ischium is shown transparent. A contraction of the funnel-shaped levator ani leads to lifting of the anus (levatore = to rise) and to forward motion caused by extension of the puborectalis. At its neutral position, the levator funnel stands at a steep angle but flattens when contracted. Because the muscle has a cone or funnel shape, during defecation, only the peripheral parts of the levator ani contract; the four areas close to the sphincter, including the puborectalis, go limp so that the anus descends, and the stool is pushed through the opened anal canal.

11.12 Pelvic Floor Muscles: Their Relation to Organs and Vessels in Males and Females

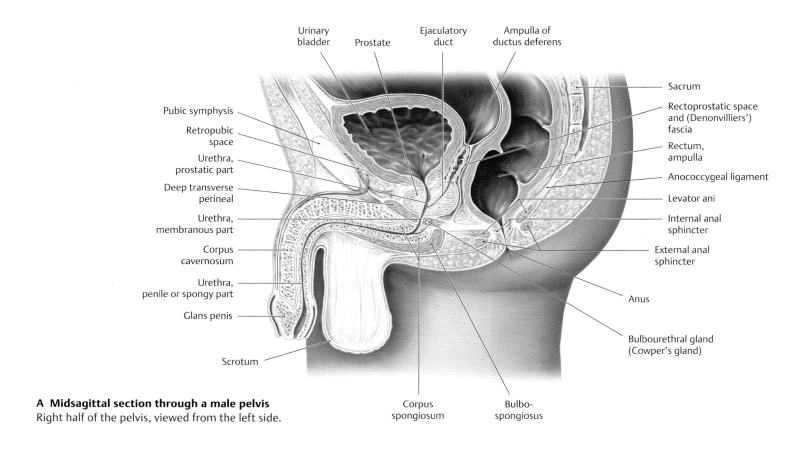

A Midsagittal section through a male pelvis
Right half of the pelvis, viewed from the left side.

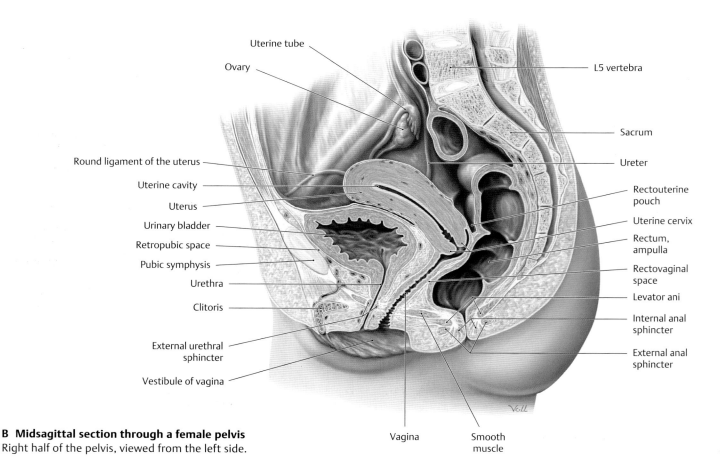

B Midsagittal section through a female pelvis
Right half of the pelvis, viewed from the left side.

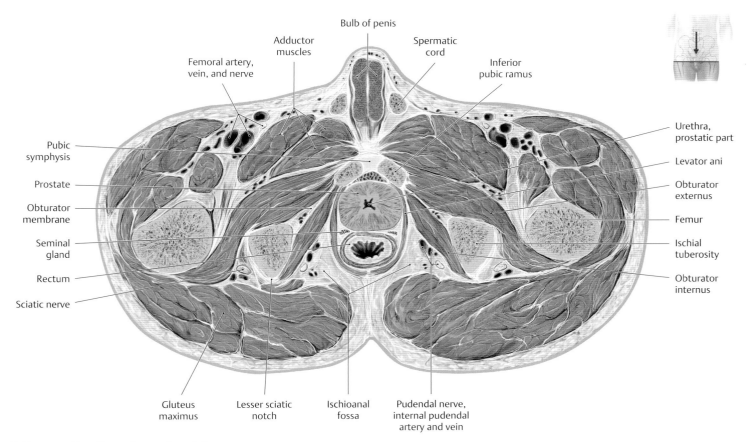

Bulb of penis

Adductor
muscles

Spermatic
cord

Femoral artery,
vein, and nerve

Inferior
pubic ramus

Pubic
symphysis

Urethra,
prostatic part

Prostate

Levator ani

Obturator
membrane

Obturator
externus

Seminal
gland

Femur

Rectum

Ischial
tuberosity

Sciatic nerve

Obturator
internus

Gluteus
maximus

Lesser sciatic
notch

Ischioanal
fossa

Pudendal nerve,
internal pudendal
artery and vein

C Cross section through a male pelvis
Superior view.

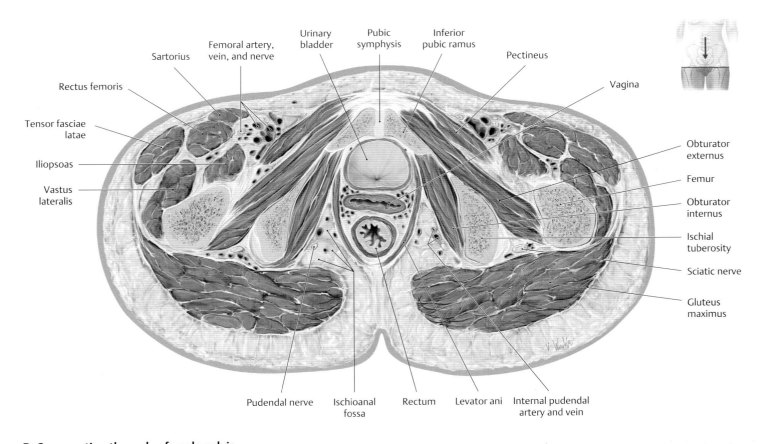

Sartorius

Femoral artery,
vein, and nerve

Urinary
bladder

Pubic
symphysis

Inferior
pubic ramus

Pectineus

Rectus femoris

Vagina

Tensor fasciae
latae

Obturator
externus

Iliopsoas

Femur

Vastus
lateralis

Obturator
internus

Ischial
tuberosity

Sciatic nerve

Gluteus
maximus

Pudendal nerve

Ischioanal
fossa

Rectum

Levator ani

Internal pudendal
artery and vein

D Cross section through a female pelvis
Superior view.

189

12.1 The Arteries

A Overview of the arteries of the trunk wall

The arrangement of the neurovascular structures in the trunk reflects the segmental anatomy of the trunk wall, particularly in the thoracic region. Accordingly, each of the intercostal spaces is traversed by an intercostal artery, vein, and nerve.

The chest wall is supplied principally by the posterior intercostal arteries, which arise from the aorta, and by anterior intercostal branches arising from the internal thoracic artery:

- The first and second posterior intercostal arteries, which are given off by the superior intercostal artery (= branch of the costocervical trunk, see **D a**)
- The third through eleventh posterior intercostal arteries (each giving off a dorsal, a collateral, and a lateral cutaneous branch, see **D b**)
- The musculophrenic artery (one of the two terminal branches of the internal thoracic artery), which runs behind the costal arch, see **B**
- The subcostal artery (twelfth intercostal artery), see **B**
- The anterior intercostal arteries, which arise from the internal thoracic artery, see **B**

Many other "regional" arteries supply the anterior, lateral, and posterior trunk wall.

Anterior trunk wall

- The perforating branches (from the internal thoracic artery, e.g., the medial mammary branches that supply the breast), see **D b**
- The superior epigastric artery (continuation of the internal thoracic artery, see **B** and **C**)
- The inferior epigastric artery (from the external iliac artery, see **B** and **C**)
- The superficial epigastric artery, see **B**
- The superficial circumflex iliac artery, see **B**
- The deep circumflex iliac artery, see **B**

Posterior trunk wall

- Dorsal branches (from the posterior intercostal arteries), each with a medial, a lateral cutaneous, and a spinal branch, see **D c**
- The first through fourth lumbar arteries (each with a dorsal and spinal branch), see **B**
- The median sacral artery, see **B**

Lateral trunk wall

- The superior thoracic artery, see **B**
- The thoracoacromial artery, see **B**
- The lateral thoracic artery, see **B**
- The lateral cutaneous branches (from the intercostal arteries), which distribute branches mainly to the breast (lateral mammary branches, see **D b**)
- The iliolumbar artery (from the internal iliac artery), which gives off an iliac, a lumbar, and a spinal branch, see **B**

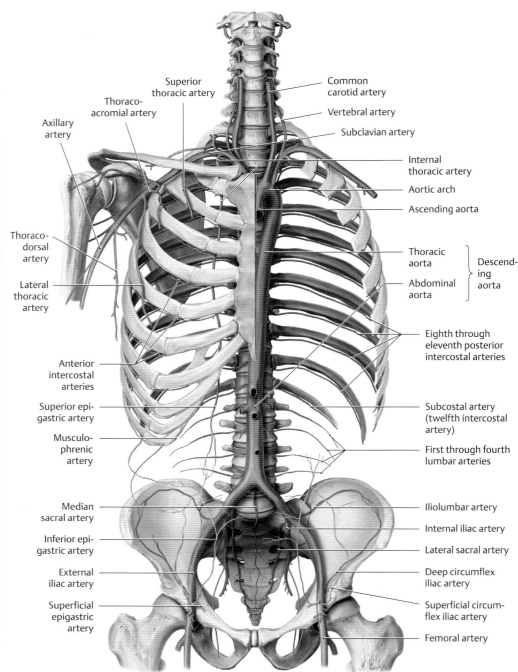

B Arteries of the trunk wall

Anterior view. The anterior portions of the ribs have been removed on the left side.

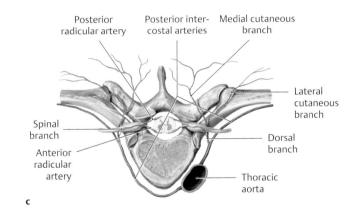

C Arteries of the trunk wall
Right lateral view.

D Course and branches of the intercostal arteries

a Anterior view of the superior intercostal artery, which gives off the first two intercostal arteries.

Note: The first and second posterior intercostal arteries are not branches of the thoracic aorta but arise from the superior intercostal artery (branch of the costocervical trunk), which are branches of the subclavian artery.

b Anterior view of the posterior intercostal arteries that are segmental branches of the thoracic aorta.

Note: The *anterior* intercostal arteries arise from the subclavian artery (via the internal thoracic artery), while the *posterior* intercostal arteries arise directly from the thoracic aorta.

c Branches of the posterior intercostal arteries, viewed from the superior view.

12.2 The Veins

A Overview of the veins of the trunk wall

The veins of the trunk wall drain into both the vena caval and azygos systems (see **B**). Within the vena caval system, we can distinguish between the tributary regions of the inferior vena cava and the superior vena cava. Connections between the superior and inferior vena cavae are called *cavocaval anastomoses* (collateral channels).

Tributaries of the superior vena cava
- Superior intercostal vein (brachiocephalic vein) (see **B**)
- Anterior intercostal veins (internal thoracic vein, subclavian vein) (see **D**)
- Superior epigastric vein (internal thoracic vein, subclavian vein)
- Lateral thoracic vein (axillary vein) (see **C**)
- Thoracoepigastric vein (axillary vein) (see **C**)

Tributaries of the inferior vena cava (see **B**)
- Posterior intercostal veins ⎫
- Subcostal vein ⎬ Ascending lumbar vein
- First through fourth lumbar veins ⎭

- Iliolumbar vein ⎫
- Median sacral vein ⎬ Common iliac vein

- Deep circumflex iliac vein ⎫
- Inferior epigastric vein ⎬ External iliac vein

- Lateral sacral vein ⎫
- Obturator vein (see p. 212) ⎬ Internal iliac vein
- Internal pudendal vein (see p. 230) ⎭

- External pudendal veins ⎫
- Superficial circumflex iliac vein ⎬ Femoral vein
- Superficial epigastric vein ⎭

Tributaries of the azygos vein (see **B**)
- Superior intercostal veins
- Posterior intercostal veins
- Hemiazygos vein
- Accessory hemiazygos vein
- Veins of the vertebral column, see **Ea**

B Major veins in the trunk
Anterior view.

C Superficial veins of the anterior trunk wall

Anterior view. Normally, these veins are not palpable, but they are of key importance in the development of portocaval anastomoses, in which the former umbilical vein connects the portal vein of the liver to the superior and inferior venae cavae. In cases where portal hypertension develops as a result of liver disease (hepatic cirrhosis due to alcohol abuse), the portal venous blood must partially bypass the liver, flowing through the paraumbilical veins (see p. 210) to the superficial truncal veins in the umbilical region (periumbilical veins) and finally to the heart. Since the superficial veins must carry considerably more blood in this situation, they undergo varicose dilation, becoming visible and palpable on the abdomen. This is also called a "Medusa's head" (*caput medusae*) because the serpentine, dilated veins around the umbilicus resemble the snake-haired head of the Gorgon.

Internal
jugular vein

Subclavian vein

Right
brachiocephalic
vein

Azygos vein

Superior
vena cava

Internal
thoracic vein

Posterior
intercostal
veins

Anterior
intercostal
veins

Superior
epigastric vein

Musculophrenic
vein

Inferior
vena cava

Subcostal vein

Lumbar veins

Inferior
epigastric vein

External iliac vein

Femoral vein

D Veins of the trunk wall
Right lateral view.

Posterior
intercostal veins

Anterior external
vertebral
venous plexus

Veins of
vertebral
column

Azygos vein

Sternum

a

Anterior
intercostal veins

Internal
thoracic veins

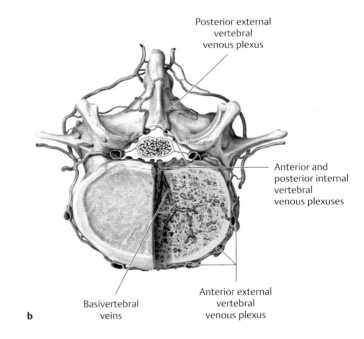

Posterior external
vertebral
venous plexus

Anterior and
posterior internal
vertebral
venous plexuses

Anterior external
vertebral
venous plexus

Basivertebral
veins

b

E Intercostal veins and venous plexuses of the vertebral canal
a Vertebral column and rib segment, anterosuperior view.
b Lumbar vertebra, superior view.

12.3 The Lymphatic Vessels and Lymph Nodes

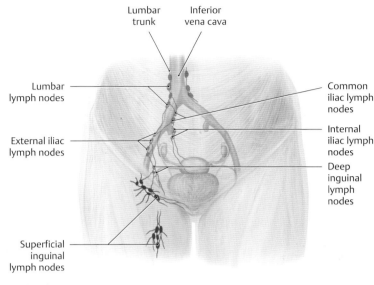

a

b

A Regional lymph nodes and their associated lymphatics
Anterior view.

a Axillary, parasternal, and cervical lymph nodes (right thoracic and axillary region with the arm abducted). The lymph node levels are described on p. 209.

b Lymph nodes of the inguinal region and lesser pelvis.

B Left and right venous angles
Anterior view. The approximately 1-cm-long *right lymphatic duct* collects lymph from the right upper quadrant of the body (see **Ca**) and empties into the **right venous angle** at the junction of the right internal jugular vein with the right subclavian vein. Its major tributaries are

- the right jugular trunk (right half of the head and neck),
- the right subclavian trunk (right upper limb, right side of the chest and back wall), and
- the right bronchomediastinal trunk (organs of the right thoracic cavity).

The *thoracic duct* is approximately 40 cm long and transports lymph from the entire lower half of the body and left upper quadrant. It empties into the **left venous angle** between the left internal jugular vein and left subclavian vein. Its main tributaries are

- the left jugular trunk (left half of the head and neck),
- the left subclavian trunk (left upper limb, left side of the chest and back wall),
- the left bronchomediastinal trunk (organs of the left thoracic cavity),
- the intestinal trunks (abdominal organs), and
- the right and left lumbar trunks (right and left lower limb; pelvic viscera; right and left pelvic, abdominal, and back wall).

The intercostal lymphatic vessels transport lymph from the upper left and right intercostal spaces to the corresponding ipsilateral lymphatic duct. The lower intercostal spaces from both sides drain to the cisterna chyli.

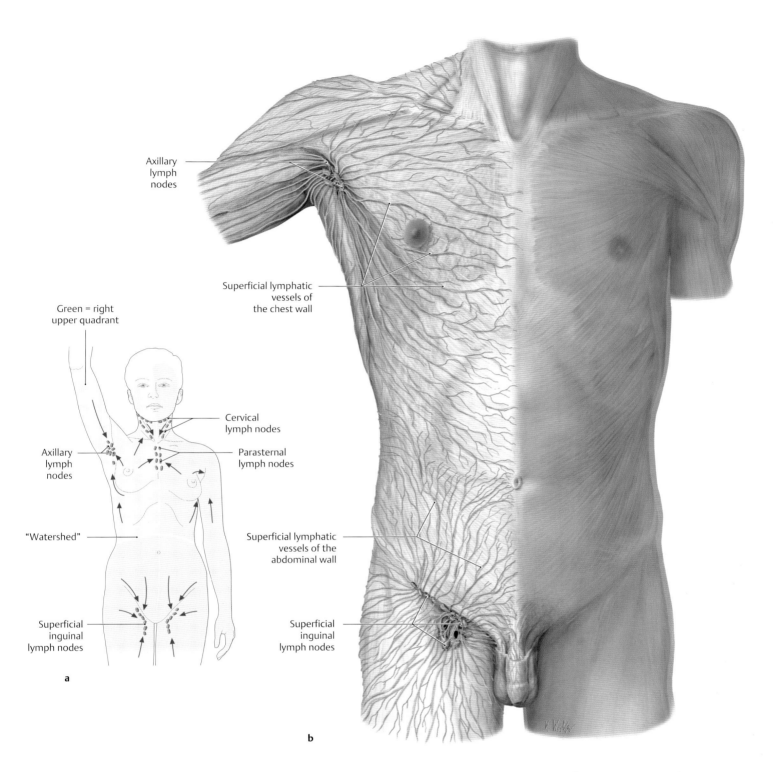

Axillary
lymph
nodes

Superficial lymphatic
vessels of
the chest wall

Green = right
upper quadrant

Cervical
lymph nodes

Axillary
lymph
nodes

Parasternal
lymph nodes

"Watershed"

Superficial lymphatic
vessels of the
abdominal wall

Superficial
inguinal
lymph nodes

Superficial
inguinal
lymph nodes

a

b

C Areas drained by the superficial lymphatic vessels of the anterior trunk wall

Anterior view.

a Lymphatic pathways and regional lymph nodes of the anterior trunk wall (arrows indicate the direction of lymph flow).
b Superficial network of lymphatic vessels in the right anterior trunk wall.

Lymph from the skin of the trunk wall is collected mainly by the axillary and superficial inguinal lymph nodes, following the general pattern of venous drainage in the anterior trunk wall. The "watershed" zone between the two drainage regions is defined by a curved line above the umbilicus and below the costal arch. Lymph from the regional axillary and inguinal lymph nodes is finally collected by two lymphatic trunks, each of which drains into the jugulosubclavian venous junction on the corresponding side of the body (right or left venous angle, see **B**). Lymphatic fluid from the right upper quadrant (green) is returned to the venous system by the *right lymphatic duct*, while lymph from the other three body quadrants (violet) is returned to the veins by the *thoracic duct*.

195

12.4 The Nerves

A Anterior and posterior branches (rami) of the spinal nerves

The trunk wall receives most of its sensory nerve supply from the anterior and posterior rami of the T1–T12 spinal cord segments (intercostal nerves and posterior rami of the spinal nerves) (see also p. 200).

Spinal cord segment	Anterior branches (anterior rami)	Posterior branches (posterior rami)
C1		Suboccipital nerve
C2	Cervical plexus	Greater occipital nerve
C3		Third occipital nerve (see p. 200)
C4		
C5		
C6	Brachial plexus	
C7		
C8		
T1		
T2		
T3		
T4		
T5		
T6		
T7	Intercostal nerves and subcostal nerve	Posterior rami*
T8		
T9		
T10		
T11		
T12		
L1		
L2	Lumbar plexus	
L3		
L4		
L5		
S1		
S2	Sacral plexus	
S3		
S4		
S5		
Co1	Coccygeal plexus (see p. 542)	
Co2		

* The posterior rami of the L1–L3 spinal nerves are also known as the superior clunial nerves, those from S1–S3 as the middle clunial nerves (see **C**).

Note: The *inferior* clunial nerves are anterior rami from the sacral plexus; see also p. 536.

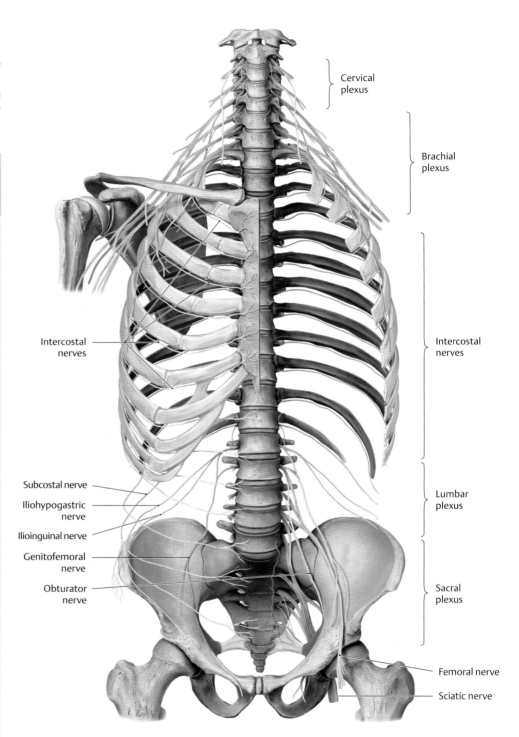

- Cervical plexus
- Brachial plexus
- Intercostal nerves
- Intercostal nerves
- Subcostal nerve
- Iliohypogastric nerve
- Ilioinguinal nerve
- Genitofemoral nerve
- Obturator nerve
- Lumbar plexus
- Sacral plexus
- Femoral nerve
- Sciatic nerve

B Nerves of the trunk wall

Anterior view. The anterior part of the left half of the thoracic cage has been removed. The trunk wall receives most of its motor and sensory innervation from the 12 thoracic spinal nerves. Of all the spinal nerves, these 12 pairs most clearly reflect the original segmental (metameric) organization of the body. The anterior rami run forward in the intercos-tal spaces to become the intercostal nerves, while the posterior rami are distributed to the intrinsic back muscles and to the skin of the back. Portions of the trunk wall are also supplied by nerves from the cervical plexus (supraclavicular nerves), brachial plexus (e.g., the long thoracic nerve), and lumbar plexus (e.g., the ilioinguinal nerve).

D Course of the intercostal nerves
Right side, anterior view.

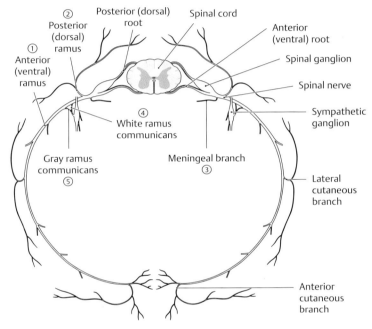

C Course of the nerves on the lateral trunk wall
Right lateral view.
Note the segmental arrangement of the intercostal nerves (compare with the segmental arrangement of the arteries and veins, pp. 190 and 192).

E Branches of a spinal nerve
Formed by the union of the posterior (sensory) and anterior (motor) roots, the approximately 1-cm-long spinal nerve courses through the intervertebral foramen and divides into five branches after exiting the vertebral canal (see **F**).

F Spinal nerve branches and the territories they supply

Spinal nerve branch	Motor or visceromotor territory	Sensory territory
① Anterior (ventral) ramus	All somatic muscles except for the intrinsic back muscles	Skin of the lateral and anterior trunk wall and of the upper and lower limbs
② Posterior (dorsal) ramus	Intrinsic back muscles	Posterior skin of the head and neck, skin of the back and buttock
③ Meningeal branch		Spinal meninges, ligaments of the spinal column, capsules of the facet joints
④ White ramus communicans	Carries preganglionic fibers from the spinal nerve to the sympathetic trunk ("white" because the preganglionic fibers are myelinated)	
⑤ Gray ramus communicans*	Carries postganglionic fibers from the sympathetic trunk back to the spinal nerve ("gray" because the fibers are unmyelinated)	

*Strictly speaking, the gray ramus communicans is not a spinal nerve branch but a branch passing from the sympathetic trunk to the spinal nerve.

197

13.1 Anterior Trunk Wall: Surface Anatomy and Superficial Nerves and Vessels

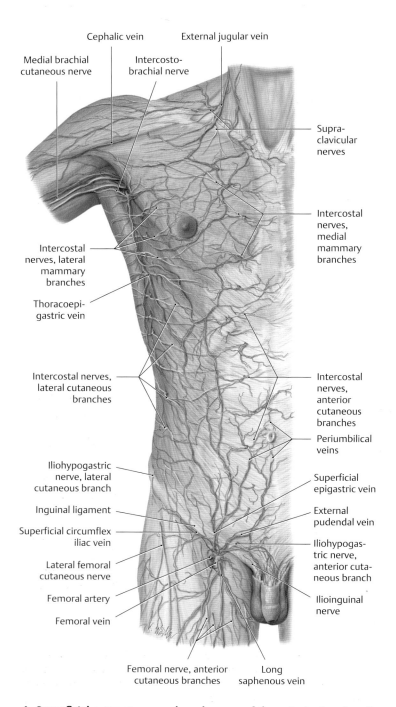

A Superficial cutaneous vessels and nerves of the anterior trunk wall
Anterior view.

Superficial vessels: Most of the *arterial supply* to the anterior trunk wall comes from two sources: the internal thoracic artery and the superficial epigastric artery. The superficial *veins* drain chiefly into the axillary vein (via the thoracoepigastric vein) and into the femoral vein (via the superficial epigastric and superficial circumflex iliac veins). The peri- and paraumbilical veins provide the main communication between the superficial veins of the trunk wall and the portal veins (portocaval anastomoses).

Superficial nerves: The *sensory supply* to the anterior trunk wall has a largely segmental arrangement (provided, for example, by lateral and anterior cutaneous branches from the intercostal nerves). The cervical plexus (supraclavicular nerves) is additionally involved in the thoracic region, as is the lumbar plexus (e.g., iliohypogastric and ilioinguinal nerves) in the lower abdominal region.

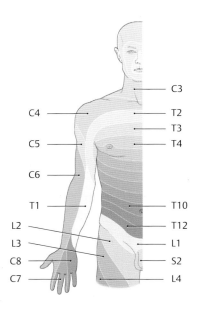

B Segmental (radicular) cutaneous innervation of the anterior trunk wall (dermatomes)
Right half of the trunk and adjacent upper limb, anterior view. Every sensory nerve root (dorsal root) innervates a specific skin area with its fibers. These "dermatomes" (see p. 86), then, correspond to associated spinal cord segments. The dermatomes are arranged in bandlike patterns that encircle the chest wall and upper abdomen. Below the umbilicus, the dermatomes become angled slightly downward toward the median plane. A "segmental gap" exists between the C4 and T2 dermatomes because the phylogenetic outgrowth of the human upper limb has removed the sensory fibers of C5–C8 and T1 from the trunk wall (after Mumenthaler).

C Peripheral sensory cutaneous innervation of the anterior trunk wall
Right half of the trunk and adjacent upper limb, anterior view. The color-coded map of the peripheral cutaneous nerve territories follows the branching pattern of the cutaneous nerves in the subcutaneous connective tissue. Besides the cutaneous branches of the intercostal nerves (anterior and lateral cutaneous branches), it is chiefly the supraclavicular nerves and the iliohypogastric and ilioinguinal nerves that supply the skin of the anterior trunk wall (after Mumenthaler).

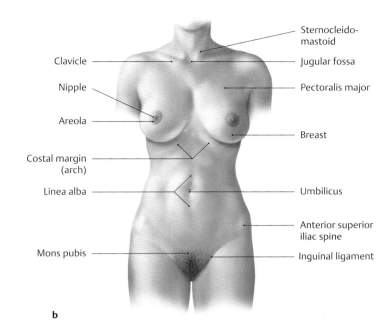

Thyroid cartilage

Delto-pectoral groove

Deltoid

Serratus anterior

Xiphoid process

Tendinous intersection

Rectus abdominis

Semilunar line

External oblique

Iliac crest

Inguinal ligament

Sartorius

Sternocleido-mastoid

Clavicle

Jugular fossa

Nipple

Pectoralis major

Areola

Breast

Costal margin (arch)

Linea alba

Umbilicus

Anterior superior iliac spine

Mons pubis

Inguinal ligament

a

b

D Surface anatomy of the anterior trunk wall
a Male, **b** female.

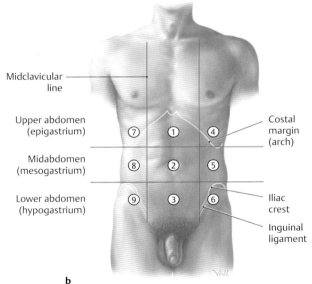

Costal margin (arch)

Right upper quadrant

Left upper quadrant

Right lower quadrant

Left lower quadrant

Periumbilical region

Midclavicular line

Upper abdomen (epigastrium)

Costal margin (arch)

Midabdomen (mesogastrium)

Lower abdomen (hypogastrium)

Iliac crest

Inguinal ligament

① Epigastric region
② Umbilical region
③ Pubic region
④ Left hypo-chondriac region
⑤ Left lateral (lumbar) region
⑥ Left inguinal region
⑦ Right hypo-chondriac region
⑧ Right lateral (lumbar) region
⑨ Right inguinal region

a

b

E Criteria for dividing the abdomen into regions
a The abdomen is divided into four quadrants by two perpendicular lines that intersect at the umbilicus.
b Coordinate system composed of two vertical and two horizontal lines. They divide the abdomen into nine regions, each located in either the upper, middle, or lower abdomen. The two vertical lines represent the left and right midclavicular lines. The two horizontal lines pass through the lowest point of the tenth ribs or the summit of the two iliac crests (see p. 35).

a   **b**   **c**

F Projection of the abdominal organs onto the four quadrants of the anterior abdominal wall
a Organs of the anterior layer, **b** organs of the middle layer,
c organs of the posterior layer.
The organs of the *anterior* layer abut the anterior abdominal wall. The organs of the *middle* layer are located in the posterior part of the abdominal cavity (some are partially retroperitoneal), and those of the *posterior* layer are located outside or behind the actual abdominal cavity (i.e., they are retroperitoneal).

199

13.2 Posterior Trunk Wall: Surface Anatomy and Superficial Nerves and Vessels

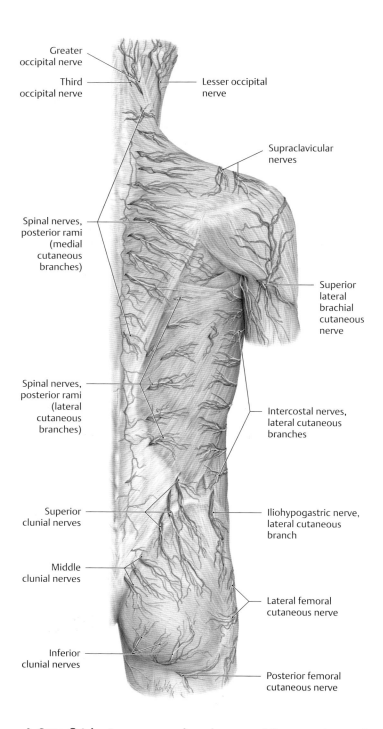

Labels (left figure):
- Greater occipital nerve
- Third occipital nerve
- Lesser occipital nerve
- Supraclavicular nerves
- Spinal nerves, posterior rami (medial cutaneous branches)
- Superior lateral brachial cutaneous nerve
- Spinal nerves, posterior rami (lateral cutaneous branches)
- Intercostal nerves, lateral cutaneous branches
- Superior clunial nerves
- Iliohypogastric nerve, lateral cutaneous branch
- Middle clunial nerves
- Lateral femoral cutaneous nerve
- Inferior clunial nerves
- Posterior femoral cutaneous nerve

A Superficial cutaneous vessels and nerves of the posterior trunk wall

Posterior view. Except for the lower buttocks and lateral portions of the trunk wall, the posterior trunk wall derives its sensory innervation from posterior rami of the spinal nerves and from lateral cutaneous branches of the intercostal nerves. This is a predominantly segmental innervation pattern, analogous to that described in the anterior trunk wall. Both the medial and lateral cutaneous nerve branches pass with the cutaneous vessels through the intrinsic back muscles to the skin of the back. The skin of the buttocks is supplied by lateral branches from the three cranial lumbar and sacral nerves (superior and middle clunial nerves).

Note: The lower part of the buttock is supplied by the inferior clunial nerves, which are branches of the sacral plexus; thus, they are derived from the *anterior* rami of the spinal nerves.

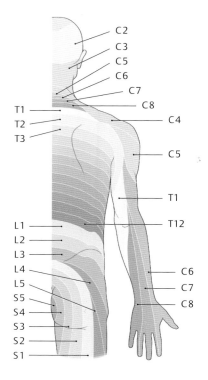

Labels (right upper figure):
- C2, C3, C5, C6, C7, C8, C4
- T1, T2, T3
- C5
- T1
- T12
- L1, L2, L3, L4, L5
- S5, S4, S3, S2, S1
- C6, C7, C8

B Segmental (radicular) cutaneous innervation of the posterior trunk wall (dermatomes)

Right half of the trunk and adjacent upper limb, posterior view (after Mumenthaler).

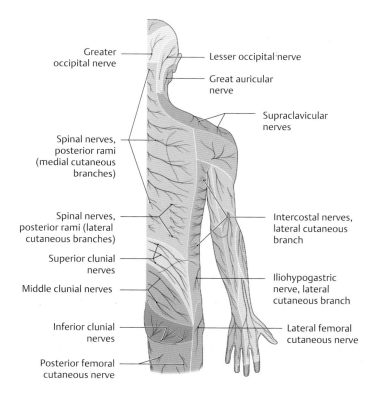

Labels (right lower figure):
- Greater occipital nerve
- Lesser occipital nerve
- Great auricular nerve
- Supraclavicular nerves
- Spinal nerves, posterior rami (medial cutaneous branches)
- Spinal nerves, posterior rami (lateral cutaneous branches)
- Intercostal nerves, lateral cutaneous branch
- Superior clunial nerves
- Middle clunial nerves
- Iliohypogastric nerve, lateral cutaneous branch
- Inferior clunial nerves
- Lateral femoral cutaneous nerve
- Posterior femoral cutaneous nerve

C Peripheral sensory cutaneous innervation of the posterior trunk wall

Right half of the trunk and adjacent upper limb, posterior view (after Mumenthaler).

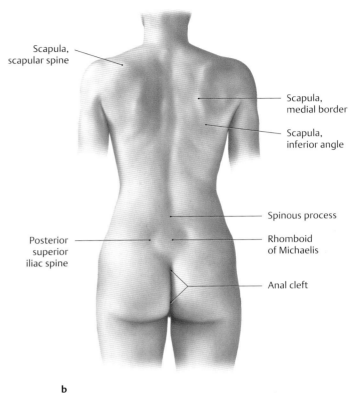

a

b

D Surface anatomy of the posterior trunk wall
a Male, **b** female.
In both sexes a *spinal furrow* runs vertically in the posterior midline of the trunk below the C 7 spinous process. It is formed by the fixation of the subcutaneous tissue to the corresponding spinous processes. At

the sacral level in males, the furrow widens to form the *sacral triangle* (bounded by the right and left posterior superior iliac spines and the upper part of the anal cleft). The corresponding diamond-shaped area in females is called the *rhomboid of Michaelis* (see **F**).

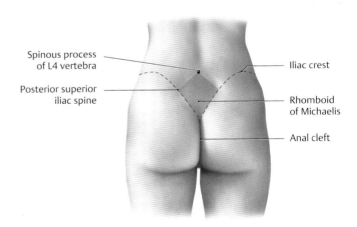

E Segmental and peripheral cutaneous innervation of the male perineal region
Lithotomy position. The segments or dermatomes have been mapped on the left side of the body, and the areas supplied by the peripheral cutaneous nerves are shown on the right side (after Mumenthaler).

F Anatomic boundaries of the Michaelis rhomboid
Female gluteal region, posterior view. In women the sacral triangle is expanded to form a diamond-shaped figure with the following boundaries: the left and right posterior superior iliac spines, the spinous process of the L 4 vertebra, and the upper part of the anal cleft. With a normal female pelvis, the vertical and horizontal dimensions of the rhomboid are approximately equal. The shape of the Michaelis rhomboid (named for the German gynecologist G. A. Michaelis, 1798–1848) reflects the width of the female pelvis, providing an indirect indicator of the size of the birth canal.

13.3 Posterior Trunk Wall, Posterior View

A Neurovascular structures of the posterior trunk wall and nuchal region

Posterior view. The segmentally arranged neurovascular structures of the posterior trunk wall (posterior rami of the spinal nerves and posterior branches of the posterior intercostal and lumbar vessels) are demonstrated on the left side of the trunk (all muscle fasciae have been removed except for the superficial layer of the thoracolumbar fascia). On the right side, the trapezius muscle has been detached from its origins and reflected laterally to show the course of the transverse cervical artery in the deep scapular region (compare with **B**).

Note: On the posterior trunk wall, only the lateral nuchal region (lesser occipital nerve, see **C**) and the lower gluteal region (inferior clunial nerves) receive their sensory supply from anterior spinal nerve rami.

The latissimus dorsi muscle has been partially removed on the right side to demonstrate the upper costolumbar triangle (of Grynfeltt). The fibrous lumbar triangle (boundaries: twelfth rib, intrinsic back muscles, and internal oblique) is similar to the lower iliolumbar triangle (of Petit, bounded by the iliac crest, latissimus dorsi, and external oblique) in that it creates a site of predilection for rare, usually acquired lumbar hernias (Grynfeltt or Petit hernia, see also p. 221).

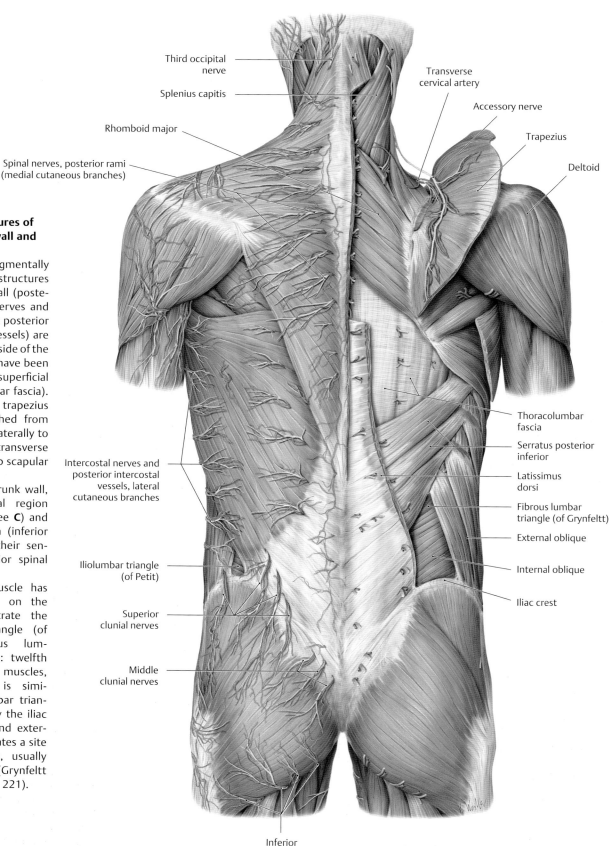

Third occipital nerve

Splenius capitis

Rhomboid major

Spinal nerves, posterior rami (medial cutaneous branches)

Transverse cervical artery

Accessory nerve

Trapezius

Deltoid

Thoracolumbar fascia

Serratus posterior inferior

Latissimus dorsi

Fibrous lumbar triangle (of Grynfeltt)

External oblique

Internal oblique

Iliac crest

Intercostal nerves and posterior intercostal vessels, lateral cutaneous branches

Iliolumbar triangle (of Petit)

Superior clunial nerves

Middle clunial nerves

Inferior clunial nerves

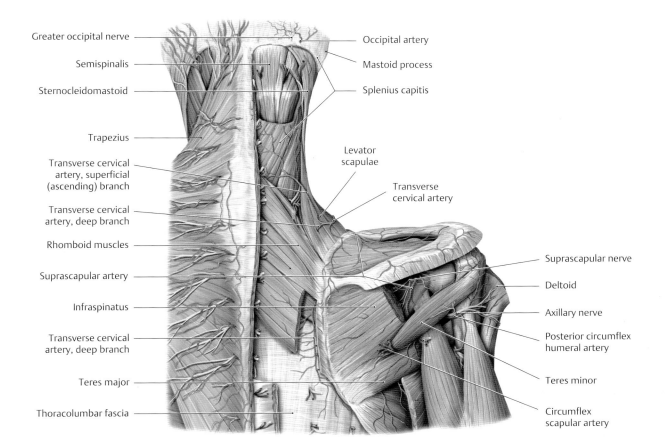

Greater occipital nerve
Semispinalis
Sternocleidomastoid
Trapezius
Transverse cervical artery, superficial (ascending) branch
Transverse cervical artery, deep branch
Rhomboid muscles
Suprascapular artery
Infraspinatus
Transverse cervical artery, deep branch
Teres major
Thoracolumbar fascia

Occipital artery
Mastoid process
Splenius capitis
Levator scapulae
Transverse cervical artery
Suprascapular nerve
Deltoid
Axillary nerve
Posterior circumflex humeral artery
Teres minor
Circumflex scapular artery

B Arteries of the deep scapular region
Right scapular region, posterior view. The trapezius, splenius capitis, deltoid, infraspinatus, and rhomboid major and minor muscles have been completely or partially removed on the right side. The deep scapular region is supplied by the transverse cervical artery, deep cervical artery (see **C**), suprascapular artery, circumflex scapular artery, and posterior circumflex humeral artery. All of these vessels arise directly or indirectly—via the thyrocervical trunk—from the subclavian artery

(neither is visible here). The suprascapular, circumflex scapular, dorsal scapular, and thoracodorsal arteries form the *"scapular arcade"* (see p. 389). Medial to the mastoid process, the occipital artery appears below the tendon of insertion of the sternocleidomastoid muscle and runs upward with the sensory greater occipital nerve to the skin of the occiput. The greater occipital nerve pierces both the trapezius and semispinalis capitis muscles in the area of their firm tendinous attachments. It may become compressed at these sites, leading to *occipital neuralgia.*

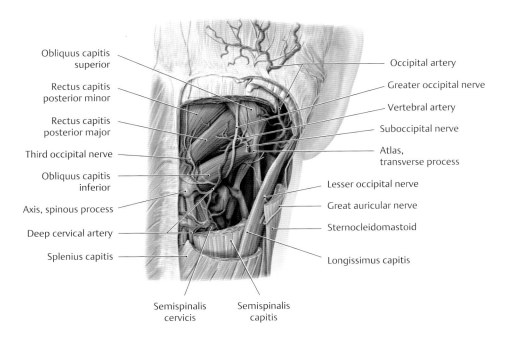

Obliquus capitis superior
Rectus capitis posterior minor
Rectus capitis posterior major
Third occipital nerve
Obliquus capitis inferior
Axis, spinous process
Deep cervical artery
Splenius capitis

Occipital artery
Greater occipital nerve
Vertebral artery
Suboccipital nerve
Atlas, transverse process
Lesser occipital nerve
Great auricular nerve
Sternocleidomastoid
Longissimus capitis

Semispinalis cervicis
Semispinalis capitis

C Suboccipital triangle (vertebral artery triangle)
Posterior view. The trapezius, sternocleidomastoid, splenius capitis, and semispinalis capitis muscles have been removed to display the suboccipital region on the right side. The suboccipital triangle is bounded by the suboccipital muscles (rectus capitis posterior major and the obliquus capitis superior and inferior). In the deep portion of the triangle, the vertebral artery runs through its groove in the atlas. The suboccipital nerve (C 1), which is purely motor, emerges above the posterior arch of the atlas to supply the short muscles of the head. The greater occipital nerve (C 2) and, at a lower level, the third occipital nerve (C 3) wind posteriorly as they pass the lower margin of the obliquus capitis inferior. The deep cervical artery, a branch of the costocervical trunk, runs between the semispinalis capitis and cervicis muscles.

13.4 Posterior Trunk Wall, Anterior View

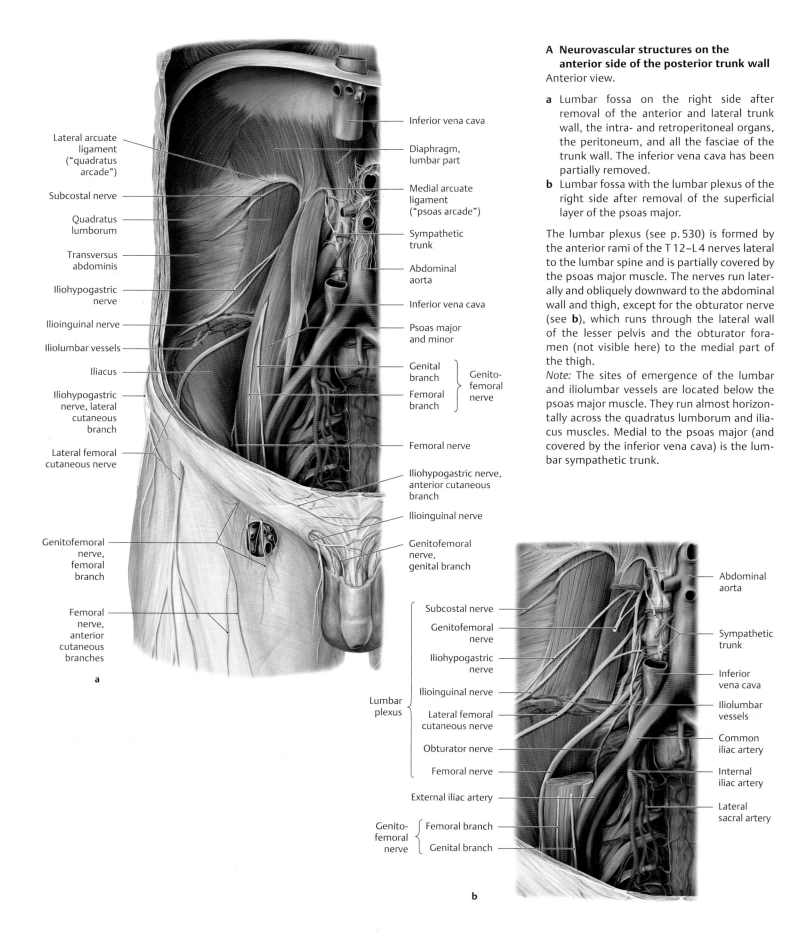

Lateral arcuate
ligament
("quadratus
arcade")

Subcostal nerve

Quadratus
lumborum

Transversus
abdominis

Iliohypogastric
nerve

Ilioinguinal nerve

Iliolumbar vessels

Iliacus

Iliohypogastric
nerve, lateral
cutaneous
branch

Lateral femoral
cutaneous nerve

Genitofemoral
nerve,
femoral
branch

Femoral
nerve,
anterior
cutaneous
branches

a

Inferior vena cava

Diaphragm,
lumbar part

Medial arcuate
ligament
("psoas arcade")

Sympathetic
trunk

Abdominal
aorta

Inferior vena cava

Psoas major
and minor

Genital
branch

Femoral
branch

} Genito-
femoral
nerve

Femoral nerve

Iliohypogastric nerve,
anterior cutaneous
branch

Ilioinguinal nerve

Genitofemoral
nerve,
genital branch

**A Neurovascular structures on the
anterior side of the posterior trunk wall**
Anterior view.

a Lumbar fossa on the right side after
removal of the anterior and lateral trunk
wall, the intra- and retroperitoneal organs,
the peritoneum, and all the fasciae of the
trunk wall. The inferior vena cava has been
partially removed.
b Lumbar fossa with the lumbar plexus of the
right side after removal of the superficial
layer of the psoas major.

The lumbar plexus (see p. 530) is formed by
the anterior rami of the T 12–L 4 nerves lateral
to the lumbar spine and is partially covered by
the psoas major muscle. The nerves run laterally and obliquely downward to the abdominal
wall and thigh, except for the obturator nerve
(see **b**), which runs through the lateral wall
of the lesser pelvis and the obturator foramen (not visible here) to the medial part of
the thigh.
Note: The sites of emergence of the lumbar
and iliolumbar vessels are located below the
psoas major muscle. They run almost horizontally across the quadratus lumborum and iliacus muscles. Medial to the psoas major (and
covered by the inferior vena cava) is the lumbar sympathetic trunk.

Lumbar
plexus
{

Subcostal nerve

Genitofemoral
nerve

Iliohypogastric
nerve

Ilioinguinal nerve

Lateral femoral
cutaneous nerve

Obturator nerve

Femoral nerve

External iliac artery

Genito-
femoral
nerve
{ Femoral branch

Genital branch

Abdominal
aorta

Sympathetic
trunk

Inferior
vena cava

Iliolumbar
vessels

Common
iliac artery

Internal
iliac artery

Lateral
sacral artery

b

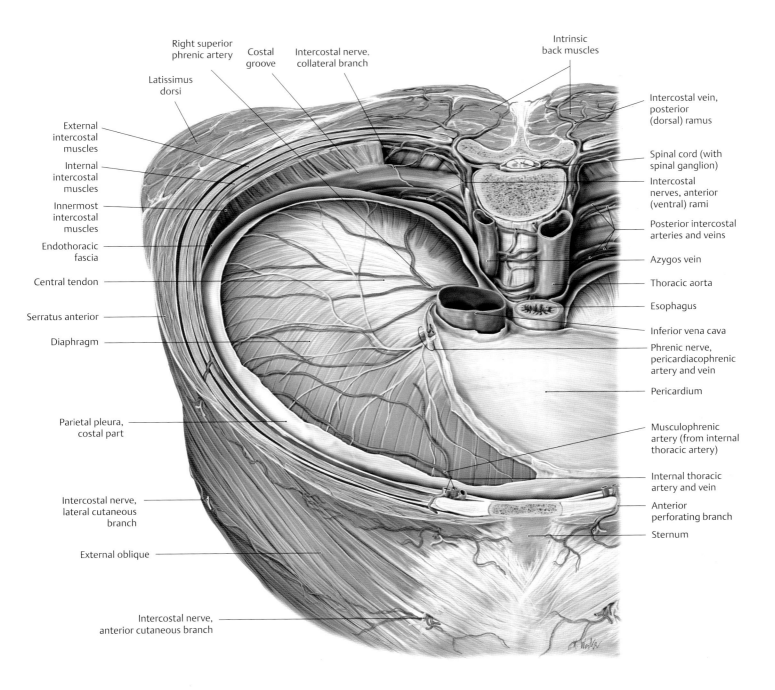

Right superior phrenic artery

Costal groove

Intercostal nerve, collateral branch

Latissimus dorsi

Intrinsic back muscles

External intercostal muscles

Internal intercostal muscles

Innermost intercostal muscles

Endothoracic fascia

Central tendon

Serratus anterior

Diaphragm

Parietal pleura, costal part

Intercostal nerve, lateral cutaneous branch

External oblique

Intercostal nerve, anterior cutaneous branch

Intercostal vein, posterior (dorsal) ramus

Spinal cord (with spinal ganglion)

Intercostal nerves, anterior (ventral) rami

Posterior intercostal arteries and veins

Azygos vein

Thoracic aorta

Esophagus

Inferior vena cava

Phrenic nerve, pericardiacophrenic artery and vein

Pericardium

Musculophrenic artery (from internal thoracic artery)

Internal thoracic artery and vein

Anterior perforating branch

Sternum

B Neurovascular structures of the posterior trunk wall at the thoracic level

Transverse section through the thorax after removal of the thoracic organs, parietal pleura, and part of the endothoracic fascia, anterosuperior view. The chest wall receives its arterial blood supply from the posterior intercostal arteries and is drained by the intercostal veins, which empty into the azygos system. The intercostal vessels run with the intercostal nerves along the inferior border of the associated rib, lodged in the costal sulcus.

13.5 Anterior Trunk Wall: Overview and Location of Clinically Important Nerves and Vessels

Lateral thoracic
artery and vein

Internal thoracic
artery and vein

Intercostal vein,
artery, and nerve

Internal
oblique

Rectus
abdominis

External
oblique

Transversus
abdominis

Inferior epigastric
artery and vein

Transversalis fascia

Superficial circumflex
iliac artery and vein

Fascia lata

Cephalic vein

Thoracoepigastric
vein

Superior epigastric
artery and vein

Rectus sheath,
posterior layer

Umbilicus

Arcuate line

Superficial
epigastric vein

Inguinal ligament

Superficial epigastric
artery and vein

Great
saphenous vein

A Neurovascular structures on the anterior side of the anterior trunk wall

Anterior view. The superficial (subcutaneous) neurovascular structures are demonstrated on the left side of the trunk and the deep neurovascular structures on the right side. For this purpose the pectoralis major and minor muscles have been completely removed on the right side, and the external and internal oblique muscles have been partially removed. Portions of the right rectus abdominis muscle have been removed or rendered transparent to demonstrate the inferior epigastric vessels. Finally, the intercostal spaces have been exposed to display the course of the intercostal vessels and nerves.

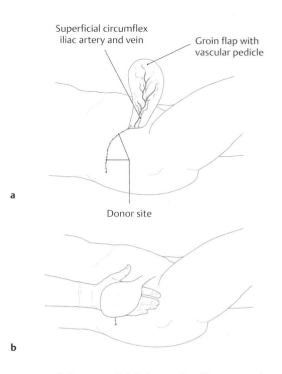

a

Donor site

b

B The arterial supply of the anterior trunk wall

Anterior view. The anterior trunk wall receives its blood supply from two main sources: the internal thoracic artery, which arises from the subclavian artery, and the inferior epigastric artery, which arises from the external iliac artery. It is also supplied by smaller vessels arising from the axillary artery (superior thoracic artery, thoracodorsal artery, and lateral thoracic artery) and from the femoral artery (superficial epigastric artery and superficial circumflex iliac artery).

C Importance of the superficial circumflex iliac artery in harvesting skin flaps for plastic surgery

a Dissection of a skin flap based on the superficial circumflex iliac artery.

b The groin flap transferred to the dorsum of the right hand (after Weber).

a

b

c

d

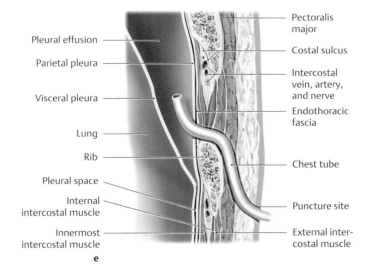

e

D Preserving the intercostal vein, artery, and nerve during the insertion of a chest tube

A chest tube may be inserted to drain an abnormal fluid collection from the pleural space, such as a pleural effusion due to bronchial carcinoma. The best site for placing the chest tube can be determined by percussion or ultrasound examination. Generally, one optimum puncture site in the sitting patient is at the level of the seventh or eighth intercostal space on the posterior axillary line (see **e** and p. 34). The drain should always be introduced at the *upper margin of a rib* to avoid injuring the intercostal vein, artery, and nerve. For additional puncture sites, see textbooks on surgery.

a–d Steps in the placement of a chest tube (anterior view; after Henne-Bruns, Dürig, and Kremer):

a A skin incision is made under local anesthesia, and the drainage tube is introduced perpendicular to the chest wall.

b On reaching the ribs, the tube is angled 90° and advanced cephalad in the subcutaneous plane, parallel to the chest wall.

c On reaching the next higher intercostal space, the tube is passed through the intercostal muscles above the rib.

d The tube is then advanced into the pleural cavity.

e Longitudinal section through the chest wall at the level of the posterior axillary line, after placement of the chest tube in the presence of pleural effusion.

207

13.6 Anterior Trunk Wall: Nerves, Blood Vessels, and Lymphatics in the Female Breast

a

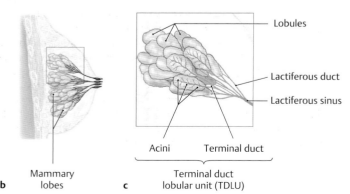

b Mammary lobes c Terminal duct lobular unit (TDLU)

A Shape and appearance of the female breast

Right breast, anterior view. The female breast is shaped like a cone that is more rounded in its lower half than in the upper quadrants. It consists of the glandular tissue (mammary gland) and a fibrous stroma that contains fatty tissue. The excretory ducts of the glandular tissue open on the cone-shaped nipple, which lies at the center of the more heavily pigmented areola. Numerous small protuberances mark the openings of apocrine sweat glands and free sebaceous glands (areolar glands).

B The mammary ridges

The rudiments of the mammary glands form in both sexes along the mammary ridges, appearing as an epidermal ridge extending from the axilla to the inguinal region on each side. Although rarely the mammary ridges may persist in humans to form accessory nipples (polythelia), normally all the rudiments disappear except for the thoracic pair. By the end of fetal development, lactiferous ducts have sprouted into the subcutaneous tissue from the two remaining epithelial buds. After menarche, breast development in females is marked by growth of the fibrous stroma and proliferation of the glandular tree in response to stimulation by sex hormones.

C Gross and microscopic anatomy of the breast

a The base of the adult female breast extends from the second to the sixth rib along the midclavicular line and directly overlies the pectoralis major, serratus anterior, and external oblique muscles. It is loosely attached to the pectoralis fascia and adjacent fascial planes (axillary and superficial abdominal fascia) by connective tissue. The breast is additionally supported, especially in its upper portion, by permeating bundles of connective tissue (the suspensory ligaments of the breast, or *Cooper's ligaments*). The glandular tissue is composed of 10 to 20 individual lobes, each of which has its lactiferous major duct that opens on the nipple by way of a dilated segment, the lactiferous sinus (structure of the lobe shown in **b**). The glands and lactiferous ducts are surrounded by firm, fibrofatty tissue that has a rich blood supply.

b Sagittal section of the duct system and portions of a lobe. A mammary lobe resembles a tree composed of branching lactiferous ducts, which terminate in smaller lobules (approximately 0.5 mm in diameter). In the *nonlactating breast* (as shown here), these lobules contain rudimentary acini that are arranged in clusters of small epithelial buds without a visible lumen.

c The terminal duct lobular unit (TDLU). One lobule and its terminal duct make up the basic secretory unit of the female breast. Each lobule is composed of acini that empty into a terminal ductule. The associated intralobular connective tissue (mantle tissue) contains stem cells that give rise to the tremendous cell growth (proliferation of the duct system and differentiation of the acini) that occurs during the transformation to the *lactating breast*. The TDLU is of key importance in pathohistology because it is the site where most malignant breast tumors originate (after Lüllmann).

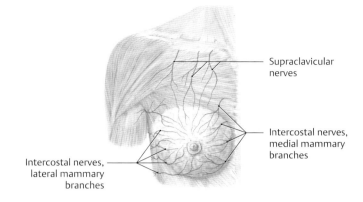

D Blood supply to the breast

The breast derives its blood supply from perforating branches of the internal thoracic artery (= medial mammary branches from the second through fourth intercostal spaces), branches of the lateral thoracic artery (lateral mammary branches), and direct branches from the second through fifth intercostal arteries (mammary branches). The breast is drained by the internal and lateral thoracic veins.

E Nerve supply to the breast

The sensory innervation of the breast has a segmental arrangement and is supplied by branches of the second through sixth intercostal nerves (lateral and medial mammary branches). Branches of the cervical plexus (supraclavicular nerves) also supply the upper portion of the breast.

G Distribution of malignant tumors by quadrant in the female breast

The numbers indicate the average percentage location of malignant breast tumors.

F Lymphatic drainage of the breast

The lymphatic vessels of the breast can be divided into a superficial, subcutaneous, and deep system. The deep system begins with lymphatic capillaries at the acinar level (see **Cb** and **c**) and is particularly important as a route for tumor metastasis. The main regional filtering stations are the axillary and parasternal lymph nodes, the approximately 30 to 60 axillary lymph nodes receiving most of the lymphatic drainage. They are the first nodes to be affected by metastasis (see **G**) and therefore have major oncological significance. The axillary lymph nodes are subdivided into levels (see p. 358):

- **Level I: lower axillary group** (lateral to the pectoralis minor):
  - Pectoral axillary lymph nodes
  - Subscapular axillary lymph nodes
  - Lateral axillary lymph nodes
  - Paramammary lymph nodes
- **Level II: middle axillary group** (at the level of the pectoralis minor):
  - Interpectoral axillary lymph nodes
  - Central axillary lymph nodes
- **Level III: upper infraclavicular group** (medial to the pectoralis minor):
  - Apical axillary lymph nodes

The *parasternal lymph nodes,* which are distributed along the thoracic vessels, chiefly drain the medial portion of the breast. From there,

tumor cells may spread across the midline to the opposite side. The survival rate in breast cancer patients correlates most strongly with the number of involved lymph nodes at the various *axillary* nodal levels. The parasternal lymph nodes are rarely important in this regard. According to Henne-Bruns, Dürig, and Kremer, the 5-year survival rate is approximately 65% with metastatic involvement of level I, 31% with involvement of level II, but approaches 0% in patients with level III involvement. This explains the key prognostic importance of a *sentinel lymphadenectomy* (removal of the sentinel lymph node). This technique is based on the assumption that every point in the integument drains via specific lymphatic pathways to a particular lymph node, rarely draining to more than one. Accordingly, the lymph node that is the first to receive lymph from the primary tumor will be the first node to contain tumor cells that have spread from the primary tumor by lymphogenous metastasis. The specific lymphatic drainage path, and thus the sentinel node, can be identified by scintigraphic mapping with radiolabeled colloids (^{99m}TC sulfur microcolloid), which has superseded the older technique of patent blue dye injection. The first lymph node to be visualized is the sentinel node. That node is selectively removed and histologically examined for the presence of tumor cells. If the sentinel node does not contain tumor cells, generally the rest of the axillary nodes will also be negative. This method is 98% accurate in predicting the level of axillary nodal involvement prior to surgery.

13.7 Anterior Trunk Wall: The Inguinal Canal

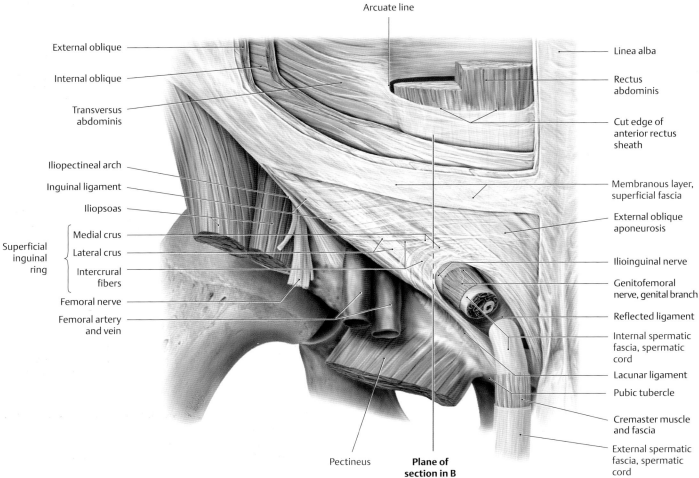

Arcuate line

External oblique

Internal oblique

Transversus abdominis

Iliopectineal arch

Inguinal ligament

Iliopsoas

Superficial inguinal ring
- Medial crus
- Lateral crus
- Intercrural fibers

Femoral nerve

Femoral artery and vein

Linea alba

Rectus abdominis

Cut edge of anterior rectus sheath

Membranous layer, superficial fascia

External oblique aponeurosis

Ilioinguinal nerve

Genitofemoral nerve, genital branch

Reflected ligament

Internal spermatic fascia, spermatic cord

Lacunar ligament

Pubic tubercle

Cremaster muscle and fascia

External spermatic fascia, spermatic cord

Pectineus

Plane of section in B

A Location of the inguinal canal in the male

Right inguinal region, anterior view. Approximately 4 to 6 cm long, the inguinal canal passes obliquely forward, downward, and medially above the inguinal ligament to pierce the anterior abdominal wall. It begins internally at the deep inguinal ring (**D** and **E**) in the lateral inguinal fossa (see p. 212) and opens externally at the superficial inguinal ring, lateral to the pubic tubercle. With the superficial abdominal fascia removed, this "external opening" of the canal can be identified as a slit-like orifice in the aponeurosis of the external oblique muscle (external oblique aponeurosis). It is bounded by the *medial crus* superomedially and by the *lateral crus* inferolaterally. Both crura are interconnected by the *intercrural fibers*. The superficial inguinal ring is completed internally by arched fibers from the inguinal ligament (reflex ligament), forming a deep groove. The inguinal canal in the male provides a pathway for the descent of the testis during fetal life (see p. 224). Its contents in the male (after testicular descent) include the spermatic cord, and its contents in the female include the round ligament of the uterus.

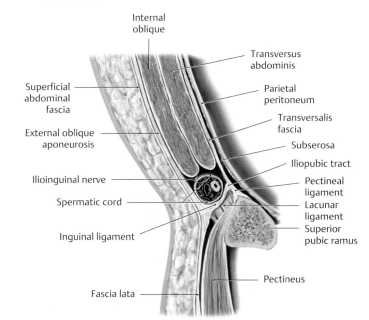

Internal oblique

Superficial abdominal fascia

External oblique aponeurosis

Ilioinguinal nerve

Spermatic cord

Inguinal ligament

Fascia lata

Transversus abdominis

Parietal peritoneum

Transversalis fascia

Subserosa

Iliopubic tract

Pectineal ligament

Lacunar ligament

Superior pubic ramus

Pectineus

B Sagittal section through the inguinal canal in the male

Medial view. *Note* the structures that form the walls of the inguinal canal above and below the spermatic cord and on the anterior and posterior sides (compare with **C**). The openings and wall structures of the inguinal canal bear an important relationship to the pathophysiology of hernias (after Schumpelick).

C Openings and wall structures of the inguinal canal

The inguinal canal resembles a flattened tube with an internal and external opening (see below), a floor, a roof, and anterior and posterior walls. A lumen is present only after its contents have been removed (the spermatic cord in males, the uterine round ligament and its artery in females, the ilioinguinal nerve and lymphatic vessels in both sexes). The inguinal canal remains patent for life, especially in males, and thus forms a path for potential herniation through the abdominal wall (see p. 213).

Openings of the inguinal canal (see A)

Superficial inguinal ring	Opening in the external oblique aponeurosis bounded by the medial crus, lateral crus, intercrural fibers, and reflected inguinal ligament
Deep inguinal ring	Opening between the interfoveolar ligament, inguinal ligament, and lateral umbilical fold; formed by an outpouching of the transversalis fascia (becomes the internal spermatic fascia) (see p. 212)

Wall structures of the inguinal canal (see B)

Floor	Inguinal ligament (densely interwoven fibers of the lower external oblique aponeurosis and adjacent fascia lata of the thigh)
Roof	Transversus abdominis and internal oblique muscles
Anterior wall	External oblique aponeurosis
Posterior wall	Transversalis fascia and peritoneum (partially thickened by the interfoveolar ligament)

a

b

c

D Contribution of the oblique abdominal muscles to the structure of the male inguinal canal

Right inguinal region, anterior view.
a–c Progressive removal of the abdominal wall muscles.

a

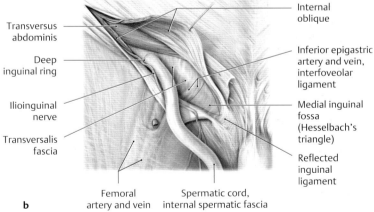

b

E The inguinal canal, progressively opened to expose the spermatic cord

a Division of the external oblique aponeurosis reveals the internal oblique muscle, some of whose fibers are continued onto the spermatic cord as the cremaster muscle. The genital branch of the genitofemoral nerve runs with it below the cremasteric fascia (see p. 532). The ilioinguinal nerve runs through the inguinal canal on the spermatic cord. Its sensory fibers pass through the superficial inguinal ring to the skin over the pubic symphysis and are distributed to the lateral portion of the scrotum or labia majora and medial thigh.

b With the internal oblique muscle divided and the cremaster muscle split, the full course of the spermatic cord through the inguinal canal can be displayed. The spermatic cord appears at the deep inguinal ring, where the transversalis fascia is invaginated into the inguinal canal (and encloses the spermatic cord on its way to the testis as the internal spermatic fascia). It runs below the transversus abdominis along the posterior wall of the inguinal canal (transversalis fascia and peritoneum). The wall at the midportion of the canal is formed by the interfoveolar ligament and is reinforced medially by the reflected inguinal ligament. Medial to the interfoveolar ligament, deep to which run the epigastric vessels, and superior to the inguinal ligament is the medial inguinal fossa, a weak spot in the abdominal wall that is a common site for direct inguinal hernias (after Schumpelick; see also p. 213).

211

13.8 Anterior Abdominal Wall: Anatomy and Weak Spots

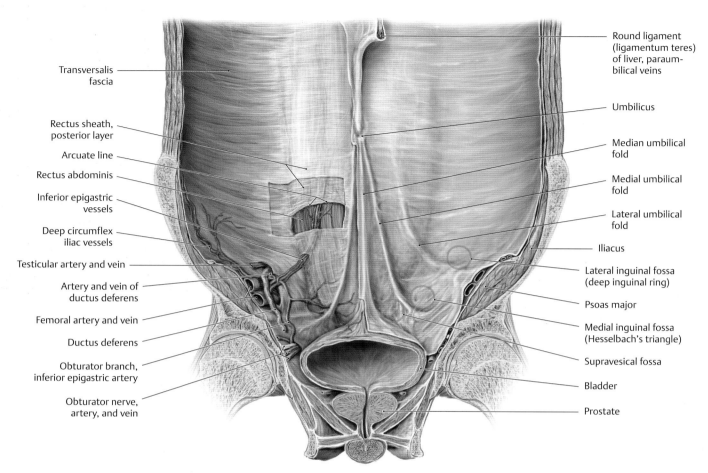

Round ligament (ligamentum teres) of liver, paraumbilical veins

Transversalis fascia

Rectus sheath, posterior layer

Arcuate line

Rectus abdominis

Inferior epigastric vessels

Deep circumflex iliac vessels

Testicular artery and vein

Artery and vein of ductus deferens

Femoral artery and vein

Ductus deferens

Obturator branch, inferior epigastric artery

Obturator nerve, artery, and vein

Umbilicus

Median umbilical fold

Medial umbilical fold

Lateral umbilical fold

Iliacus

Lateral inguinal fossa (deep inguinal ring)

Psoas major

Medial inguinal fossa (Hesselbach's triangle)

Supravesical fossa

Bladder

Prostate

A Internal surface anatomy of the anterior abdominal wall in the male

Coronal section through the abdominal and pelvic cavity at the level of the hip joints, posterior view. All of the abdominal and pelvic organs have been removed except for the urinary bladder and prostate. Portions of the peritoneum and transversalis fascia have also been removed on the left side. The internal surface anatomy of the lower abdominal wall is marked by five peritoneal folds, which extend toward the umbilicus:

- An unpaired *median umbilical fold* on the midline (contains the obliterated urachus)
- Paired left and right *medial umbilical folds* (contain the left and right obliterated umbilical artery)

- Paired left and right *lateral umbilical folds* (contain the left and right inferior epigastric vessels)

Located between the peritoneal folds on each side are three more or less distinct fossae, which are sites of potential herniation through the anterior abdominal wall:

- The *supravesical fossa,* located between the median and medial umbilical folds above the apex of the bladder
- The *medial inguinal fossa* (Hesselbach's triangle), located between the medial and lateral umbilical folds
- The *lateral inguinal fossa,* located lateral to the lateral umbilical fold (site of the deep inguinal ring)

B Internal and external openings for abdominal hernias

Above the inguinal ligament, the median, medial, and lateral umbilical folds (see **A**) form three sites of weakness on each side of the abdominal wall where indirect and direct inguinal hernias and suprapubic hernias typically occur. Another weak spot is located *below the inguinal ligament* and medial to the femoral vein in the femoral ring. At that site the femoral ring is covered only by loose, compliant connective tissue, the femoral septum, which is permeated by numerous lymphatic vessels. The sharp-edged lacunar ligament forms the medial border of the femoral ring and can contribute to the incarceration of a femoral hernia (see p. 215).

Hernia	Internal opening*	External opening*
	Above the inguinal ligament:	
Supravesical hernia	Supravesical fossa	Superficial inguinal ring
Direct inguinal hernia	Medial inguinal fossa (Hesselbach's triangle)	Superficial inguinal ring
Indirect inguinal hernia	Lateral inguinal fossa (deep inguinal ring)	Superficial inguinal ring
	Below the inguinal ligament:	
Femoral hernia	Femoral ring	Saphenous opening

* The internal opening is where the hernia starts and the external opening is where it is observed clinically.

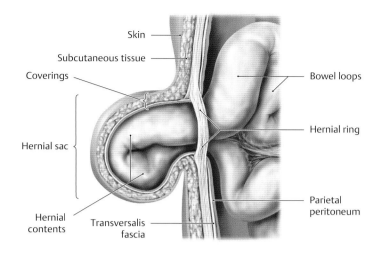

of greatest weakness (least resistance) in the abdominal wall. Occasionally, these weak spots cannot withstand a rise of intra-abdominal pressure, and openings are created for the herniation of abdominal viscera. The term "hernia" (L. *hernia* = "rupture") refers to the protrusion of parietal peritoneum through an anatomic opening (e.g., inguinal or femoral hernia) or a secondary defect (e.g., umbilical hernia). An *external hernia* is one that protrudes from the abdominal cavity and is visible on the body surface, while an *internal hernia* protrudes into a peritoneal pouch that is contained within the abdomen. Hernias are also classified by the time of their occurrence as *congenital* (e.g., umbilical hernia, indirect inguinal hernia through a patent processus vaginalis) or *acquired* (e.g., direct inguinal hernia, femoral hernia). The following components of a hernia are important in terms of surgical treatment:

Hernial opening: the orifice or defect through which the viscus herniates.

Hernial sac: the pouch, generally lined by parietal peritoneum, that contains the herniated viscus. Its size is highly variable, depending on the extent of the hernia.

Hernial contents: may be almost any intra-abdominal viscus but usually consist of greater omentum or loops of small bowel.

Coverings: the tissue layers surrounding the hernial sac. The composition of the coverings depends on the location and mechanism of the hernia.

C Definition, occurrence, and structure of an abdominal hernia

Between the thorax and bony pelvis is an extended skeletal gap that is covered by multiple abdominal wall layers composed of broad muscles, fasciae, aponeuroses, and peritoneum. The muscular foundation is deficient at certain locations, and the abdominal wall at those sites is formed entirely by connective-tissue structures. These are the areas

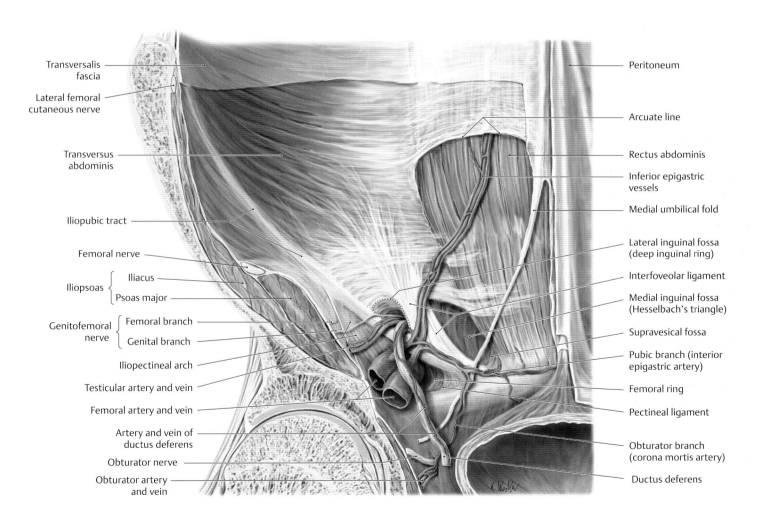

D Internal hernial openings in the male inguinal and femoral region

Detail from **A**, posterior view. The peritoneum and transversalis fascia have been partially removed to reveal the hernial openings more clearly. The internal openings (see **A** and **B**) for indirect and direct inguinal hernias, femoral hernias, and suprapubic (= supravesical) hernias are indicated by color shading.

13.9 Inguinal and Femoral Hernias

A Hernias of the groin region: inguinal and femoral hernias*

Hernia	Openings and course
• **Direct (medial) inguinal hernia** Always acquired	• *Internal opening:* medial inguinal fossa (Hesselbach's triangle), i.e., above the inguinal ligament and medial to the inferior epigastric artery and vein • *Course:* sac is perpendicular to the abdominal wall • *External opening:* superficial inguinal ring
• **Indirect (lateral) inguinal hernia** Congenital (patent processus vaginalis) or acquired	• *Internal opening:* deep inguinal ring, i.e., above the inguinal ligament and lateral to the inferior epigastric artery and vein • *Course:* sac passes through the inguinal canal • *External opening:* superficial inguinal ring
• **Femoral hernia** Always acquired	• *Internal opening:* femoral ring and septum, i.e., below the inguinal ligament and medial to the femoral artery and vein • *Course:* sac passes through the femoral canal below the fascia lata • *External opening:* saphenous opening

* 80% of all hernias are inguinal hernias (90% of which occur in males), and approximately 10% are femoral hernias (more common in females) (see also p. 216). Inguinal hernias are among the most common structural defects in humans, accounting for some 20% of all surgical operations.

Deep inguinal ring

Inguinal ligament

Location of inguinal canal

Femoral vessels

Inferior epigastric vessels

Superficial inguinal ring

Peritoneum of hernial sac

Transversalis fascia (= internal spermatic fascia)

Cremaster muscle and spermatic cord

B Congenital or acquired indirect inguinal hernia
Right male inguinal region with the skin and superficial body fascia removed, anterior view. The fascia lata of the thigh is shown transparent, and the spermatic cord is windowed. Regardless of the location of the *internal* opening, both *indirect (lateral)* and *direct (medial)* inguinal hernias (see **C**) emerge from the superficial inguinal ring above the inguinal ligament. Indirect inguinal hernias may be congenital (due to a patent processus vaginalis) or acquired and follow a tract parallel to the abdominal wall. The hernial sac enters the expanded deep inguinal ring (internal opening), which is lateral to the epigastric vessels, and passes medially and obliquely along the inguinal canal. Invested by the fascia enclosing the spermatic cord, it finally emerges at the superficial inguinal ring and descends into the scrotum. The coverings of all indirect inguinal hernias include the peritoneum and the transversalis fascia (internal spermatic fascia).

Inferior epigastric vessels

Inguinal ligament

Superficial inguinal ring

Femoral vessels

Cremasteric fascia

Sartorius and pectineus muscles, fascia lata

External oblique aponeurosis

Location of medial inguinal fossa (Hesselbach's triangle)

Transversalis fascia

Peritoneum of hernial sac

Cremaster muscle and spermatic cord

C Acquired direct inguinal hernia

Right inguinal region in the male with the skin and superficial fascia removed, anterior view. The fascia lata of the thigh is lightly shaded. Direct inguinal hernias are always acquired and follow a tract that is perpendicular to the abdominal wall. The hernia will leave the abdominal cavity medial to the inferior epigastric vessels within medial inguinal fossa (see p. 217). Such hernias may pass through the superficial inguinal ring, and in such instances the hernial sac is medial to the spermatic cord.

Rosenmüller lymph nodes (deep inguinal lymph nodes)

Femoral vessels in the saphenous opening

Peritoneum of hernial sac

Transversalis fascia

Fascia lata

Inferior epigastric vessels

Inguinal ligament

Superficial inguinal ring

Uterine round ligament

Lacunar ligament

Hernial sac

Great saphenous vein

D Acquired femoral hernia

Right female inguinal region with the skin and superficial fascia removed, anterior view. Femoral hernias are always acquired and are more common in women (broader pelvis and larger femoral ring). They always pass inferior to the inguinal ligament and medial to the femoral vein, extending through the femoral ring to enter the femoral canal (not visible here). The funnel-shaped canal begins at the femoral ring (the internal opening of the hernia, not visible here), ends approximately 2 cm inferiorly at the saphenous opening, and lies anterior to the pectineal fascia. The sharp-edged lacunar ligament forms the medial boundary of the femoral ring (risk of incarceration). Typically, the femoral canal is occupied by loose fatty and connective tissue and deep inguinal lymph nodes. Femoral hernias may emerge at the saphenous opening (external opening), which is covered by the thin cribriform fascia, and thus become subcutaneous.

13.10 Topographic Anatomy of Inguinal Hernias

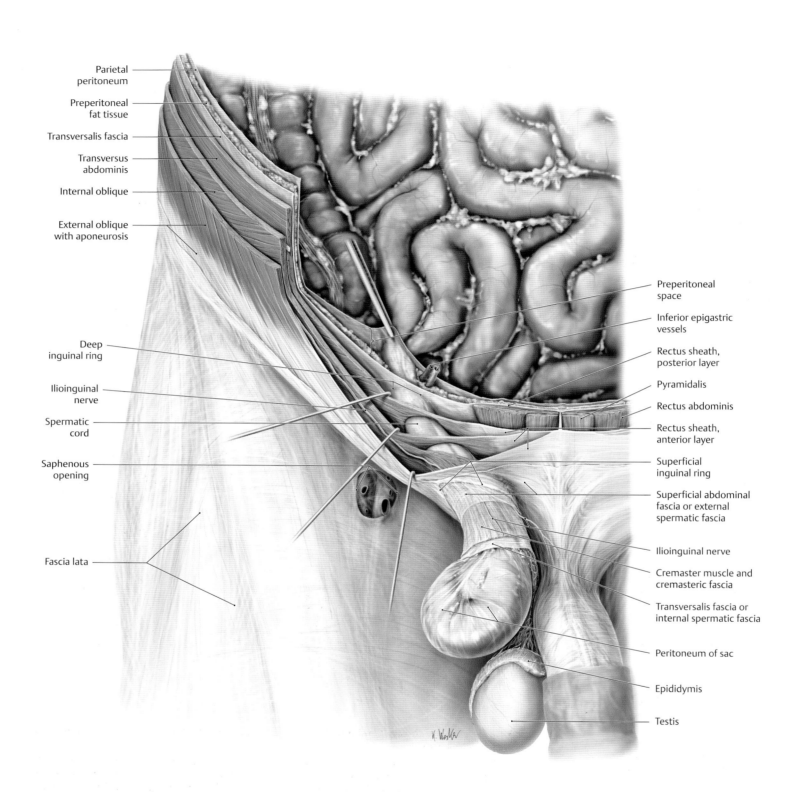

Parietal peritoneum
Preperitoneal fat tissue
Transversalis fascia
Transversus abdominis
Internal oblique
External oblique with aponeurosis
Deep inguinal ring
Ilioinguinal nerve
Spermatic cord
Saphenous opening
Fascia lata

Preperitoneal space
Inferior epigastric vessels
Rectus sheath, posterior layer
Pyramidalis
Rectus abdominis
Rectus sheath, anterior layer
Superficial inguinal ring
Superficial abdominal fascia or external spermatic fascia
Ilioinguinal nerve
Cremaster muscle and cremasteric fascia
Transversalis fascia or internal spermatic fascia
Peritoneum of sac
Epididymis
Testis

A Acquired, indirect inguinal hernia in a male (right side)
Anterior view, skin and abdominal walls largely removed. In the area of the inguinal canal that runs from upper lateral to lower medial, the individual abdominal wall muscles have been spread apart to reveal the relationship of structures. The hernial sac of the indirect inguinal hernia (a hernia that runs through the inguinal canal) containing an intestinal loop is visible. Because the hernial sac is within the spermatic cord, the hernia is covered by parietal peritoneum, transversalis fascia, and the cremaster muscle and cremasteric fascia.

B Schematic representation of the inguinal canal, the abdominal wall layers, and their continuation into the covering of the testes

Anterior view; several section planes have been combined in this schematic. The two arrows point to the lateral inguinal fossa (= deep inguinal ring) and the medial inguinal fossa (Hesselbach's triangle). The inferior epigastric vessels extend between them in the lateral umbilical fold. The lateral inguinal fossa is the internal hernial orifice for indirect inguinal hernias (see **Da**); the medial inguinal fossa, for direct inguinal hernias (see **Db**). Both types of inguinal hernias use the superficial inguinal ring as the external hernial orifice. *Note:* The tunica vaginalis with its visceral layer and parietal layer is the remnant of the obliterated processus vaginalis (**b**) (compare p. 224).

b   a

C Comparison of layers of the abdominal wall and the corresponding coverings of the spermatic cord and testes

The coverings of the spermatic cord and testes are derivatives of muscles and fasciae of the abdominal wall and envelop the spermatic cord and testes in a sac (scrotum), whose superficial layer is formed from the abdominal skin.

Abdominal wall layers	Coverings of the spermatic cord and testes
• Abdominal skin and membranous layer of superficial fascia	→ Scrotal skin with tunica dartos
• External oblique fascia	→ External spermatic fascia
• Internal oblique muscle and fascia	→ Cremaster muscle with cremasteric fascia
• Transversalis fascia	→ Internal spermatic fascia
• Peritoneum	→ Tunica vaginalis, parietal layer and visceral layer

a   b

D Comparison of indirect and direct inguinal hernias

a **Indirect inguinal hernia** (congenital or acquired): The inner hernial orifice (lateral inguinal fossa = deep inguinal ring) is lateral to the inferior epigastric vessels. The hernial contents (e.g., intestinal loops), which are enclosed by the parietal peritoneum, either push through the inguinal canal to the scrotum (acquired hernia) or move through the still-open processus vaginalis (see **Bb**) to the scrotum (congenital hernia). The hernial sac is made of the same elements in both cases: parietal peritoneum, transversalis fascia, and cremaster muscle.

b **Direct inguinal hernia** (acquired): The inner hernial orifice (medial inguinal fossa = Hesselbach's triangle) is medial to the inferior epigastric vessels. The hernial contents push directly through the abdominal wall and via the superficial inguinal ring to the scrotum. In comparison to indirect inguinal hernias, the hernial sac consists only of parietal peritoneum and transversalis fascia.

217

13.11 Diagnosis and Treatment of Hernias

a

b

A Technique for the examination of inguinal and femoral hernias
Hernias of the groin region, like most hernias, are typically precipitated by a rise of intra-abdominal pressure (e.g., due to coughing, sneezing, or straining) and present as a palpable bulge or swelling in the inguinal region. Usually this swelling regresses spontaneously when the patient lies down; thus, the clinical examination is performed with the patient in a standing position. Spontaneous pain is generally absent with an uncomplicated hernia, and a foreign body sensation is more common. Persistent pain accompanied by a feeling of pressure at the hernia site, nausea, and vomiting are signs of incarceration (see **C**). In patients with a bulge in the inguinal region or a scrotal mass (see p. 227), the differential diagnosis should include hydrocele, varicocele, ectopic testis, lymphoma, and other tumors of the testis or epididymis. Since inguinal and femoral hernias are of the external type and are easily accessible to inspection and palpation, the diagnosis is generally made clinically.

a Palpation from the iliac spine (the three-finger rule): The "three-finger rule" makes it easier to appreciate the topographical anatomy of inguinal and femoral hernias and differentiate among direct and indirect inguinal hernias and femoral hernias. When the examiner places the thenar eminence on the anterior superior iliac spine, the index finger points to a direct hernia, the middle finger to an indirect hernia, and the ring finger to a femoral hernia. Thus, when a hernia is felt below the index finger, for example, this means that the patient has a direct inguinal hernia.
Caution: The hernial sac protrudes through the superficial inguinal ring in both direct and indirect hernias, so there is no difference between them based on inspection or palpation.

b Palpation from the scrotum: This technique is particularly useful for palpating smaller inguinal hernias in the standing patient. By invaginating the scrotum and groin skin, the examiner palpates along the spermatic cord to the superficial inguinal ring and touches the posterior wall of the inguinal canal with the pad of the finger. When the patient coughs, an experienced examiner can distinguish a direct hernia, which strikes the pad of the finger, from an indirect hernia, which strikes the distal tip of the finger.

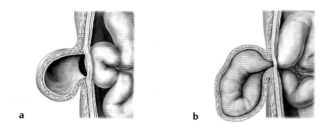

a   b

B Complete reduction of a hernia and an incarcerated hernia (strangulation)

a When the herniated viscus can move freely within the hernial sac

and at the hernial opening, generally the hernia can be reduced spontaneously (e.g., by lying down) or by manual manipulation. As a result, there is no risk of acute incarceration.

b Incarceration is the most serious complication of a hernia. Strangulation at the neck of the hernia restricts blood flow to the herniated bowel, with effects ranging from ischemia to necrosis. The patient may develop symptoms of a functional or mechanical bowel obstruction with a life-threatening interruption of intestinal transit due to narrowing or obstruction of the bowel lumen. Given the risk of bowel perforation and peritonitis in these cases, immediate surgery is indicated (see **C**).

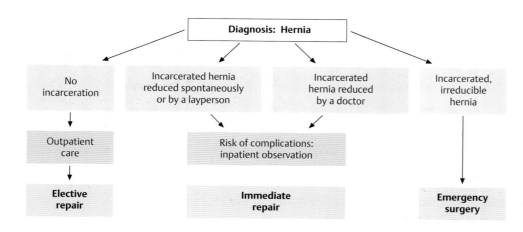

C Hernia symptoms and timing of the repair (after Henne-Bruns, Dürig, and Kremer)
As a rule, hernias do not respond definitively to conservative treatment (e.g., trusses or binders), and a permanent reduction is achieved only by surgical closure of the hernial opening (see **E**). The timing of the repair is based on the clinical presentation, i.e., the presence of a reducible, irreducible, or incarcerated hernia.

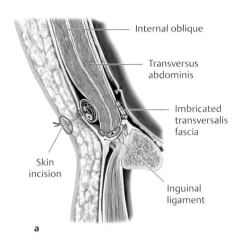

Internal oblique
Transversus abdominis
External oblique aponeurosis
Parietal peritoneum
Transversalis fascia
Subserosa
Ilioinguinal nerve
Pectineal ligament
Spermatic cord
Lacunar ligament
Inguinal ligament
Superior pubic ramus
Fascia lata
Pectineus

a

Hernial defect (Hesselbach's triangle)

b

D Condition after direct, acquired inguinal hernia
Sagittal sections through the male inguinal region: **a** normal; **b** direct, acquired inguinal hernia.

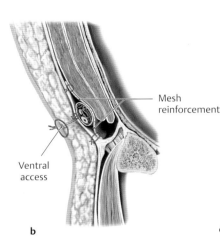

Internal oblique
Transversus abdominis
Imbricated transversalis fascia
Skin incision
Inguinal ligament

a

Mesh reinforcement
Ventral access

b

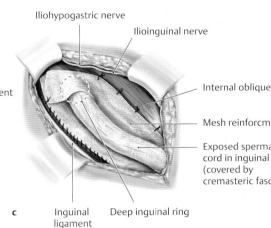

Iliohypogastric nerve
Ilioinguinal nerve
Internal oblique
Mesh reinforcment
Exposed spermatic cord in inguinal canal (covered by cremasteric fascia)
Inguinal ligament
Deep inguinal ring

c

E Inguinal hernia repair

Sagittal section through the male inguinal region.

Various surgical methods are available for hernia repair. They differ mainly in the technique used to reinforce the posterior wall of the inguinal canal. In all methods, the steps are as follows:
- Expose the hernial sac.
- Reduce the hernial contents.
- Close the hernial orifice and thus restore the stablility of the abdominal walls.

In younger patients, in which there is a strong relationship between fascia and muscle, reconstruction usually is performed without the use of foreign material to reinforce the abdominal wall (e.g., the Shouldice technique). In older patients or in the case of a recurring hernia, the abdominal wall is usually reinforced with a mesh patch (e.g., the Lichtenstein technique) during surgery.

a Shouldice technique: The posterior wall of the inguinal canal is reinforced by overlapping the transversalis fascia and suturing the internal oblique and transversus abdominis muscles to the inguinal ligament in two layers.

b, c Lichtenstein technique: With this tension-free repair, the abdominal wall is reinforced by placing a synthetic mesh patch posterior to the internal oblique and transversus abdominis.

d–f Mesh reinforcement through totally extraperitoneal (TEP) or transabdominal preperitoneal (TAPP) repair. The abdominal wall is reinforced by placing a mesh patch through a peritoneal incision anterior to the internal oblique and transversus abdominis in the preperitoneal space between the transversalis fascia and parietal peritoneum (**d**). Whereas in TEP the peritoneal cavity is not entered (extraperitoneal, **e**), in TAPP the parietal peritoneum has to be entered from inside the peritoneal cavity (transabdominal, **f**).

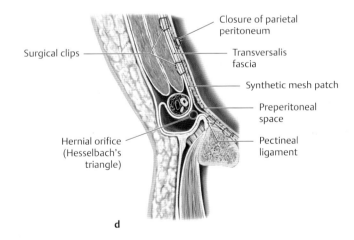

Surgical clips
Closure of parietal peritoneum
Transversalis fascia
Synthetic mesh patch
Preperitoneal space
Hernial orifice (Hesselbach's triangle)
Pectineal ligament

d

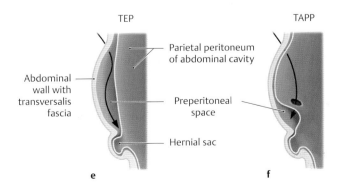

TEP
TAPP
Parietal peritoneum of abdominal cavity
Abdominal wall with transversalis fascia
Preperitoneal space
Hernial sac

e

f

219

13.12 Rare External Hernias

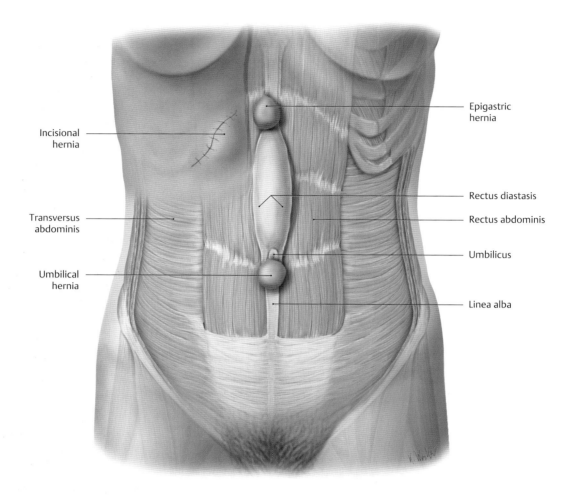

Incisional hernia

Transversus abdominis

Umbilical hernia

Epigastric hernia

Rectus diastasis

Rectus abdominis

Umbilicus

Linea alba

A Location of hernias in the anterior abdominal wall

B Hernias of the anterior abdominal wall*

Hernia	Location, occurrence, and typical features

• **Umbilical hernia**	• Umbilical region, passing through the umbilical ring:
	  – Congenital umbilical hernia: incomplete regression of the normal fetal umbilical hernia due to scarring of the umbilical papilla (hernial sac: amnion and peritoneum)
	  – Acquired umbilical hernia: common after multiple pregnancies, also in association with obesity, hepatic cirrhosis, or ascites (secondary widening of the umbilical ring)

• **Omphalocele**	• Congenital persistence (1:6000) of an abdominal wall defect with an incomplete reduction of abdominal viscera during fetal life; unlike an umbilical hernia, the omphalocele is not covered by skin or subcutaneous tissue but only by peritoneum, mucous connective tissue (Wharton jelly), and amniotic epithelium (so the contents are easily recognized)
• **Epigastric hernia**	• The hernial openings are gaps in the linea alba excluding the umbilicus (on a continuum with rectus diastasis, see below)
• **Rectus diastasis**	• The rectus muscles separate at the linea alba when the abdominal muscles are tightened, creating a site for potential herniation (the hernia reduces on relaxation, and complaints are rare)
• **Incisional hernia**	• Occurs at a previous incision site (usually in the upper abdominal midline)

*Umbilical and epigastric hernias comprise approximately 10% of all hernias.

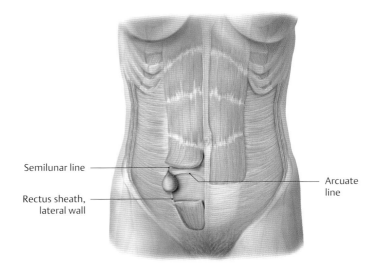

Semilunar line

Rectus sheath, lateral wall

Arcuate line

D Spigelian hernia

C Other rare hernias occurring elsewhere on the trunk*

Hernia	Location
• **Spigelian hernia**	• Anterior abdominal wall between the semilunar line and lateral rectus sheath, usually at the level of the arcuate line
• **Lumbar hernia**	• Between the twelfth rib and iliac crest: – Superior lumbar hernia (superior costolumbar triangle, Grynfeltt's triangle): between the twelfth rib and iliocostalis – Inferior lumbar hernia (inferior iliolumbar triangle, Petit's triangle): between the iliac crest, latissimus dorsi, and externus oblique muscles
• **Obturator hernia**	• Through the obturator foramen and then between the pectineus, adductor longus, and obturator externus muscles
• **Sciatic hernia**	• Through the greater sciatic foramen: – Suprapiriform hernia (above the piriformis muscle) – Infrapiriform hernia (below the piriformis muscle) – Spinotuberous hernia (in front of the sacrotuberous ligament)
• **Perineal hernia**	• Through the pelvic floor: – Anterior perineal hernia (in front of the deep transverse perineal) – Posterior perineal hernia (behind the deep transverse perineal) – Ischiorectal hernia (through the levator ani into the ischioanal fossa)

*Less than 1% of all hernias, generally acquired (after Schumpelick).

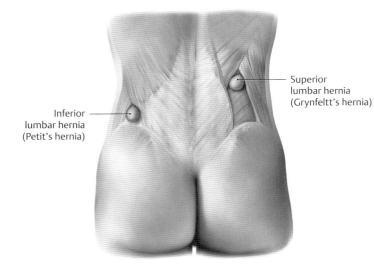

Inferior lumbar hernia (Petit's hernia)

Superior lumbar hernia (Grynfeltt's hernia)

E Lumbar hernia

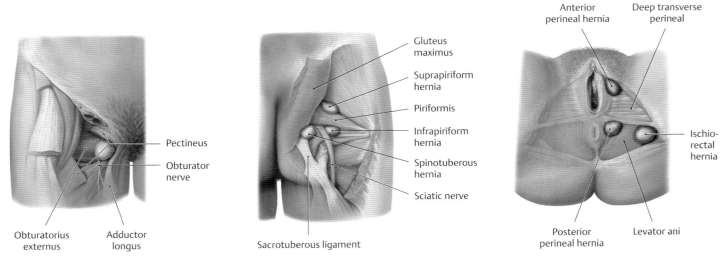

Pectineus

Obturator nerve

Obturatorius externus

Adductor longus

F Obturator hernia

Gluteus maximus

Suprapiriform hernia

Piriformis

Infrapiriform hernia

Spinotuberous hernia

Sciatic nerve

Sacrotuberous ligament

G Sciatic hernia

Anterior perineal hernia

Deep transverse perineal

Ischio-rectal hernia

Posterior perineal hernia

Levator ani

H Perineal hernia

13.13 Development of the External Genitalia

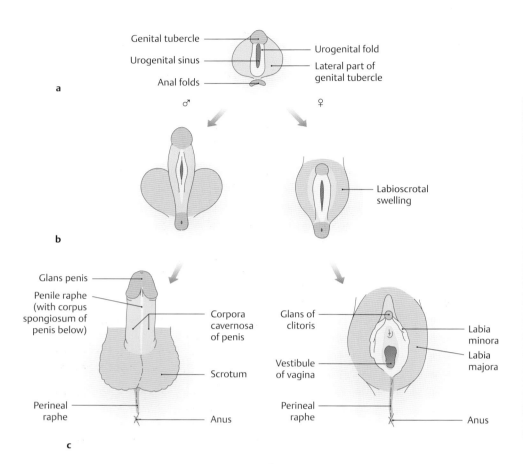

B Derivatives of the undifferentiated embryonic genital anlage (primordia) during development of the external genital organs (after Starck)*

Undiffe-rentiated anlage	Male	Female
Genital tubercles	Glans penis, corpora caver-nosa of penis	Clitoris, glans of clitoris
Urogenital folds	Penile raphe, corpus spongiosum of penis	Labia minora
Genital swellings	Scrotum	Labia majora
Urogenital sinus	Spongy part of urethra	Vestibule of vagina
Anal folds	Perineal raphe	Perineal raphe

*Details on the development of the gonads and genital tracts can be found in text-books of embryology.

A Development of the external genitalia

a Rudimentary, undifferentiated external genitalia in a 6-week-old embryo.

b Differentiation of the external genitalia along male or female lines in a 10-week-old fetus.

c Differentiated external genitalia in the newborn.

The external genital organs develop from an undifferentiated mesoder-mal primordium in the *cloaca* and, like the gonads, pass through an ini-tial **indifferent stage**. The anorectal area and urogenital sinus (cloaca) are not yet separated from each other and are closed externally by a common cloacal membrane. The following elevations develop around the cloacal membrane due to intensive mesodermal cell divisions:

- Anterior: the genital tubercles
- Lateral: the urogenital folds
- Posterior: the anal folds
- Lateral to the urogenital folds: the genital swellings (labioscrotal swellings)

Later, between the sixth and seventh weeks of development, the uro-rectal septum divides the cloaca into an anterior part (urogenital sinus) and a posterior part (anus and rectum). The cloacal membrane disap-pears, and the urogenital ostium forms anteriorly. The early perineum forms at the level of the urorectal septum (by fusion of the paired anal folds to the perineal raphe). **Differentiation of the genital organs** begins approximately in the eighth to ninth week of fetal development. Sexual differentiation is clearly evident by the 13th week and is fully developed by the 16th week.

- In the *male fetus,* the genital tubercles enlarge *under the influence of testosterone* to form the phallus and future penis. The urogenital sinus closes completely by fusion of the genital folds and forms the spongy part of the urethra. The genital (scrotal) swellings unite to form the scrotum.
- In the *female fetus (absence of testosterone),* the genital tubercles give rise to the clitoris. The urogenital sinus persists as the vestibule of the vagina, and the two genital folds form the labia minora. The genital swellings enlarge to form the labia majora.

Male sex organs develop only in the presence of the factors listed below:

- A functionally competent *SRY (sex-determining region of the Y) gene* on the Y chromosome (otherwise, ovaries and a female phenotype will develop). The SRY gene ensures that anti-müllerian hormone and Leydig cells are produced (see below).
- Among its other functions, the *anti-müllerian hormone* induces regression of the müllerian ducts. It is formed in the somatic cells of the testicular cords (future Sertoli cells) starting in the eighth week of fetal life.
- *Leydig cells* begin to form in the fetal testes by the ninth week and produce large amounts of androgens (testosterone) until birth. They stimulate differentiation of the *wolffian duct* into seminiferous tubules and the development of the male external genitalia.

Alteration or interruption of this process of differentiation at any stage can lead to incomplete midline fusion, which leaves persistent clefts (hypospadias, epispadias, see **C**), or to more extensive external genital anomalies (see **E**) (after Starck).

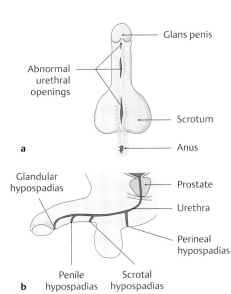

a

b

Glans penis

Abnormal urethral openings

Scrotum

Anus

Glandular hypospadias

Prostate

Urethra

Perineal hypospadias

Penile hypospadias

Scrotal hypospadias

C Hypospadias: a urethral anomaly in boys

a Cleft anomalies affecting the underside of the penis and scrotum.

b Possible sites of emergence of the urethra in hypospadias (penis viewed from the lateral view).

If the genital folds do not fuse completely during sexual differentiation (see **A**), the result is a cleft anomaly of the urethra, which may open on the underside of the penis (*hypospadias*) or on its dorsal surface (*epispadias*). Hypospadias is much more common, with an incidence of 1:3000 compared to 1:100,000 for epispadias. It is most common to find an abnormal urethral orifice in the glans region of the penis (glandular hypospadias). Additionally, the shaft of the penis is usually shortened and angled downward by the presence of ventral fibrous bands. Surgical correction is generally performed between the sixth month and second year of life (after Sökeland, Schulze, and Rübben).

Clitoris

Vagina

Anus

Urethral orifice

D External genitalia of a woman with adrenogenital syndrome

Anterior view. The external genitalia show definite signs of masculinization. The clitoris is markedly enlarged. The labia majora and minora are partially fused, and the urogenital sinus forms an undersized vestibule (see **E**, female pseudohermaphroditism).

E Various forms of intersexuality*

Condition	Features
• **True hermaph-roditism****	• Very rare form of hermaphroditism (approximately 70% of cases have a female karyotype: 46,XX). The gonads contain both testicular and ovarian tissue *(ototestis)*, but with a preponderance of ovarian tissue. Hence the external genitalia tend to have a female appearance with a markedly enlarged clitoris. A uterus is frequently present. Most hermaphrodites are raised as girls.
• **Pseudohermaph-roditism**	• The pseudohermaphrodite has a definite chromosomal sex (female: 46,XX or male: 46,XY) but a phenotype of the *opposite* gender. The condition is termed male pseudohermaphroditism when a testis is present and female pseudohermaphroditism when an ovary is present.
– *Male pseudo-hermaphroditism* → Chromosomal sex: male (46,XY) → Phenotype: female	• **Etiology and pathogenesis** The female phenotype results from a lack of fetal androgen exposure: 1. Disturbance of testosterone synthesis 2. Disturbance of testosterone conversion 3. Androgen receptor defect 4. Testicular dysgenesis • **Example: testicular feminization** (1:20,000 live births): – 46,XY chromosome complement – Individual has a female phenotype (estrogen synthesis present) but lacks pubic and axillary hair ("hairless woman"). The upper vagina and uterus are also absent. – *Cause:* androgen receptor defect or a disturbance of androgen metabolism (5α-reductase-2 defect) – *Result:* absence of spermatogenesis – *Treatment:* removal of the testes, which are usually in the inguinal region (risk of malignant transformation) and estrogen replacement for life
– *Female pseudo-hermaphroditism* → Chromosomal sex: female (46,XX) → Phenotype: male	• **Etiology and pathogenesis** The male phenotype results from fetal androgen exposure: 1. Congenital enzyme defect 2. Diaplacental androgen exposure • **Example: congenital adrenogenital syndrome** (1:5000 live births): – 46,XX chromosome complement – Female internal genital organs with masculinized *external* genitalia (enlarged clitoris, partial fusion of the labia majora, small urogenital sinus, see **D**) – *Cause:* adrenocortical hyperplasia with impaired steroid synthesis based on a genetic enzyme defect (most commonly a 21-hydroxylase deficiency). The low hormone level causes increased adrenocorticotropic hormone secretion, leading to the overproduction of androgens. – *Treatment:* hydrocortisone therapy for life, which may be combined with a mineralocorticoid.

* Intersexuality refers to a condition marked by contradictions in the development of general external sex characteristics, the gonads, and the chromosomal sex.
** Named after Hermaphroditos, the androgynous son of Hermes and Aphrodite from Greek mythology.

13.14 Male External Genitalia: Testicular Descent and the Spermatic Cord

a Second month, **b** third month, **c** at birth, **d** after obliteration of the processus vaginalis of the peritoneum.

A Overview of the male genital organs

The internal and external male genitalia are distinguished by their *origins*. The internal reproductive organs originate from the two urogenital ridges located above the pelvic floor (except for the prostate and bulbourethral glands, which develop from urethral epithelium and thus are derivatives of the urogenital sinus). By contrast, the external genital organs develop around the urogenital sinus from a genital anlage (primordium) located below the pelvic floor (see p. 222).

Male internal genital organs	Male external genital organs

• Testes
• Epididymis
• Ductus deferens (vas deferens)
• Accessory sex glands
  – Prostate
  – Seminal glands
  – Bulbourethral glands
  (Cowper's glands)
	• Penis
	• Scrotum
	• Coverings of the testis

Topographically, however, the testis, epididymis, and a portion of the ductus deferens are classified among the external genital organs because they migrate from the abdominal cavity into the scrotum during fetal development (testicular descent).

C Anomalous position of the testes

Abnormalities in the descent of the tests occur in approximately 3% of all newborns. A testis may be retained in the abdominal cavity or in the inguinal canal (cryptorchidism or retained testis). A deficiency of androgen production is the presumed cause. An ectopic testis is one that strays from the normal tract and occupies an abnormal position. The principal results are infertility due to the higher ambient temperature and an increased risk of malignant transformation.

B Descent of a testis

Lateral view.

a Second month, **b** third month, **c** at birth, **d** after obliteration of the processus vaginalis of the peritoneum.

Near the end of the second month of development, the gonads and the rest of the mesonephros lie in a common peritoneal fold (urogenital fold), from which the "gonadal ligaments" are derived after regression of the mesonephros. The lower gonadal ligament, called the gubernaculum, is important for the descent of the testis. It passes below the genital ducts, pierces the abdominal wall in the area of the inguinal canal, and ends in the labioscrotal swelling, an outpouching of the anterior abdominal wall. Traction from this gonadal ligament (a consequence of body growth, which is more rapid than the growth of the genital organs) causes the testis and epididymis to slide downward along the posterior trunk wall external to the peritoneum **(transabdominal descent)**. By the start of the third month, the testis has already reached the entrance of the future inguinal canal. The processus vaginalis, a funnel-shaped outpouching of peritoneum, forms anterior to the gubernaculum and is continued into the scrotal swelling with the other layers of the abdominal wall. It gives rise to the coverings of the spermatic cord and testis after the testis has completed its descent. A second phase, which is completed shortly before birth **(transinguinal descent)**, culminates in passage of the testis through the inguinal canal into the scrotum. After testicular descent is completed (by birth), the processus vaginalis is obliterated except for a small space that partially surrounds the testis as the scrotal cavity (tunica vaginalis of the testis with a visceral layer and a parietal layer, see p. 226). Failure of this process of obliteration results in a persistent communication between the abdominal cavity and testicular cavity (congenital indirect inguinal hernia, see p. 214) (after Starck).

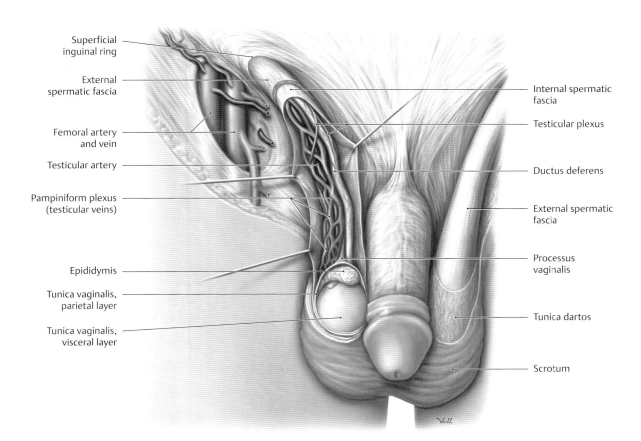

Superficial inguinal ring

External spermatic fascia

Femoral artery and vein

Testicular artery

Pampiniform plexus (testicular veins)

Epididymis

Tunica vaginalis, parietal layer

Tunica vaginalis, visceral layer

Internal spermatic fascia

Testicular plexus

Ductus deferens

External spermatic fascia

Processus vaginalis

Tunica dartos

Scrotum

D The penis, scrotum, and spermatic cord

Anterior view. The skin has been partially removed from over the scrotum and spermatic cord. The tunica dartos and external spermatic fascia are exposed on the left side, and the spermatic cord on the right side has been opened in layers. The skin of the scrotum differs in many respects from the skin of the abdominal wall. It is more pigmented, markedly thinner, more mobile, and devoid of subcutaneous fat. It also contains a network of myofibroblasts (tunica dartos), whose contraction causes a wrinkling of the skin. This reduces the surface area of the scrotum and, when accompanied by vasoconstriction of the cutaneous vessels, reduces heat loss from the testes. This mechanism regulates the temperature to optimize spermatogenesis.

E Contents of the spermatic cord

Cross section through the spermatic cord. The neurovascular structures that supply the testes converge at the level of the deep inguinal ring, forming a bundle the thickness of the small finger that is held together by loose connective tissue and by the coverings of the spermatic cord and testes. The coverings consist of the following structures:

- Cremasteric fascia with the cremaster muscle
- Genital branch of the genitofemoral nerve
- Cremasteric artery and vein
- Ductus deferens
- Artery and vein of the ductus deferens
- Testicular artery
- Testicular veins (pampiniform plexus)
- Autonomic nerve fibers (testicular plexus)
- Lymphatic vessels
- The obliterated processus vaginalis

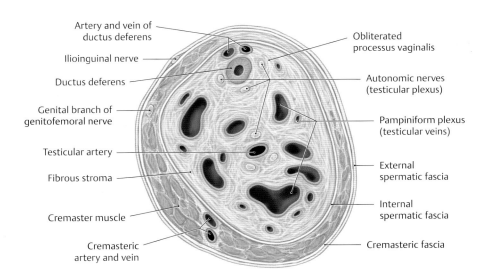

Artery and vein of ductus deferens

Ilioinguinal nerve

Ductus deferens

Genital branch of genitofemoral nerve

Testicular artery

Fibrous stroma

Cremaster muscle

Cremasteric artery and vein

Obliterated processus vaginalis

Autonomic nerves (testicular plexus)

Pampiniform plexus (testicular veins)

External spermatic fascia

Internal spermatic fascia

Cremasteric fascia

Special features: The large veins of the pampiniform plexus are exceptionally thick-walled, with a three-layered structure, and hence are easily mistaken for arteries. In life the ductus deferens, with its compact muscular wall, is palpable through the skin as a firm cord the thickness of a knitting needle. The ease of surgical access to this site is utilized in *vasectomy,* or ligation of the ductus deferens, to interrupt the transport of sperm (sterilization).

13.15 Male External Genitalia: The Testis and Epididymis

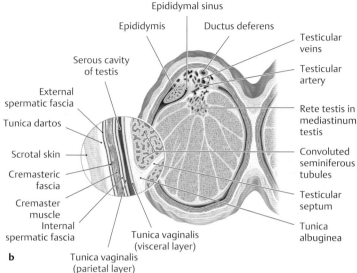

a

b

A Tunica vaginalis and serous cavity of the testis

a Opened tunica vaginalis of the left testis, lateral view.
b Cross section through the testis, epididymis, and scrotum, superior view.

The tunica vaginalis (unobliterated end of the processus vaginalis, see p. 224) forms a serous coat surrounding the testis and epididymis. Its visceral layer is fused to the tunica albuginea of the testis. At the mediastinum testis (a suspensory ligament where nerves and vessels enter and leave the testis), the tunica vaginalis is reflected to form the parietal layer, which is covered externally by the internal spermatic fascia. Between the two layers is a slitlike mesothelium-lined space (serous cavity of the testis) that contains a scant amount of fluid and is partially continuous between the testis and epididymis (epididymal sinus). An abnormal fluid collection in this cavity is called a *testicular hydrocele* (see **Fb**) (after Rauber and Kopsch).

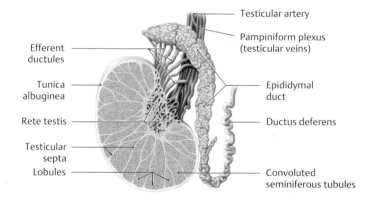

B Surface anatomy of the testis and epididymis

Left testis and epididymis, lateral view. The combined weight of the testis and epididymis at sexual maturity is approximately 20 to 30 g. The *testis* has an ovoid shape (approximately 5 cm long and 3 cm wide) and an average volume of approximately 18 mL (12–20 mL). The testicular tissue is enclosed in a tough fibrous capsule (tunica albuginea) and has a rubbery consistency. The *epididymis* consists of a head, which is attached to the upper pole of the testis, and a body and tail that curve down along the mediastinum on the posterior side of the testis. The tail of the epididymis becomes continuous with the ductus deferens at the lower pole of the testis.

C Structure of the testis and epididymis

Section through the testis (epididymis intact), lateral view. Fibrous testicular septa extend radially from the tunica albuginea of the testis toward the mediastinum testis, subdividing the testicular tissue into approximately 370 wedge-shaped lobules. Each lobule contains one or more convoluted seminiferous tubules, in whose epithelium the spermatocytes are formed (spermatogenesis, see p. 5) and which open into the rete testis. From there, approximately 10 to 15 efferent ductules pass to the head of the epididymis, where the epididymal duct begins. This single duct is continuous distally with the ductus deferens, which passes through the inguinal canal in the spermatic cord to enter the abdominal cavity and opens into the prostatic part of the urethra via a short intervening segment, the ejaculatory duct (see p. 229).

a

b

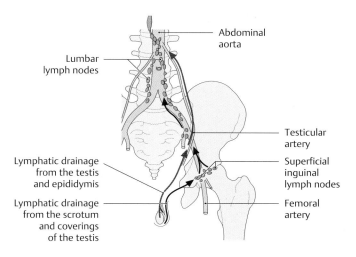

D Blood supply of the testis

a Arterial supply: The testis, epididymis, and their coverings are supplied by three different arteries, which anastomose with one another (after Hundeiker and Keller, quoted in Rauber and Kopsch):

- Testicular artery: arises directly from the aorta
- Artery of the ductus deferens: arises from the internal iliac artery
- Cremasteric artery: arises from the inferior epigastric artery

The vessels supplying the scrotum arise from the internal pudendal artery (see p. 556).

b Different venous drainage patterns of the right and left testes: Venous blood from the testis and epididymis flows into the testicular veins in the area of the mediastinum testis. These veins form an elongated venous network, especially distally, called the pampiniform plexus. It surrounds the branches of the testicular artery and ascends with it through the inguinal canal into the retroperitoneum. There the *right* testicular vein empties into the inferior vena cava, while the *left* testicular vein opens into the left renal vein. This asymmetry of venous drainage has major clinical relevance: the left testicular vein enters the left renal vein at a right angle. This creates a physiologically significant constriction that can obstruct venous outflow from the left testicular vein and thus from the pampiniform plexus (varicocele, see **Fd**). In this case, the pampiniform plexus can no longer perform its "thermostat" function (cooling venous blood returning from the testicular artery), resulting in a local heat buildup that may compromise the fertility of the left testis.

E Lymphatic drainage and regional lymph nodes of the testis, the epididymis, the coverings of the testis, and the scrotum

The lymphatic vessels of the testis and epididymis drain to the lumbar lymph nodes, accompanied by the testicular vessels. The lymphatic vessels from the scrotum and the coverings of the testis drain to the superficial inguinal nodes (see p. 528).

Note: Advanced testicular tumors tend to metastasize to retroperitoneal lymph nodes because they serve as the primary lymphatic conduit from the testis and epididymis.

F Abnormal findings on clinical examination of the external genitalia

a–f Diseases that may present with scrotal swelling: a inguinal hernia, **b** testicular hydrocele (serous fluid collection in the serous cavity of the testis), **c** spermatocele (retention cyst in the epididymis), **d** varicocele (painful, varicose dilation of the pampiniform plexus), **e** epididymitis (painful bacterial inflammation of the epididymis), **f** testicular tumor (painless, usually unilateral induration of the testis).

g Bimanual examination of the testis and epididymis: Clinical examination of the external genitalia should include palpation of the testis and epididymis (bimanual examination). Based on the disease features noted above, the following questions should be addressed during the clinical examination:

- Is the mass confined to the scrotum?
- Is there transient enlargement of the mass when the patient coughs?
- Is the mass translucent when examined by *transillumination* (illumination with a flashlight)?
- Is the mass painless or tender to pressure?

Note: A painless induration of the testis, especially in young men, should always raise suspicion of a testicular tumor (after Sökeland, Schulze, and Rübben).

13.16 Male External Genitalia: The Fasciae and Erectile Tissues of the Penis

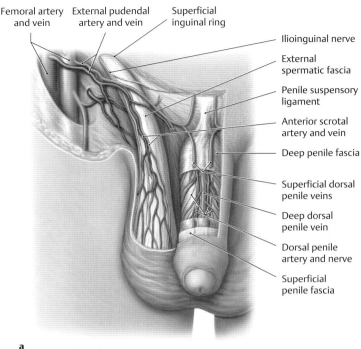

Femoral artery and vein — External pudendal artery and vein — Superficial inguinal ring

Ilioinguinal nerve

External spermatic fascia

Penile suspensory ligament

Anterior scrotal artery and vein

Deep penile fascia

Superficial dorsal penile veins

Deep dorsal penile vein

Dorsal penile artery and nerve

Superficial penile fascia

a

A Arrangement of the penile fasciae
a Anterior view of the penis (skin and fasciae partially removed).
b Right lateral view of the penis (skin and fasciae partially removed).
c Cross section through the shaft of the penis.

The penis is covered by thin, mobile skin that is devoid of fatty tissue. The skin over the glans penis is duplicated to form the prepuce (foreskin), which is attached to the undersurface of the glans by the median fold of the frenulum (see **b**). The erectile tissues of the penis are surrounded by a common, strong envelope of collagenous fibers, the *tunica albuginea*. The two layers of the penile fascia (superficial and deep) also surround the corpus spongiosum and corpora cavernosa. The erectile tissues, their fibrous sheaths, and the way in which the vessels are incorporated into these fibrous sheaths are of key interest in understanding the function of the penis (see p. 231).

Superficial penile fascia — Superficial dorsal penile vein — Dorsal penile artery and nerve, branch of the deep dorsal penile vein — Prepuce

Corona of glans

Glans penis

External urethral orifice

Frenulum

Penile skin — Deep penile fascia — Corpus cavernosum and corpus spongiosum with tunica albuginea

b

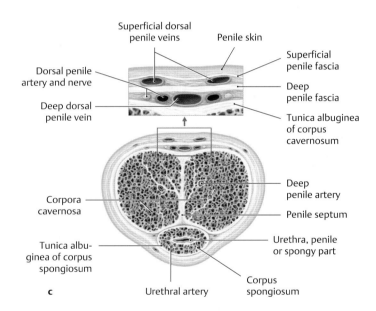

Superficial dorsal penile veins — Penile skin

Dorsal penile artery and nerve

Deep dorsal penile vein

Superficial penile fascia

Deep penile fascia

Tunica albuginea of corpus cavernosum

Corpora cavernosa

Deep penile artery

Penile septum

Tunica albuginea of corpus spongiosum

Urethra, penile or spongy part

Urethral artery

Corpus spongiosum

c

B Constriction of the prepuce (phimosis)
a Constriction of the prepuce in a 3-year-old boy.
b Appearance following circumcision.

The epithelium of the inner layer of the prepuce is adherent to the surface epithelium of the glans penis in newborns and infants. Because of this, the distal junction of the outer and inner layers of the prepuce is normally constricted, a condition characterized as **physiological phimosis**. During the first 2 years of life, the epithelial attachments become separated due to enlargement of the glans and the secretion of smegma (cellular debris sloughed from the stratified keratinized epithelium). If the prepuce still cannot slide over the glans by 3 years of age due to a functional stenosis (e.g., persistent epithelial attachments due to an absence of smegma secretion), the phimosis should be surgically corrected by circumcision. This procedure may be conservative or radical, resecting all the foreskin (as shown here), depending on the severity of the phimosis. Immediate surgical intervention (before 3 years of age) is necessary for **paraphimosis**—an emergency situation in which the glans is strangulated by the narrowed foreskin (painful, livid swelling of the glans due to decreased blood flow, with risk of necrosis) (after Sökeland, Schulze, and Rübben).

a

b

C The erectile tissues and erectile muscles of the penis

a Inferior view. The corpus spongiosum is partially mobilized, and the skin and fasciae have been removed. The ischiocavernosus and bulbospongiosus muscles have been removed on the left side, along with the inferior fascia of the urogenital diaphragm.

b Cross section through the root of the penis. The root of the penis is firmly attached to the perineal membrane and pelvic skeleton. It is distinguished from the freely mobile shaft (body) of the penis, with its dorsal and urethral surfaces, and from the glans penis, which bears the external urethral orifice. The penis contains two types of erectile tissue:

- The paired corpora cavernosa
- The unpaired corpus spongiosum

At the root of the penis, each of the corpora cavernosa tapers to form a crus penis. Between the two crura lies the thickened end of the corpus spongiosum, the bulb of the penis. The glans penis forms the distal end of the corpus spongiosum. Its posterior margin is broadened to form the corona, which is turned over the ends of the corpora cavernosa. The erectile tissues receive their blood supply from branches of the internal pudendal artery, which branches in the deep perineal space (see pp.183 and 230).

a

b

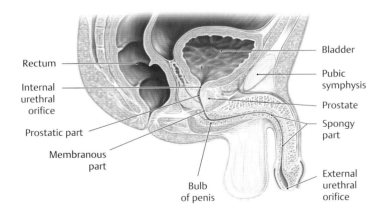

D Course of the male urethra

Midsagittal section through a male pelvis. The male urethra consists of a prostatic part, a membranous part, and a penile or spongy part named for different regions of the pelvis and external genitalia (see p. 224). The spongy part begins where it enters the bulb of the penis and terminates at the external urethral orifice.

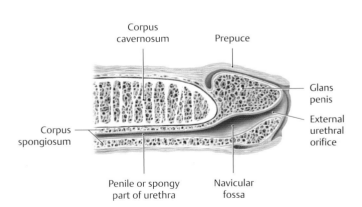

E Midsagittal section through the distal penis

The spongy part of the urethra undergoes an approximately 2-cm-long fusiform dilation within the glans penis. In this area, the navicular fossa, the stratified columnar epithelium of the urethra, gives way to stratified, nonkeratinized squamous epithelium. The upper cell layers of this epithelium are rich in glycogen, which—as in the vaginal milieu in females—provides a culture medium for the lactic acid bacteria that thrive there (acidic pH protects against pathogenic organisms).

229

13.17 Male External Genitalia: Nerves and Vessels of the Penis

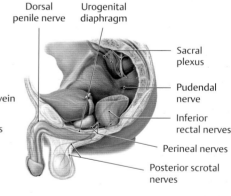

A Neurovascular structures of the male perineal region

Lithotomy position with the scrotum removed, inferior view. The superficial perineal space on the right side has been opened by removing the superficial perineal fascia. The erectile muscles and root of the penis have been removed on the left side, and the deep perineal space is partially exposed. The penis has been transected across the shaft, and the spermatic cords have been divided.

B Dorsal vessels and nerves of the penis

The prepuce, skin, and superficial fascia have been completely removed from the penile shaft. The deep penile fascia has also been removed from the left dorsum.

C Arterial supply to the penis and scrotum

Left lateral view. The penis and scrotum derive their arterial supply from the internal pudendal artery. This vessel enters the ischioanal fossa and, after giving off the inferior rectal artery to the anus, courses to the posterior border of the urogenital diaphragm. Then, after giving off the perineal artery, it passes through the deep perineal space into the superficial perineal space (see p.183), where it divides into its terminal branches: the dorsal penile artery, deep penile artery, bulbar penile artery, and urethral artery.

D Venous drainage of the penis and scrotum

Left lateral view. The veins of the penis (especially the deep dorsal penile vein and its tributaries, the deep penile and bulbar penile veins) open initially into the internal pudendal vein and then into the prostatic venous plexus. Exceptions are the superficial dorsal penile veins (not seen here), which drain via the external pudendal veins into the long saphenous vein. On its way to the prostatic venous plexus, the deep dorsal penile vein passes through a narrow space just below the symphysis between the arcuate pubic ligament and the transverse perineal ligament (see ligaments in **A**).

E Nerve supply to the penis and scrotum

Left lateral view. The pudendal nerve enters the ischioanal fossa and, after giving off the inferior rectal nerves, courses to the external anal sphincter and to the skin of the anus at the posterior border of the urogenital diaphragm. There it divides into its terminal branches, the perineal nerves. The superficial branches pass through the superficial perineal space to the skin of the perineum and posterior scrotum (posterior scrotal branches). The deep branches course in the deep perineal space. They innervate the erectile muscles (via muscular branches), the skin of the penis, and the erectile bodies (via the dorsal penile nerve). The course of the autonomic fibers is shown in **F**.

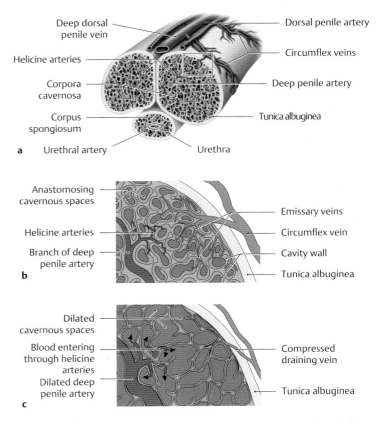

F Overview of the male sexual reflexes

The sexual reflexes in males are evoked by a variety of stimuli (e.g., tactile, visual, olfactory, acoustic, and psychogenic). Somatic and autonomic nerve pathways transmit the stimulus to the erection and ejaculation centers in the thoracolumbar and sacral spinal cord, from which it is relayed to higher centers (e.g., the hypothalamus and limbic system). For example, *tactile cutaneous stimuli* to the genitalia are transmitted to the sacral cord by *afferent somatic* fibers (dorsal penile nerve from the pudendal nerve, shown in green) and are relayed in the erection center (S2–S4) to *efferent parasympathetic* fibers (pelvic splanchnic nerves, shown in blue). These impulses, which stimulate vasodilation of the arteries supplying the erectile tissues (see **G**), are critically influenced by descending pathways from higher centers. Conversely, the excitatory impulses evoked by increasing mechanical stimulation of the glans penis ascend from the sacral cord to the ejaculation center located at the T12–L2 levels. There they are relayed to *efferent sympathetic* fibers (hypogastric nerves, shown in purple) and stimulate smooth muscle contractions in the epididymis, ductus deferens, prostate, and seminal glands. Simultaneous stimulation of the erectile muscles by efferent *somatic* nerve fibers (perineal nerves from the pudendal nerve, shown in red) produces rhythmic contractions that expel the ejaculate from the urethra (emission). Failure to achieve an erection despite an active libido (psychological interest in sexual activity) is defined as erectile dysfunction. The recent development of successful medical treatment of *erectile dysfunction* with sildenafil (Viagra [Pfizer]) is based on its modulation of the second messenger cyclic guanosine monophosphate (cGMP). When the primary messenger nitrous oxide (NO) is released by neural stimulation, it activates the enzyme guanylate cyclase in penile erectile tissues. This enzyme generates cGMP as a second messenger, which in turn induces vasodilation and produces an erection. Sildenafil selectively inhibits cGMP breakdown by a specific phosphodiesterase (PDE5) that is prominent in erectile tissue. cGMP accumulates, vessels remain dilated, and penile erection is sustained. Sildenafil treatment thus effectively amplifies the initial neural stimuli, with the potential of prolonging normal erections and overcoming other, inhibitory physiological problems (after Klinke and Silbernagl).

G Mechanism of penile erection (after Lehnert)

a Penis in cross section, showing the blood vessels involved in erection (enlarged views in **b** and **c**).
b Corpus cavernosum in the flaccid state.
c Corpus cavernosum in the erect state.

Penile erection is based essentially on *maximum engorgement* and pressure elevation in the cavities (cavernous spaces) of the corpora cavernosa combined with a *constriction of venous outflow*. This mechanism raises the intracavernous blood pressure to approximately 10 times the normal systolic blood pressure (approximately 1200 mmHg in youngmen). Microscopically, the erectile tissue of the penis consists of an arborized trabecular meshwork of connective-tissue and smooth-muscle cells that is connected to the tunica albuginea. Among the trabeculae are interanastomosing cavities that are lined with endothelium. Branches of the deep penile artery, called the helicine arteries, open into these cavities. In the flaccid state, the helicine arteries are more or less occluded by "intimal pads." When an erection occurs, the afferent arteries dilate, and the helicine arteries open under the influence of the autonomic nervous system. The result is that with each pulse wave, blood is forced into the cavernous spaces, increasing the volume of the erectile tissue and raising the intracavitary pressure. The tunica albuginea, which has a limited capacity for distension, becomes taut and compresses the veins that pass through it. This mechanism, aided by the occlusion of emissary veins, causes a constriction of venous outflow, enabling the penis to remain stiff and hard. Meanwhile, the dense venous plexuses in the corpus spongiosum and glans prevent excessive compression of the urethra. The flaccid phase begins with vasoconstriction of the afferent arteries. An undesired, prolonged, and painful erection is called *priapism* (from Priapus, the Greco-Roman god of procreation) and may occur, for example, in certain blood diseases or metabolic disorders. The initial treatment of this condition is medical; one option is the use of vasoconstrictors (etilefrine or norepinephrine). Surgical treatment involves making "punch anastomoses" to promote the outflow of blood.

13.18 Female External Genitalia: Overview and Episiotomy

a

b

A Overview of the female genital organs
a Internal and some external genital organs.
b External genitalia, lithotomy position with the labia minora separated.

As in males, a distinction is drawn between the development and the topography of the female internal and external reproductive organs. The homology in the development of the male and female genital organs is reflected chiefly in the comparable histological features of the corresponding parts (see textbooks of histology). The female external genitalia (pudendum) is also known in clinical parlance as the *vulva*. It is separated from the internal genital organs by the *hymen* (not shown here). The outer boundaries of the vulva are formed by the mons pubis, a fatty-fleshy prominence over the pubic symphysis, and the labia majora, two pigmented ridges of skin that contain smooth muscle cells as well as sebaceous glands, sweat glands, and scent glands. The labia majora are interconnected anteriorly and posteriorly by a bridge of tissue called the anterior or posterior labial commissure. The area between the posterior commissure and anus is the perineal raphe. Specific structures are listed in the table at right.

Female internal genital organs	Female external genital organs (vulva)

• Ovary
• Uterine tube
• Uterus
• Vagina
	• Mons pubis
	• Labia majora
	• Labia minora
	• Vestibule of vagina
	• Vestibular bulb
	• Clitoris
	• Vestibular glands
	  – Greater vestibular glands
	    (Bartholin's glands)
	  – Lesser vestibular glands

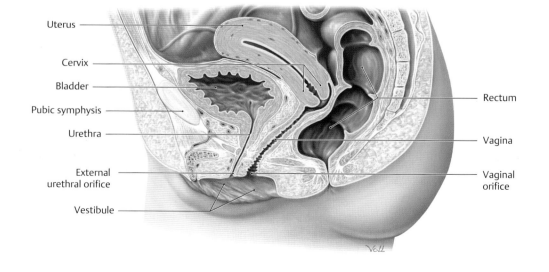

B Midsagittal section through a female pelvis
Left lateral view.
Note the close proximity of the external urethral orifice to the vaginal orifice, which opens into the vestibule.

a

C Episiotomy: indications and technique
a Pelvic floor with crowning of the fetal head.
b Types of episiotomy: midline, mediolateral, lateral.
c Mediolateral episiotomy performed at the height of a contraction.

Episiotomy is a common obstetric procedure utilized to enlarge the birth canal during the expulsive stage of labor (see p. 542). When the fetal head crowns through the pelvic floor, the levator ani muscle in particular is passively stretched, forced downward, and rotated approximately 90°. The "levator plate" thus helps to form the wall of the distal birth canal along with the urogenital diaphragm and bulbospongiosus muscle. As such, it comes under considerable tension at the perineal body during the pushing stage of labor. To protect the perineal muscles from tearing, the obstetrician counteracts this tension by supporting the perineum with two fingers *(perineal protection)*. An *episiotomy* is often performed to prevent uncontrolled laceration of the perineum (maternal indication). There is an imminent danger of perineal laceration during the delivery when the perineal skin is stretched to the point that it turns white, indicating diminished blood flow. The primary purpose of an episiotomy, however, is to expedite the delivery of a baby

that is at risk for hypoxia during the expulsive stage. An *early episiotomy* is one that is made before the head crowns (the head is visible with contractions and pushing but recedes between contractions). A *timely episiotomy* is made after the head has crowned, when there is maximum tension on the perineal skin. Three types of episiotomy are available (see **D** for advantages and disadvantages):

- **Midline episiotomy:** straight down from the vagina toward the anus
- **Mediolateral episiotomy:** oblique incision from the posterior commissure
- **Lateral episiotomy:** lateral incision from the lower third of the vulva

After the placenta is delivered, the episiotomy is usually closed in at least three layers (vaginal suture, deep perineal suture, and cutaneous suture). Local anesthesia is generally required, especially when an early episiotomy has been done. If the episiotomy was made at the height of a contraction after crowning of the head, anesthesia is unnecessary. Local infiltration anesthesia and the pudendal block (PDB) are described on p. 542.

D Advantages and disadvantages of the different types of episiotomy (after Goerke)

Episiotomy	Divided muscles	Advantages	Disadvantages
• Midline	• None	• Easy to repair • Heals well	• May lengthen to a grade III perineal laceration
• Mediolateral	• Bulbospongiosus • Superficial transverse perineal	• Gains more room • Low risk of laceration	• Heavier bleeding • More difficult to repair • More difficult healing
• Lateral*	• Bulbospongiosus • Superficial transverse perineal • Levator ani (puborectalis)	• Gains the most room	• Heaviest bleeding • Potential complications (e.g., anal incontinence) • Greatest postpartum complaints

*Very rarely used.

233

13.19 Female External Genitalia: Neurovascular Structures, Erectile Tissues, Erectile Muscles, and Vestibule

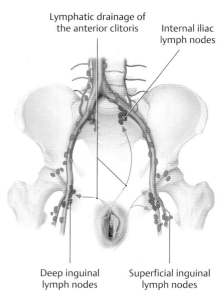

A Nerves and vessels of the female perineal region

Lithotomy position. The labia majora, skin, superficial perineal fascia, and fatty tissue in the ischioanal fossa have been removed to demonstrate the neurovascular structures. The bulbospongiosus and ischiocavernosus muscles and the perineal membrane have also been dissected away on the left side.

B Lymphatic drainage of the female external genitalia

Female pelvis, anterior view. Lymph from the female external genitalia drains to the superficial inguinal lymph nodes. The only exceptions are the anterior portions of the clitoris (body and glans), which drain to the deep inguinal and internal iliac lymph nodes.

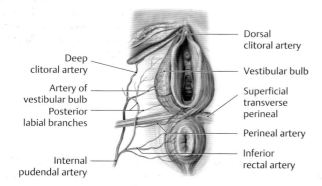

C Arterial supply to the female external genitalia

Perineal region, inferior view. The female external genitalia, like the penis and scrotum, are supplied by the internal pudendal artery, which enters the ischioanal fossa (not seen here). After giving off the inferior rectal artery to the anus, the internal pudendal artery passes anteriorly into the superficial perineal space. Another branch, the perineal artery, supplies the perineal region, the erectile muscles, and the *posterior part* of the labia majora (posterior labial branches). In the superficial perineal space (not visible here, see p.183), the internal pudendal artery divides into its terminal branches, the artery of the vestibular bulb and the deep and dorsal clitoral arteries (which supply the corpus cavernosum of the clitoris). The *anterior part* of the labia majora is supplied by the external pudendal arteries (anterior labial branches), which arise from the femoral artery (not seen here).

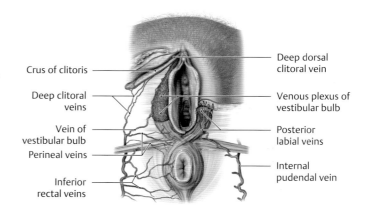

D Venous drainage of the female external genitalia

Venous drainage is handled by the following vessels:

- The deep clitoral veins, posterior labial veins, and vein of the vestibular bulb, which drain into the *internal pudendal vein*
- The superficial dorsal clitoral veins and anterior labial veins, which drain into the *external pudendal veins* (not seen here)
- The deep dorsal clitoral vein, which drains into the *vesical venous plexus*

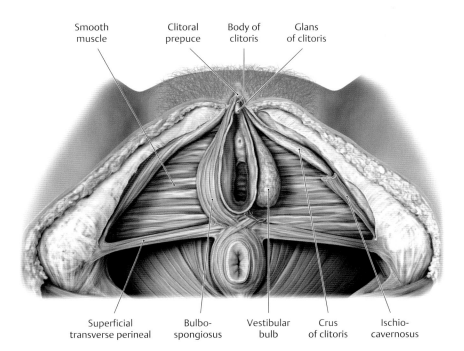

Smooth muscle · Clitoral prepuce · Body of clitoris · Glans of clitoris

Superficial transverse perineal · Bulbo-spongiosus · Vestibular bulb · Crus of clitoris · Ischio-cavernosus

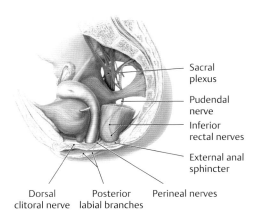

Sacral plexus · Pudendal nerve · Inferior rectal nerves · External anal sphincter · Perineal nerves

Dorsal clitoral nerve · Posterior labial branches

E Erectile tissues and erectile muscles in the female

Perineal region, lithotomy position. The labia majora and minora, skin, and superficial perineal fascia have been removed, as well as the erectile muscles on the left side.

Erectile tissues: The erectile tissues of the *clitoris* are distributed around both of its crura and its short shaft (body). They correspond to the erectile tissues in the male and are named accordingly: the right and left *corpora cavernosa of the clitoris,* homologous to the corpora cavernosa of the penis. The swelling at the end of the clitoral shaft is called the glans of clitoris, homologous to the glans penis. Its sensory innervation is like that of the penile glans, and it is mostly covered by a clitoral prepuce. The erectile tissue of the *labia minora* is located in the hairless, fat-free skin folds of the labia minora and is termed the *vestibular bulb,* which is the homologue of the corpus spongiosum in the male.

Erectile muscles: The two crura of the clitoris, one on each side, by which the clitoris arises from the inferior pubic ramus are covered by the *ischiocavernosus* muscle, and the dense erectile venous plexus at the base of the labia is covered by the *bulbospongiosus.*

F Nerve supply to the female external genitalia

Lesser pelvis, left lateral view. The pudendal nerve enters the ischioanal fossa. After giving off the inferior rectal nerves to the external anal sphincter and anal skin, it courses to the posterior border of the urogenital diaphragm, where it divides into its terminal branches (perineal nerves). The *superficial branches* pass through the superficial perineal space (not seen here) to the skin of the perineum and the posterior portions of the labia majora (posterior labial branches). The *deep branches* course in the deep perineal space, distributing muscular branches to the erectile muscles and the dorsal clitoral nerve to the clitoris. The anterior portions of the labia majora are supplied by anterior labial branches from the ilioinguinal nerve (not seen here).

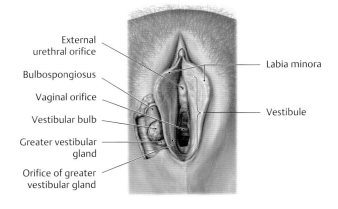

External urethral orifice · Bulbospongiosus · Vaginal orifice · Vestibular bulb · Greater vestibular gland · Orifice of greater vestibular gland

Labia minora · Vestibule

G The vestibule and vestibular glands

Lithotomy position with the labia separated. The vestibule, bounded by the labia minora, contains the external openings of the urethra and vagina (external urethral orifice and vaginal orifice) and the vestibular glands. The *lesser vestibular glands* (not seen here) have numerous openings near the external urethral orifice, while the paired *greater vestibular glands* each open by a 1-cm-long duct at the posterior border of the vestibular bulb on the inner surface of the labia minora. The lesser vestibular glands are homologous to the urethral glands in the male, and the greater vestibular glands to the bulbourethral glands. The vestibular glands produce a mucous secretion that moistens the vestibule and reduces friction during coitus, preventing epithelial injury. Next to the external urethral orifice are two short, blind, rudimentary excretory ducts called paraurethral ducts (not shown here). They correspond developmentally to the male prostate but have no known function in the female. Like the vestibular glands, however, they are susceptible to bacterial colonization. Bacterial colonization of the greater vestibular glands (Bartholin's glands) can lead to *bartholinitis,* a painful inflammation with swelling and redness. An inflammation that occludes the excretory ducts of the glands can produce a painful *retention cyst,* which should be opened or removed.

The Upper Limb

14.1 The Upper Limb as a Whole

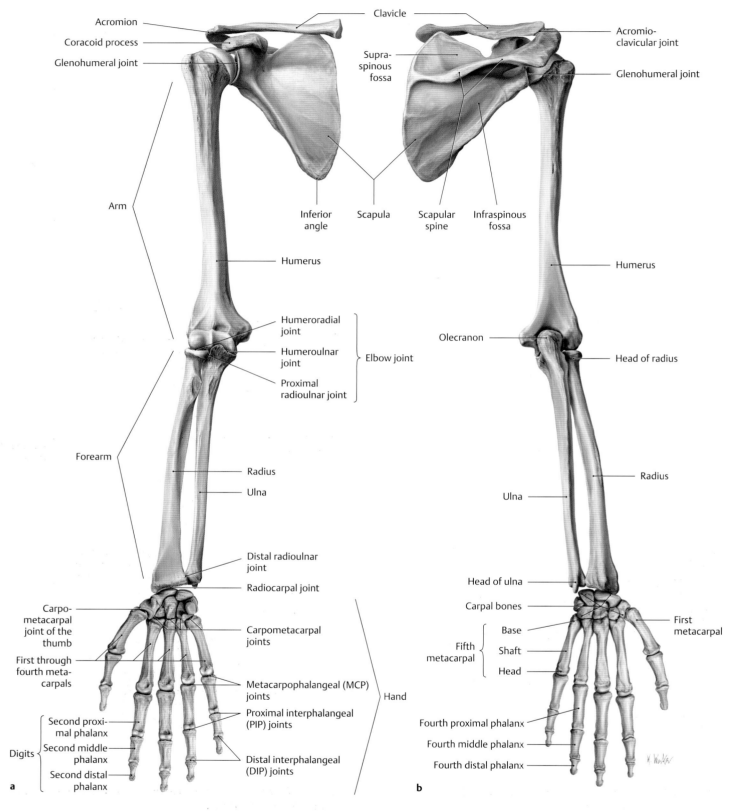

A Skeleton of the right upper limb

a Anterior view, **b** posterior view.

The skeleton of the upper limb consists of the shoulder girdle, arm, forearm, wrist, and hand. The shoulder girdle (clavicle and scapula) is joined to the upper limb at the shoulder joint, and it joins the upper limb to the thorax at the sternoclavicular joint (see p. 259). The limb itself consists of the

- arm,
- forearm, and
- hand.

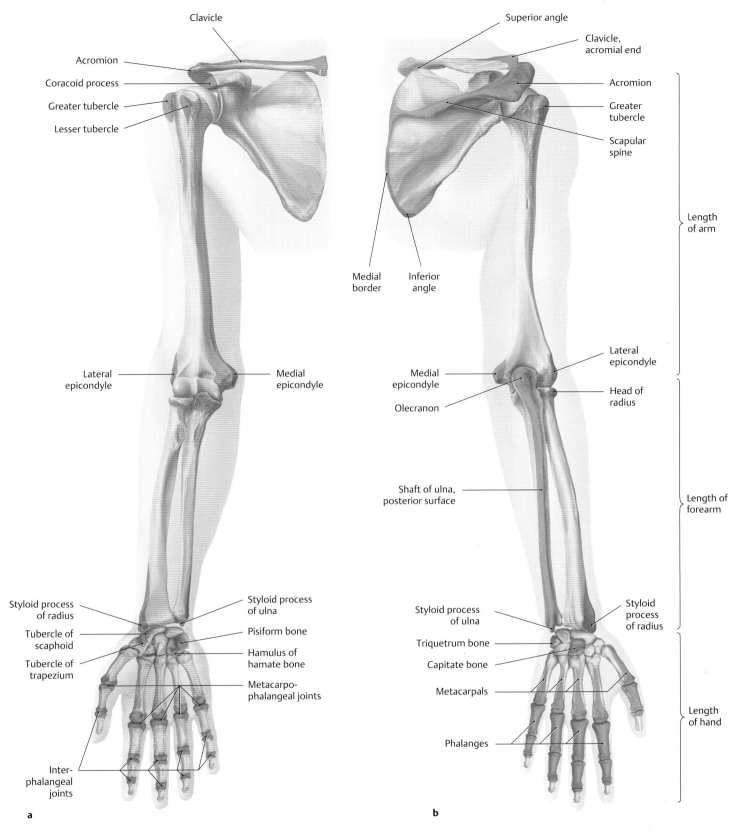

a **b**

B Palpable bony prominences on the right upper limb
a Anterior view, **b** posterior view.
Except for the lunate and trapezoid bones, all of the bones in the upper limb are palpable to some degree through the skin and soft tissues. By consensus, standard reference points have been defined for use in measuring the lengths of the segments of the dependent limb (with the palm turned forward):

• Length of the arm = distance from the acromion to the lateral epicondyle

• Length of the forearm = distance from the lateral epicondyle to the styloid process of the radius
• Length of the hand = distance from the styloid process of the radius to the tip of the third finger

The segment lengths of the limb may be measured, for example, to aid in the precise evaluation of isolated pediatric growth disturbances that are confined to a particular bone.

239

14.2 Integration of the Shoulder Girdle into the Skeleton of the Trunk

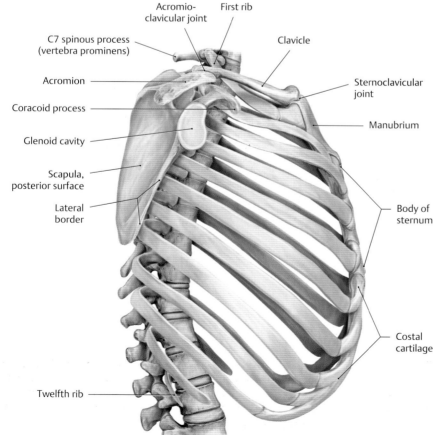

A Bones of the right shoulder girdle in relation to the trunk

a Anterior view, **b** posterior view, **c** lateral view.

The two bones of the shoulder girdle (the clavicle and scapula) are connected at the acromioclavicular joint (see p. 259). In its normal anatomic position, the scapula extends from the second to the seventh rib. The inferior angle of the scapula is level with the spinous process of the seventh thoracic vertebra, and the scapular spine is level with the spinous process of the third thoracic vertebra. When the scapula occupies a normal position, its long axis is angled slightly laterally, and its medial border forms a 3 to 5° angle with the midsagittal plane.

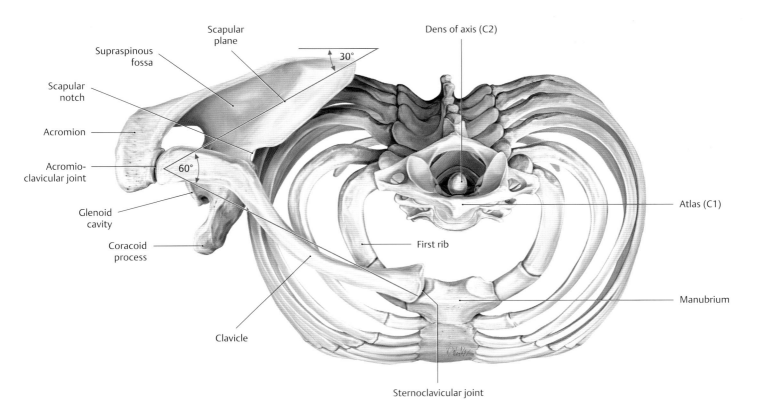

Scapular plane

Supraspinous fossa

Scapular notch

Acromion

Acromio-clavicular joint

Glenoid cavity

Coracoid process

Clavicle

Dens of axis (C2)

30°

60°

First rib

Sternoclavicular joint

Atlas (C1)

Manubrium

B Right shoulder girdle

Superior view. With the transition to a bipedal mode of locomotion, the human scapula moved from the more lateral placement in quadruped mammals to a more *posterior* position, and also a more frontal orientation, on the back of the thorax. Viewed from above, the scapula forms a 30° angle with the coronal plane. The scapula and clavicle sub-

tend an angle of approximately 60°. Because of this arrangement, the two shoulder joints are angled slightly forward, shifting the range of arm movements forward into the field of vision and action. This reorientation in humans creates the opportunity for visual control of manual manipulations (hand–eye coordination).

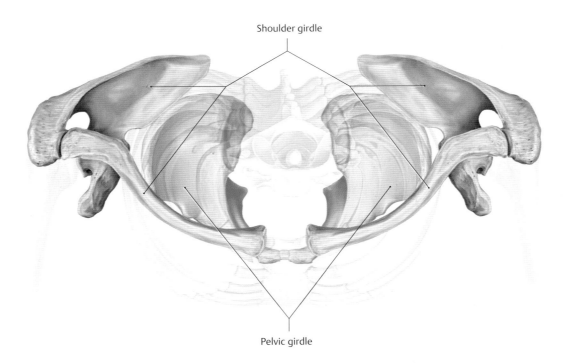

Shoulder girdle

Pelvic girdle

C Comparison of the shoulder girdle and pelvic girdle in their relation to the skeleton of the trunk

Superior view. Unlike the very mobile shoulder girdle, the pelvic girdle, consisting of the paired hip (coxal) bones, is firmly integrated into the axial skeleton. As the trunk assumes an upright position, the pelvis moves over the weight-bearing surface of the feet, making it necessary

for the pelvis to support the total weight of the trunk. This basically limits the lower limbs to functions of locomotion and support while freeing the upper limbs from these tasks and making them a versatile organ of movement and expression that is particularly useful for touching and grasping.

14.3 The Bones of the Shoulder Girdle

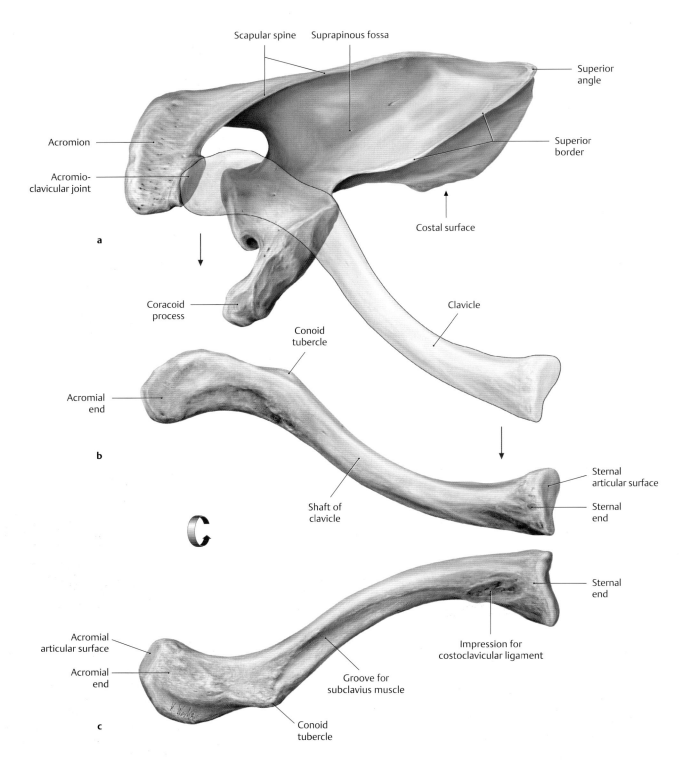

A Position and shape of the right clavicle
a Clavicle in its normal relation to the scapula, superior view.
b Isolated clavicle, superior view.
c Isolated clavicle, inferior view.

The clavicle is an S-shaped bone, approximately 12 to 15 cm long in adults, that is visible and palpable beneath the skin along its entire length. The medial or *sternal end* of the clavicle bears a saddle-shaped articular surface, while the lateral or *acromial end* has a flatter, more vertical articular surface. The clavicle is the *only* bone in the limbs that is not preformed in cartilage during embryonic development; instead, it ossifies directly from *connective tissue* (membranous ossi-

fication). A congenital failure or abnormality in the development of this connective tissue results in an anomaly called *cleidocranial dysostosis*. There may be associated ossification defects in the cranial vault, which are also formed by membranous ossification (*craniofacial dysostosis*). Besides fractures due to obstetric trauma (1–2% of all newborns), fractures of the middle third of the clavicle are one of the most common fractures that are sustained by children and adults (in children, some 50% of all clavicular fractures occur before 6 years of age).

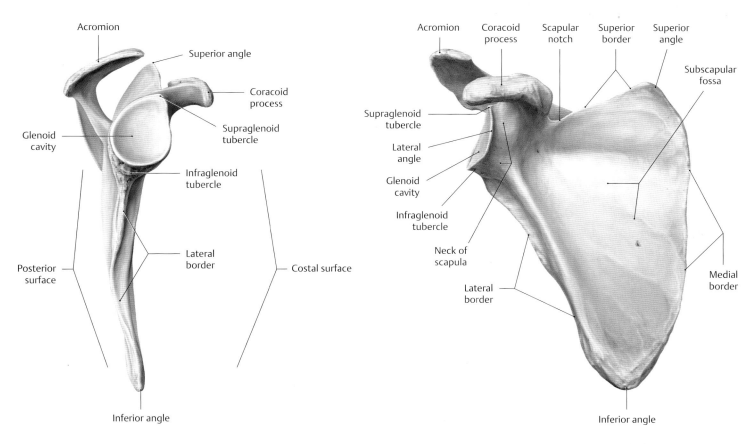

B The right scapula. Lateral view

C The right scapula. Anterior view

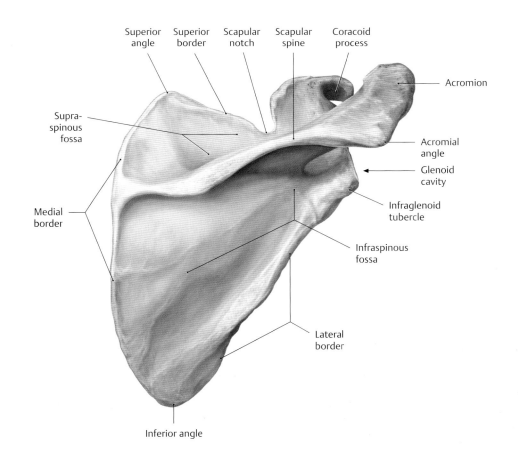

D The right scapula. Posterior view

E The scapular foramen

The superior transverse ligament of the scapula (see p. 267) can become ossified, transforming the scapular notch into an anomalous bony canal referred to as a *scapular foramen*. This can lead to compression of the suprascapular nerve as it passes through this canal (see p. 388). Active rotational movements of the shoulder aggravate the nerve, leading to significant symptoms (*scapular notch syndrome*). A common result is weakness and atrophy of the muscles—the supraspinatus and infraspinatus—that the suprascapular nerve innervates (see p. 303).

14.4 The Bones of the Upper Limb: The Humerus

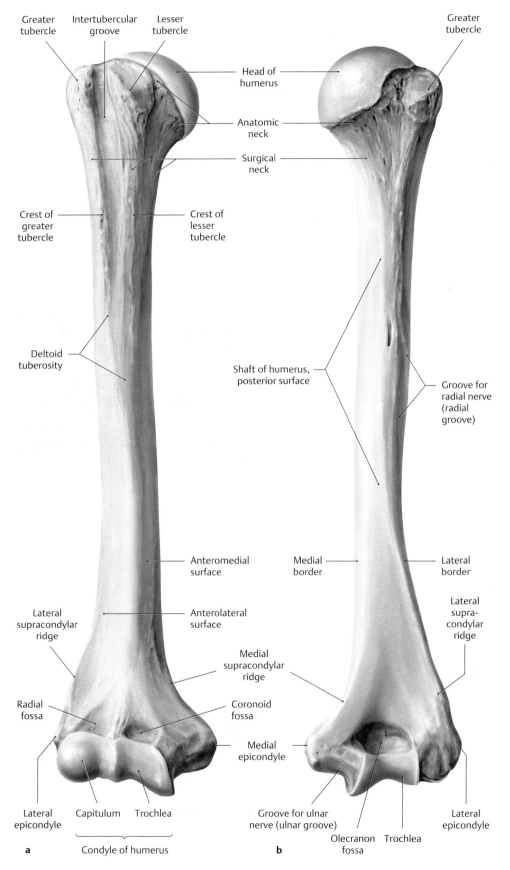

Greater tubercle

Intertubercular groove

Lesser tubercle

Head of humerus

Anatomic neck

Surgical neck

Crest of greater tubercle

Crest of lesser tubercle

Deltoid tuberosity

Shaft of humerus, posterior surface

Groove for radial nerve (radial groove)

Anteromedial surface

Medial border

Lateral border

Lateral supracondylar ridge

Anterolateral surface

Lateral supra- condylar ridge

Medial supracondylar ridge

Radial fossa

Coronoid fossa

Medial epicondyle

Lateral epicondyle

Capitulum

Trochlea

Groove for ulnar nerve (ulnar groove)

Lateral epicondyle

Olecranon fossa

Trochlea

a

Condyle of humerus

b

A The right humerus
a Anterior view, **b** posterior view.

Supracondylar process

B Supracondylar process
An anomaly sometimes found on the distal humerus above the medial epicondyle is referred to as a supracondylar process. This bony outgrowth is a relatively rare atavistic feature in humans that corresponds to a normal structure in other vertebrates, in which it forms part of a supracondylar canal (see p. 393).

Supratrochlear foramen

C The supratrochlear foramen
The presence of a supratrochlear foramen is another rare variant in which the two opposing olecranon and coronoid fossae communicate through an opening.

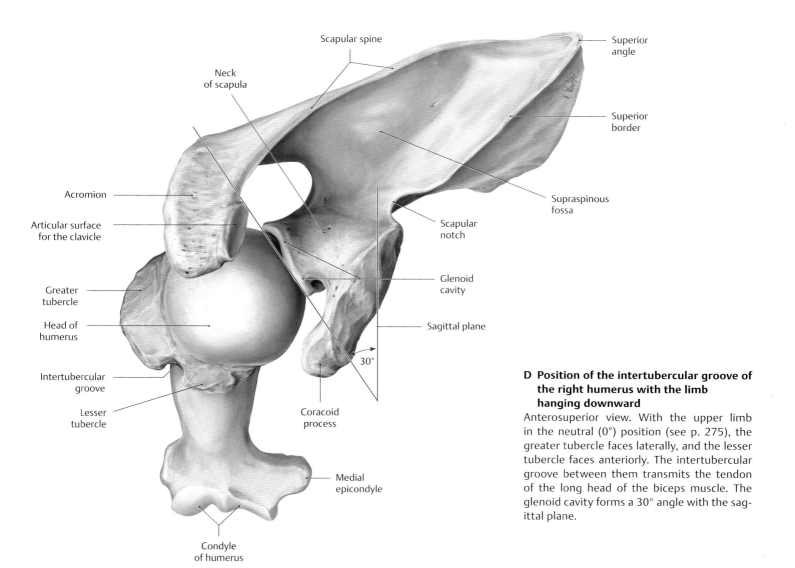

Scapular spine

Neck of scapula

Acromion

Articular surface for the clavicle

Greater tubercle

Head of humerus

Intertubercular groove

Lesser tubercle

Condyle of humerus

Superior angle

Superior border

Supraspinous fossa

Scapular notch

Glenoid cavity

Sagittal plane

30°

Coracoid process

Medial epicondyle

D Position of the intertubercular groove of the right humerus with the limb hanging downward

Anterosuperior view. With the upper limb in the neutral (0°) position (see p. 275), the greater tubercle faces laterally, and the lesser tubercle faces anteriorly. The intertubercular groove between them transmits the tendon of the long head of the biceps muscle. The glenoid cavity forms a 30° angle with the sagittal plane.

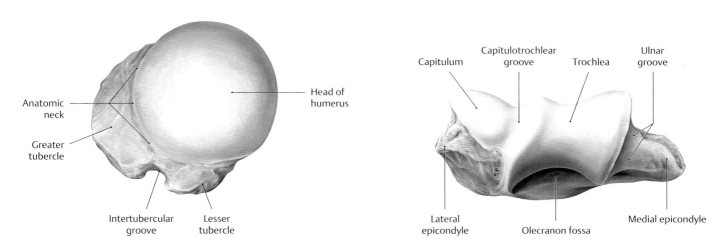

Anatomic neck

Greater tubercle

Head of humerus

Intertubercular groove

Lesser tubercle

Capitulum

Capitulotrochlear groove

Trochlea

Ulnar groove

Lateral epicondyle

Olecranon fossa

Medial epicondyle

E The proximal right humerus. Superior view

F The distal right humerus. Inferior view

14.5 The Bones of the Upper Limb: Torsion of the Humerus

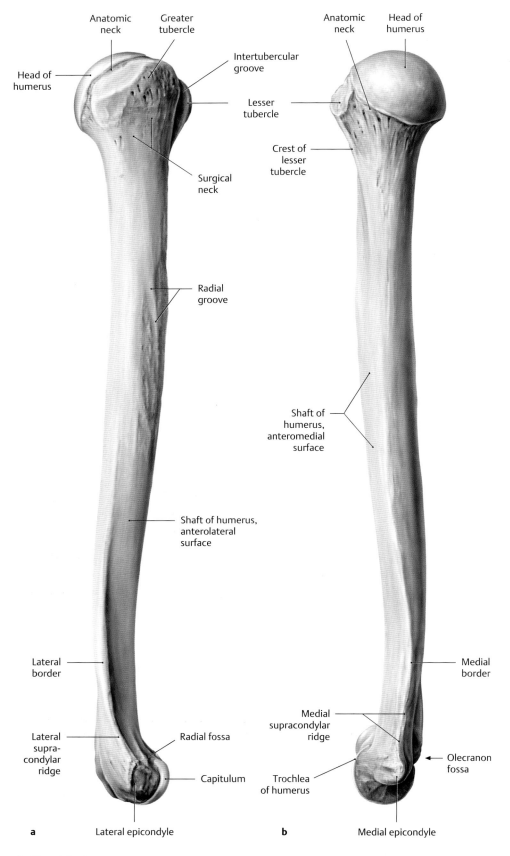

A The right humerus
a Lateral view, **b** medial view.

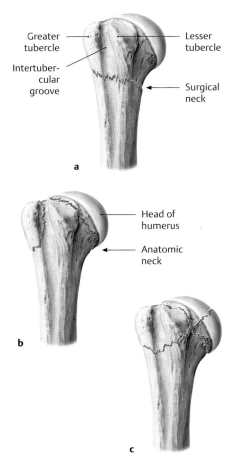

B Fractures of the proximal humerus

Anterior view. Fractures of the proximal humerus comprise approximately 4 to 5% of all fractures. They occur predominantly in older patients who sustain a fall onto the outstretched arm or directly onto the shoulder. Three main types are distinguished:

- Extra-articular fractures (**a**)
- Intra-articular fractures (**b**)
- Comminuted fractures (**c**)

Not infrequently, extra-articular fractures at the level of the *surgical neck* (site of predilection for extra-articular fractures of the proximal humerus) and intra-articular fractures at the level of the *anatomic neck* are accompanied by injuries of the blood vessels that supply the humeral head (anterior and posterior circumflex humeral arteries, see p. 355), with an associated risk of post-traumatic avascular necrosis. Besides proximal humeral fractures, other important injuries are fractures of the humeral shaft and fractures of the distal humerus (e.g., supracondylar fractures). Fractures of the humeral shaft are frequently associated with damage to the radial nerve in its groove (see p. 369 for neurologic deficits following a radial nerve lesion).

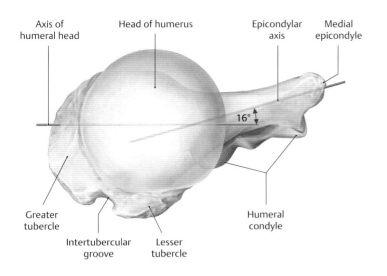

C Torsion of the humerus

Right humerus, superior view. The shaft of the adult humerus normally exhibits some degree of torsion, i.e., the proximal end of the humerus is rotated relative to its distal end. The degree of this torsion can be assessed by superimposing the axis of the humeral head (from the center of the greater tubercle to the center of the humeral head) over the epicondylar axis of the elbow joint. This *torsion angle* equals approximately 16° in an adult, compared to about 60° in a newborn. The decrease in the torsion angle with body growth correlates with the change in the position of the scapulae. Thus, while the glenoid cavity in the newborn still faces anteriorly, it is directed much more laterally in the adult (see p. 241). As the position of the scapula changes, there is a compensatory decrease in the torsion angle to ensure that hand movements will remain within the visual field of the adult.

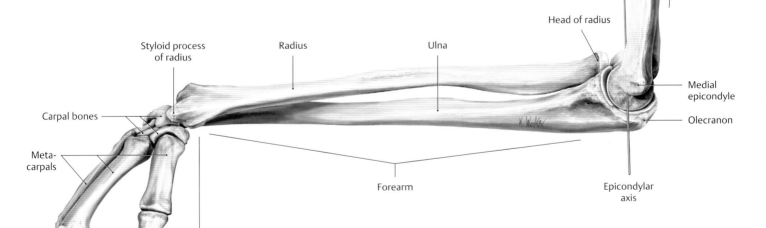

D Comparison of the humeral head axis and epicondylar axis

Skeleton of the right arm, viewed from the medial view with the forearm pronated.

14.6 The Bones of the Upper Limb: The Radius and Ulna

Trochlear notch

Articular fovea

Head of radius, articular circumference

Neck of radius

Coronoid process

Radial notch

Radial tuberosity

Ulnar tuberosity

Anterior border

Shaft of ulna, anterior surface

Interosseous border

Interosseous border

Shaft of radius, anterior surface

Articular circum-ference

Head of ulna

Styloid process of radius

Carpal articular surface

Styloid process of ulna

a

Olecranon

Head of radius, articular circumference

Radial notch

Neck of radius

Coronoid process

Radial tuberosity

Posterior border

Medial surface

Interosseous border

Posterior surface

Posterior surface

Posterior border

Lateral surface

Dorsal tubercle (Lister's tubercle)

Head of ulna

Styloid process of ulna

Styloid process of radius

b

A The radius and ulna of the right forearm
a Anterior view, **b** posterior view.
The radius and ulna are not shown in their normal relationship; they have been separated to demonstrate the articular surfaces of the proximal and distal radioulnar joints.

Humerus

Capitulum

Trochlea

Head of radius

Coronoid process

Radial tuberosity

Ulnar tuberosity

Radius

Ulna

Carpometa-carpal joint of the thumb

Radiocarpal joint

Carpometacarpal joints

a

Humerus

Lateral epicondyle

Humeroulnar joint

Medial epicondyle

Humeroradial joint

Elbow joint

Proximal radioulnar joint

Radius

Ulna

Distal radioulnar joint

Carpal bones

Styloid process of radius

First metacarpal

Metacarpo-phalangeal (MCP) joints

First proximal phalanx

First distal phalanx

Proximal interphalangeal (PIP) joints

Second metacarpal

Second proximal phalanx

Distal interphalangeal (DIP) joints

Second middle phalanx

Second distal phalanx

b

B The radius and ulna of the right arm in (a) supination and (b) pronation
The radius and ulna are parallel to each other in supination, whereas in pronation the radius crosses over the ulna. The movement of turning the palm upward or downward (supination/pronation) takes place at the proximal and distal radioulnar joints (see p. 280).

249

14.7 The Bones of the Upper Limb: The Articular Surfaces of the Radius and Ulna

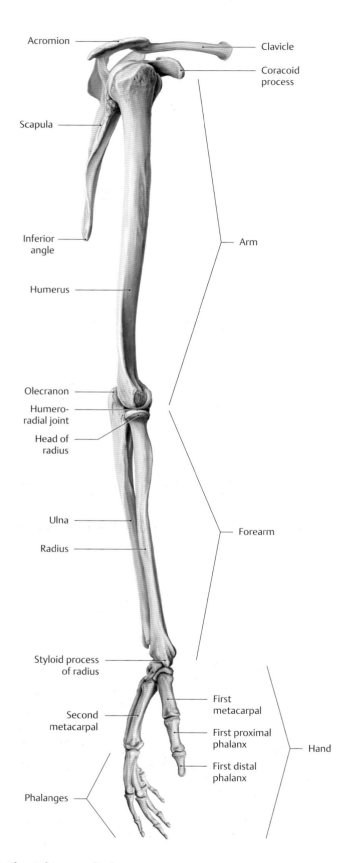

Acromion

Clavicle

Coracoid process

Scapula

Inferior angle

Arm

Humerus

Olecranon

Humero-radial joint

Head of radius

Ulna

Radius

Forearm

Styloid process of radius

First metacarpal

Second metacarpal

First proximal phalanx

Hand

First distal phalanx

Phalanges

Trochlear notch

Olecranon

Radial notch

Coronoid process

Supinator crest

Head of radius

Neck of radius

Interosseous border

Lateral surface

Anterior surface

Styloid process of ulna

Head of ulna

Dorsal tubercle

Styloid process of radius

A The right upper limb
Lateral view. The forearm is supinated (the radius and ulna are parallel).

B Right forearm
Lateral view. The radius and ulna are shown in a disarticulated position to demonstrate the articular surfaces of the ulna for the proximal and distal radioulnar joints (see **C**).

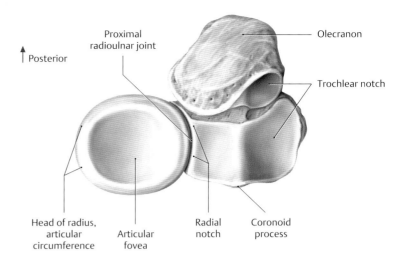

D The proximal articular surfaces of the radius and ulna of the right forearm. Proximal view

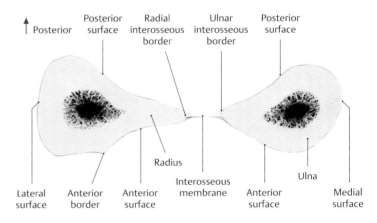

E Cross section through the right radius and ulna. Proximal view

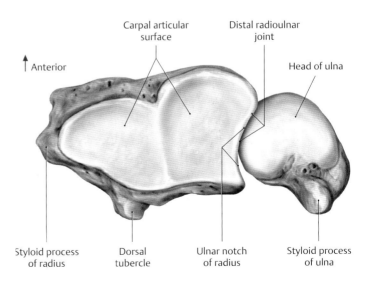

C The radius and ulna of the right forearm

Anterosuperior view. The proximal and distal radioulnar joints are functionally interlinked by the interosseous membrane between the radius and ulna. As a result, motion in one joint is invariably combined with motion in the other (see p. 282).

F The distal articular surfaces of the radius and ulna of the right forearm. Distal view

14.8 The Bones of the Upper Limb: The Hand

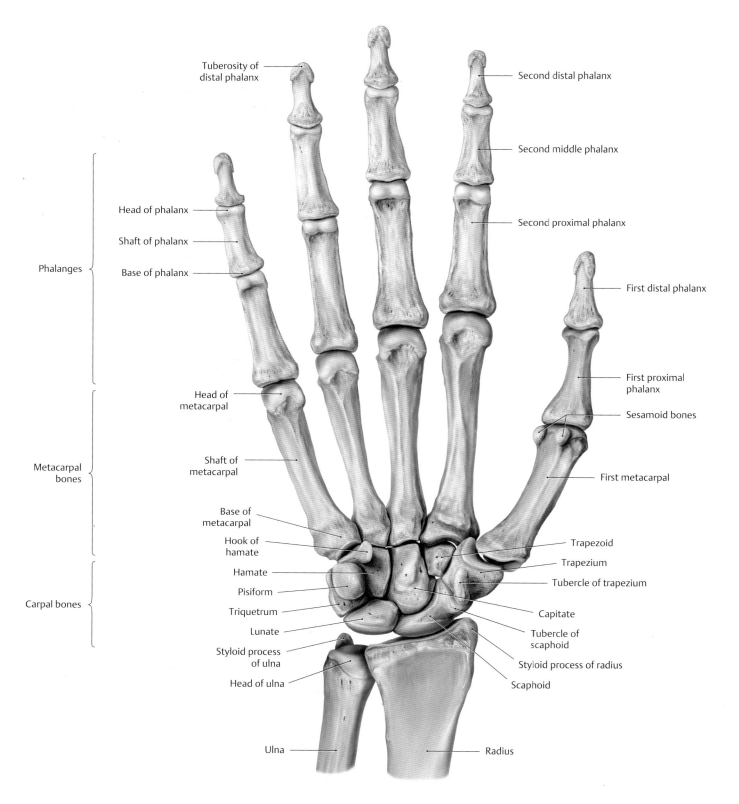

A The bones of the right hand. Palmar view

The skeleton of the hand consists of

- the carpal bones,
- the metacarpal bones, and
- the phalanges.

The palm refers to the anterior (flexor) surface of the hand, the dorsum to the posterior (extensor) surface. The terms of anatomic orientation in the hand are palmar or volar (toward the anterior surface), dorsal (toward the posterior surface), ulnar (toward the ulna or small finger), and radial (toward the radius or thumb).

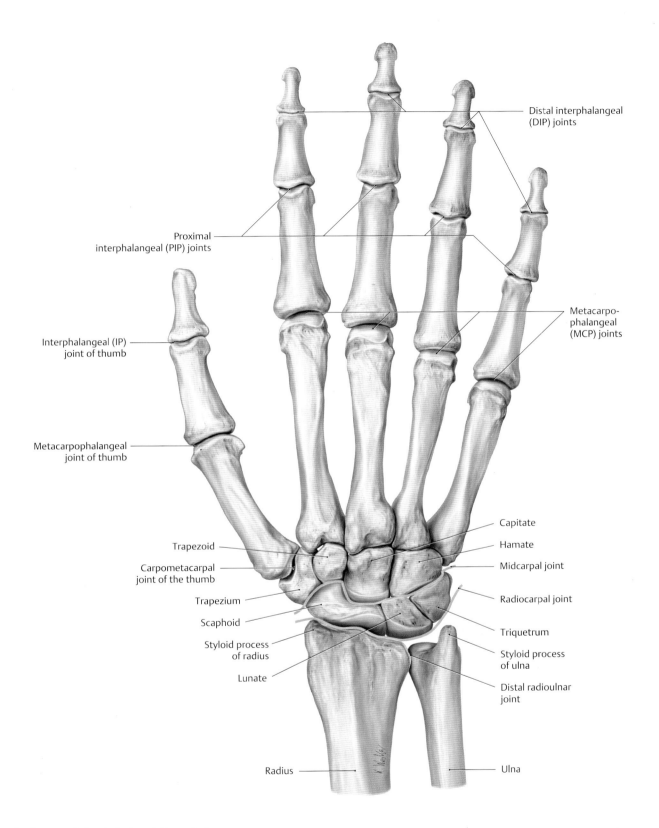

Distal interphalangeal
(DIP) joints

Proximal
interphalangeal (PIP) joints

Metacarpo-
phalangeal
(MCP) joints

Interphalangeal (IP)
joint of thumb

Metacarpophalangeal
joint of thumb

Trapezoid

Carpometacarpal
joint of the thumb

Trapezium

Scaphoid

Styloid process
of radius

Lunate

Capitate

Hamate

Midcarpal joint

Radiocarpal joint

Triquetrum

Styloid process
of ulna

Distal radioulnar
joint

Radius

Ulna

B The bones of the right hand. Dorsal view
The radiocarpal and midcarpal joints are indicated by blue lines.

14.9 The Bones of the Upper Limb: The Carpal Bones

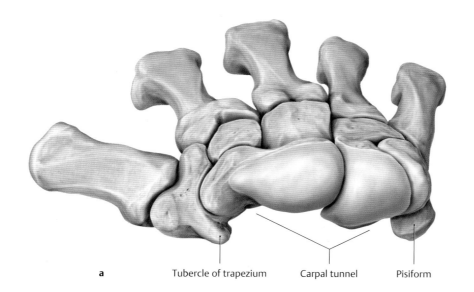

a   Tubercle of trapezium   Carpal tunnel   Pisiform

b

    ▨ Scaphoid column

    ▨ Lunate column

    ▨ Triquetral column

First through
fifth metacarpals

Capitate

Hamate

Triquetrum

Scaphoid

Lunate

Styloid process
of ulna

Trapezoid

Trapezium

Styloid process of radius

Dorsal
tubercle

Radius

Ulna

A Carpal bones of the right hand

a After removal of radius and ulna, proximal view; **b** column model of the hand, dorsal view; **c** with the wrist in flexion, proximal view.

The carpal bones are arranged in two rows of four bones each—one proximal row and one distal row (see also **B**). From a biomechanical and clinical standpoint, the carpal bones do not form two transverse rows but are arranged in three longitudinal columns: a radial scaphoid column (consisting of the scaphoid, trapezium, and trapezoid bones), a central lunate column (consisting of the lunate and capitate), and an ulnar triquetral column (consisting of the triquetrum and hamate). In this functional classification, the pisiform is regarded as a sesamoid bone embedded in the tendon of the flexor carpi ulnaris muscle (see p. 404). The bones in each row are interconnected by tight joints, their surfaces exhibiting a palmar concavity and a dorsal convexity. This creates the carpal tunnel on the palmar surface (see p. 288), which is bounded by a bony eminence on the radial and ulnar sides.

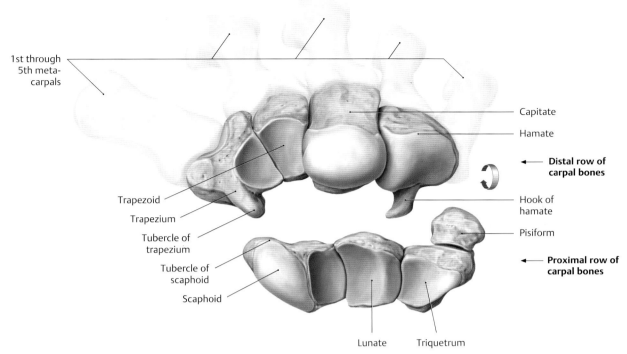

1st through
5th meta-
carpals

Capitate

Hamate

**← Distal row of
carpal bones**

Trapezoid

Trapezium

Tubercle of
trapezium

Hook of
hamate

Pisiform

**← Proximal row of
carpal bones**

Tubercle of
scaphoid

Scaphoid

Lunate   Triquetrum

B Articular surfaces of the midcarpal joint of the right hand
The *distal* row of carpal bones is shown from the *proximal* view. The
proximal row is shown from the *distal* view.

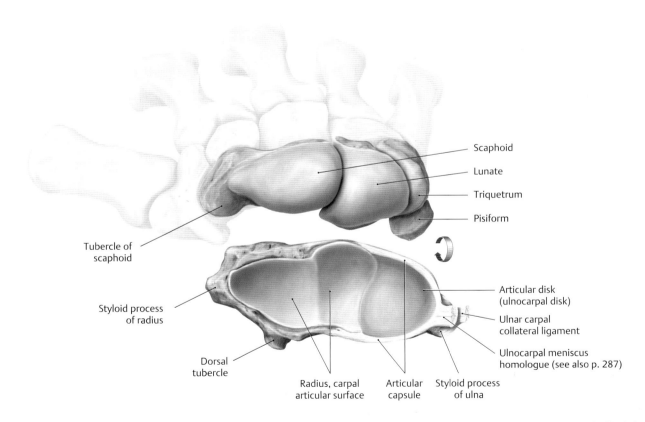

Scaphoid

Lunate

Triquetrum

Pisiform

Tubercle of
scaphoid

Styloid process
of radius

Articular disk
(ulnocarpal disk)

Ulnar carpal
collateral ligament

Ulnocarpal meniscus
homologue (see also p. 287)

Dorsal
tubercle

Radius, carpal
articular surface

Articular
capsule

Styloid process
of ulna

C Articular surfaces of the radiocarpal joint of the right hand
The proximal row of carpal bones is shown from the proximal view.
The articular surfaces of the radius and ulna and the articular disk
(ulnocarpal disk) are shown from the distal view.
Clinically, the radiocarpal joint is subdivided into a radial compartment
and an ulnar compartment. This takes into account the presence of the
interposed ulnocarpal disk, which creates a second, ulnar half of the
radiocarpal joint in addition to the radial half. Accordingly, the radius
articulates with the proximal row of carpal bones in the radial compartment, while the head of the ulna and ulnocarpal disk articulate with the
proximal row of carpal bones in the ulnar compartment.

255

14.10 Architecture of the Radiocarpal Junction and the Metacarpus; Distal Radius and Scaphoid Fractures

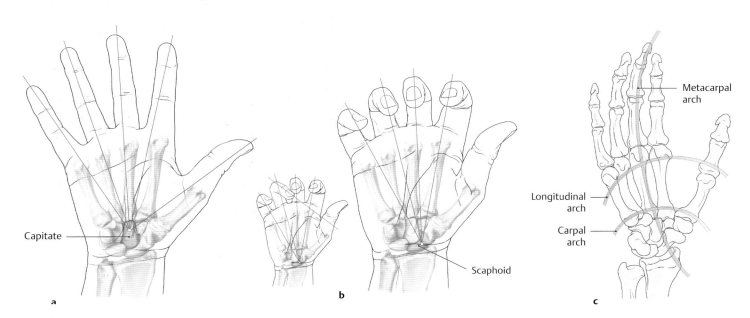

Capitate

Scaphoid

Metacarpal arch

Longitudinal arch

Carpal arch

a   b   c

A Architecture of the metacarpus

The metacarpus is the key region for the architecture of the hand. It is where the five digital rays form and then develop into the thumb and fingers. While in neutral position, the longitudinal axis of each finger is parallel, and the longitudinal axis of the abducted thumb and the spread fingers converge to an intersection point in the capitate (**a**). However, when bending the finger joints, the axes converge to an intersection point in the scaphoid (**b**). Only the knowledge of these de-

fined basic anatomic positions allows for the diagnosis of mal-alignments caused by injury (most notably rotational mal-alignments of the fingers, meaning "twisting" of phalanges as a result of a fracture (see inset). The five digital rays are connected by three functionally significant arches (**c**): a longitudinal arch along the third ray, a metacarpal arch, and a transverse carpal arch.

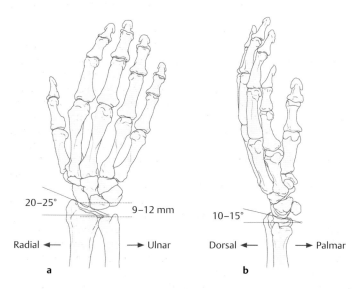

20–25°   9–12 mm

Radial ← → Ulnar

10–15°

Dorsal ← → Palmar

a   b

c

d

B Inclination angle of the articulating surfaces along the distal radius

a   Radioulnar inclination angle, right hand, dorsal view.
b   Dorsopalmar inclination angle, right hand, ulnar view.
c   X-ray image of carpal region, dorsopalmar beam path and
d   radioulnar beam path (**c** and **d** from Schmidt HM, Lanz U. Chirurgische Anatomie der Hand. 2nd ed. Stuttgart: Thieme; 2003).

The distal radius helps form the radiocarpal and distal radioulnar joints. In addition, it supports the ulnocarpal disk and the strong dorsal and palmar extrinsic ligaments (see p. 284). It is primarily responsible for carpal load transmission within the longitudinally arranged columns (scaphoid column, lunate column, and triquetrum, see p. 254) and thus

is prone to injury (see **C**). For a harmonious relationship between the parts forming the radiocarpal joint in terms of optimal mobility of the hand, the position of the part of the socket formed by the radius is of importance. The carpal articulating surface of the ulna is not vertical to the longitudinal axis of the forearm, but in a radioulnar inclination angle of 20 to 25° (ulnar inclination) and a dorsopalmar inclination angle of 10 to 15° (palmar inclination). The distal radial length relative to the ulna (tip of the styloid process of the radius to the carpal articulating surface of the ulna) is approximately 9 to 12 mm (important for optimal mobility of the hand).

a

Styloid process
of radius   Dorsal

b   Extension fracture
       = "Colles' fracture"

c

Styloid process
of radius   Dorsal

d   Bending fracture
       = "Smith fracture"

e

"Chinese
finger trap"

f

C Distal radius fractures

Accounting for 20 to 25% of all fractures, the distal (or near the wrist) radius fracture as a result of falling on the hand is the most common fracture in humans. Affected are almost 80% of women over the age of 50 (main cause: postmenopausal osteoporosis). Depending on the position of the carpus relative to the distal radius at the moment of impact, 90% of falls result in extension fractures (Colles' fracture; see **a** and **b**), and 10%, in flexion fractures (see **e**, from Henne-Bruns D, Dürig M, Kremer B. Chirurgie. 2nd ed. Stuttgart: Thieme; 2003).

In distal radius fractures, one generally differentiates between extra- and intra-artciular fractures, with the extra-articular fractures typically located 3 to 4 cm proximal to the radiocarpal joint. The standard criteria for such a diagnosis are determined by taking conventional X-ray images of the wrists in two planes (see **e** lateral view). The therapeutic procedure (conservatively using casts or surgically through osetosynthesis) depends on the angle and direction of dislocation (fracture stability), the course of the fracture line (intra-/extra-articular), and the severity of accompanying injuries (e.g., involvement of the ulna, most notably the styloid process). Less complicated (nondislocated, easy-to-reposition) and primarily stable fractures are conservatively treated using "Chinese finger traps" (**f**) with the help of an image intensifier. Axial alignment, most notably of the original radial length and angle (ulnar and palmar inclination angles, see **Ba** and **Bb**), are being restored through vertical extension and joint immobilization with the help of a dorsopalmar splint. With intra-artciular fractures involving large articular fragments, osteosynthetic stabilization is generally recommended.

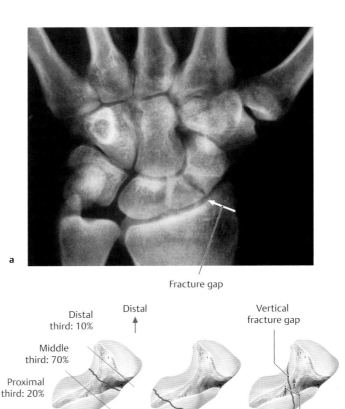

a   Fracture gap

Distal
third: 10%   Distal   Vertical
                               fracture gap
Middle
third: 70%

Proximal
third: 20%

b   **c**   **d**
   Proximal   "Shear forces"

D Scaphoid fractures

a Scaphoid fracture as seen on X-ray, dorsopalmar view (from Matzen P. Praktische Orthopädie. 3rd ed. Stuttgart: J. A. Barth Verlag Thieme; 2002).
b Frequency and distribution of scaphoid fractures.

Carpal fractures, most notably scaphoid fractures (accounting for two thirds of all cases), are another injury caused by falling on the outstretched hand extended in the dorsal direction. Unlike distal radial fractures (see **C**), young people are predominantly affected by scaphoid fractures (typical sports injury). During physical examination, the symptoms can be relatively discrete. Usually the symptoms include tenderness on palpation of the area around the anatomic snuff box with simultaneous radial or ulnar abduction and compressive pain around the thumb and index finger. In the case of a suspected scaphoid fracture, conventional radiographs of the wrist in four different planes (so-called scaphoid quartet series) should be taken (see **a**, white arrow), in order to determine the direction of the fracture gap. If the X-ray image fails to confirm the suspected diagnosis 10 to 14 days after initially stabilizing the fracture, a follow-up X-ray must be taken (if needed using CT scans). At this point, the process of resorption in the fracture hematoma is usually completed so that the fracture gap is wider and thus more clearly visible. Depending on the location, scaphoid fractures are classified into fractures of the proximal third, central third, or distal third (see **b**). The healing process is especially lengthy in fractures of the proximal third (up to 3 months in an upper arm cast for stabilization with inclusion of the thumb basal joint, see **c**) because this part of the bone has few blood vessels (the scaphoid receives the majority of its blood supply via distal vessels). The healing process is just as lengthy in slanted or vertical fractures due to the resulting shearing forces pushing in opposite directions (see **d**).

Note: The scaphoid bone is involved in all movements of the hand, which makes long-term stabilization rather difficult. Thus, pseudo-osteoarthritis is a typical complication of scaphoid fracture (= false joint after failed fracture healing, see p. 88).

14.11 The Joints of the Shoulder: Overview and Clavicular Joints

A The five joints of the shoulder
Right shoulder, anterior view. A total of five joints contribute to the wide range of arm motions at the shoulder joint. There are three true shoulder joints and two functional articulations:

- **True joints:**
  1. Sternoclavicular joint
  2. Acromioclavicular joint
  3. Glenohumeral joint
- **Functional articulations:**
  4. Subacromial space: a space lined with bursae (subacromial and subdeltoid bursae) that allows gliding between the acromion and the rotator cuff (= muscular cuff of the glenohumeral joint, consisting of the supraspinatus, infraspinatus, subscapularis, and teres minor muscles, which press the head of the humerus into the glenoid cavity; see p. 303).
  5. Scapulothoracic joint: loose connective tissue between the subscapularis and serratus anterior muscles that allows gliding of the scapula on the chest wall.

Besides the true joints and functional articulations, the two ligamentous attachments between the clavicle and first rib (costoclavicular ligament) and between the clavicle and coracoid process (coracoclavicular ligament) contribute to the mobility of the upper limb. All of these structures together comprise a functional unit, and free mobility in all the joints is necessary to achieve a full range of motion. This expansive mobility is gained at the cost of stability, however. Since the shoulder has a loose capsule and weak reinforcing ligaments, it must rely on the stabilizing effect of the rotator cuff tendons. As the upper limb changed in mammalian evolution from an organ of support to one of manipulation, the soft tissues and their pathology assumed increasing importance. As a result, a large percentage of shoulder disorders involve the soft tissues.

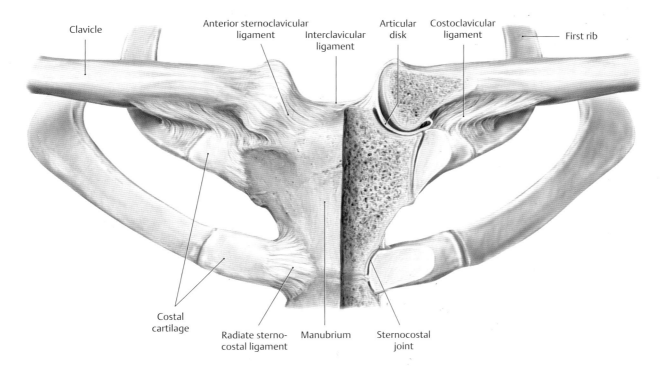

Clavicle — Anterior sternoclavicular ligament — Interclavicular ligament — Articular disk — Costoclavicular ligament — First rib

Costal cartilage — Radiate sterno-costal ligament — Manubrium — Sternocostal joint

B The sternoclavicular joint and its ligaments

Anterior view. The sternoclavicular joint (also called the *medial* clavicular joint) and the acromioclavicular joint (the *lateral* clavicular joint, see below) together make up the true joints within the shoulder girdle itself. In the figure, a coronal section has been made through the sternum and adjacent clavicle to demonstrate the inside of the left sternoclavicular joint. A fibrocartilaginous articular disk compensates for the mismatch of surfaces between the two saddle-shaped articular faces of the clavicle and manubrium.

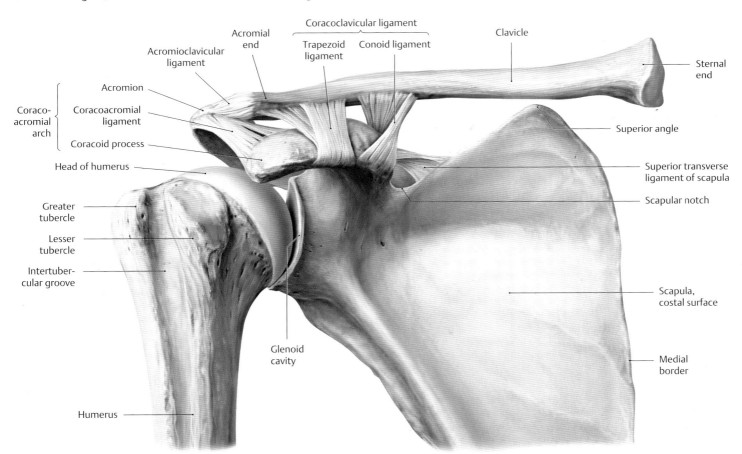

Coracoclavicular ligament — Acromial end — Trapezoid ligament — Conoid ligament — Clavicle

Acromioclavicular ligament — Sternal end

Coraco-acromial arch — Acromion — Coracoacromial ligament — Coracoid process — Head of humerus — Superior angle — Superior transverse ligament of scapula — Scapular notch

Greater tubercle — Lesser tubercle — Intertubercular groove — Scapula, costal surface

Glenoid cavity — Medial border

Humerus

C The acromioclavicular joint and its ligaments

Right shoulder, anterior view. The acromioclavicular joint (the *lateral* clavicular joint) has the form of a *plane joint*. Because the articulating surfaces are flat, they must be held in place by strong ligaments (acromioclavicular, coracoacromial, and coracoclavicular ligaments). This greatly limits the mobility of the acromioclavicular joint. In some individuals the acromioclavicular joint has a variably shaped articular disk that gives the joint greater mobility.

259

14.12 The Joints of the Shoulder: Ligaments of the Clavicular and Scapulothoracic Joints

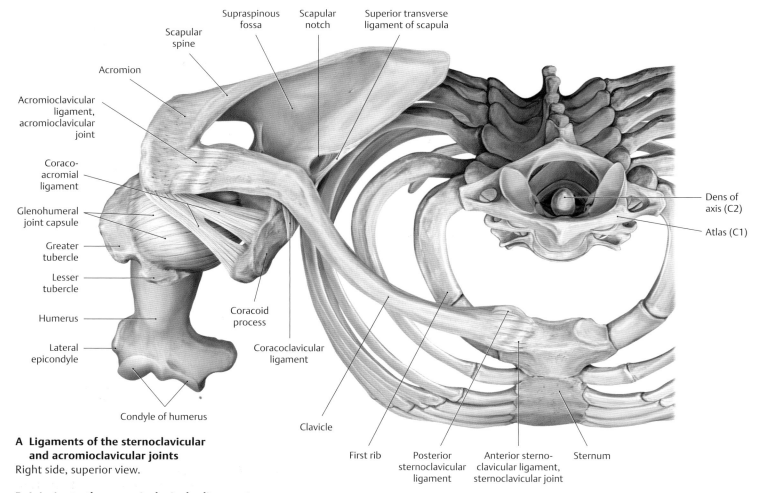

A Ligaments of the sternoclavicular and acromioclavicular joints

Right side, superior view.

B Injuries to the acromioclavicular ligaments

These injuries often result from falling on a shoulder or an outstretched arm. According to Tossy, they can be classified into three types:

Tossy I The acromioclavicular and coracoclavicular ligaments are stretched but still intact.

Tossy II The acromioclavicular ligament is ruptured, with subluxation of the joint.

Tossy III Ligaments are all disrupted, with complete dislocation of the acromioclavicular joint.

Rockwood added three more types that occur less frequently:

Rockwood IV: Dislocation of the clavicle shifts dorsally, due to the clavicular part of the deltoid being pulled off the clavicle.

Rockwood V: Dislocation of lateral end of the clavicle is increased in the cranial direction, due to the deltoid and trapezius being pulled off the clavicle.

Rockwood VI: The lateral end of the clavicle underneath the acromion or the coracoid is dislocated (very rare).

Depending on the extent of the injury, the so-called piano-key phenomenon can be triggered through palpation (caution: painful!). The lateral end of the clavicle, which is elevated due to the injury, can be reduced by applying pressure from the cranial direction, but it pops back up when pressure is released. Radiographs in different planes will show widening of the space in the acromioclavicular joint. Comparative-stress radiographs with the patient holding approximately 10-kg weights in each hand will reveal the extent of upward displacement of the lateral end of the clavicle on the affected side (is not performed in cases of visible partial rupture of ligaments in order to avoid further damage).

260

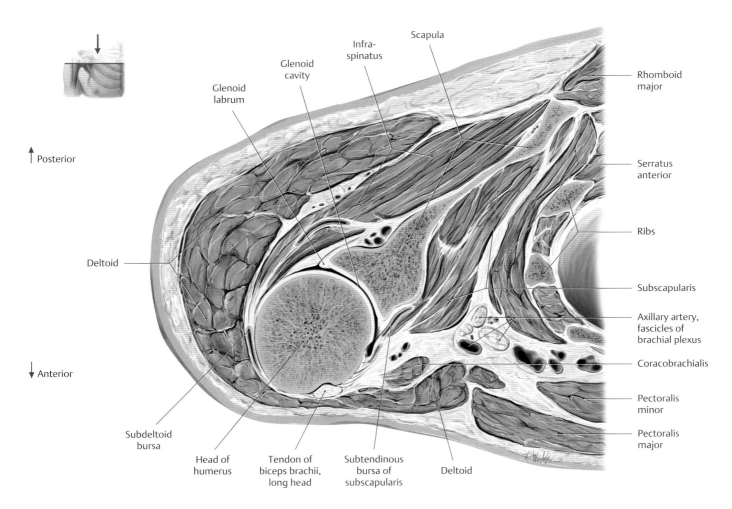

Labels (clockwise): Scapula · Infra-spinatus · Glenoid cavity · Glenoid labrum · Rhomboid major · Serratus anterior · Ribs · Subscapularis · Axillary artery, fascicles of brachial plexus · Coracobrachialis · Pectoralis minor · Pectoralis major · Deltoid · Subtendinous bursa of subscapularis · Tendon of biceps brachii, long head · Head of humerus · Subdeltoid bursa · Deltoid · Posterior · Anterior

C Transverse section through the right shoulder joint

Superior view. In all movements of the shoulder girdle, the scapula glides on a curved surface of loose connective tissue between the serratus anterior and subscapularis muscles (see **D**). This surface can be considered a "scapulothoracic" joint that allows the scapula not only to change the position of the shoulder (translational motion), but also to pivot, with the glenohumeral joint maintained in a relatively stable position on the thorax (rotational motion) (see p. 274) (drawing based on a specimen from the Anatomical Collection at the University of Kiel).

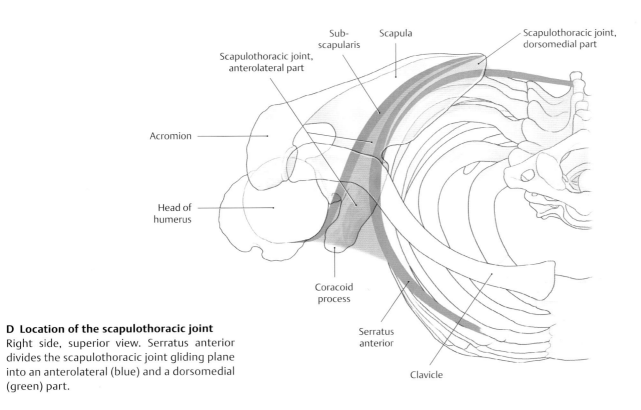

Labels: Sub-scapularis · Scapula · Scapulothoracic joint, dorsomedial part · Scapulothoracic joint, anterolateral part · Acromion · Head of humerus · Coracoid process · Serratus anterior · Clavicle

D Location of the scapulothoracic joint

Right side, superior view. Serratus anterior divides the scapulothoracic joint gliding plane into an anterolateral (blue) and a dorsomedial (green) part.

14.13 The Joints of the Shoulder: Articular Surfaces, Articular Capsule, and Articular Cavity of Glenohumeral Joint

a

b

A Articulating bony elements of the right shoulder joint (glenohumeral joint) and shoulder dislocation

a Anterior view.
b Posterior view.
c Lateral view.
d Articulating surfaces

c

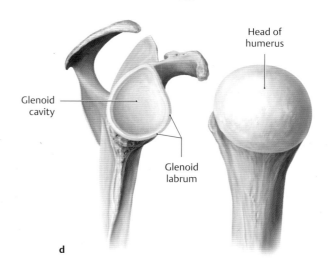

d

In the shoulder joint—the most mobile joint in the human body but also the most susceptible to injury—the head of the humerus articulates with the glenoid cavity of the scapula to form a spheroidal type of joint. The articular surface of the scapula, which is three to four times smaller than the head of the humerus, is enlarged by a rim of fibrocartilage, the glenoid labrum, which is approximately 5 mm wide at its base (see **d**). While this size discrepancy of the articulating surfaces serves to increase the range of shoulder motion, it compromises the stability of the joint. Since the joint capsule and ligaments are weak, the rotator cuff tendons are the primary stabilizers of the glenohumeral joint (see p. 304).

Dislocations of the shoulder joint are notoriously common. Approximately 45% of all dislocations involve the shoulder joint. In typical cases the head of the humerus dislocates anteriorly or anteroinferiorly in response to forcible external rotation of the raised arm. Whereas considerable trauma is generally needed to cause the initial dislocation, certain movements of the shoulder (e.g., excessive arm rotation during sleep) may be sufficient to redislocate the humeral head from the glenoid cavity (recurrent shoulder dislocation).

In addition to physical examination (based on postion of the arm, occurring pain, and palpation of shoulder contour), diagnostic procedures for a dislocated shoulder include x-rays in two planes. In injuries caused by dislocation, especially anterior luxation, which account for most cases, mainly the rim of the socket (torn-off labrum, so-called Bankert lesion) and humeral head (impression fracture caused by rim of socket, so-called Hill-Sachs lesion) are affected. Additional important complications include simultaneous damage to the axillary nerve (test sensitivity in the autonomous zone), the axillary artery (test capillary refill time of the radial artery), and, particularly in older patients, the rotator cuff (rupture).

B Repositioning of shoulder dislocation
a Repositioning according to Arlt; **b** repositioning according to Hippocrates
There are several techniques to reduce a dislocated shoulder. In all cases, the repositioning should be performed with the patient under sedation or analgesia, possibly even anesthesia. According to the Arlt method, the patient sits in a chair with the affected arm hanging downward over the upholstered armrest. Reposition is achieved through longitudinal traction, with the armrest serving as a support. The method as described by Hippocrates requires the patient to lie on the floor. Here, too, reduction is performed through longitudinal traction of the arm, with the doctor's foot placed in the axilla, thereby serving as a counter bearing.

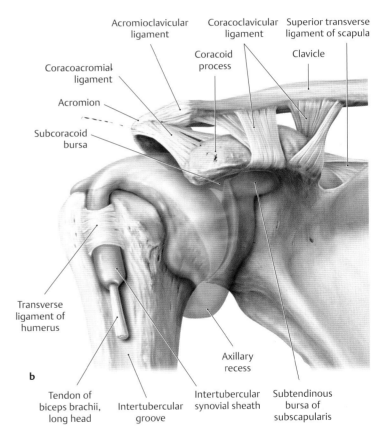

C Capsule, ligaments, and joint cavity of the right shoulder
a Anterior view.
b Joint cavity with capsule removed, anterior view.

The capsule of the shoulder joint is broad and very thin posteriorly, where it is not reinforced by ligaments. But it is strengthened anteriorly by three ligaments (the superior, medial, and inferior glenohumeral ligaments; see p. 264) and superiorly by the coracohumeral ligament. The coracoacromial ligament, acromion, and coracoid process together form the *coracoacromial arch*, which helps stabilize the humeral head in the glenoid cavity but also limits upward movement of the humerus. When the arm is hanging at the side, the lower part of the joint capsule, which is not reinforced by muscle, sags to form the axillary recess. This redundant fold provides a reserve capacity that is particularly useful during abduction movements of the arm. With prolonged disuse of the arm, the axillary recess may become atrophic or obliterated by adhesions, causing significant limitation of arm motion.

The cavity of the shoulder joint is connected to the adjacent bursae. The subtendinous bursa of the subscapularis muscle and the subcoracoid bursa consistently communicate with the joint cavity. The tendon sheath of the long head of the biceps brachii also communicates with the joint cavity in its passage through the intertubercular groove.

Note: The glenohumeral ligaments are usually clearly visible only at the inner side of the capsule.

14.14 The Joints of the Shoulder: Ligaments, Reinforcing Capsule, and Rotator Interval of the Glenohumeral Joint

a

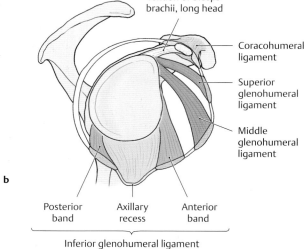

b

A Coracohumeral ligament
Right shoulder joint, superior view
The coracohumeral ligament arises from the base of the coracoid process as a strong, broad band. Its two parts pass from there to the greater and lesser tubercles of the humerus. The coracohumeral ligament stabilizes the tendon of the long head of the biceps brachii as it passes posterior to the coracohumeral ligament and before it passes through the intertubercular groove.

B Ligaments reinforcing capsules
a Right shoulder joint, anterior view; **b** schematic representation of the ligaments reinforcing the capsule after removal of the humeral head and cutting through both the capsule and the tendons of insertion of the rotator cuff muscles, lateral view; **c** origin and insertion of ligaments reinforcing capsule, lateral view.

The capsule of the shoulder joint is relatively loose and thin posteriorly. Anteriorly, it is reinforced by the glenohumeral ligaments, which differ significantly in shape and are usually clearly visible only when viewed arthroscopically (see p. 270).

- **Superior glenohumeral ligament:** It passes from the upper margin of the glenoid cavity to the intertubercular groove and to the lesser tubercle, forming, together with the coracohumeral ligament, the rotator interval (see **D**).

- **Middle glenohumeral ligament:** It passes at almost a right angle to the tendon of insertion of the subscapularis, from the upper margin of the glenoid cavity to the anatomic neck of the humerus.

- **Inferior glenohumeral ligament:** It consists of three parts, an anterior and posterior band and the axillary recess located between the bands. All three parts extend from the inferior margin of the glenoid cavity to the middle of the anatomic neck of the humerus, with the middle part (axillary recess) extending down to the surgical neck. The inferior glenohumeral ligament forms a hammock, especially during abduction, and is of particular significance to the anterior-inferior stability of the shoulder.

c

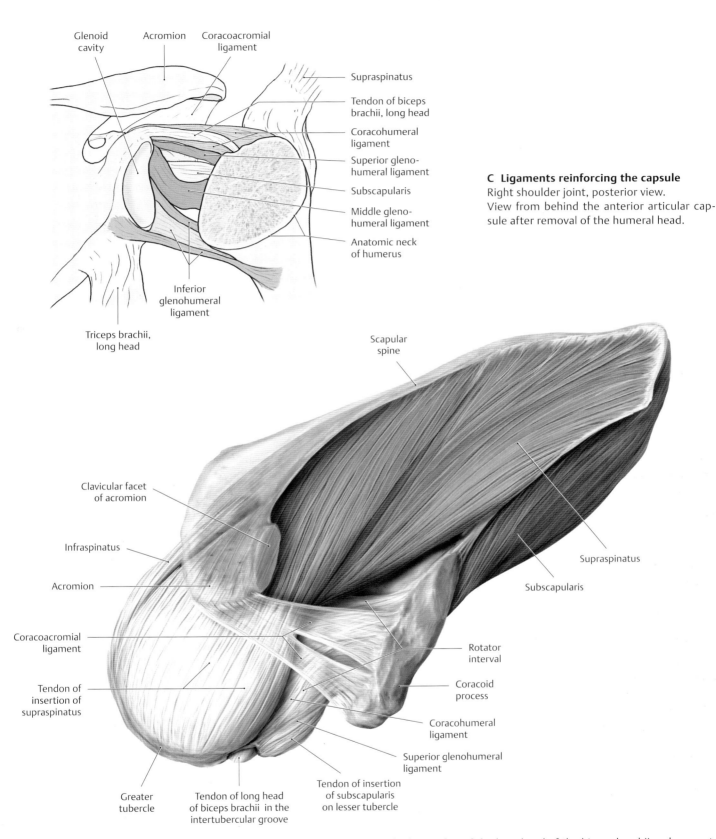

Glenoid cavity

Acromion

Coracoacromial ligament

Supraspinatus

Tendon of biceps brachii, long head

Coracohumeral ligament

Superior gleno-humeral ligament

Subscapularis

Middle gleno-humeral ligament

Anatomic neck of humerus

Inferior glenohumeral ligament

Triceps brachii, long head

C Ligaments reinforcing the capsule
Right shoulder joint, posterior view.
View from behind the anterior articular capsule after removal of the humeral head.

Scapular spine

Clavicular facet of acromion

Infraspinatus

Acromion

Coracoacromial ligament

Tendon of insertion of supraspinatus

Greater tubercle

Tendon of long head of biceps brachii in the intertubercular groove

Tendon of insertion of subscapularis on lesser tubercle

Supraspinatus

Subscapularis

Rotator interval

Coracoid process

Coracohumeral ligament

Superior glenohumeral ligament

D Rotator interval
Right shoulder, superior view; clavicle and deltoid have been removed. The rotator interval is the capsular area or gap between the superior edge of the subscapularis and the anterior edge of the supraspinatus. The glenohumeral and coracohumeral ligaments are primarily responsible for reinforcing the articular capsule. The ligaments join together in the rotator interval to form the so-called biceps pulley, which sur-

rounds the tendon of the long head of the biceps brachii and prevents it from being dislocated in an anterior-medial direction. The superior glenohumeral ligament forms the bottom and the coracohumeral ligament forms the top of this "sling" or "pulley" (see **Bb**). In addition, fibers from the tendons of insertion of the subscapularis and supraspinatus are interwoven in the rotator interval.

14.15 The Joints of the Shoulder: The Subacromial Space

A Subacromial space, right shoulder
Lateral view. The deltoid muscle has been removed to demonstrate the following structures:

- The attachments of the rotator cuff muscles (supraspinatus, infraspinatus, teres minor, and subscapularis) to the proximal humerus (see also **B**)
- The tendons of origin of the biceps brachii muscle
- The subacromial space with the subacromial bursa, which consistently communicates with the subdeltoid bursa

The two bursae allow frictionless gliding between the humeral head and the rotator cuff tendons (especially the supraspinatus and the upper part of the infraspinatus) beneath the coracoacromial arch during abduction and elevation of the arm (see p. 275).

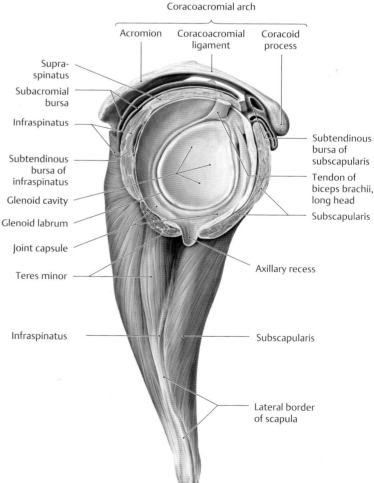

B Subacromial bursa and glenoid cavity of the right shoulder joint
Lateral view. The humeral head has been removed and the rotator cuff tendons of insertion have been divided to demonstrate the glenoid cavity of the shoulder joint. The *glenoid labrum* enlarges and deepens the glenoid only very slightly. Just before inserting into the humeral head, the muscles of the rotator cuff send tendinous expansions to the joint capsule that help to press the humeral head into the glenoid cavity. The subacromial bursa is located between the coracoacromial arch and the tendons that insert on the humeral head (see **D**).

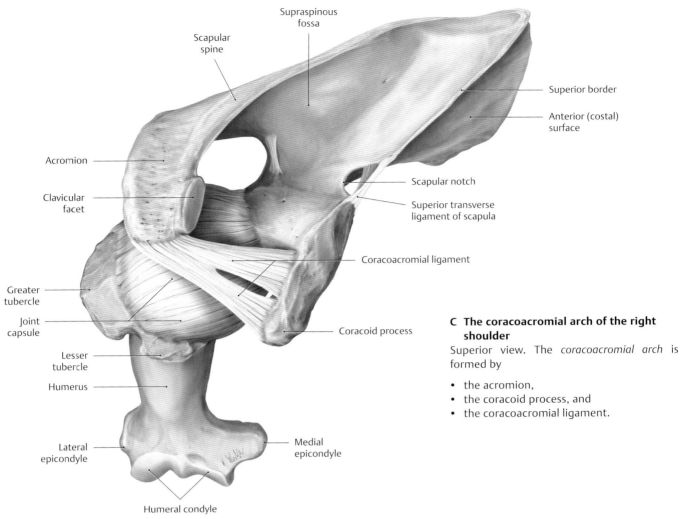

Supraspinous fossa

Scapular spine

Acromion

Clavicular facet

Greater tubercle

Joint capsule

Lesser tubercle

Humerus

Lateral epicondyle

Humeral condyle

Medial epicondyle

Superior border

Anterior (costal) surface

Scapular notch

Superior transverse ligament of scapula

Coracoacromial ligament

Coracoid process

C The coracoacromial arch of the right shoulder

Superior view. The *coracoacromial arch* is formed by

- the acromion,
- the coracoid process, and
- the coracoacromial ligament.

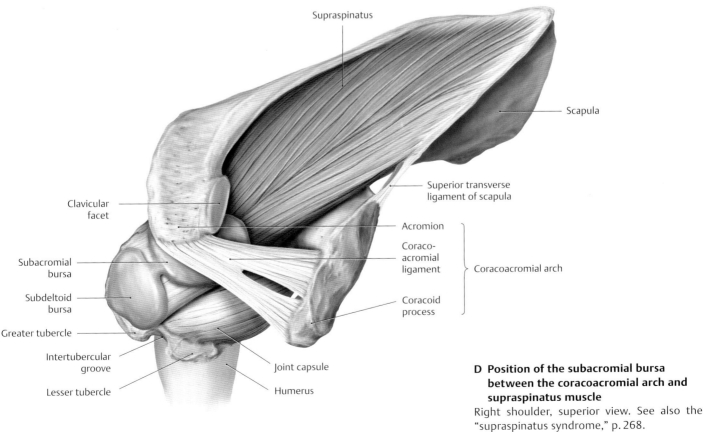

Supraspinatus

Scapula

Clavicular facet

Subacromial bursa

Subdeltoid bursa

Greater tubercle

Intertubercular groove

Lesser tubercle

Joint capsule

Humerus

Superior transverse ligament of scapula

Acromion

Coraco-acromial ligament

Coracoid process

Coracoacromial arch

D Position of the subacromial bursa between the coracoacromial arch and supraspinatus muscle

Right shoulder, superior view. See also the "supraspinatus syndrome," p. 268.

267

14.16 **The Subacromial and Subdeltoid Bursae**

Coracoacromial arch

Coracoacromial ligament

Acromion

Coracoid process

Subacromial bursa

Subdeltoid bursa

Glenohumeral joint capsule

Deltoid

Tendon sheath in intertubercular groove

Subcutaneous acromial bursa

Acromioclavicular ligament

Trapezius

Coracoclavicular ligament

Clavicle

Superior transverse ligament of scapula

First rib

Subtendinous bursa of subscapularis

Subscapularis

Biceps brachii, long head

Biceps brachii, short head

Coraco-brachialis

Teres major

A Location of bursae in the right shoulder
Anterior view. The pectoralis major and minor and serratus anterior muscles have been removed. The location of the bursae can be seen through the deltoid muscle, which is lightly shaded.
Note in particular the coracoacromial arch and the underlying subacromial bursa.

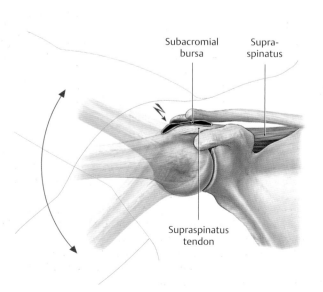

Subacromial bursa

Supraspinatus

Supraspinatus tendon

B Supraspinatus (impingement) syndrome
A supraspinatus tendon that has been thickened by calcification or other degenerative changes can be caught underneath the acromion, impinging upon the subacromial bursa, when the arm is abducted (see **D**). Pain from this *supraspinatus*, or *impingement*, *syndrome* occurs in an arc of motion between 60 and 120° of abduction.

Labels for figure C:
- Skin and subcutaneous tissue
- Trapezius
- Subacromial bursa
- Supraspinatus
- Scapula, glenoid cavity
- Subscapularis
- Glenoid labrum
- Axillary recess
- Teres major
- Latissimus dorsi
- Acromion
- Supraspinatus tendon
- Head of humerus
- Subdeltoid bursa
- Deltoid
- Humerus

C Coronal section through the right shoulder joint

Anterior view. The tendon of insertion of the supraspinatus muscle differs structurally from ordinary traction tendons. Its distal course gives it the function of a gliding tendon, which passes over the fulcrum of the humeral head (arrows). In that area, located approximately 1 to 2 cm proximal to its insertion on the greater tubercle, the tendon tissue in contact with the humeral head is composed of fibrocartilage. This fibrocartilage zone is avascular, representing an adaptation of the tendon to the pressure loads imposed by the bony fulcrum (drawing based on a specimen from the Anatomical Collection at the University of Kiel).

Labels for figure D:
- Subdeltoid bursa
- Calcification
- Subacromial bursa
- Acromion
- Supraspinatus

a   b   c   d   e

D Damage to the supraspinatus tendon

a Calcification of the tendon of insertion of the supraspinatus, resulting from degenerative changes in the area surrounding the fibrocartilaginous zone (see also **C**); **b–d** partial defects in the supraspinatus tendon (**b** bursal-sided, **c** intratendinous, and **d** articular-sided); **e** complete defect (tear) of the supraspinatus tendon (also called rotator cuff rupture).

Degenerative changes of the rotator cuff, primarily the supraspinatus tendon, together with the clinical effects on the tendon of the long head of the biceps brachii, as well as the subacromial and subdeltoid bursa, generally lead to a painful functional disorder in the shoulder area. The cause of this so-called subacromial syndrome (or subacromial pain syndrome) is the pathologic contact of the calcified and thickened supraspinatus tendon with the acromion, or subacromial impingement syndrome. After a complete rotator cuff rupture (in 95% of all cases, the supraspinatus tendon is involved), the subacromial and subdeltoid bursae communicate with the articular cavity. The supraspinatus normally contributes significantly to the first 10° of abduction (the "starter function"; see p. 302).

269

14.17 Shoulder Arthroscopy

A Overview of arthroscopy of the shoulder joint
Arthroscopy of the shoulder joint has taken on an increasingly important role in the field of arthroscopic surgery. Initially, it was predominantly a diagnostic procedure. Over time, as a result of technical advances, it has become a surgical technique for resection and reconstruction of the shoulder joint, increasingly replacing open shoulder surgeries. Arthroscopy is now considered primarily a therapeutic surgical procedure, which also allows a dynamic functional evaluation of the capsule ligament structures, e.g., in case of instability. Currently, all surgeries are possible as part of arthroscopy of the shoulder joint, with the exception of endoprothesis. Indications for arthroscopy of the shoulder joint can be classified into three groups:

- Shoulder instability, e.g., labral lesion (Bankert lesion), osteochondral lesion (Hill-Sachs lesion);
- Degenerative changes, e.g., partial or complete rotator cuff rupture, subacromial impingement syndrome (tendonitis calcarea), biceps brachii tendon; and
- Inflammatory changes, e.g., synovialitis, adhesive capsulitis.

B Patient positioning
Two standard positions are available:

- Lateral position
- Half-sitting position (so-called beach-chair position)

In the half-sitting position, the patient sits upright with the back flexed at 60°. The advantage of this position is that it allows full rotation and abduction of the arm during surgery. In addition, in case the operation needs to be converted to an open procedure, there is no need to repostion the patient, nor does it require additional washing or surgical drapes. Furthermore, the arm can be extended using traction weights in order to get a better view inside the joint.

C Shoulder arthroscopy portals
a Right shoulder joint, lateral view; for better orientation, the most important anatomic landmarks have been marked: coracoid process, lateral end of the clavicle, acromion, and acromioclavicular joint; **b** arthroscopic portals, right shoulder joint (humeral head removed), lateral view. With the arthroscopic portals, one differentiates between

- Instrument portals (through which instruments are inserted) and
- Optical portals.

The standard portal for the 30°-angled arthroscope is created by making a stab incision 1 cm inferior and 1.5 cm medial to the posterolateral acromial margin (dorsal portal). Afterward, a blunt trocar is used to perforate first the subcutaneous tissue followed by the deltoid and the dorsal capsule in the direction of the coracoid process. Then, the trocar is replaced by a camera, and the articular cavity is washed. The anterior and anterior-superior portals are commonly used to insert the instruments. Depending on the type of surgery, additional portals can be created, e.g., the lateral portal for access to the subacromial space. Whereas the anterior portal is created by incising the skin lateral to the tip of the coracoid process and accessing the joint above the subscapularis tendon, the anterior-superior portal is made just in front of the anterolateral angle of the acromion with the joint being accessed just behind the tendon of the long head of the biceps brachii. Moving the arthroscope to different portals allows for a complete overview of the articular space.

a

b

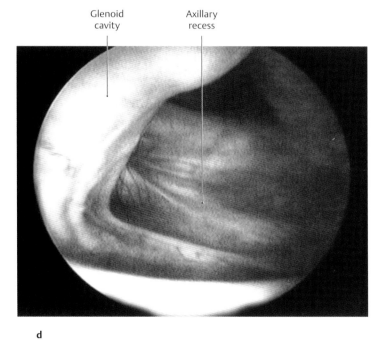

c

d

D Arthroscopic anatomy of the shoulder joint

a Schematic representation of the arthroscopically visible fields of sight; right shoulder, dorsal view; **b-d** corresponding arthroscopy images (from Merk H, Jerosch J, Hrsg. Arthroskopie des Schultergelenks. Stuttgart: Thieme; 2000).

For the arthroscopic evaluation of the intra-articular structures, a standardized test using examining hooks is recommended. The goal of this examination is the inspection of the entire articular space. In the beach-chair position (see **B**) with dorsal view, the glenoid cavity is oriented vertically. Over the opposite humeral head, the tendon of the long head of the biceps brachii passes horizontally through the superior articular space to the supraglenoid tubercle and is clearly visible as an anatomic landmark. The tendon of the long head of the biceps brachii together with the glenoid cavity and head of the humerus form the anterior triangle with the subscapularis tendon and the transverse humeral ligament (**b, c**). By tilting the lens upward, the insertion of the tendon of the long head of the biceps brachii into the intertubercular groove in the rotator interval becomes visible at the anterior edge of the supraspinatus tendon. The superior glenohumeral ligament and the anterior edge of the supraspinatus tendon form a U-shaped sling, which crosses underneath the tendon of the long head of the biceps brachii. Furthermore, the undersurface of the supraspinatus and infraspinatus tendons can be made visible. The inferior glenohumeral ligament can be best evaluated from the anterior portal looking toward the axillary recess. It extends—with its anterior and posterior fibers as well as the axillary recess located between them—to the inferior edge of the glenoid cavity.

14.18 X-ray and Cross-sectional Anatomy of the Shoulder

A Conventional diagnostic radiology of the right shoulder joint

In primary diagnosis, clinical assessments and sonographic examinations (see **B**) are followed by X-ray radiography. Additionally, complicated injuries can be examined with the help of computed tomography and magnetic resonance imaging (see **C**). Similar to the X-ray radiography in evaluating bones and joints, it is recommended to take two images of two perpendicular planes:

- Anteroposterior image (**a** and **b**) and
- Axial (transverse) image (**c** and **d**).

In order to avoid overlap in X-ray images, the glenoid cavity needs to be placed at a 30° angle when taking an anteroposterior image. At slight external rotation, the head of the humerus and the glenoid cavity are shown without overlap; the greater tubercle forms the lateral contour. In the axial image, the patient lies on his or her back with the arm slightly rotated outward and abducted. The X-ray cassette is positioned superior to the shoulder with the beam hitting the axilla inferiorly. As a result, the head of the humerus and glenoid cavity are shown at a right angle to the anteroposterior image (enhancing the detection of fractures).

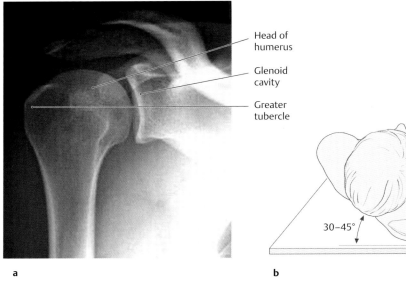

Head of humerus
Glenoid cavity
Greater tubercle

a

b

30–45°

Glenoid cavity
Greater tubercle
Coracoid process

c

d

a

Tendon of biceps brachii, long head
Subscapularis tendon
Lesser tubercle

Greater tubercle
Deltoid

c

Deltoid
Tendon of biceps brachii, long head
Greater tubercle
Lesser tubercle

b

B Diagnostic ultrasound of the anterior region of the left shoulder

a Sonogram; **b** position of the transducer at the level of the intertubercular groove of the left shoulder joint; **c** schematic representation of the sonogram (caudal view of the transverse section) (**a** and **b** from Konermann W, Gruber G. Ultraschalldiagnostik der Bewegungsorgane. 2nd ed. Stuttgart: Thieme; 2006).

Like diagnostic x-rays, in standardized sonographic examination of joints, two almost perpendicular planes (transverse and longitudinal) are used. Rotation of the arm, combined with different positions of the transducer, allows for an all-encompassing examination of the shoulder joint.

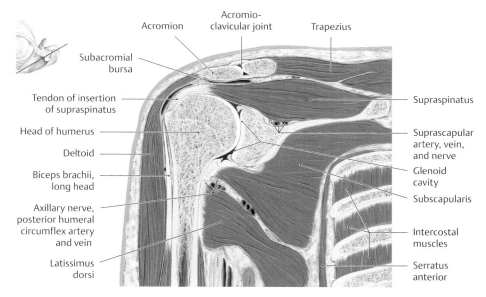

a Coronal, T1-weighted image (cross section parallel to the supraspinatus and perpendicular to the glenoid cavity)

b Sagittal, T1-weighted image (cross section parallel to the glenoid cavity)

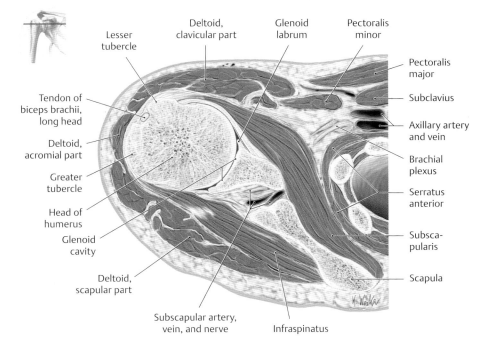

c Axial (transverse), T1-weighted image

C MRI examination of the right shoulder joint in three planes
(From Möller TB, Reif E. Taschenatlas der Schnittbildanatomie, Band III. Stuttgart: Thieme; 2007.) *Note:* Axial images are always viewed inferiorly.

14.19 Movements of the Shoulder Girdle and Shoulder Joint

A Movements of the scapula
The sternoclavicular and acromioclavicular joints are mechanically linked in such a way that all movements of the clavicle are accompanied by movements of the scapula. The scapula moves by gliding on the chest wall in the scapulothoracic joint. Both its movement and its fixation are effected by muscular slings. The following types of scapular movement are distinguished:

a Elevation and depression (during elevation and depression of the shoulder girdle): translation of the scapula in the craniocaudal direction.

b Abduction and adduction (during protraction and retraction of the shoulder girdle): horizontal translation of the scapula in the postero-medial-to-anterolateral direction.

c Lateral rotation of the inferior angle (during abduction or elevation of the arm): rotation of the scapula about an anteroposterior axis through the center of the scapula. With an approximately 60° range of rotation, the inferior angle of the scapula moves about 10 cm laterally, while the superior angle moves about 2 to 3 cm inferomedially.

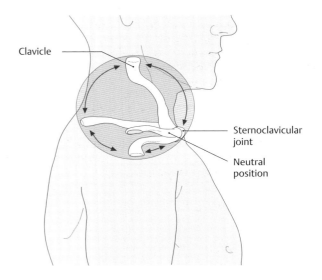

B Movements (and range of motion) in the sternoclavicular joint
a Elevation and depression of the shoulder about a parasagittal axis.
b Protraction and retraction of the shoulder about a longitudinal (vertical) axis.

C Range of motion of the clavicle
Right clavicle, lateral view. Viewing the range of motion of the clavicle in the sternoclavicular joint from the lateral view, we find that the clavicle moves roughly within a conical shell whose apex is directed toward the sternum, and with a slightly oval base approximately 10 to 13 cm in diameter. The clavicle also rotates about its own axis, particularly during elevation of the shoulder girdle, where its S shape significantly increases the range of shoulder elevation. The range of this rotation is approximately 45° and creates a third degree of freedom that gives the sternoclavicular joint the function of a spheroidal joint.

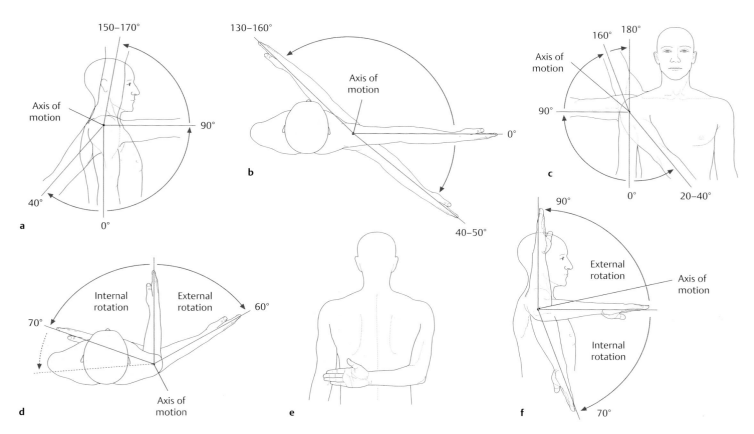

D Movements in the shoulder joint

As a typical spheroidal joint, the shoulder joint has three mutually perpendicular cardinal axes with three degrees of freedom and a total of six main directions of movement. In a very basic sense, all movements in the shoulder girdle can be classified as vertical, horizontal, or rotational. In *vertical movements*, the arm is elevated in various directions from a neutral adducted position. In *horizontal movements*, the arm is moved forward or backward while in 90° of abduction. *Rotational movements* can be performed with the arm in any position. The maximum *range* of these various movements can be achieved only by concomitant movement of the shoulder girdle, however.

a Flexion and extension occur about a horizontal axis.
b Flexion and extension of the arm raised to 90° abduction are also described as horizontal movements.

c Abduction and adduction occur about a sagittal axis, with movements past 90° often referred to as elevation. In clinical parlance, however, the term "elevation" is generally applied to all vertical movements. Past 80 to 90° of abduction, an automatic external rotation occurs that keeps the greater tubercle from impinging on the coracoacromial arch. When the arm is abducted while internally rotated, the range of abduction is decreased to approximately 60°.
d–f Internal and external rotation of the arm occurs about the longitudinal (shaft) axis of the humerus. When the arm is flexed at the elbow during these movements, the forearm can be used as a pointer. When the arm is hanging at the side, the maximum range of internal rotation is limited by the trunk. Placing the arm behind the back is equivalent to 95° of internal rotation (**e**). When the arm is abducted 90°, the range of external rotation is increased, while the maximum range of internal rotation is slightly reduced (**f**).

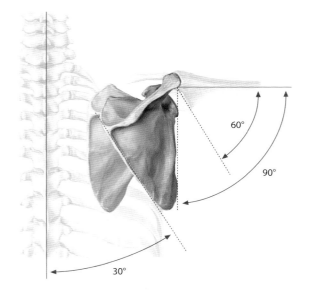

E Humeroscapular rhythm

The arm and scapula move in a 2 : 1 ratio during abduction. This means that when the arm is abducted 90°, for example, 60° of that movement occurs in the glenohumeral joint, while 30° is accomplished by concomitant movement of the shoulder girdle. This "humeroscapular rhythm" is dependent upon freedom of movement of the scapula during abduction. Diseases of the shoulder joint can alter this rhythm, often causing the scapula to begin its rotation considerably earlier. This is best illustrated by cases involving ankylosis or arthrodesis of the glenohumeral joint (pathological or intentional operative stiffening or fixation), in which movements in the shoulder girdle alone still permit the arm to be abducted 40 to 60° and still allow for one third the normal range of flexion/extension.

275

14.20 The Elbow Joint as a Whole

a Anterior view

b Posterior view

c Lateral view

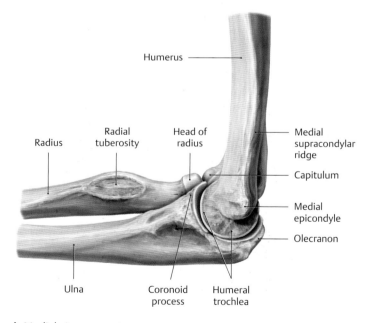

d Medial view

A The articulating skeletal elements of the right elbow joint

The *humerus*, *radius*, and *ulna* articulate with one another at the elbow (cubital) joint. The elbow consists of three articulations:

- The humeroulnar joint between the humerus and ulna
- The humeroradial joint between the humerus and radius
- The proximal radioulnar joint between the proximal ends of the ulna and radius

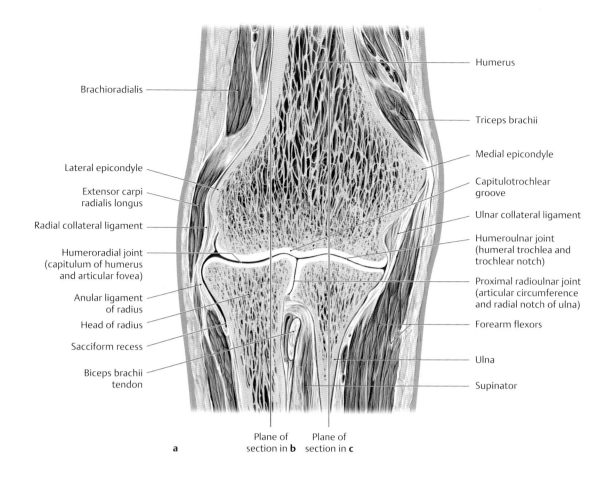

Brachioradialis

Lateral epicondyle

Extensor carpi radialis longus

Radial collateral ligament

Humeroradial joint (capitulum of humerus and articular fovea)

Anular ligament of radius

Head of radius

Sacciform recess

Biceps brachii tendon

Humerus

Triceps brachii

Medial epicondyle

Capitulotrochlear groove

Ulnar collateral ligament

Humeroulnar joint (humeral trochlea and trochlear notch)

Proximal radioulnar joint (articular circumference and radial notch of ulna)

Forearm flexors

Ulna

Supinator

Plane of section in **b**   Plane of section in **c**

a

Brachialis   Humerus   Triceps brachii

Capitulum

Brachio-radialis

Articular fovea

Head of radius

Fat pad

Articular circum-ference

Radial notch of ulna

Anconeus

Supinator

b   Radius   Ulna

Brachialis   Humerus   Triceps brachii

Fat pad

Coronoid fossa

Olecranon fossa

Olecranon bursa

Humeral trochlea

Olecranon

Trochlear notch

c   Coronoid process   Ulna

B Skeletal and soft-tissue elements of the right elbow joint

a Coronal section viewed from the front (*note* the planes of section shown in **b** and **c**).

b Sagittal section through the humeroradial joint and proximal radio-ulnar joint, medial view.

c Sagittal section through the humeroulnar joint, medial view.

(Drawings based on specimens from the Anatomical Collection at the University of Kiel.)

277

14.21 The Elbow Joint: Capsule and Ligaments

a

c

Humerus

Olecranon fossa

Medial epicondyle

Ulnar groove

Ulnar collateral ligament

Olecranon

Lateral supracondylar ridge

Lateral epicondyle

Radial collateral ligament

Humerus

Lesser tubercle, supracondylar ridge

Lateral epicondyle

Sacciform recess

Radius

Olecranon

Radial collateral ligament

Anular ligament of radius

Neck of radius

Ulna

Radius

Radial tuberosity

Anular ligament of radius

Humerus

Ulnar collateral ligament, anterior part

Medial epicondyle

Ulnar collateral ligament, posterior part

Ulnar collateral ligament, transverse part

Ulna

Coronoid process

Olecranon

b

a   **b**   **c**

A The capsule and ligaments of the right elbow joint in 90° flexion

a Posterior view, **b** medial view, **c** lateral view with forearm pronated. Both the humeroradial and humeroulnar joints are stabilized by powerful collateral ligaments that strengthen the lateral portions of the joint capsule. These structures, called the *ulnar collateral ligament* and *radial collateral ligament*, have a fan-shaped arrangement that can give lateral stability to the joint in any position. The *anular ligament* of the radius (see also **D**) stabilizes the proximal radioulnar joint.

B The Hueter line and triangle

a Extension, posterior view; **b** flexion, medial view; **c** flexion, posterior view.

The epicondyles and the olecranon lie on a straight line when viewed from the posterior view in the extended elbow. They also lie on a straight line when viewed from the lateral view in the flexed elbow. But when the flexed elbow is viewed from behind, the two epicondyles and the tip of the olecranon form an equilateral triangle. Fractures and dislocations alter the shape of the triangle.

C The capsule and ligaments of the right elbow joint in extension
a Anterior view, **b** Anterior view with the ventral portions of the capsule removed.
The joint capsule of the elbow encloses all three articulations in the elbow joint complex. While the capsule is thin anteriorly and posteriorly, it is reinforced on each side by the collateral ligaments (see **A**).

Over the end of the radius, the joint capsule is expanded below the annular ligament to form the sacciform recess—a redundant tissue fold that provides a reserve capacity during pronation and supination of the forearm. During flexion and extension, the brachialis and anconeus muscles tighten the joint capsule to prevent entrapment of the capsule between the articular surfaces (see p. 312).

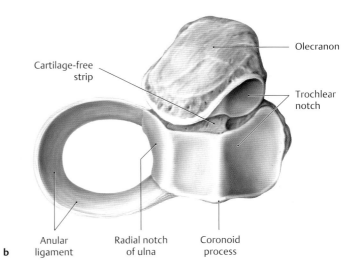

D Course of the anular ligament in the right proximal radioulnar joint
a View of the proximal articular surfaces of the radius and ulna after removal of the humerus. **b** Same view as in **a** with the radius also removed.
The anular ligament is of key importance in stabilizing the proximal radioulnar joint. It runs from the anterior to the posterior border of the

radial notch of the ulna (= cartilage-covered articular surface on the ulna), wrapping around the radial head and pressing it into the ulnar articular surface. Histologically, the inner surface of the anular ligament has the fibrocartilaginous structure of a gliding tendon, enabling it to withstand the compressive loads that are transmitted to the ligament.

14.22 The Forearm: Proximal and Distal Radioulnar Joints

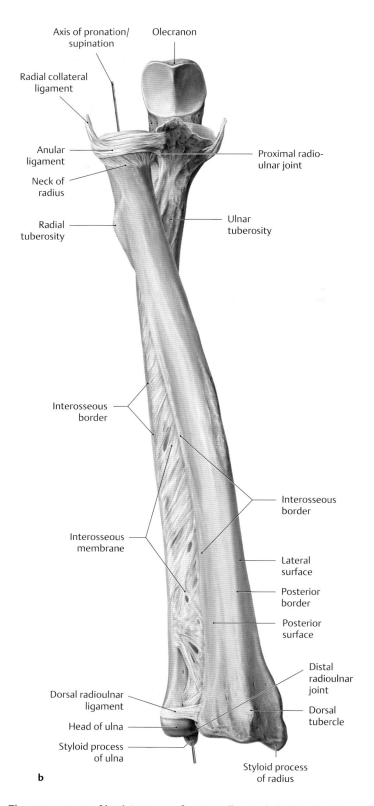

a

b

A Ligaments and axes for pronation and supination in the proximal and distal radioulnar joints
Right forearm, anterior view.

a Supination (the radius and ulna are parallel to each other).
b Pronation (the radius crosses over the ulna).

The proximal radioulnar joint functions together with the distal radioulnar joint to enable pronation and supination movements of the hand.

The movements of both joints are functionally interlinked by the interosseous membrane, so that the movement of one is necessarily associated with movement of the other. The axis for pronation and supination runs obliquely from the center of the humeral capitulum (not shown) through the center of the radial articular fovea down to the styloid process of the ulna.

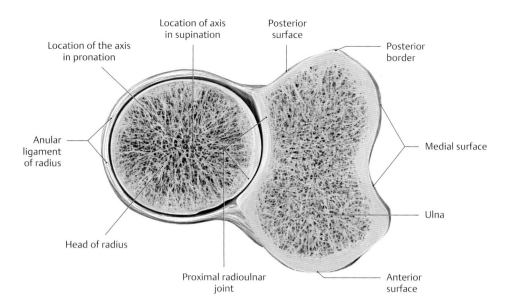

B Cross section through the right proximal radioulnar joint in pronation

Distal view. Owing to the slightly oval shape of the radial head, the pronation/supination axis that runs through the radial head moves approximately 2 mm radially during pronation (the long diameter of the radial head is transverse when pronation is reached). This ensures that when the hand is pronated, there will be sufficient space for the radial tuberosity within the interosseous space (= the space between the radial tuberosity and oblique cord; see **Aa**, for example).

Note the thicker articular cartilage of the radial articular circumference on the pronation side. This thickening occurs as an adaptation to the greater articular pressure in the proximal radioulnar joint in the pronated position.

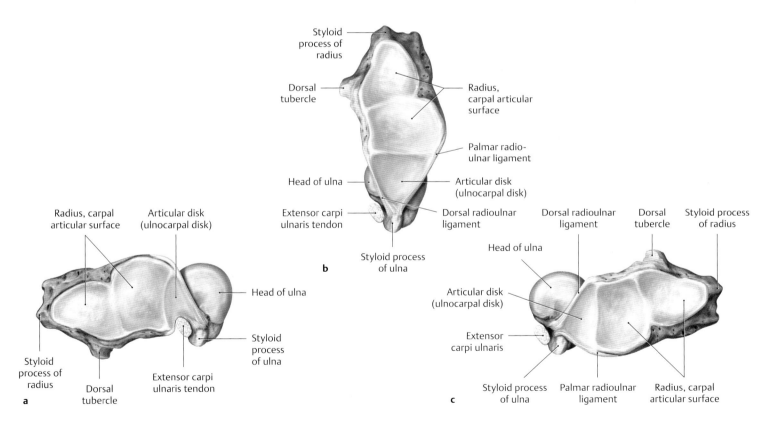

C Rotation of the radius and ulna during pronation and supination

View of the distal articular surfaces of the radius and ulna of the right forearm. For clarity, the ulnocarpal disk is not shown.

a Supination
b Semipronation
c Pronation

The dorsal and palmar radioulnar ligaments are part of the "ulnocarpal complex," which serves to stabilize the distal radioulnar joint. The mode of contact between the two distal articular surfaces varies with the position of the radius and ulna. They are in close apposition only in an intermediate (semipronated or neutral) position (after Schmidt and Lanz).

14.23 Movements of the Elbow and Radioulnar Joints

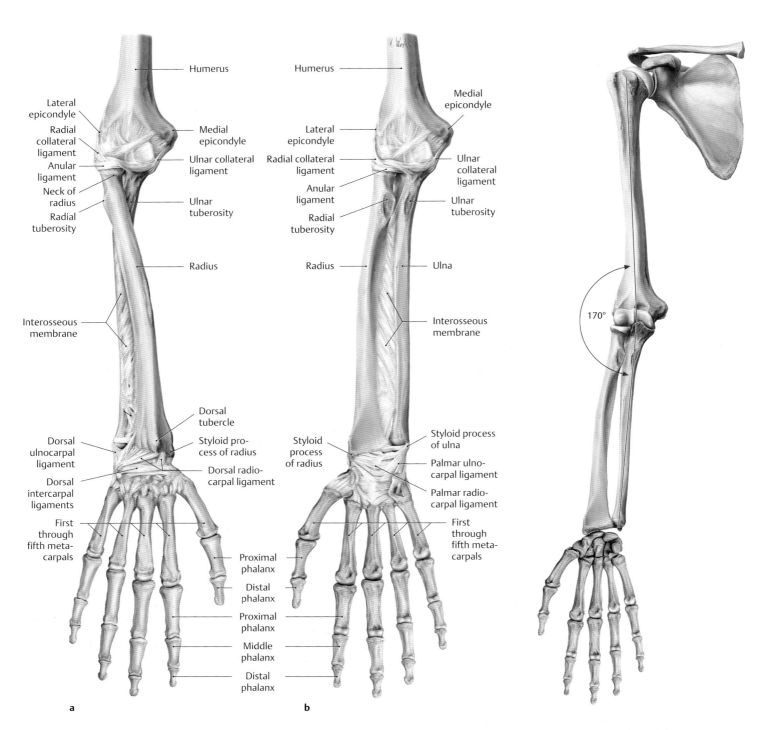

Humerus

Lateral epicondyle

Radial collateral ligament

Anular ligament

Neck of radius

Radial tuberosity

Medial epicondyle

Ulnar collateral ligament

Ulnar tuberosity

Radius

Interosseous membrane

Dorsal ulnocarpal ligament

Dorsal intercarpal ligaments

Dorsal tubercle

Styloid process of radius

Dorsal radio-carpal ligament

First through fifth meta-carpals

Proximal phalanx

Distal phalanx

Proximal phalanx

Middle phalanx

Distal phalanx

a

Humerus

Medial epicondyle

Lateral epicondyle

Radial collateral ligament

Anular ligament

Radial tuberosity

Ulnar collateral ligament

Ulnar tuberosity

Radius

Ulna

Interosseous membrane

Styloid process of radius

Styloid process of ulna

Palmar ulno-carpal ligament

Palmar radio-carpal ligament

First through fifth meta-carpals

b

170°

A Pronation and supination of the right hand
Anterior view.
a Pronation, **b** supination.
Pronation and supination of the hand make it possible to raise an object to the mouth for eating and to touch any area of the body for protection or cleaning. Pronation and supina-

tion are also essential for the working hand in actions such as turning a screwdriver, screwing in a light bulb, emptying a bucket, and unlocking a door. The range of hand movements can be further increased by adding movements of the shoulder girdle and trunk. This may be done, for example, to enable a full 360° twisting movement of the hand.

B Normal valgus of the elbow joint
Skeleton of the right upper limb with the forearm supinated. Anterior view.
The shape of the humeral trochlea (see p. 276) results in a normal valgus angulation between the humeral shaft and ulna (*cubitus valgus*) [valgus = bend or twist outward, away from the body axis]). This applies particularly during extension and supination. This "cubital angle" equals approximately 170°.

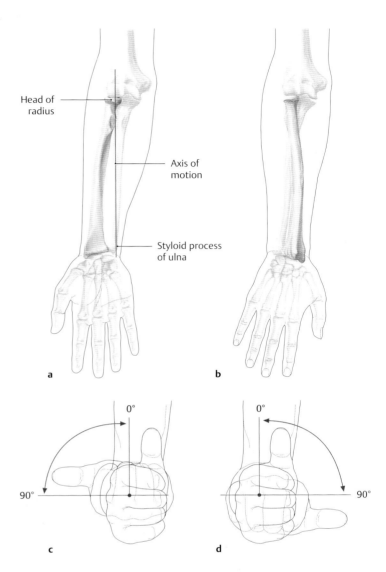

C Range of motion in the humeroradial and humeroulnar joints of the elbow

The flexion/extension axis of the forearm runs below the epicondyles through the capitulum and trochlea of the humerus. Starting from the neutral (0°) position, both joints have a maximum range of 150° in flexion and approximately 10° in extension. Both movements are constrained either by soft tissues (muscles, fat, etc. = soft-tissue restraint) or by bone (olecranon = bony restraint).

D Range and axis of pronation/supination of the right hand

The neutral (0°) position of the hand and forearm is also called semi-pronation. The axis of pronation/supination extends through the head of the radius and the styloid process of the ulna.

a Supination (the radius and ulna are parallel to each other).
b Pronation (the radius crosses over the ulna).
c Supination of the hand with the elbow flexed, viewed from the front (the palmar surface of the hand is up).
d Pronation of the hand with the elbow flexed, viewed from the front (the palmar surface of the hand is down).

E Pulled elbow, or nursemaid's elbow

Pilled elbow is a very common injury in children (5- to 7-year-olds; with increasing age, ligaments become stronger, reducing the risk of injuries). The head of the radius slips under the anular ligament (radial head subluxation), which results from a sudden pull on a child's arm. As a result, the anular ligament gets stuck between the radius and the capitulum, the elbow joint is locked in a slighly bent position, the arm remains turned inward (pronated position). Due to subluxation and accompanying pain, the child keeps the arm immobile and allows it to hang downward, which makes the arm appear to be paralyzed (pseudoparesis; so-called Chassaignac's paralysis). The clinical findings and the required X-ray examination in two planes to rule out any bone injuries (epiphyseal fracture of the head of the radius) confirm the diagnosis. After reduction, during which the bent elbow joint is extended while firmly supinating the wrist, the child is symptom-free within minutes.

283

14.24 **Overview of the Ligaments of the Hand**

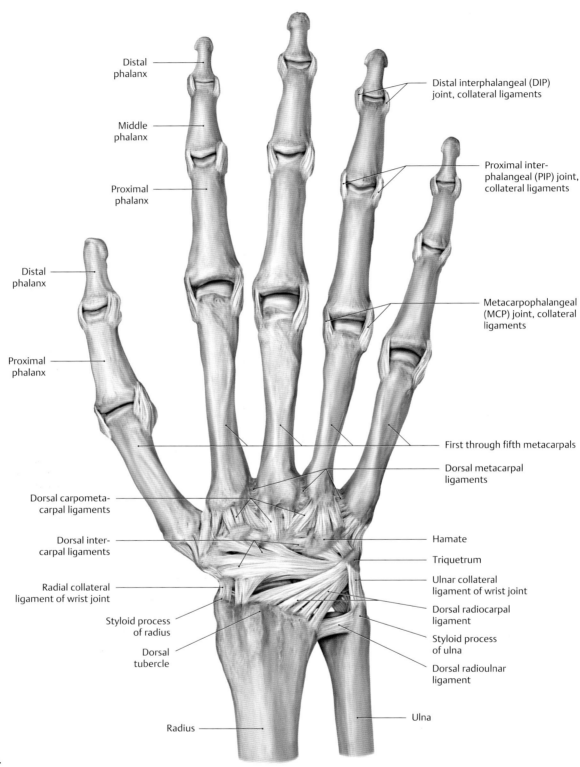

Distal phalanx

Middle phalanx

Proximal phalanx

Distal interphalangeal (DIP) joint, collateral ligaments

Proximal inter-phalangeal (PIP) joint, collateral ligaments

Distal phalanx

Proximal phalanx

Metacarpophalangeal (MCP) joint, collateral ligaments

First through fifth metacarpals

Dorsal metacarpal ligaments

Dorsal carpometa-carpal ligaments

Dorsal inter-carpal ligaments

Hamate

Triquetrum

Radial collateral ligament of wrist joint

Ulnar collateral ligament of wrist joint

Styloid process of radius

Dorsal radiocarpal ligament

Styloid process of ulna

Dorsal tubercle

Dorsal radioulnar ligament

Ulna

Radius

a Dorsal view.

A   The ligaments of the right hand.
Carpal ligaments connect adjacent bones, limiting excess movement and providing stability to the wrist. Their courses vary. They are closely interwoven, and so they are difficult to dissect. The so-called extrinsic carpal ligaments, which run closer to the surface, are interwoven with the articular capsule and primarily act to stabilize it. Deeper, the so-called intrinsic carpal ligaments (see p. 286), divide the joint space into individual compartments.

Distal inter-phalangeal (DIP) joint capsule

Distal phalanx

Proximal inter-phalangeal (PIP) joint capsule

Middle phalanx

Proximal phalanx

Deep transverse metacarpal ligament

Metacarpo-phalangeal (MCP) joint, collateral ligaments

Palmar metacarpal ligaments

Hook of hamate

Ulnar collateral ligament

Pisiform bone

Flexor carpi ulnaris tendon of insertion

Ulnotriquetral ligament (palmar ulnocarpal ligament)

Styloid process of ulna

Ulna

Palmar ligaments

Distal phalanx

Proximal phalanx

First through fifth meta-carpals

Palmar carpometa-carpal ligaments

Palmar intercarpal ligaments

Tubercle of trapezium

Radial collateral ligament

Styloid process of radius

Palmar radiocarpal ligament

Palmar radioulnar ligament

Distal radioulnar joint

Radius

b Palmar view.

Aside from the common classification as extrinsic and intrinsic, the carpal ligaments are also classified according to their location and arrangement:

- The ligaments between the forearm and carpal bones (radiocarpal and ulnocarpal ligaments, collateral ligaments)
- The ligaments between individual carpal bones (intercarpal liga-ments)

- The ligaments between the carpal and metacarpal bones (carpo-metacarpal ligaments)
- The ligaments between the bases of the metacarpals (metacarpal ligaments)

285

14.25 Intrinsic Ligaments of the Hand, Compartments of the Joint, and Ulnocarpal Complex

A Interosseous ligaments and compartments within the carpus
a Coronal section of the right carpus, dorsal view (drawing based on a specimen from the Anatomical Collection of the University of Kiel); **b** schematic representation of compartments (dorsal view of right hand); **c** arthrography of the radiocarpal joint (courtesy of Dr. J. Koebke, Anatomical Institute, University of Cologne); **d** and **e** CT arthrography of the radiocarpal joint (from Bohndorf K, Imhof H, Fischer W. Radiologische Diagnostik der Knochen und Gelenke. 2nd ed. Stuttgart: Thieme; 2006): **d** intact compartment; **e** lesion of the ulnocarpal disk with contrast agent crossing over into the radioulnar joint.

In addition to the extrinsic ligaments of the carpus (see p. 284), which reinforce the articular capsule, there are intrinsic ligaments. These interosseous ligaments, along with the ulnocarpal disk (triangular disk), divide the intra-articular space into compartments, some of which are completely enclosed. These compartments include (see **b**)

- distal radioulnar joint,
- radiocarpal joint,
- medial carpal compartment,
- carpometacarpal joint,
- intermetacarpal compartment, and
- thumb saddle joint.

Knowledge of these compartments is clinically significant for conducting and interpreting arthrographies (**c** to **e**).

The main intrinsic interosseous ligaments are those of the distal carpal row (capitohamate and trapeziocapitate ligaments), the proximal carpal row (lunotriquetral and scapholunate ligaments) (see **a**), and the ulnocarpal disk, the most important structure of the ulnocarpal complex (see **b**). These ligament structures often succumb to degeneration or are affected in cases of carpal injuries. Degenerative changes in the ulnocarpal disk can already be detected in people in their 20s, but degeneration of the interosseous ligaments of the proximal carpal row are more commonly seen in older patients (in 30% of all cases).

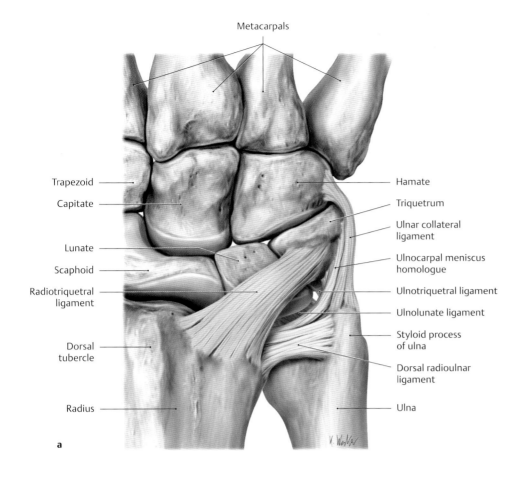

Metacarpals

Trapezoid

Capitate

Lunate

Scaphoid

Radiotriquetral
ligament

Dorsal
tubercle

Radius

Hamate

Triquetrum

Ulnar collateral
ligament

Ulnocarpal meniscus
homologue

Ulnotriquetral ligament

Ulnolunate ligament

Styloid process
of ulna

Dorsal radioulnar
ligament

Ulna

a

Hamate

Midcarpal
joint

Lunate

Lunotriquetral
ligament

Ulnocarpal disk

Radiocarpal joint

Distal radio-
ulnar joint

Radius

Ulnar collateral
ligament

Triquetrum

Ulnocarpal
meniscus
homologue

Extensor carpi
ulnaris tendon and
tendon sheath

Styloid process
of ulna

b

Articular
surface

Ulnolunate
ligament

Ulnotriquetral
ligament

Palmar radioulnar
ligament

Articular disk
(ulnocarpal disk)

Ulnar collateral
ligament

Ulnocarpal meniscus
homologue

Styloid process
of ulna

Styloid process
of radius

Dorsal
tubercle

Radiotriquetral
ligament

Dorsal radioulnar
ligament

c

B The ulnocarpal complex

a Ulnocarpal complex of the right hand, dorsal view; **b** schematic representation of a histologic specimen of an ulnocarpal complex (from Schmidt HM, Lanz U. Chirurgische Anatomie der Hand. 2nd ed. Stuttgart: Thieme; 2003); **c** ulnocarpal complex of the right hand, distal view.

The ulnocarpal complex, which appears triangular in shape (synonym: triangular fibrocartilage complex, TFCC), is a combination of ligaments and disks and serves as a connection between the distal ulna, the distal radioulnar joint, and the proximal carpal row. In the case of injuries to the ulnocarpal complex, patients usually report ulnar-sided wrist pain. Functionally, the ulnocarpal complex is divided into

- Ulnocarpal disk (triangular disk)
- Dorsal and palmar radioulnar ligaments
- Ulnolunate and ulnotriquetral ligaments
- Ulnocarpal meniscus
- Ulnar collateral ligament
- Radiotriquetral ligament (a component of the dorsal radiocarpal ligament)

The ulnocarpal disk, which consists of fibrocartilage, extends transversely and is located between the distal ulna and the triquetrum or the lunate. It arises from the distal edge of the radius of the ulnar notch in the hyaline cartilage, and two of its fibrous bands (often) extend both to the styloid process of the ulna and the base of the distal ulna. The outer margins of the disk are attached to the dorsal and palmar radioulnar ligaments. The central and radial parts of the fibrocartilaginous disk are slightly vascular and thus take considerably longer to heal following injuries. Degenerative changes, too, are a common occurrence in this area. The ulnocarpal disk is not to be confused with the ulnocarpal meniscus, the collagen fibers of which extend from the dorsal and ulnar edges of the ulnocarpal disk to the palmar side of the triquetrum. The ulnocarpal meniscus bridges the ulnar intra-articular space of the proximal wrist, which is wide in humans and especially in ulnar abduction helps to increase the force-transmitting surface.

287

14.26 **The Carpal Tunnel**

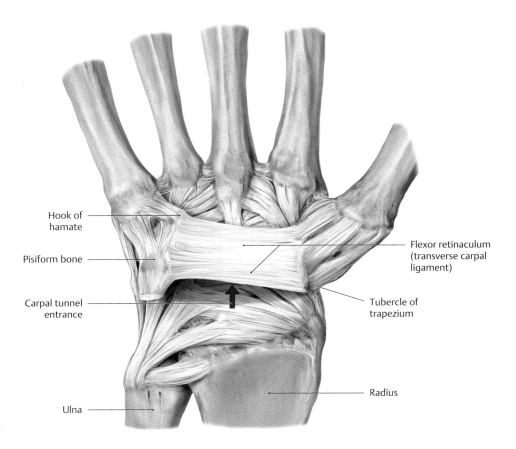

A Flexor retinaculum (transverse carpal ligament) and carpal tunnel, right hand

Anterior view. The bony elements of the wrist form a concave groove on the palmar side (see also **C**), which is closed by the flexor retinaculum (referred to clinically as the transverse carpal ligament) to form a fibro-osseous tunnel called the carpal tunnel or carpal canal. The narrowest part of this canal is located approximately 1 cm beyond the midline of the distal row of carpal bones (see **D**). The cross-sectional area of the tunnel at that site measures only about 1.6 cm². The carpal tunnel is traversed by a total of *nine flexor tendons* (enclosed in tendon sheaths and embedded in connective tissue) and the *median nerve* (see

p. 372). The tight fit of sensitive neurovascular structures with closely apposed, frequently moving tendons in this narrow space often causes problems when any of the structures swell or degenerate, leading to *carpal tunnel syndrome*. Narrowing of the tunnel can entrap or compress the median nerve, altering its function both by direct mechanical action and by restricting the blood flow within the nerve sheath. With chronic compression, the median nerve itself begins to degenerate beyond the site of entrapment, causing progressive pain and paresthesia and, ultimately, denervation and wasting of the muscles it serves, particularly the abductor pollicis brevis (see p. 372).

B Axial magnetic resonance image (T1-weighted) of the right hand at the level of the carpal tunnel

Proximal view. The flexor retinaculum (transverse carpal ligament) can be recognized as a band of low signal intensity (red arrow). Just below it toward the radial side is the median nerve (small arrow), whose water and lipid contents cause it to display a higher signal intensity than the superficial and deep flexor tendons. The primary diagnosis of carpal tunnel syndrome is based on clinical signs and electrophysiological measurements such as nerve conduction velocity. While conventional radiographs and CT scans can detect bony causes of the syndrome, magnetic resonance imaging can also demonstrate soft-tissue causes (e.g., edema or swelling of the median nerve, fibrosis, neuroma).

H = Hamate
K = Capitate
T = Trapezium
Ti = Trapezoid

(From Vahlensieck M, Reiser M. MRT des Bewegungsapparates. 3rd ed. Stuttgart: Thieme; 2006.)

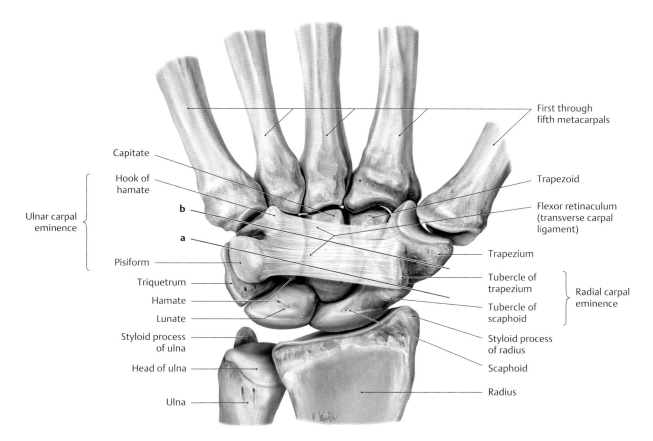

C Bony boundaries of the carpal tunnel of the right hand

Anterior view. The carpal bones form a convex arch on the dorsal side of the wrist and a concave arch on the palmar side. This creates a *carpal tunnel* on the palmar side, which is bounded by bony elevations on the radial and ulnar sides (the radial and ulnar carpal eminences). The tubercles of the trapezium and scaphoid form the palpable eminence on the radial side, while the hook of the hamate and the pisiform bone form the eminence on the ulnar side. Stretched between them is the flexor retinaculum (transverse carpal ligament), which closes the carpal tunnel on the palmar side (the planes of section marked **a** and **b** correspond to the cross sections in Fig. **D**).

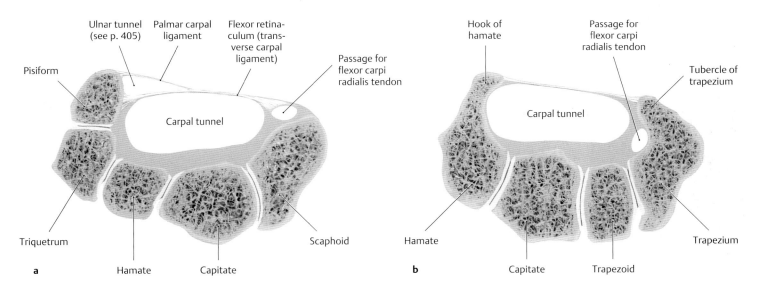

D Cross sections through the carpal tunnel

a Cross section through the proximal part of the carpal tunnel (plane **a** in **C**).

b Cross section through the distal part of the carpal tunnel (plane **b** in **C**).

Note: The carpal tunnel is narrowest over the center of the distal row (approximately 10 mm) of carpal bones (**b**) (after Schmidt and Lanz). In all, the carpal tunnel has a median cross-sectional area of approximately 1.6 to 1.7 cm².

14.27 **The Ligaments of the Fingers**

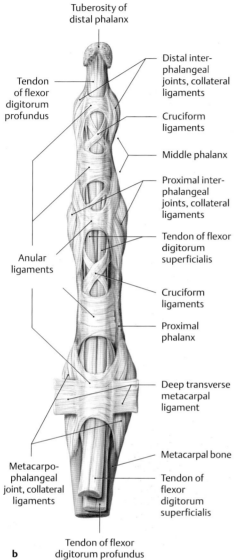

A The joint capsules, ligaments, and digital tendon sheath of the right middle finger
a Lateral view, **b** Palmar view.

The long flexor tendons (flexor digitorum superficialis and profundus) run in a strong, common synovial tendon sheath (not shown here) on the palmar side of the fingers. The *tendon sheaths* are guide mechanisms that allow for frictionless gliding of the long flexor tendons. The outer fibrous layer of the tendon sheaths, the stratum fibrosum, is strengthened by *anular ligaments* and *cruciform ligaments* (see **B**), which also bind the sheaths to the palmar surface of the phalanx and prevent palmar deviation of the sheaths during flexion. The gaps between the anular and cruciform ligaments are necessary to allow flexion of the fingers (see also p. 344, Musculature: Topographical Anatomy).

B Ligaments reinforcing the digital tendon sheath
a Lateral view in extension, **b** lateral view in flexion.
A1–5 = anular ligaments, C1–3 = cruciate ligaments.

- First anular ligament (A1): at the level of the metacarpophalangeal joint
- Second anular ligament (A2): on the shaft of the proximal phalanx
- Third anular ligament (A3): at the level of the proximal interphalangeal joint
- Fourth anular ligament (A4): on the shaft of the middle phalanx
- Fifth anular ligament (A5): at the level of the distal interphalangeal joint

The cruciform ligaments are highly variable in their course.

C Longitudinal section through the distal part of a finger
In the metacarpophalangeal joint, as well as the proximal and distal interphalangeal joints, the palmar articular surfaces of the phalanges are enlarged proximally by a fibrocartilaginous plate called the palmar ligament (volar plate). The palmar ligaments also form the floor of the digital tendon sheaths at these locations (after Schmidt and Lanz).

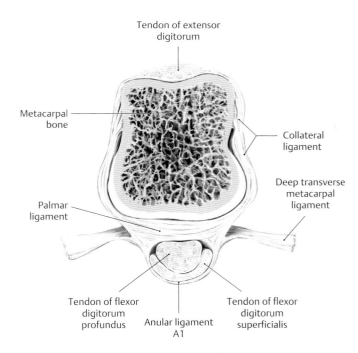

D The capsule and ligaments of the metacarpophalangeal joint
a Extension, **b** flexion. Lateral view.
Note: The collateral ligament is lax in extension and taut in flexion. For this reason, the finger joints should always be placed in a "functional position" (e.g., with the metacarpophalangeal joints flexed approximately 50 to 60°, see p. 295) if the hand is to be immobilized (e.g., in a cast) for a long period of time. If this is not done and the finger joints remain extended for a prolonged period, the collateral ligaments will shorten and create an extension deformity after the cast is removed. The accessory collateral ligament and phalangoglenoid ligament are taut in both flexion and extension and act mainly as restraints to limit extension.

E Cross section through the head of the third metacarpal of the right hand
Proximal view. At the level of the second through fifth metacarpal heads, the volar fibrocartilage plates (palmar ligaments) are interconnected by transverse bands, the deep transverse metacarpal ligaments. By binding the palmar ligaments to the A 1 anular ligaments (see **B**) of the flexor tendon sheaths, they also strengthen the distal metacarpus and stabilize the transverse metacarpal arch (after Schmidt and Lanz).

14.28 The Carpometacarpal Joint of the Thumb

Tuberosity of distal phalanx

Head of phalanx

Shaft of phalanx

Base of phalanx

Distal phalanx

Middle phalanx

First distal phalanx

Proximal phalanx

First proximal phalanx

First metacarpal

Head of meta-carpal

Shaft of meta-carpal

Base of metacarpal

Trapezoid

a

Trapezium

Capitate

b

Lunate

Scaphoid

Styloid process of radius

Styloid process of ulna

Radius

Ulna

A Axes of motion of the carpometacarpal joint of the thumb
Skeleton of the right hand, radial view. The first metacarpal bone has been moved slightly distally to facilitate orientation. The saddle-shaped articular surfaces of the trapezium and first metacarpal allow movements about two cardinal axes:

- An abduction/adduction axis (**a**)
- A flexion/extension axis (**b**)

While the axis for abduction/adduction runs approximately on a dorso-palmar line, the axis for flexion/extension runs transversely through the sellar limb of the trapezium. When the thumb is moved toward the small finger (opposition), a rotary movement takes place about a longitudinal axis through the first metacarpal bone (third degree of freedom). This oppositional movement of the thumb—essential for precision grasping movements of the hand—is made possible by the natural mismatch of the articular surfaces (see **F**).

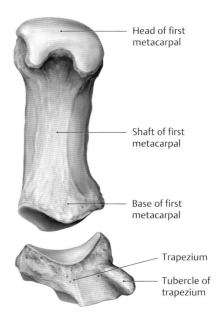

Head of first metacarpal

Shaft of first metacarpal

Base of first metacarpal

Trapezium

Tubercle of trapezium

B Articulating surfaces of the carpometacarpal joint of the thumb
Palmar-ulnar view. The articular surface of the trapezium is convex in the dorsopalmar direction and concave in the radioulnar direction. This is opposite to the curvatures found in the corresponding articular surface of the first metacarpal bone.

a

b

c

d

C Types of grip
Normal hand actions can be reduced to four primary types of grip:
a Pinch or precision grip, **b** power grip, **c** key grip, **d** hook grip.
The clinical examination should include function testing of the hand, giving particular attention to disturbances of fine motor skills and gross strength. It is important, for example, to evaluate the pinch grip and key grip, the pinch grip between the thumb and index finger having fundamental importance for the function of the hand. This is why, in issues pertaining to workers' compensation, loss of the thumb or index finger is considered to have a more serious impact on occupational capacity than the loss of the other long fingers.

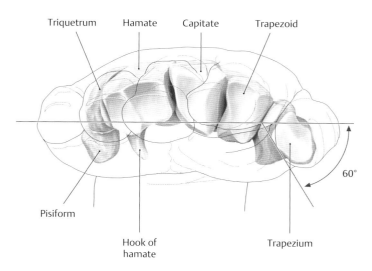

E Relationship of the thumb to the fingers in the neutral (0°) position

Right hand, distal view. Owing to the concave arch of the carpal bones, the scaphoid and trapezium have a markedly radiopalmar orientation. As a result, the metacarpus of the thumb is not placed in line with the other fingers but is rotated approximately 60° toward the palm.

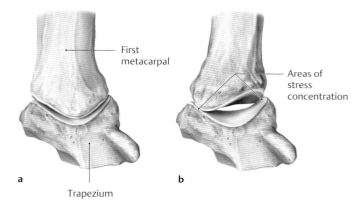

F Rotation-induced incongruity of the carpometacarpal joint during opposition of the thumb

a Neutral (0°) position, **b** the thumb in opposition.

As a sellar (saddle-shaped) joint, the carpometacarpal joint of the thumb is subjected to functional stresses that may promote osteoarthritis (after Koebke). The potentially harmful stresses are created by rotation of the first metacarpal bone during opposition of the thumb. When the thumb is maximally opposed, this rotation greatly reduces the surface area available for stress transfer across the joint (contrast this with the large area available in **a**). This concentration of stresses in a localized area predisposes to degenerative changes in the ascending sellar limb of the first metacarpal bone and the articular surface of the trapezium (first carpometacarpal osteoarthritis).

D Movements in the carpometacarpal joint of the thumb

Right hand. Palmar view.

a The neutral (0°) position.
b Axes of motion in the carpometacarpal joint of the thumb.
c Adduction.
d Abduction.
e Flexion.
f Extension.
g Opposition.
h Axis for opposition of the thumb. As the first metacarpal rotates, its area of contact with the articular surface of the trapezium is greatly diminished (see **F**).

14.29 Movements of the Hand and Finger Joints

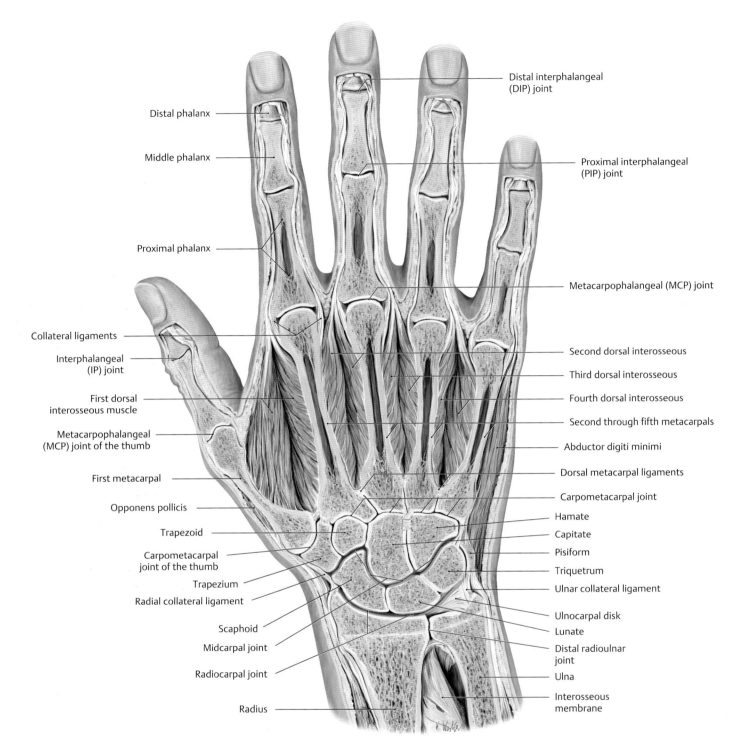

Distal interphalangeal (DIP) joint

Distal phalanx

Middle phalanx

Proximal interphalangeal (PIP) joint

Proximal phalanx

Metacarpophalangeal (MCP) joint

Collateral ligaments

Second dorsal interosseous

Interphalangeal (IP) joint

Third dorsal interosseous

First dorsal interosseous muscle

Fourth dorsal interosseous

Second through fifth metacarpals

Metacarpophalangeal (MCP) joint of the thumb

Abductor digiti minimi

First metacarpal

Dorsal metacarpal ligaments

Opponens pollicis

Carpometacarpal joint

Trapezoid

Hamate

Carpometacarpal joint of the thumb

Capitate

Pisiform

Triquetrum

Trapezium

Radial collateral ligament

Ulnar collateral ligament

Ulnocarpal disk

Scaphoid

Lunate

Midcarpal joint

Distal radioulnar joint

Radiocarpal joint

Ulna

Radius

Interosseous membrane

A Transverse section through the right hand
Posterior view. The hand and forearm are connected at the **radiocarpal and midcarpal joints** (both indicated by blue lines in the drawing). Morphologically, the *radiocarpal joint* is an ovoid or ellipsoidal joint, while the *midcarpal joint* is an interdigitating hinge joint (with an approximately S-shaped joint space between the proximal and distal rows of carpal bones). Except for the carpometacarpal joint of the thumb, the joints between the distal row of carpal bones and the bases of the metacarpals (the carpometacarpal joints) are *amphiarthroses* (joined by fibrocartilage) that permit very little motion.

The **finger joints** are classified as follows:

- *Metacarpophalangeal joints* between the metacarpal bones and the proximal phalanges (MCP joints, spheroidal type)
- *Proximal interphalangeal joints* between the proximal and middle phalanges (PIP joints, hinge type)
- *Distal interphalangeal joints* between the middle and distal phalanges (DIP joints, hinge type)

Since the *thumb* lacks a middle phalanx, it has only two joints: a metacarpophalangeal joint and an interphalangeal joint (drawing based on a specimen from the Anatomical Collection at the University of Kiel).

B Movements of the radiocarpal and midcarpal joints

Starting from the neutral (0°) position, palmar flexion and dorsal extension are performed about a transverse axis (**a**), while radial and ulnar deviation occurs about a dorsopalmar axis (**b**). The *transverse* axis runs through the lunate bone for the radiocarpal joint and through the capitate bone for the midcarpal joint. The *dorsopalmar* axis runs through the capitate bone. Thus, while palmar flexion and dorsal extension can occur in both the radiocarpal and midcarpal joints, radial and ulnar deviation can occur only in the radiocarpal joint.

C Functional position of the hand

For postoperative immobilization of the hand, the desired position of the wrist and fingers should be considered when the cast, splint, or other device is applied. Otherwise the ligaments may shorten, and the hand can no longer assume a normal resting position.

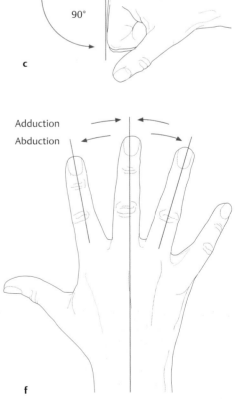

D Range of motion of the finger joints

The proximal interphalangeal (PIP) and distal interphalangeal (DIP) joints are pure hinge joints with only one degree of freedom (flexion extension). The metacarpophalangeal (MCP) joints of the second through fifth fingers are shaped like spheroidal joints with three theretcal degrees of freedom, but rotation is so limited by the collateral ligaments that only two degrees of freedom exist: flexion/extension and abduction/adduction. The following specific movements of the finger joints are distinguished:

a Flexion in the DIP joint.
b Flexion in the PIP joint.
c Flexion in the MCP joint.

d Extension in the DIP joint.
e Extension in the MCP joint.
f Abduction and adduction in the MCP joints (spreading the fingers apart and bringing them together about a dorsopalmar axis through the heads of the metacarpals).

Abduction/adduction movements are described in relation to the middle finger: all movements away from the middle finger are classified as abduction, all movements toward the middle finger as adduction.

295

15.1 Functional Muscle Groups

A Principles used in classification of the muscles of the upper limb

The muscles of the upper limb can be classified according to various criteria. An optimum system for classification should be logical and clear. The following criteria are suitable for classifying muscles:

• Origin
• Topography
• Function
• Innervation

While function and topography in the upper limb are often interrelated (muscles with the same action on a joint are often located close together), muscles that have similar actions in the shoulder region (e.g., muscles of the shoulder joint and shoulder girdle) vary considerably in their location. The following classification (**B**), then, is a compromise between topographical and functional considerations. In section **C**, a different muscle classification system, based on innervation, is presented.

The grouping of muscles by the pattern of their innervation reveals features of their embryological and phylogenetic origin and provides clinical insights into the clusters of consequences from damage to particular nerves.

B Functional-topographical classification of the muscles of the upper limb

Muscles of the shoulder girdle

Shoulder girdle muscles that have migrated from the head
• Trapezius
• Sternocleidomastoid
• Omohyoid

Posterior muscles of the trunk and shoulder girdle
• Rhomboid major
• Rhomboid minor
• Levator scapulae

Anterior muscles of the trunk and shoulder girdle
• Subclavius
• Pectoralis minor
• Serratus anterior

Muscles of the shoulder joint

Posterior shoulder muscles
• Supraspinatus
• Infraspinatus
• Teres minor
• Subscapularis
• Deltoid
• Latissimus dorsi
• Teres major

Anterior shoulder muscles
• Pectoralis major
• Coracobrachialis

Muscles of the arm

Posterior arm muscles
• Triceps brachii
• Anconeus

Anterior arm muscles
• Brachialis
• Biceps brachii

Muscles of the forearm

Posterior forearm muscles
• Superficial extensors
  – Extensor digitorum
  – Extensor digiti minimi
  – Extensor carpi ulnaris

• Deep extensors
  – Supinator
  – Abductor pollicis longus
  – Extensor pollicis brevis
  – Extensor pollicis longus
  – Extensor indicis

Anterior forearm muscles
• Superficial flexors
  – Pronator teres
  – Flexor digitorum superficialis
  – Flexor carpi radialis
  – Flexor carpi ulnaris
  – Palmaris longus

• Deep flexors
  – Flexor digitorum profundus
  – Flexor pollicis longus
  – Pronator quadratus

Radial forearm muscles
• Radialis group
  – Brachioradialis
  – Extensor carpi radialis longus
  – Extensor carpi radialis brevis

Muscles of the hand

Metacarpal muscles
• First through fourth lumbricals
• First through fourth dorsal interossei
• First through third palmar interossei

Thenar muscles
• Abductor pollicis brevis
• Adductor pollicis
• Flexor pollicis brevis
• Opponens pollicis

Hypothenar muscles
• Abductor digiti minimi
• Flexor digiti minimi
• Opponens digiti minimi
• Palmaris brevis

C Classification of the muscles of the upper limb by their innervation

Almost all the muscles of the upper limb are innervated by the brachial plexus arising from spinal cord segments C5–T1. Exceptions are the trapezius, sternocleidomastoid, and omohyoid; originating in vertebrate evolution as muscles of the head, they are supplied by cranial nerve XI (accessory nerve) and the cervical plexus (ansa cervicalis).

Nerve	Innervated muscles
Accessory nerve	Trapezius Sternocleidomastoid
Ansa cervicalis	Omohyoid
Dorsal scapular nerve	Levator scapulae Rhomboid major Rhomboid minor
Suprascapular nerve	Supraspinatus Infraspinatus
Long thoracic nerve	Serratus anterior
Nerve to the subclavius	Subclavius
Subscapular nerves	Subscapularis (upper and lower) Teres major (upper)
Thoracodorsal nerve	Latissimus dorsi
Medial and lateral pectoral nerves	Pectoralis major Pectoralis minor
Musculocutaneous nerve	Coracobrachialis Biceps brachii Brachialis
Axillary nerve	Deltoid Teres minor
Radial nerve	Triceps brachii Anconeus Supinator Brachioradialis Extensor carpi radialis longus Extensor carpi radialis brevis Extensor digitorum Extensor digiti minimi Extensor carpi ulnaris Extensor pollicis longus Extensor pollicis brevis Extensor indicis Abductor pollicis longus
Median nerve	Pronator teres Pronator quadratus Palmaris longus Flexor carpi radialis Flexor pollicis longus Flexor digitorum profundus (half) Flexor digitorum superficialis Abductor pollicis brevis Opponens pollicis Flexor pollicis brevis (superficial head) First and second lumbricals
Ulnar nerve	Flexor carpi ulnaris Flexor digitorum profundus (half) Palmaris brevis Flexor digiti minimi brevis Abductor digiti minimi Opponens digiti minimi Adductor pollicis Flexor pollicis brevis (deep head) Palmar and dorsal interossei Third and fourth lumbricals

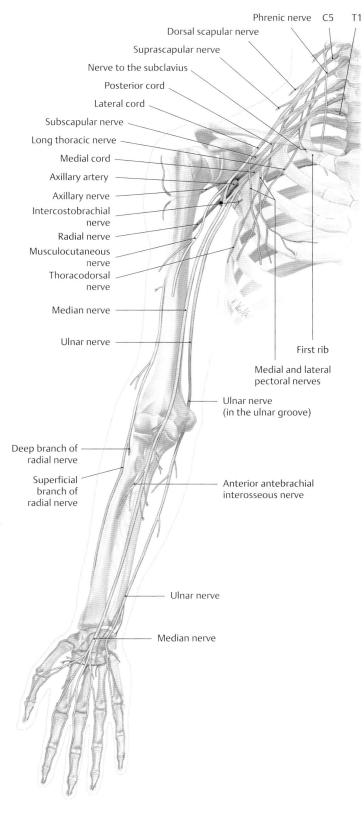

D Overview of the motor branches of the brachial plexus that supply the muscles of the upper limb

With the outgrowth of the limb buds from the trunk during embryonic development, the branches of the brachial plexus follow the genetically determined *posterior* extensor muscles and *anterior* flexor muscles. The nerves for the *extensors* (radial and axillary nerves) arise from the three *posterior* divisions of the brachial plexus, while the nerves for the *flexors* (musculocutaneous nerve, ulnar nerve, median nerve) arise from the three *anterior* divisions of the plexus (see p. 394, Neurovascular Systems: Topographical Anatomy).

297

15.2 The Muscles of the Shoulder Girdle: Trapezius, Sternocleidomastoid, and Omohyoid

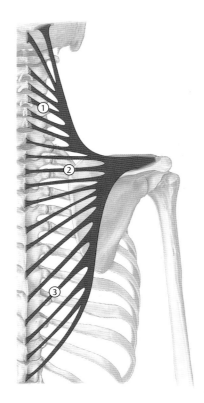

A Schematic of the trapezius

Trapezius

Origin:
① Descending part1[1]:
- Occipital bone (superior nuchal line and external occipital protuberance)
- The spinous processes of all cervical vertebrae via the nuchal ligament

② Transverse part:
Broad aponeurosis at the level of the T 1–T 4 spinous processes

③ Ascending part:
Spinous processes of T 5–T 12

Insertion:
- Lateral third of the clavicle (descending part)
- Acromion (transverse part)
- Scapular spine (ascending part)

Actions:
- Descending part:
  – Draws the scapula obliquely upward and rotates the glenoid cavity inferiorly (acting with the inferior part of the serratus anterior)
  – Tilts the head to the same side and rotates it to the opposite side (with the shoulder girdle fixed)
- Transverse part: draws the scapula medially
- Ascending part: draws the scapula medially downward (supports the rotating action of the descending part)
- Entire muscle: steadies the scapula on the thorax

Innervation: Accessory nerve (CN XI) and cervical plexus (C2, C4)

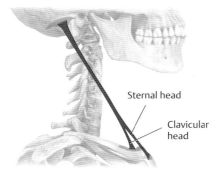

Sternal head

Clavicular head

B Schematic of the sternocleidomastoid

Sternocleidomastoid

Origin:
- Sternal head: manubrium
- Clavicular head: medial third of the clavicle

Insertion: Mastoid process and superior nuchal line

Actions:
- Unilateral: – Tilts the head to the same side
  – Rotates the head to the opposite side
- Bilateral: – Extends the head
  – Assists in respiration when the head is fixed

Innervation: Accessory nerve (CN XI) and the cervical plexus (C2, C3)

Intermediate tendon

C Schematic of the omohyoid

Omohyoid

Origin: Superior border of the scapula

Insertion: Body of the hyoid bone

Actions:
- Depresses (fixes) the hyoid bone
- Moves the larynx and hyoid bone downward (for phonation and the final phase of swallowing)
- Tenses the cervical fascia with its intermediate tendon and maintains patency of the internal jugular vein

Innervation: Ansa cervicalis (C 1–C 3) from the cervical plexus

[1]The tables and associated diagrams above are intended to give a systematic overview of the named muscles and their actions, while the drawings on p. 299 are intended to display the muscles as they would appear in a dissection. Not all structures listed in the tables are shown in the drawings on p. 299 because they are not all visible in those views.

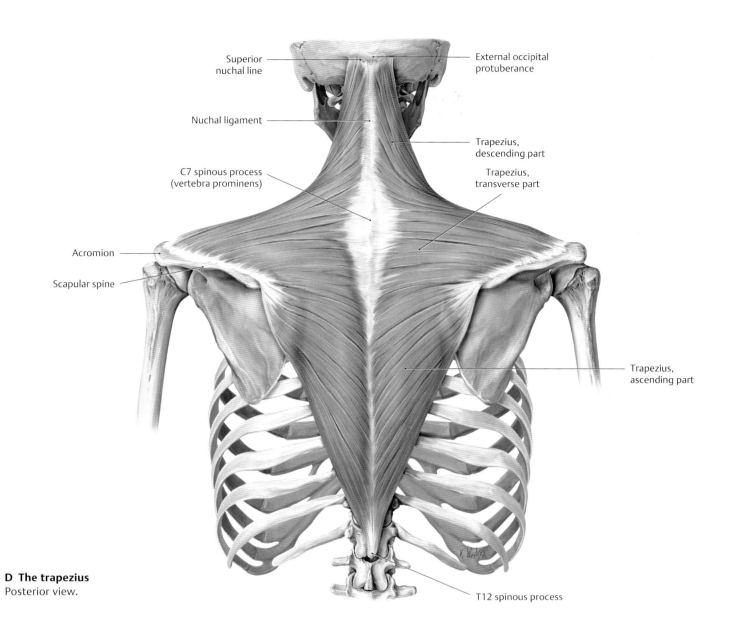

Superior nuchal line

External occipital protuberance

Nuchal ligament

Trapezius, descending part

Trapezius, transverse part

C7 spinous process (vertebra prominens)

Acromion

Scapular spine

Trapezius, ascending part

T12 spinous process

D The trapezius
Posterior view.

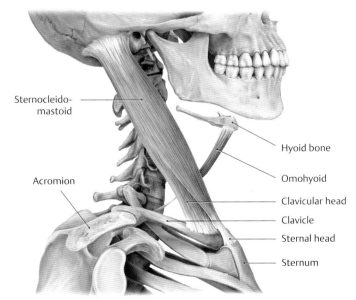

Sternocleido-mastoid

Acromion

Hyoid bone

Omohyoid

Clavicular head

Clavicle

Sternal head

Sternum

E The sternocleidomastoid and omohyoid
Right side, lateral view.

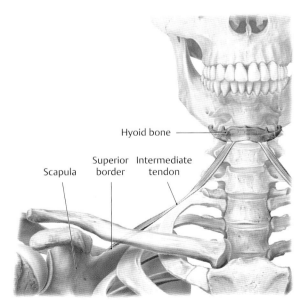

Hyoid bone

Scapula

Superior border

Intermediate tendon

F The omohyoid
Right side, anterior view.

15.3 The Muscles of the Shoulder Girdle: Serratus Anterior, Subclavius, Pectoralis Minor, Levator Scapulae, and Rhomboids Major and Minor

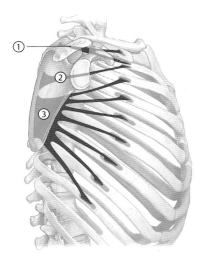

A Schematic of the serratus anterior

Serratus anterior

Origin:	First through ninth ribs
Insertion:	Scapula: ① Superior part (costal and dorsal surfaces of superior angle)
	② Intermediate part (costal surface of medial border)
	③ Inferior part (costal and dorsal surfaces of inferior angle and costal surface of medial border)
Actions:	• Entire muscle: draws the scapula laterally forward, elevates the ribs when the shoulder girdle is fixed (assists in respiration)
	• Inferior part: rotates the scapula and draws its inferior angle laterally forward (rotates glenoid cavity superiorly), allowing for arm to be elevated above 90°
	• Superior part: lowers the raised arm (antagonist to the inferior part)
Innervation:	Long thoracic nerve (C5–C7)

① Subclavius

Origin:	First rib (chondro-osseous junction)
Insertion:	Inferior surface of the clavicle (lateral third)
Action:	Steadies the clavicle in the sternoclavicular joint
Innervation:	Nerve to the subclavius (C5, C6)

② Pectoralis minor

Origin:	Third through fifth ribs
Insertion:	Coracoid process of the scapula
Actions:	• Draws the scapula downward, causing its inferior angle to move posteromedially (lowers the raised arm), rotates glenoid inferiorly
	• Assists in respiration
Innervation:	Medial and lateral pectoral nerves (C8, T1)

B Schematic of the subclavius and pectoralis minor

① Levator scapulae

Origin:	Transverse processes of the C1–C4 vertebrae
Insertion:	Superior angle of the scapula
Actions:	• Draws the scapula medially upward while moving the inferior angle medially (returns the raised arm to the neutral [0°] position)
	• Inclines the neck toward the same side (when the scapula is fixed)
Innervation:	Dorsal scapular nerve and cervical spinal nerves (C3, C4)

② Rhomboid minor

Origin:	Spinous processes of the C6 and C7 vertebrae
Insertion:	Medial border of the scapula (above the scapular spine)
Actions:	• Steadies the scapula
	• Draws the scapula medially upward (returns the raised arm to the neutral [0°] position)
Innervation:	Dorsal scapular nerve (C4, C5)

③ Rhomboid major

Origin:	Spinous processes of the T1–T4 vertebrae
Insertion:	Medial border of the scapula (below the scapular spine)
Actions:	• Steadies the scapula
	• Draws the scapula medially upward (returns the raised arm to the neutral [0°] position)
Innervation:	Dorsal scapular nerve (C4, C5)

C Schematic of the levator scapulae and rhomboids minor and major

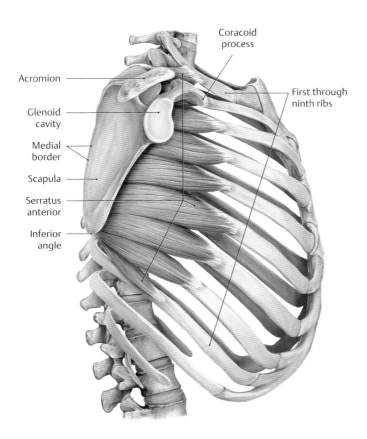

Coracoid
process

Acromion

Glenoid
cavity

Medial
border

Scapula

Serratus
anterior

Inferior
angle

First through
ninth ribs

D The serratus anterior
Right side, lateral view.

Clavicle

First rib

Acromion

Coracoid
process

Subclavius

Pectoralis
minor

Third
through
fifth ribs

E The pectoralis minor and subclavius
Right side, anterior view.

C1 (atlas)

C2 (axis)

C1–C4
transverse processes

Levator scapulae

Rhomboid
minor

Superior
angle

Clavicle

C7 (vertebra
prominens)
spinous process

T1–T4
spinous processes

Rhomboid
major

Acromion

Scapular spine

Medial border

Scapula,
posterior
surface

Inferior
angle

**F The levator scapulae, rhomboid major,
and rhomboid minor**
Right side, posterior view.

301

15.4 The Posterior Muscles of the Shoulder Joint: The Rotator Cuff

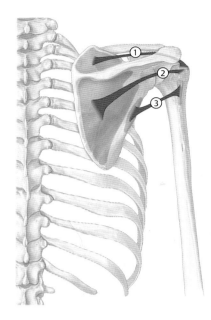

① Supraspinatus

Origin:	Supraspinous fossa of the scapula
Insertion:	Greater tubercle of the humerus
Action:	Abduction
Innervation:	Suprascapular nerve (C4–C6)

② Infraspinatus

Origin:	Infraspinous fossa of the scapula
Insertion:	Greater tubercle of the humerus
Action:	External rotation
Innervation:	Suprascapular nerve (C4–C6)

③ Teres minor

Origin:	Lateral border of the scapula
Insertion:	Greater tubercle of the humerus
Action:	External rotation, weak adduction
Innervation:	Axillary nerve (C5, C6)

A Schematic of the supraspinatus, infraspinatus, and teres minor

④ Subscapularis

Origin:	Subscapular fossa of the scapula
Insertion:	Lesser tubercle of the humerus
Action:	Internal rotation
Innervation:	Upper and lower subscapular nerves (C5, C6)

B Schematic of the subscapularis

C Muscles of the rotator cuff: supraspinatus, infraspinatus, teres minor, and subscapularis
Right shoulder joint.

a Anterior view.
b Posterior view.
c Lateral view.

15.5 The Posterior Muscles of the Shoulder Joint: The Deltoid

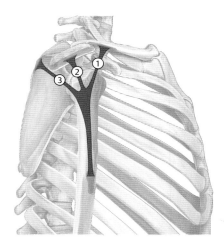

Deltoid

Origin:	① Clavicular part: lateral third of the clavicle
	② Acromial part: acromion
	③ Spinal part: scapular spine
Insertion:	Deltoid tuberosity on the humerus
Actions:	• Clavicular part: flexion (moves the arm and shoulder forward), internal rotation, adduction
	• Acromial part: abduction
	• Spinal part: extension (moves the arm and shoulder backward), external rotation, adduction

Between 60° and 90° of abduction, the clavicular and spinal parts of the deltoid assist the acromial part of the muscle with abduction.

Innervation: Axillary nerve (C5, C6)

A Schematic of the deltoid

a

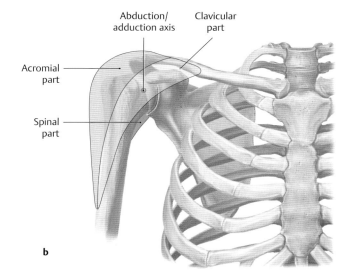

b

B The variable actions of the deltoid components
a Cross section through the right shoulder joint.
b Right shoulder joint in the neutral (0°) position, anterior view.
c Right shoulder joint in 60° of abduction, anterior view.

The actions of the three parts of the deltoid muscle (clavicular, acromial, and spinal) depend on their relationship to the position of the humerus and its axis of motion. As a result, the parts of the deltoid can act antagonistically as well as synergistically. At *less than 60°* abduction, the clavicular and spinal parts of the deltoid act as antagonists to the acromial part, but at *more than 60°* abduction, the acromial part assists in the abduction. Starting from the neutral (0°) position, the acromial part of the deltoid abducts the arm and steadies it in any position it assumes. When the arm is abducted past approximately 60°, the clavicular and spinal parts also become active as they move past the sagittal motion axis (abduction/adduction axis, **c**). This alters the action of these parts: they act as adductors below 60°, but when the arm passes 60°, they become abductors.

c

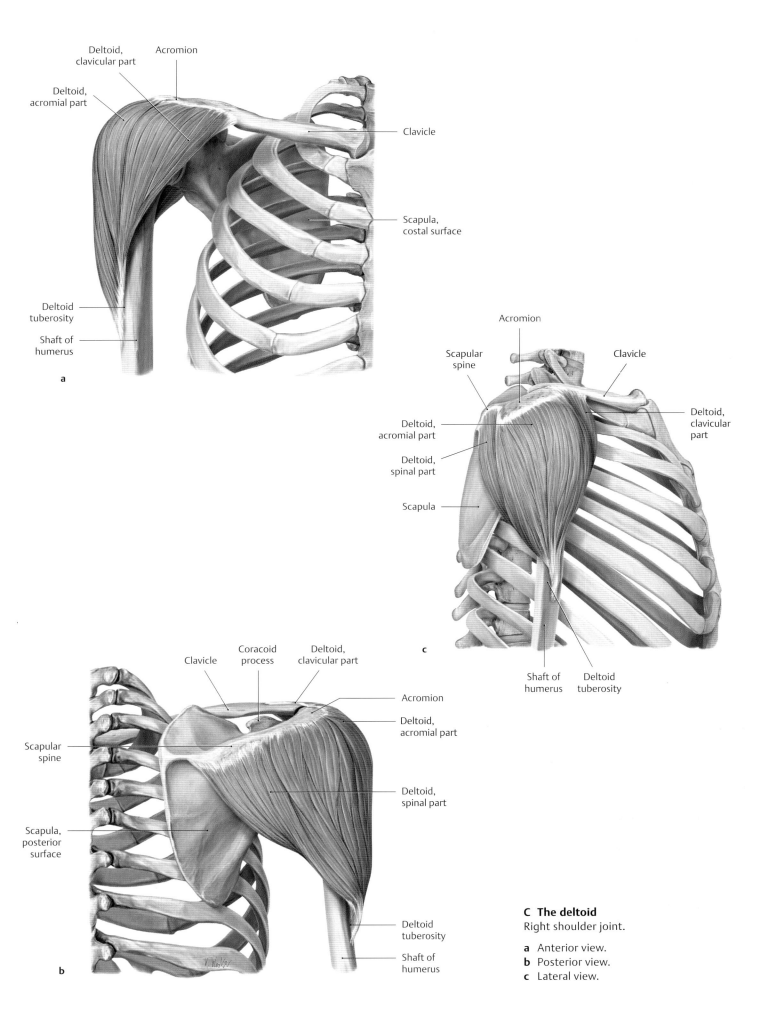

Deltoid,
clavicular part

Acromion

Deltoid,
acromial part

Clavicle

Scapula,
costal surface

Deltoid
tuberosity

Shaft of
humerus

a

Acromion

Scapular
spine

Clavicle

Deltoid,
acromial part

Deltoid,
clavicular
part

Deltoid,
spinal part

Scapula

Shaft of
humerus

Deltoid
tuberosity

c

Clavicle

Coracoid
process

Deltoid,
clavicular part

Acromion

Scapular
spine

Deltoid,
acromial part

Scapula,
posterior
surface

Deltoid,
spinal part

Deltoid
tuberosity

Shaft of
humerus

b

C The deltoid
Right shoulder joint.

a Anterior view.
b Posterior view.
c Lateral view.

305

15.6 The Posterior Muscles of the Shoulder Joint: Latissimus Dorsi and Teres Major

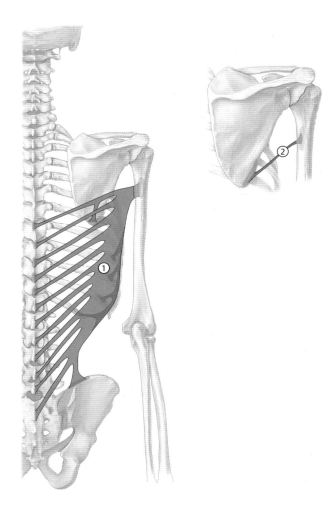

A Schematic of the latissimus dorsi and teres major

① **Latissimus dorsi**

Origin:	• Vertebral part:
	– Spinous processes of the T7–T12 vertebrae
	– Thoracolumbar fascia of the spinous processes of all lumbar vertebrae and the sacrum
	• Iliac part: posterior third of the iliac crest
	• Costal part: Ninth through twelfth ribs
	• Scapular part: inferior angle of the scapula
Insertion:	Floor of the intertubercular groove of the humerus
Actions:	Internal rotation, adduction, extension (moves the arm backward), respiration (expiration, "cough muscle")
Innervation:	Thoracodorsal nerve (C6–C8)

② **Teres major**

Origin:	Inferior angle of the scapula
Insertion:	Crest of the lesser tubercle of the humerus
Action:	Internal rotation, adduction, extension
Innervation:	Lower subscapular nerve (C5, C6)

B Course of the tendon of insertion of the latissimus dorsi in the neutral position and in elevation

Posterior view. The latissimus dorsi muscle is most active in the abducted or elevated arm. Raising the arm untwists the muscle fibers in the area of insertion, increasing the muscle's stretch and maximizing the force it can exert. When the position of the arm is fixed, the latissimus dorsi can pull the body upward, as in the act of climbing, or can depress the arm against a resistance. This makes the latissimus dorsi an important muscle for paraplegics, for example, who can use that muscle to raise themselves from wheelchairs.

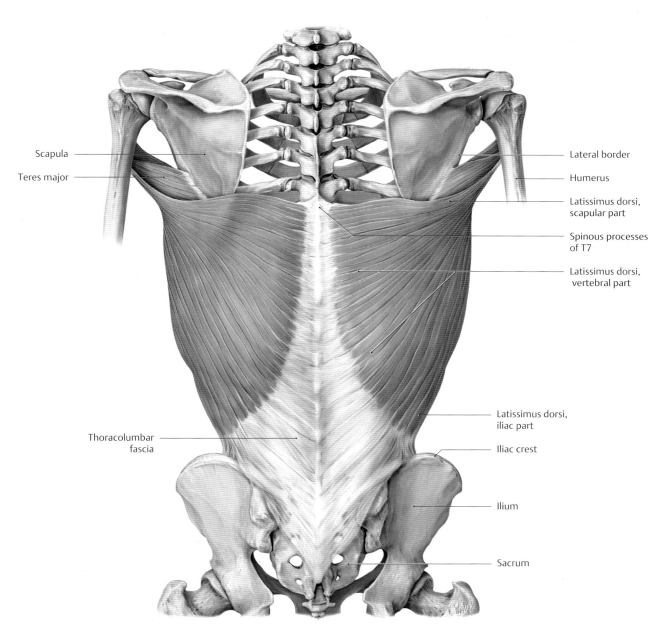

Scapula

Teres major

Lateral border

Humerus

Latissimus dorsi, scapular part

Spinous processes of T7

Latissimus dorsi, vertebral part

Thoracolumbar fascia

Latissimus dorsi, iliac part

Iliac crest

Ilium

Sacrum

C The latissimus dorsi and teres major
Posterior view.

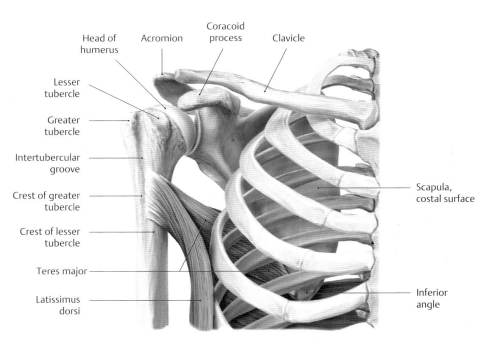

Head of humerus

Acromion

Coracoid process

Clavicle

Lesser tubercle

Greater tubercle

Intertubercular groove

Crest of greater tubercle

Scapula, costal surface

Crest of lesser tubercle

Teres major

Inferior angle

Latissimus dorsi

D Insertion of the latissimus dorsi on the floor of the intertubercular groove and the teres major on the crest of the lesser tubercle
Right side, anterior view.

15.7 The Anterior Muscles of the Shoulder Joint: Pectoralis Major and Coracobrachialis

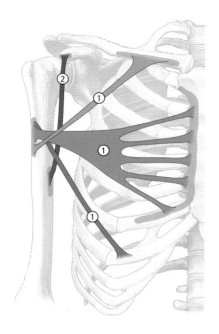

① **Pectoralis major**

Origin:
- Clavicular part: medial half of the clavicle
- Sternocostal part: sternum and the second through sixth costal cartilages
- Abdominal part: anterior layer of the rectus sheath

Insertion: Crest of the greater tubercle of the humerus

Actions:
- Adduction and internal rotation (entire muscle)
- Flexion (clavicular and sternocostal parts)
- Assists respiration when the shoulder girdle is fixed

Innervation: Medial and lateral pectoral nerves (C5–T1)

② **Coracobrachialis**

Origin: Coracoid process of the scapula
Insertion: Humerus (in line with the crest of the lesser tubercle)
Actions: Flexion, adduction, internal rotation
Innervation: Musculocutaneous nerve (C5–C7)

A **Schematic of the pectoralis major and coracobrachialis**

B Twisting of the tendon of insertion of the pectoralis major

Anterior view. The three parts of the pectoralis major (clavicular, sternocostal, and abdominal) converge laterally and insert on the crest of the greater tubercle by a broad tendon that has a horseshoe-shaped cross section. The tendon fiber bundles are twisted on themselves in such a way that the clavicular part inserts lower on the humerus than the sternocostal part, which inserts lower than the abdominal part. As with the latissimus dorsi, the muscle fibers of the pectoralis major become untwisted and stretched with increasing elevation of the arm, increasing the force that the muscle can exert.

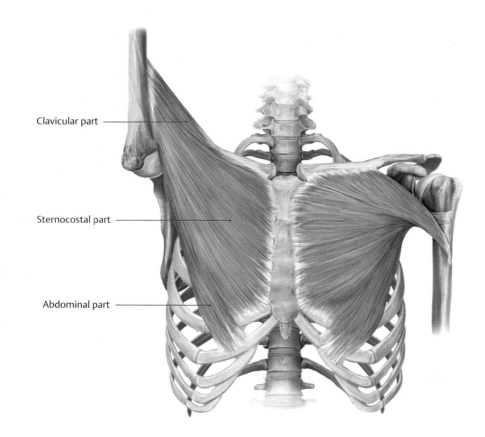

Clavicular part

Sternocostal part

Abdominal part

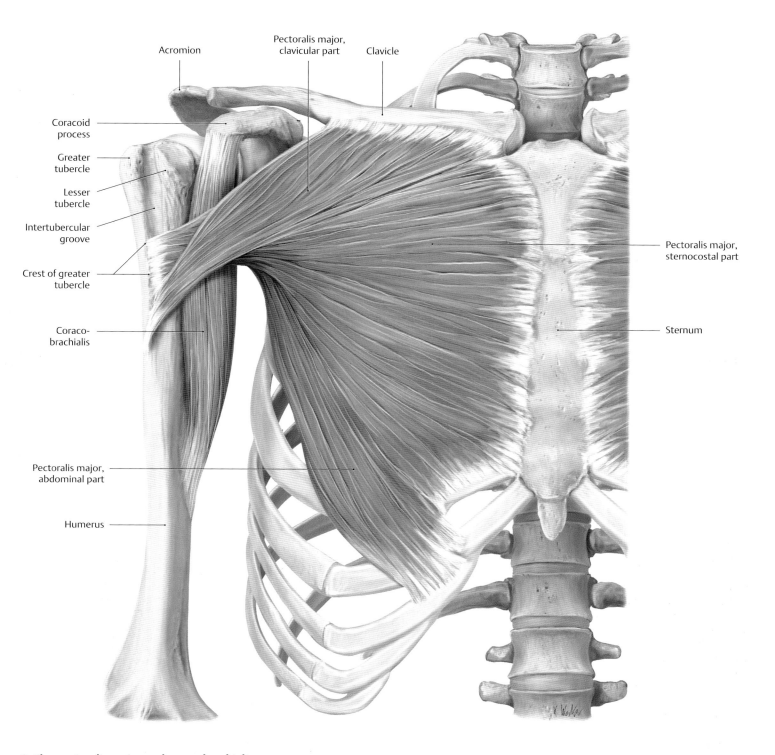

Acromion

Pectoralis major, clavicular part

Clavicle

Coracoid process

Greater tubercle

Lesser tubercle

Intertubercular groove

Crest of greater tubercle

Coraco-brachialis

Pectoralis major, abdominal part

Humerus

Pectoralis major, sternocostal part

Sternum

C The pectoralis major and coracobrachialis
Right side, anterior view.

15.8 The Anterior Muscles of the Arm: Biceps Brachii and Brachialis

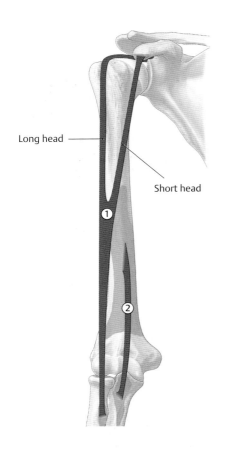

Long head

Short head

① **Biceps brachii**

Origin:
- Long head: supraglenoid tubercle of the scapula
- Short head: coracoid process of the scapula

Insertion: Radial tuberosity and antebrachial fascia via bicipital aponeurosis

Actions:
- Elbow joint:
  – Flexion, supination (with the elbow flexed)
- Shoulder joint:
  – Flexion (forward motion of humerus)
  – Stabilization of humeral head during deltoid contraction
  – Abduction and internal (medial) rotation of the humerus (long head)

Innervation: Musculocutaneous nerve (C5–C7)

② **Brachialis**

Origin: Distal half of the anterior surface of the humerus, also the medial and lateral intermuscular septa

Insertion: Ulnar tuberosity

Action: Flexion at the elbow joint

Innervation: Musculocutaneous nerve (C5, C6) and radial nerve (C5, C7)

A Schematic of the biceps brachii and brachialis

B Supinating action of the biceps brachii with the elbow flexed

a The forearm is pronated with the elbow flexed (right arm, medial view).

b Cross section at the level of the radial tuberosity with the forearm pronated (proximal view).

c The forearm is supinated with the elbow flexed (right arm, medial view).

d Cross section at the level of the radial tuberosity with the forearm supinated (proximal view).

When the elbow is flexed, the biceps brachii acts as a powerful supinator in addition to its role as a flexor, because the lever arm in that position is almost perpendicular to the axis of pronation/supination (see p. 280). This is why *supination movements* are particularly effective when the elbow is flexed. When the forearm is *pronated* (**a**), the tendon of insertion of the biceps brachii is wrapped around the radius. When the muscle then contracts to flex the elbow, the tendon unwraps like a rope coiled around a crank (**b**).

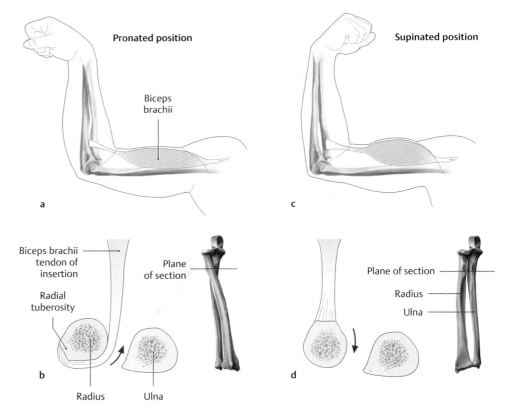

Pronated position

Supinated position

Biceps brachii

Biceps brachii tendon of insertion

Radial tuberosity

Plane of section

Plane of section

Radius

Ulna

Radius

Ulna

a

b

c

d

C The biceps brachii and brachialis
Right arm, anterior (ventral) view.

D The brachialis
Right arm, anterior (ventral) view.

15.9 The Posterior Muscles of the Arm: Triceps Brachii and Anconeus

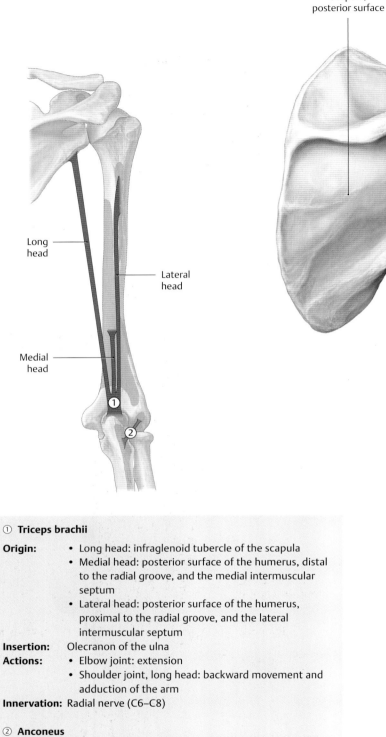

Long head

Lateral head

Medial head

Scapula, posterior surface

Scapular spine

Coracoid process

Acromion

Head of humerus

Greater tubercle

Infraglenoid tubercle

Shaft of humerus

Lateral border

Triceps brachii, medial head

Triceps brachii, long head

Triceps brachii, lateral head

Medial epicondyle

Olecranon

Lateral epicondyle

Anconeus

Ulna

Radius

① **Triceps brachii**

Origin:
- Long head: infraglenoid tubercle of the scapula
- Medial head: posterior surface of the humerus, distal to the radial groove, and the medial intermuscular septum
- Lateral head: posterior surface of the humerus, proximal to the radial groove, and the lateral intermuscular septum

Insertion: Olecranon of the ulna

Actions:
- Elbow joint: extension
- Shoulder joint, long head: backward movement and adduction of the arm

Innervation: Radial nerve (C6–C8)

② **Anconeus**

Origin: Lateral epicondyle of the humerus (and the posterior joint capsule in some cases)

Insertion: Olecranon of the ulna (radial surface)

Actions: Extends the elbow and tightens its joint capsule

Innervation: Radial nerve (C6–C8)

A Schematic of the triceps brachii and anconeus

B The triceps brachii and anconeus
Right arm, posterior (dorsal) view.

Coracoid process

Acromion

Greater tubercle

Infraglenoid tubercle

Triceps brachii, tendon of origin of the lateral head

Triceps brachii, long head

Radial groove

Triceps brachii, medial head

Triceps brachii, tendon of insertion

Medial epicondyle

Lateral epicondyle

Olecranon

Anconeus

C The triceps brachii and anconeus
Right arm, posterior (dorsal) view. The lateral head of the triceps brachii has been partially removed.

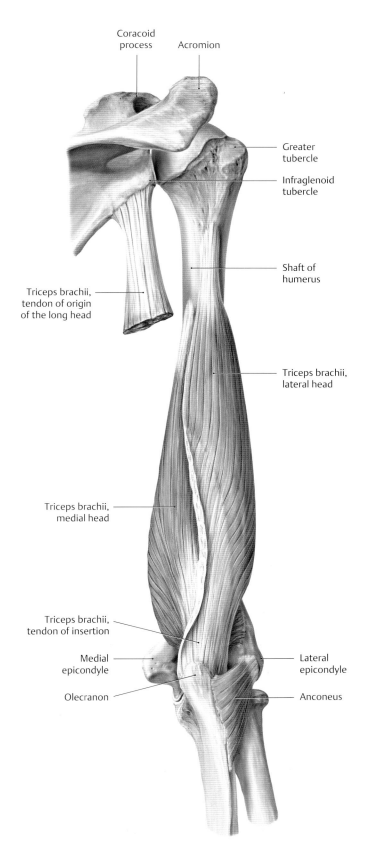

Coracoid process

Acromion

Greater tubercle

Infraglenoid tubercle

Shaft of humerus

Triceps brachii, tendon of origin of the long head

Triceps brachii, lateral head

Triceps brachii, medial head

Triceps brachii, tendon of insertion

Medial epicondyle

Lateral epicondyle

Olecranon

Anconeus

D The triceps brachii and anconeus
Right arm, posterior (dorsal) view. The long head of the triceps brachii has been partially removed.

313

15.10 The Muscles of the Anterior Forearm: The Superficial and Deep Flexors

A Schematic of the superficial flexors

B Schematic of the deep flexors

① **Pronator teres**

Origin:	• Humeral head: medial epicondyle of the humerus • Ulnar head: coronoid process of the ulna
Insertion:	Lateral surface of the radius (distal to the supinator insertion)
Actions:	• Elbow joint: weak flexion • Forearm joints: pronation
Innervation:	Median nerve (C6, C7)

② **Flexor digitorum superficialis**

Origin:	• Humero-ulnar head: medial epicondyle of the humerus and coronoid process of the ulna • Radial head: anterior border of radius distal to the radial tuberosity
Insertion:	The sides of the middle phalanges of the second through fifth digits
Actions:	Wrist joints and the MCP and PIP joints of the second through fifth digits: flexion
Innervation:	Median nerve (C8, T1)

③ **Flexor carpi radialis**

Origin:	Medial epicondyle of the humerus
Insertion:	Base of the second metacarpal (and sometimes of the third metacarpal)
Actions:	Wrist joints: flexion and abduction (radial deviation) of the hand
Innervation:	Median nerve (C6, C7)

④ **Flexor carpi ulnaris**

Origin:	• Humeral head: medial epicondyle • Ulnar head: olecranon
Insertion:	Pisiform, hook of the hamate, base of the fifth metacarpal
Actions:	Wrist joints: flexion and adduction (ulnar deviation) of the hand
Innervation:	Ulnar nerve (C8, T1)

⑤ **Palmaris longus**

Origin:	Medial epicondyle of the humerus
Insertion:	Palmar aponeurosis
Actions:	Wrist joints: flexion tightens the palmar aponeurosis for gripping
Innervation:	Median nerve (C7, C8)

① **Flexor digitorum profundus**

Origin:	Proximal two thirds of the flexor surface of the ulna and the adjacent interosseous membrane
Insertion:	Palmar surface of the distal phalanges of the second through fifth digits
Actions:	Wrist joints and the MCP, PIP, and DIP joints of the second through fifth digits: flexion
Innervation:	• Median nerve (radial part, second and third digits), C8, T1 • Ulnar nerve (ulnar part, fourth and fifth digits), C8, T1

② **Flexor pollicis longus**

Origin:	Mid-anterior surface of the radius and the adjacent interosseous membrane
Insertion:	Palmar surface of the distal phalanx of the thumb
Actions:	• Wrist joints: flexion and radial abduction of the hand • Carpometacarpal joint of the thumb: opposition • MCP and IP joints of the thumb: flexion
Innervation:	Median nerve (C8, T1)

③ **Pronator quadratus**

Origin:	Distal one fourth of the anterior surface of the ulna
Insertion:	Distal one fourth of the anterior surface of the radius
Actions:	Pronates the hand, stabilizes the distal radioulnar joint
Innervation:	Median nerve (C8, T1)

DIP, distal interphalangeal; IP, interphalangeal; MCP, metacarpophalangeal; PIP, proximal interphalangeal.

Medial epicondyle, common head of flexors

Radial tuberosity

Pronator teres

Flexor carpi radialis

Palmaris longus

Flexor carpi ulnaris

Flexor digitorum superficialis

Flexor digitorum superficialis

Second metacarpal, base

Pisiform bone

Hook of hamate

Fifth metacarpal, base

Palmar aponeurosis

Second through fifth middle phalanges

C The superficial flexors (pronator teres, flexor digitorum superficialis, flexor carpi radialis, flexor carpi ulnaris, and palmaris longus)
Right forearm, anterior view.

Humerus, medial epicondyle

Coronoid process

Radial tuberosity

Ulnar tuberosity

Interosseous membrane

Radius

Flexor digitorum profundus

Flexor pollicis longus

Pronator quadratus

Tubercle of trapezium

Trapezium

Pisiform bone

Hook of hamate

First distal phalanx, base

Fourth distal phalanx

D The deep flexors (flexor digitorum profundus, flexor pollicis longus, and pronator quadratus)
Right forearm, anterior view.

315

15.11 The Muscles of the Forearm: The Radialis Muscles

A Schematic of the radialis muscles

① **Brachioradialis**

Origin:	Lateral surface of the distal humerus, lateral intermuscular septum
Insertion:	Styloid process of the radius
Actions:	• Elbow joint: flexion
	• Forearm joints: semipronation
Innervation:	Radial nerve (C5, C6)

② **Extensor carpi radialis longus**

Origin:	Lateral surface of the distal humerus (lateral supracondylar ridge), lateral intermuscular septum
Insertion:	Dorsal base of the second metacarpal
Actions:	Wrist joints: dorsal extension (assists in fist closure), abduction (radial deviation) of the hand
Innervation:	Radial nerve (C6, C7)

③ **Extensor carpi radialis brevis**

Origin:	Lateral epicondyle of the humerus
Insertion:	Dorsal base of the third metacarpal
Actions:	Wrist joints: dorsal extension (assists in fist closure), abduction (radial deviation) of the hand
Innervation:	Radial nerve (C7, C8)

B The radialis muscles (brachioradialis, extensor carpi radialis longus, and extensor carpi radialis brevis)
Right forearm.

a Lateral (radial) view.
b Posterior (dorsal) view.

15.12 The Muscles of the Posterior Forearm: The Superficial and Deep Extensors

A Schematic of the superficial extensors

B Schematic of the deep extensors

① **Extensor digitorum**

Origin:	Common head (lateral epicondyle of the humerus)
Insertion:	Dorsal digital expansion of the second through fifth digits
Actions:	• Wrist joints: extension
	• MCP, PIP, and DIP joints of the second through fifth digits: extension and abduction of the fingers
Innervation:	Radial nerve (C7, C8)

② **Extensor digiti minimi**

Origin:	Common head (lateral epicondyle of the humerus)
Insertion:	Dorsal digital expansion of the fifth digit
Actions:	• Wrist joints: extension, adduction (ulnar deviation)
	• MCP, PIP, and DIP joints of the fifth digit: extension and abduction of the fifth digit
Innervation:	Radial nerve (C7, C8)

③ **Extensor carpi ulnaris**

Origin:	Common head (lateral epicondyle of the humerus), ulnar head (dorsal surface of the ulna)
Insertion:	Base of the fifth metacarpal
Actions:	Wrist joints: extension, adduction (ulnar deviation) of the hand
Innervation:	Radial nerve (C7, C8)

① **Supinator**

Origin:	Olecranon of the ulna, lateral epicondyle of the humerus, radial collateral ligament, anular ligament of the radius
Insertion:	Radius (between the radial tuberosity and the insertion of pronator teres)
Action:	Radioulnar joint: supination
Innervation:	Radial nerve (C7, C8)

② **Abductor pollicis longus**

Origin:	Dorsal surfaces of the radius and ulna, also the interosseous membrane
Insertion:	Base of the first metacarpal
Actions:	• Radiocarpal joint: abduction (radial deviation) of the hand
	• Carpometacarpal joint of the thumb: abduction
Innervation:	Radial nerve (C7, C8)

③ **Extensor pollicis brevis**

Origin:	Posterior surface of the radius and the interosseous membrane (distal to abductor pollicis longus)
Insertion:	Base of the proximal phalanx of the thumb
Actions:	• Radiocarpal joint: abduction (radial deviation) of the hand
	• Carpometacarpal and MCP joints of the thumb: extension
Innervation:	Radial nerve (C7, C8)

④ **Extensor pollicis longus**

Origin:	Posterior surface of the ulna and the interosseous membrane
Insertion:	Base of the distal phalanx of the thumb
Actions:	• Wrist joints: extension and abduction (radial deviation) of the hand
	• Carpometacarpal joint of the thumb: adduction
	• MCP and interphalangeal joints of the thumb: extension
Innervation:	Radial nerve (C7, C8)

⑤ **Extensor indicis**

Origin:	Posterior surface of the ulna and the interosseous membrane
Insertion:	Posterior digital expansion of the second digit
Actions:	• Wrist joint: extension
	• MCP, PIP, and DIP joints of the second digit: extension
Innervation:	Radial nerve (C7, C8)

DIP, distal interphalangeal; IP, interphalangeal; MCP, metacarpophalangeal; PIP, proximal interphalangeal.

Olecranon

Lateral epicondyle

Common head of extensor digitorum, extensor digiti minimi, and extensor carpi ulnaris

Ulna

Extensor carpi ulnaris

Extensor digitorum

Extensor digiti minimi

Radius

Fifth metacarpal, base

Fifth proximal phalanx, base

Dorsal digital expansion, intertendinous connections

C The superficial extensors (extensor digitorum, extensor digiti minimi, and extensor carpi ulnaris)
Right forearm, posterior (dorsal) view.

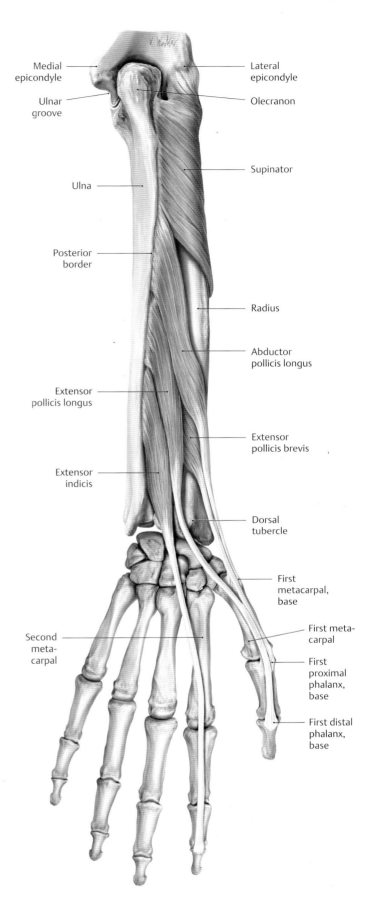

Medial epicondyle

Lateral epicondyle

Ulnar groove

Olecranon

Supinator

Ulna

Posterior border

Radius

Abductor pollicis longus

Extensor pollicis longus

Extensor pollicis brevis

Extensor indicis

Dorsal tubercle

First metacarpal, base

Second metacarpal

First metacarpal

First proximal phalanx, base

First distal phalanx, base

D The deep extensors (supinator, abductor pollicis longus, extensor pollicis brevis, extensor pollicis longus, and extensor indicis)
Right forearm, posterior (dorsal) view.

319

15.13 The Intrinsic Muscles of the Hand: The Thenar and Hypothenar Muscles

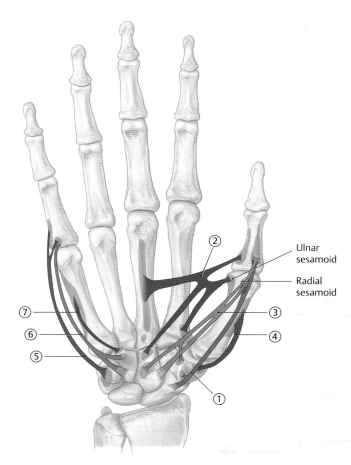

A Schematic of the thenar (①–④) and hypothenar (⑤–⑦) muscles

① **Abductor pollicis brevis**

Origin:	Scaphoid and trapezium, flexor retinaculum
Insertion:	Base of the proximal phalanx of the thumb (via the radial sesamoid)
Actions	Abduction of the thumb
Innervation:	Median nerve (C8, T1)

② **Adductor pollicis**

Origin:	• Transverse head: palmar surface of the third metacarpal • Oblique head: capitate, base of second and third metacarpals
Insertion:	Base of the proximal phalanx of the thumb (via the ulnar sesamoid)
Actions:	• CMC joint of the thumb: opposition • MCP joint of the thumb: flexion
Innervation:	Ulnar nerve (C8, T1)

③ **Flexor pollicis brevis**

Origin:	• Superficial head: flexor retinaculum • Deep head: capitate, trapezium
Insertion:	Base of the proximal phalanx of the thumb (via the radial sesamoid)
Actions:	• CMC joint of the thumb: flexion, opposition • MCP joint of the thumb: flexion
Innervation:	• Superficial head: Median nerve (C8, T1) • Deep head: Ulnar nerve (C8, T1)

④ **Opponens pollicis**

Origin:	Trapezium
Insertion:	Radial border of the first metacarpal
Action:	CMC joint of the thumb: opposition
Innervation:	Median nerve (C8, T1)

⑤ **Abductor digiti minimi**

Origin:	Pisiform
Insertion:	Ulnar base of the proximal phalanx and the dorsal digital expansion of the fifth digit
Actions:	• MCP joint of the little finger: flexion and abduction of the little finger • PIP and DIP joints of the little finger: extension
Innervation:	Ulnar nerve (C8, T1)

⑥ **Flexor digiti minimi brevis**

Origin:	Hook of the hamate, flexor retinaculum
Insertion:	Base of the proximal phalanx of the fifth digit
Action:	MCP joint of the little finger: flexion
Innervation:	Ulnar nerve (C8, T1)

⑦ **Opponens digiti minimi**

Origin:	Hook of the hamate and flexor retinaculum
Insertion:	Ulnar border of the fifth metacarpal
Action:	Draws the metacarpal in the palmar direction (opposition)
Innervation:	Ulnar nerve (C8, T1)

Palmaris brevis (not shown, see also pp. 343 and 348)

Origin:	Ulnar border of the palmar aponeurosis
Insertion:	Skin of the hypothenar eminence
Action:	Tightens the palmar aponeurosis (protective function)
Innervation:	Ulnar nerve (C8, T1)

CMC, carpometacarpal; DIP, distal interphalangeal; MCP, metacarpointerphalangeal; PIP, proximal interphalangeal.

Labels in figure: ②, Ulnar sesamoid, Radial sesamoid, ⑦, ⑥, ⑤, ③, ④, ①

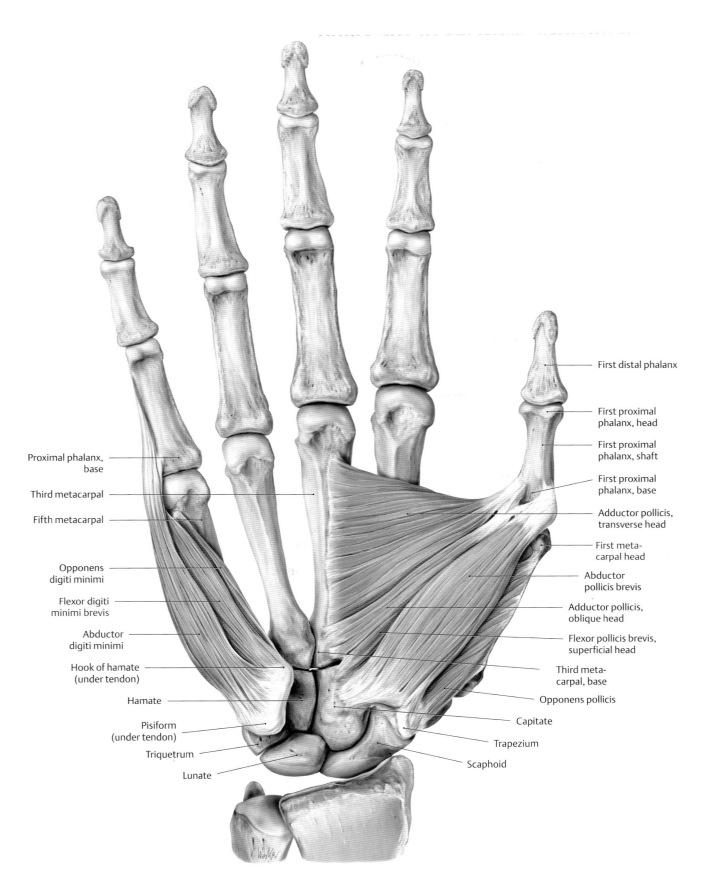

First distal phalanx

First proximal phalanx, head

First proximal phalanx, shaft

First proximal phalanx, base

Adductor pollicis, transverse head

First meta-carpal head

Abductor pollicis brevis

Adductor pollicis, oblique head

Flexor pollicis brevis, superficial head

Third meta-carpal, base

Opponens pollicis

Capitate

Trapezium

Scaphoid

Proximal phalanx, base

Third metacarpal

Fifth metacarpal

Opponens digiti minimi

Flexor digiti minimi brevis

Abductor digiti minimi

Hook of hamate (under tendon)

Hamate

Pisiform (under tendon)

Triquetrum

Lunate

B **The thenar muscles (abductor pollicis brevis, adductor pollicis, flexor pollicis brevis, and opponens pollicis) and the hypothenar muscles (abductor digiti minimi, flexor digiti minimi brevis, and opponens digiti minimi)**
Right hand, anterior (palmar) view

321

15.14 The Intrinsic Muscles of the Hand: Lumbricals and Interossei (Metacarpal Muscles)

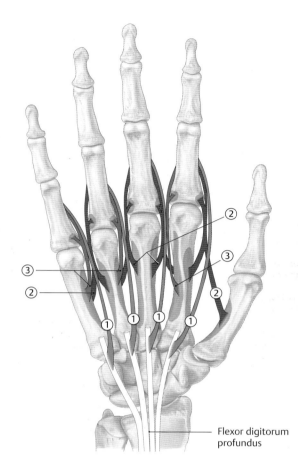

A Schematic of the metacarpal muscles

Flexor digitorum profundus

① **First through fourth lumbrical muscles**

Origin: Radial sides of the tendons of flexor digitorum profundus (variable)

Insertion:
- First lumbrical: dorsal digital expansion of the second digit (index finger)
- Second lumbrical: dorsal digital expansion of the third digit (middle finger)
- Third lumbrical: dorsal digital expansion of the fourth digit (ring finger)
- Fourth lumbrical: dorsal digital expansion of the fifth digit (little finger)

Actions:
- MCP joints of the second through fifth digits: flexion
- PIP and DIP joints of the second through fifth digits: extension

Innervation:
- Median nerve, C8, T1 (first and second lumbricals)
- Ulnar nerve, C8, T1 (third and fourth lumbricals)

② **First through fourth dorsal interossei**

Origin: By two heads from adjacent sides of the first through fifth metacarpals

Insertion:
- Dorsal digital expansion of the second through fourth digits, base of the proximal phalanx
- First interosseus: radial side of the second proximal phalanx (index finger)
- Second interosseus: radial side of the third proximal phalanx (middle finger)
- Third interosseus: ulnar side of the third proximal phalanx (middle finger)
- Fourth interosseus: ulnar side of the fourth proximal phalanx (ring finger)

Actions:
- MCP joints of the second through fourth digits: flexion
- PIP and DIP joints of the second through fourth digits: extension and abduction of the fingers (abduction of the index and ring fingers from the middle finger)

Innervation: Ulnar nerve (C8, T1)

③ **First through third palmar interossei**

Origin:
- First interosseus: ulnar side of the second metacarpal (index finger)
- Second interosseus: radial side of the fourth metacarpal (ring finger)
- Third interosseus: radial side of the fifth metacarpal (little finger)

Insertion: Dorsal digital expansion and base of the proximal phalanx of the associated finger

Actions:
- MCP joints of the second, fourth, and fifth digits: flexion
- PIP and DIP joints of the second, fourth, and fifth digits: extension and adduction of the fingers (adduction of the second, fourth, and fifth digits toward the middle finger)

Innervation: Ulnar nerve (C8, T1)

DIP, distal interphalangeal; MCP, metacarpointerphalangeal; PIP, proximal interphalangeal.

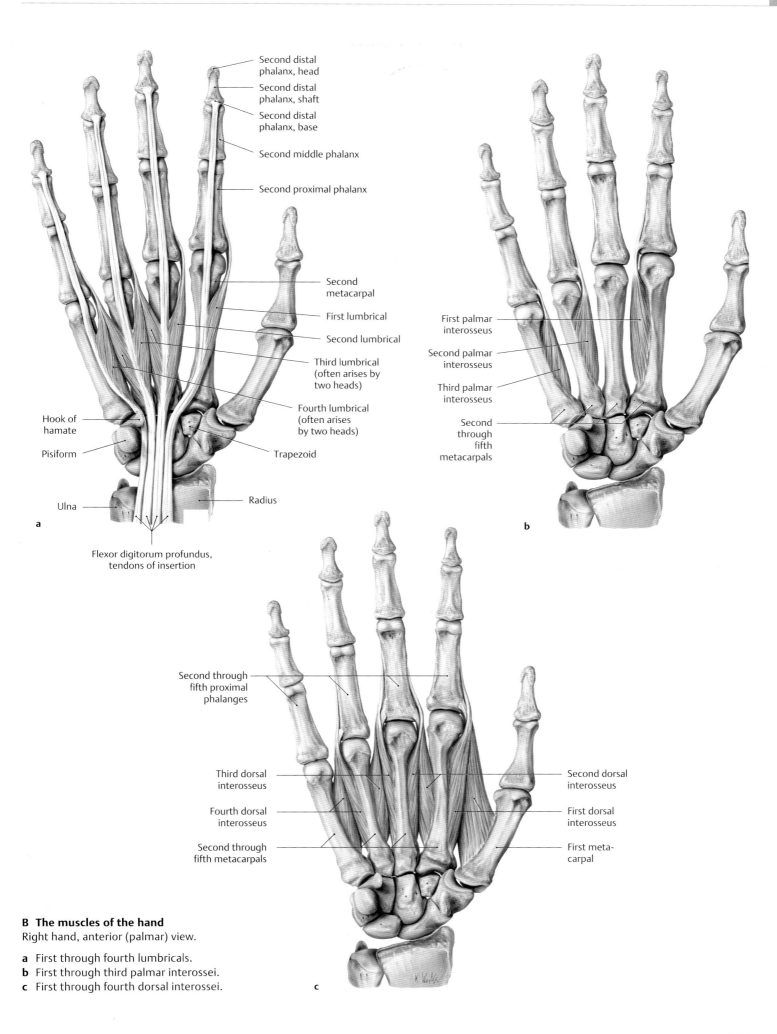

Second distal
phalanx, head

Second distal
phalanx, shaft

Second distal
phalanx, base

Second middle phalanx

Second proximal phalanx

Second
metacarpal

First lumbrical

Second lumbrical

Third lumbrical
(often arises by
two heads)

Fourth lumbrical
(often arises
by two heads)

Trapezoid

Hook of
hamate

Pisiform

Ulna

Radius

a

Flexor digitorum profundus,
tendons of insertion

First palmar
interosseus

Second palmar
interosseus

Third palmar
interosseus

Second
through
fifth
metacarpals

b

Second through
fifth proximal
phalanges

Third dorsal
interosseus

Fourth dorsal
interosseus

Second through
fifth metacarpals

Second dorsal
interosseus

First dorsal
interosseus

First meta-
carpal

c

B The muscles of the hand
Right hand, anterior (palmar) view.

a First through fourth lumbricals.
b First through third palmar interossei.
c First through fourth dorsal interossei.

15.15 Overview of Muscle Functions: Shoulder (Glenohumeral) Joint

A Movements of the shoulder (glenohumeral) joint*

Type of movement	Extent of movement	Muscle	Innervation	Responsible nerve segment
Flexion	90° (>90° = elevation)	• Deltoid (clavicular part)	• Axillary nerve	• C5, C6
		• Biceps brachii	• Musculocutaneous nerve	• C5–C7
		• Pectoralis major (clavicular and sternocostal parts)	• Medial and lateral pectoral nerves	• C5–T1
		• Coracobrachialis	• Musculocutaneous nerve	• C5–C7
Extension	40°	• Latissimus dorsi	• Thoracodorsal nerve	• C6–C8
		• Teres major	• Lower subscapular nerve	• C5, C6
		• Triceps brachii, (long head)	• Radial nerve	• C6–C8
		• Deltoid (spinal part)	• Axillary nerve	• C5, C6
Abduction	90° (>90° = elevation)	• Deltoid (acromial part), above 60°, the entire muscle	• Axillary nerve	• C5, C6
		• Supraspinatus	• Suprascapular nerve	• C5, C6
		• Biceps brachii (long head)	• Musculocutaneous nerve	• C5–C7
Adduction	20–40°	• Pectoralis major	• Medial and lateral pectoral nerves	• C5–T1
		• Latissimus dorsi	• Thoracodorsal nerve	• C6–C8
		• Triceps brachii (long head)	• Radial nerve	• C6–C8
		• Teres major	• Lower subscapular nerve	• C5, C6
		• Deltoid (clavicular and spinal parts)	• Axillary nerve	• C5, C6
		• Coracobrachialis	• Musculocutaneous nerve	• C5–C7
Internal rotation	50–95°	• Subscapularis	• Upper and lower subscapular nerve	• C5, C6
		• Pectoralis major	• Medial and lateral pectoral nerves	• C5–T1
		• Biceps brachii, (long head)	• Musculocutaneous nerve	• C5–C7
		• Deltoid (clavicular part)	• Axillary nerve	• C5, C6
		• Teres major	• Lower subscapular nerve	• C5, C6
		• Latissimus dorsi	• Thoracodorsal nerve	• C6–C8
External rotation	60–90° (depending on extent of flexion)	• Infraspinatus	• Suprascapular nerve	• C4–C6
		• Teres minor	• Axillary nerve	• C5, C6
		• Deltoid (spinal part)	• Axillary nerve	• C5, C6

* The starting point of the functional approach is movement within the joint. The muscles, which are involved in all movements, are listed in the order of their strength. Remember, however, that although individual muscles may be involved in particular movements, their functional significance may be negligible. In order to describe the many types of movement in a joint, each joint (respective of its degree of freedom) is assigned clearly defined basic movements along defined axes. Only the combination of these basic movements allows for a range of movements depending on the individual joint.

a Flexion

b Extension

c Abduction

d Adduction

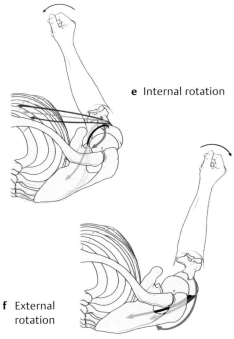

e Internal rotation

f External rotation

B Movements of the shoulder joint

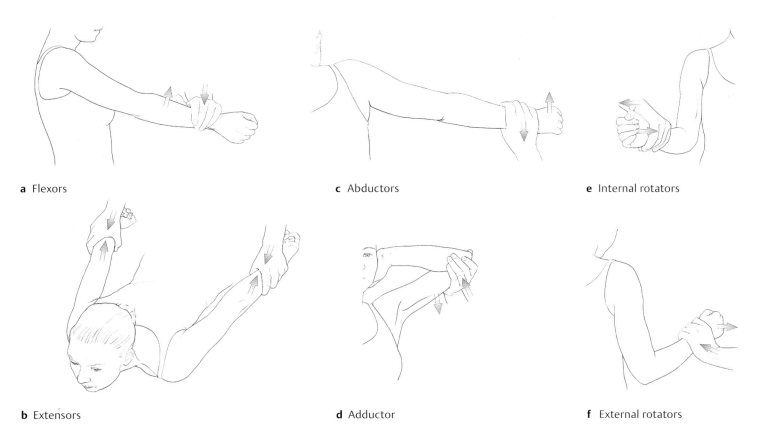

a Flexors

c Abductors

e Internal rotators

b Extensors

d Adductor

f External rotators

C Functional muscle testing in the shoulder joint

In order to test muscle strength, the patient is asked to actively move the muscle group against some resistance from the examiner. The force generated by the muscle action is measured using a scale from 0 to 5.

D Clinical symptoms of shoulder joint muscle shortening or weakness

Muscles	Symptoms of muscle shortening	Symptoms of muscle weakness
Flexors	Shoulder is commonly protracted.	In order to compensate for muscle weakness, the acromion is lifted, and the upper body, due to increased lumbar lordosis, moves posteriorly. In case of isolated weakness of the deltoid, the shoulder contours are flattened with the acromion protruding.
Extensors	Significantly impaired movements in elevation and external rotation.	Weakness in the extensors becomes apparent when extreme loads are placed on the shoulder, e.g., propping oneself up using both arms.
Abductors	Impaired movement as a result of shortened muscles (primarily supraspinatus and biceps brachii), especially in extension, adduction, and external rotation of the shoulder joint.	The arm cannot maintain the arm in abduction against gravity. Flattening of the contours of the shoulder with typical indentation below the acromion, often subluxation of the shoulder joint with the arm hanging down.
Adductors	Protracted shoulder and increased thoracic kyphosis, along with compensatory cervical lordosis. Significantly impaired arm movements in flexion and abduction above the head.	Dysfunction in sequence of abdominal muscles of the opposite side, meaning mainly hitting and chopping motions with the affected limb are impeded. Difficulty holding large or heavy objects at waist level.
Internal rotators	Significantly impaired movement when lifting the arm above the head with simultaneous external rotation.	An isolated weakness of the internal rotators is rare and is compensated for by the flexors (most of the daily chores are performed in flexion and internal rotation).
External rotators	Shortening of the external rotators is rare (mostly following long periods of immobilization) and leads to impaired internal rotation.	Insufficent inferior glide of the head of the humerus during elevation, resulting in compensatory activation of abductors (e.g., supraspinatus), pulling up of the shoulder, and increased lateral trunk flexion.

15.16 Overview of Muscle Functions: Elbow Joint

A Movements of the elbow joint*

Type of movement	Extent of movement	Muscle	Innervation	Responsible nerve segment
Flexion	130–150°	• Biceps brachii • Brachialis • Brachioradialis • Pronator teres	• Musculocutaneous nerve • Musculocutaneous nerve • Radial nerve • Median nerve	• C5–C7 • C5, C6 • C5, C6 • C6, C7
Extension	10°	• Triceps brachii • Anconeus	• Radial nerve • Radial nerve	• C6–C8 • C6–C8
*Supination**	90°	• Biceps brachii • Supinator • Brachioradialis (pronated)	• Musculocutaneous nerve • Radial nerve • Radial nerve	• C5–C7 • C7, C8 • C5, C6
*Pronation**	90°	• Pronator quadratus • Pronator teres • Brachioradialis (supinated)	• Median nerve • Median nerve • Radial nerve	• C8, T1 • C6, C7 • C5, C6

*In addition to the elbow joint, the distal radioulnar joint is involved in turning the forearm.

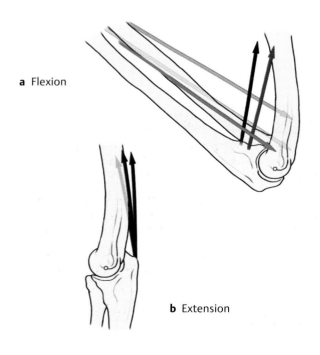

a Flexion

b Extension

B Movements of the elbow joint

c Supination

d Pronation

a Flexors

b Extensors

c Supinators
(elbow joint is flexed)

d Supinators
(elbow joint is
extended)

e Pronators

C Functional testing of muscles of the elbow joint

D Clinical symptoms of elbow joint muscle shortening and weakness

Muscles	Symptoms of muscle shortening	Symptoms of muscle weakness
Flexors	Flexion contracture of the elbow with involvement of the biceps brachii, resulting in significant functional impairment, requiring a shift from supination to pronation.	Muscle weakness, e.g., of the biceps brachii, leads to preponderance of pronation; thus, eating, for instance (moving a spoon to the mouth), is significantly impaired.
Extensors	Extension contracture of the elbow resulting in significant functional impairment in routine daily movements.	It is not possible to throw an object. The affected patient is not able to use a walking device since he or she cannot apply any weight on his or her hands due to inability to extend the elbow.
Supinators	Impaired movement when forearm is pronated. Compensated for by increased internal rotation and abduction of the shoulder joint.	Weakness in supinators becomes apparent in numerous routine daily movements: e.g., unlocking a door, turning off a faucet, or tightening a screw.
Pronators	Impaired movement when forearm is supinated. Compensated for by increased external rotation and adduction of the shoulder joint.	Routine daily movements are hampered (see above), such as unlocking a door or turning off a faucet.

327

15.17 Overview of Muscle Functions: Wrist

A Movement of the proximal and distal wrist (radiocarpal and mediocarpal joints)

Type of movement	Extent of movement	Muscle	Innervation	Responsible nerve segment
Palmar flexion	60–80°	• Flexor digitorum superficialis	• Median nerve	• C8, T1
		• Flexor digitorum profundus	• Median nerve	• C8, T1
			• Ulnar nerve	• C8, T1
		• Flexor carpi ulnaris	• Ulnar nerve	• C8, T1
		• Flexor pollicis longus	• Median nerve	• C8, T1
		• Flexor carpi radialis	• Median nerve	• C6, C7
		• Palmaris longus	• Median nerve	• C7, C8
Dorsal extension	40–60°	• Extensor digitorum	• Radial nerve	• C7, C8
		• Extensors carpi radialis longus and brevis	• Radial nerve	• C6–C8
		• Extensor carpi ulnaris	• Radial nerve	• C7, C8
		• Extensor indicis	• Radial nerve	• C7, C8
		• Extensor pollicis longus	• Radial nerve	• C7, C8
		• Extensor digiti minimi	• Radial nerve	• C7, C8
Abduction (radial deviation)	20°	• Extensors carpi radialis longus and brevis	• Radial nerve	• C6–C8
		• Abductor pollicis longus	• Radial nerve	• C7, C8
		• Extensor pollicis brevis	• Radial nerve	• C7, C8
		• Extensor pollicis longus	• Radial nerve	• C7, C8
		• Flexor pollicis longus	• Median nerve	• C8, T1
		• Flexor carpi radialis	• Median nerve	• C6, C7
Abduction (ulnar deviation)	30–40°	• Extensor carpi ulnaris	• Radial nerve	• C7, C8
		• Flexor carpi ulnaris	• Ulnar nerve	• C8, T1
		• Extensor digiti minimi	• Radial nerve	• C7, C8

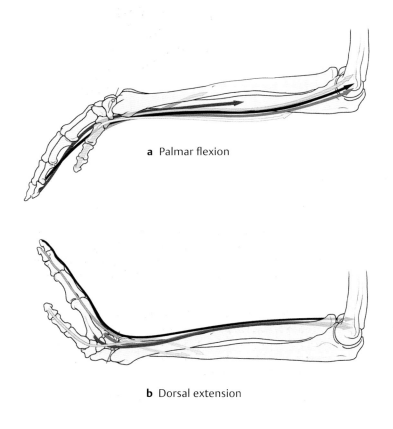

a Palmar flexion

b Dorsal extension

B Movements of the proximal and distal wrist

c Radial abduction

d Ulnar abduction

a Palmar flexion

b Dorsal extension

c Radial abduction

d Ulnar abduction

C Functional muscle testing of the proximal and distal wrist

D Clinical symptoms of muscle shortening and weakness of the proximal and distal wrist

Muscles	Symptoms of muscle shortening	Symptoms of muscle weakness
Palmar flexors	Impaired movement in dorsal extension of the wrist and finger joints, combined with constant overloading to palmar flexors, which leads to epicondylitis medialis (golfer's elbow).	When lifting heavy objects, the affected patient is not able to sufficiently stabilize the wrist with supinated forearm; thus, the wrist tilts in a dorsal direction. In the long run, this leads to injuries resulting from overload of the tendons of origin of the finger and hand flexors.
Dorsal extensors	Impaired movement in palmar flexion of wrist and finger joints, combined/accompanied by constant overloading to dorsal extensors, which leads to epicondylitis lateralis (tennis elbow).	When lifting heavy objects, the affected patient is not able to sufficiently stabilize the wrist with pronated forearm; thus, the wrist tilts in a palmar direction. In the long run, this leads to injuries resulting from overload of the tendons of origin of the finger and hand extensors.
Radial abductors	Weakening of ulnar abduction.	Always combined with weakened dorsal extension and palmar flexion.
Ulnar abductors	Weakening of radial abduction.	Loss of strength functionally less visible.

16.1 The Posterior Muscles of the Shoulder Girdle and Shoulder Joint

Semispinalis capitis

Sternocleido-mastoid

Splenius capitis

Trapezius, descending part

Scapular spine

Deltoid

Trapezius, transverse part

Trapezius, ascending part

Teres major

Triceps brachii, long head

Triceps brachii, lateral head

Latissimus dorsi

Brachioradialis

Extensor carpi radialis brevis

Extensor carpi radialis longus

Olecranon

External oblique

Anconeus

Thoracolumbar fascia

Flexor carpi ulnaris

Extensor carpi ulnaris

A Muscles of the shoulder girdle and shoulder joint
Right half of the body, posterior view. Superficial layer.

Extensor digitorum

Iliac crest

Internal oblique

Superior
nuchal line

Sternocleido-
mastoid

Semispinalis
capitis

Splenius capitis

Splenius cervicis

Rhomboid minor

Levator scapulae

Rhomboid major

Clavicle

Acromion

Supraspinatus

Scapular spine

Deltoid

Medial border of scapula

Infraspinatus

Teres minor

Teres major

Latissimus
dorsi

Serratus
anterior

Serratus
posterior inferior

Triceps brachii

External oblique

Trapezius
(cut edge)

Erector spinae,
thoracolumbar fascia

Latissimus dorsi
(cut edge)

Thoracolumbar
fascia

Internal
oblique

**B Muscles of the shoulder girdle and
shoulder joint**
Right half of the body, posterior view. Deep
layer. Portions of the trapezius and latissimus
dorsi muscles have been removed.

331

16.2 The Posterior Muscles of the Shoulder Joint and Arm

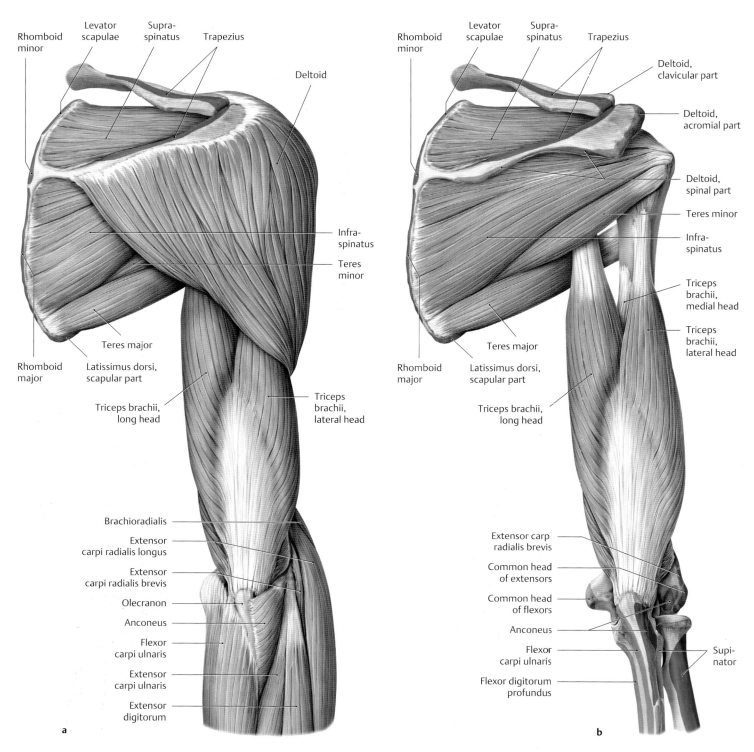

A Muscles of the shoulder and arm
Right side, posterior view. The origins and insertions of the muscles are indicated by color shading (red = origin, blue = insertion).

a After removal of the trapezius.

b After removal of the deltoid and forearm muscles.

Rhomboid minor

Levator scapulae

Supraspinatus

Trapezius

Deltoid, clavicular part

Deltoid, acromial part

Supraspinatus

Infraspinatus

Teres minor

Deltoid, spinal part

Triceps brachii, lateral head

Teres minor

Infraspinatus

Deltoid

Brachialis

Triceps brachii, medial head

Triceps brachii, lateral head (cut edge)

Teres major

Rhomboid major

Latissimus dorsi, scapular part

Triceps brachii, long head

Extensor carpi radialis longus

Extensor carpi radialis brevis

Common head of extensors

Common head of flexors

Anconeus

a

Rhomboid minor

Levator scapulae

Supraspinatus

Trapezius

Deltoid, clavicular part

Deltoid, acromial part

Supraspinatus

Infraspinatus

Teres minor

Deltoid, spinal part

Triceps brachii, long head

Triceps brachii, lateral head

Radial groove

Deltoid

Brachialis

Triceps brachii, medial head

Teres minor

Infraspinatus

Teres major

Rhomboid major

Latissimus dorsi, scapular part

Extensor carpi radialis longus

Brachioradialis

Extensor carpi radialis brevis

Common head of extensors

Common head of flexors

Triceps brachii

Anconeus

b

B Muscles of the shoulder and arm
Right side, posterior view. The origins and insertions of the muscles are indicated by color shading (red = origin, blue = insertion).

a The supraspinatus, infraspinatus, and teres minor have been

removed. The lateral head of the triceps brachii has been partially removed.
b All the muscles have been removed.

16.3 The Anterior Muscles of the Shoulder Girdle and Shoulder Joint

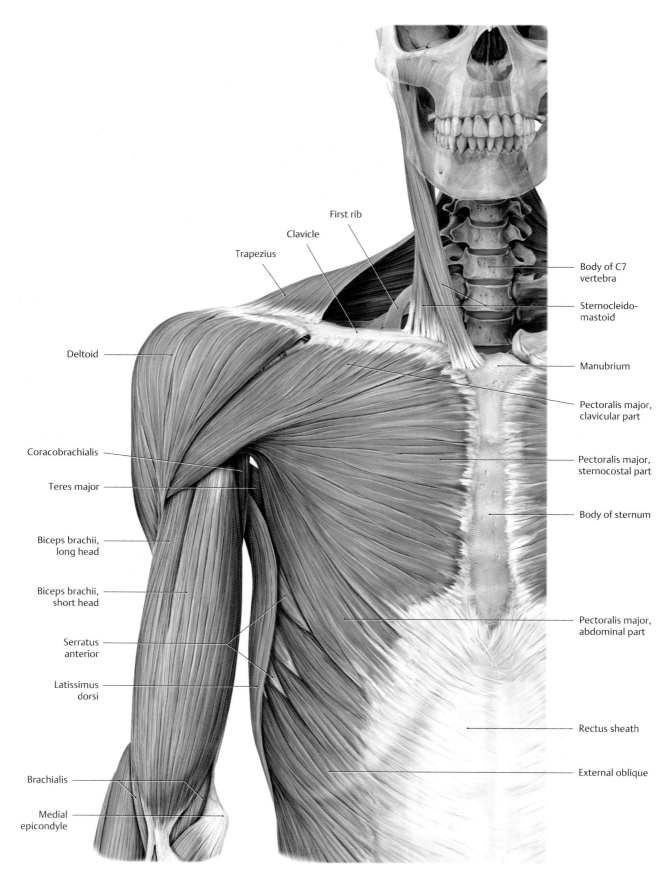

First rib

Clavicle

Trapezius

Body of C7
vertebra

Sternocleido-
mastoid

Deltoid

Manubrium

Pectoralis major,
clavicular part

Coracobrachialis

Pectoralis major,
sternocostal part

Teres major

Body of sternum

Biceps brachii,
long head

Biceps brachii,
short head

Serratus
anterior

Pectoralis major,
abdominal part

Latissimus
dorsi

Rectus sheath

Brachialis

External oblique

Medial
epicondyle

A Muscles of the shoulder and arm
Right side, anterior view.

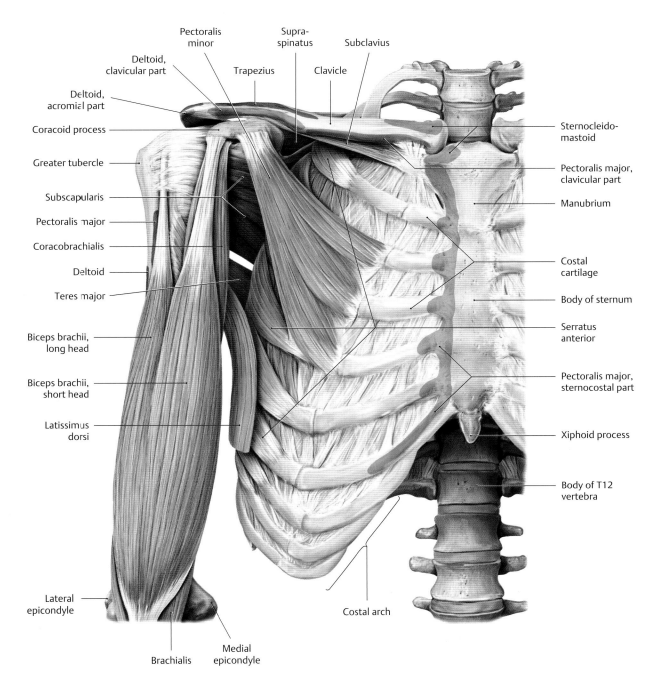

B Muscles of the shoulder and arm
Right side, anterior view. The origins and insertions of the muscles are indicated by color shading (red = origin, blue = insertion). The sternocleidomastoid, trapezius, pectoralis major, deltoid, and external oblique muscles have been completely removed. The latissimus dorsi has been partially removed.

16.4 The Muscles of the Shoulder Joint and Anterior Arm

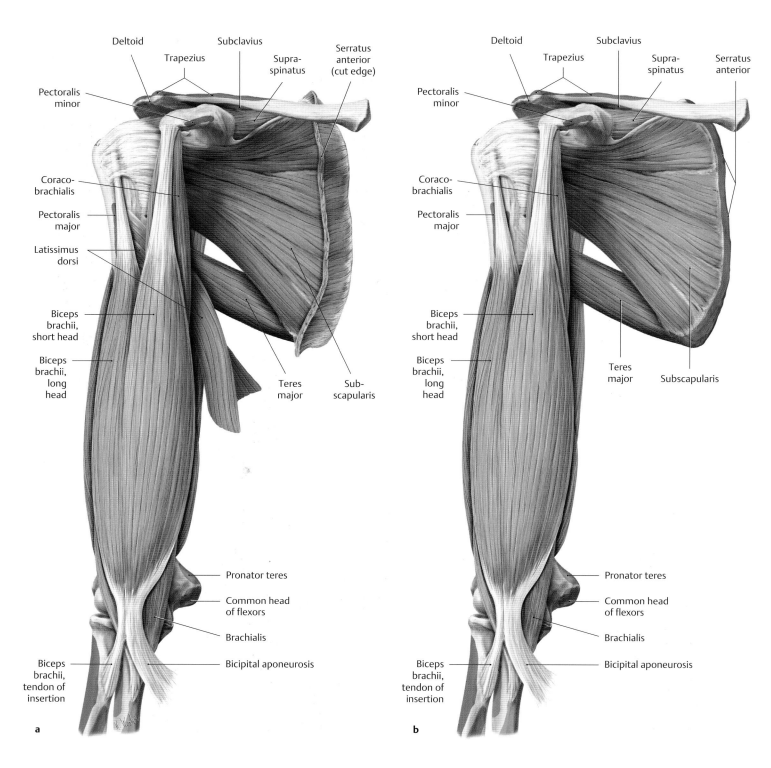

A Muscles of the shoulder and arm
Right side, anterior view. The origins and insertions of the muscles are indicated by color shading (red = origin, blue = insertion).

a After removal of the thoracic skeleton. Latissimus dorsi and serratus anterior have been removed to their insertions.
b Latissimus dorsi and serratus anterior have been completely removed.

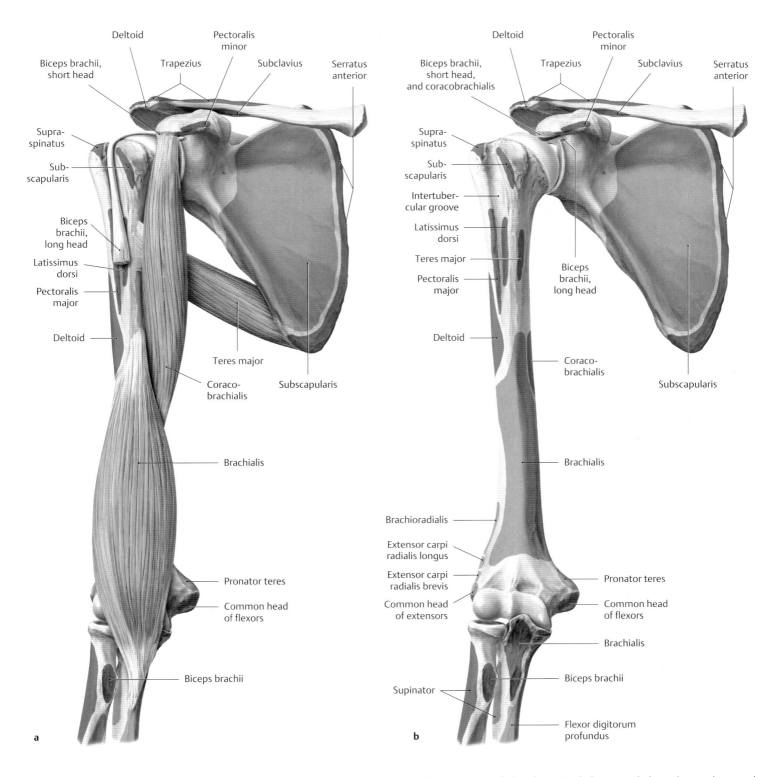

B Muscles of the shoulder and arm

Right side, anterior view. The origins and insertions of the muscles are indicated by color shading (red = origin, blue = insertion).

a After removal of the thoracic skeleton and the subscapularis and supraspinatus muscles. The biceps brachii has been removed to the tendon of origin of its long head (*note* its course through the intertubercular groove).

b All the muscles have been removed.

337

16.5   The Muscles of the Anterior Forearm

Biceps brachii

Biceps brachii, tendon of insertion

Brachioradialis

Extensor carpi radialis longus

Extensor carpi radialis brevis

Brachialis

Medial epicondyle, common head of flexors

Bicipital aponeurosis

Pronator teres

Flexor carpi radialis

Palmaris longus

Flexor carpi ulnaris

Flexor digitorum superficialis

Flexor pollicis longus

Abductor pollicis longus

Palmaris longus

Flexor digitorum superficialis, tendons of insertion

Flexor pollicis longus, tendon of insertion

Flexor digitorum profundus, tendons of insertion

a

Brachialis

Medial epicondyle, common head of flexors

Biceps brachii

Supinator

Pronator teres

Flexor digitorum superficialis

Flexor pollicis longus

Pronator quadratus

Brachioradialis

Flexor carpi ulnaris

Abductor pollicis longus

Flexor digitorum superficialis, tendons of insertion

Flexor pollicis longus, tendon of insertion

Flexor digitorum profundus, tendons of insertion

b

A Muscles of the forearm
Right forearm, anterior view. The origins and insertions of the muscles are indicated by color shading (red = origin, blue = insertion).

a The superficial flexors and the radialis group are shown.
b The radialis group (brachioradialis, extensor carpi radialis longus, extensor carpi radialis brevis) has been completely removed, along with the flexor carpi radialis, flexor carpi ulnaris, abductor pollicis longus, palmaris longus, and biceps brachii.

Brachialis

Pronator teres, humeral head

Medial epicondyle, common head of flexors

Flexor digitorum superficialis, ulnar head

Biceps brachii

Supinator

Flexor digitorum superficialis, radial head

Pronator teres

Flexor pollicis longus

Pronator quadratus

Brachioradialis

Abductor pollicis longus

Flexor carpi ulnaris

Flexor digitorum profundus

Flexor pollicis longus, tendon of insertion

Flexor digitorum profundus, tendons of insertion

a

Brachioradialis

Extensor carpi radialis longus

Extensor carpi radialis brevis

Lateral epicondyle, common head of extensors, supinator

Brachialis

Pronator teres, humeral head

Medial epicondyle, common head of flexors

Flexor digitorum superficialis, ulnar head

Pronator teres, ulnar head

Brachialis

Biceps brachii

Supinator

Flexor digitorum superficialis, radial head

Pronator teres

Flexor pollicis longus

Pronator quadratus

Brachioradialis

Abductor pollicis longus

Flexor digitorum profundus

Flexor carpi ulnaris

Flexor carpi radialis

Flexor pollicis longus

Flexor digitorum superficialis

Flexor digitorum profundus

b

B Muscles of the forearm

Right forearm, anterior view. The origins and insertions of the muscles are indicated by color shading (red = origin, blue = insertion).

a Pronator teres and flexor digitorum superficialis have been removed.
b All the muscles have been removed.

339

16.6 The Muscles of the Posterior Forearm

a

b

A Muscles of the forearm

Right forearm, posterior view. The origins and insertions of the muscles are indicated by color shading (red = origin, blue = insertion).

a The superficial extensors and the radialis group are shown.
b Triceps brachii, anconeus, flexor carpi ulnaris, extensor carpi ulnaris, and extensor digitorum have been removed.

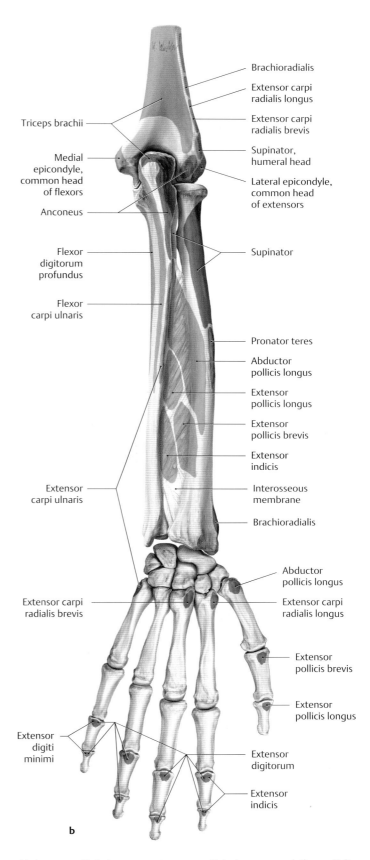

a

b

B Muscles of the forearm

Right forearm, posterior view. The origins and insertions of the muscles are indicated by color shading (red = origin, blue = insertion).
Note the interosseous membrane, which contributes to the origin of several muscles in the forearm.

a Abductor pollicis longus, extensor pollicis longus, and the radialis group have been removed.
b All the muscles have been removed.

16.7 Cross sectional Anatomy of the Arm and Forearm

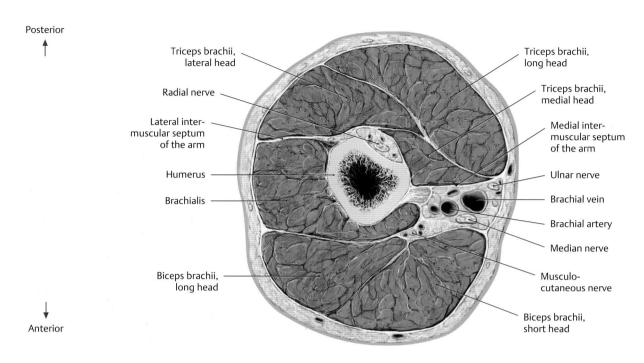

A Cross section through the right arm
Proximal view. The location of the sectional plane is shown in **C**.

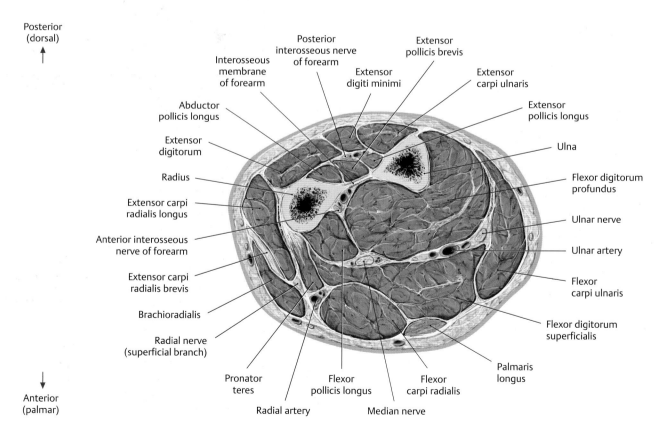

B Cross section through the right forearm
Proximal view. The location of the plane of section is shown in **D**.

Deltoid

Pectoralis
major

Coraco-
brachialis

Teres major

Biceps brachii,
long head

Biceps brachii,
short head

Humerus

Biceps
brachii

Brachio-
radialis

Brachialis

Medial
epicondyle

C "Windowed" dissection of the right arm
Anterior view.

Biceps
brachii

Brachialis

Medial
epicondyle,
common head
of flexors

Biceps brachii,
tendon of
insertion

Bicipital
aponeurosis

Brachio-
radialis

Pronator
teres

Extensor
carpi radialis
longus

Flexor
carpi radialis

Extensor
carpi radialis
brevis

Palmaris
longus

Radius

Ulna

Flexor
carpi ulnaris

Flexor digitorum
superficialis

Flexor
pollicis longus

Abductor
pollicis longus

Thenar
muscles

Palmaris
longus

Flexor retinaculum
(transverse
carpal ligament)

Palmaris
brevis

Palmar
aponeurosis

D "Windowed" dissection of the right forearm
Anterior view.

343

16.8 The Tendon Sheaths of the Hand

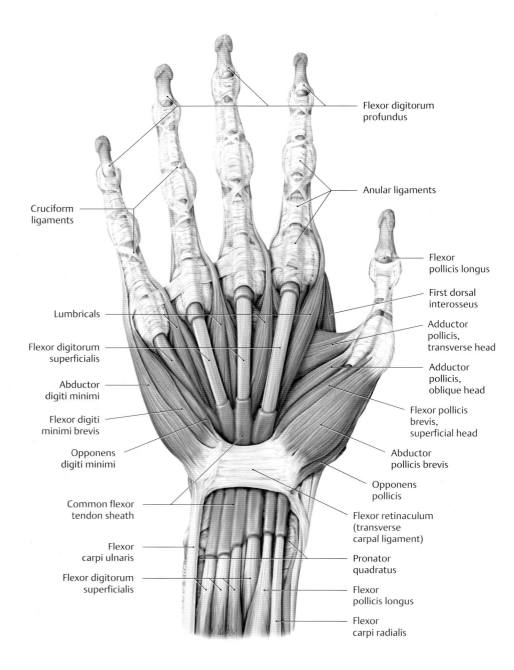

A Carpal and digital tendon sheaths on the palmar surface of the right hand

The palmar aponeurosis (see p. 348) has been removed. The tendons of the flexor pollicis longus, flexor digitorum superficialis, and flexor digitorum profundus run from the distal forearm through a fibro-osseous canal (carpal tunnel) to the palm, accompanied by the median nerve and protected by the palmar carpal tendon sheaths (see also p. 288 and p. 402). The carpal tendon sheath of the flexor pollicis longus is consistently continuous with the digital tendon sheath of the thumb, while the digital tendon sheaths of the remaining fingers show variable communication with the carpal tendon sheaths (see **B**).

Labels (figure A):
- Flexor digitorum profundus
- Anular ligaments
- Cruciform ligaments
- Flexor pollicis longus
- First dorsal interosseus
- Adductor pollicis, transverse head
- Lumbricals
- Adductor pollicis, oblique head
- Flexor digitorum superficialis
- Abductor digiti minimi
- Flexor pollicis brevis, superficial head
- Flexor digiti minimi brevis
- Abductor pollicis brevis
- Opponens digiti minimi
- Opponens pollicis
- Common flexor tendon sheath
- Flexor retinaculum (transverse carpal ligament)
- Flexor carpi ulnaris
- Pronator quadratus
- Flexor digitorum superficialis
- Flexor pollicis longus
- Flexor carpi radialis

B Communication between the digital and carpal tendon sheaths

Right hand, anterior view (after Schmidt and Lanz).

a In 71.4% of cases (Scheldrup 1951) the digital tendon sheath of the little finger communicates directly with the carpal tendon sheath, while the other tendon sheaths of the second through fourth digits extend only from the metacarpophalangeal joint to the distal interphalangeal joint.

b In 17.4% of cases the carpal tendon sheath does not communicate with the digital tendon sheath of the little finger.

c Besides the tendon sheath of the little finger, the carpal tendon sheath may occasionally be continuous with the digital tendon sheath of the index finger (3.5%) or of the ring finger (3%).

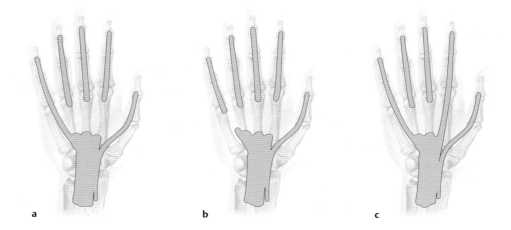

a   b   c

C Dorsal tendon compartments for the extensor tendons

First tendon compartment:	Abductor pollicis longus Extensor pollicis brevis
Second tendon compartment:	Extensor carpi radialis longus and brevis
Third tendon compartment:	Extensor pollicis longus
Fourth tendon compartment:	Extensor digitorum Extensor indicis
Fifth tendon compartment:	Extensor digiti minimi
Sixth tendon compartment:	Extensor carpi ulnaris

The location of the tendon compartments is shown in **D**.

D Extensor retinaculum and dorsal carpal tendon sheaths

Right hand, posterior view. The extensor retinaculum is part of the antebrachial (forearm) fascia. Its transverse fibers strengthen the fibrous layer of the tendon sheaths and fix them to the dorsum of the hand. Deep to the extensor retinaculum are *tendon sheath compartments*, which transmit the long extensor tendons singly or in groups. There are a total of six of these compartments, numbered 1 to 6 from the radial side to the ulnar side of the wrist (their contents are shown in **C**).

Dorsal digital expansion

Intertendinous connections

Abductor digiti minimi

Dorsal interossei

Dorsal carpal tendon sheaths

First tendon compartment: abductor pollicis longus, extensor pollicis brevis

Second tendon compartment: extensor carpi radialis longus and brevis

Third tendon compartment: extensor pollicis longus

Fourth tendon compartment: extensor digitorum, extensor indicis

Plane of section in **E**

Fifth tendon compartment: extensor digiti minimi

Sixth tendon compartment: extensor carpi ulnaris

Dorsal tubercle

Extensor retinaculum

E Schematic cross section through the forearm at the level of the distal radioulnar joint

Right forearm, proximal view. (Location of the sectional plane is shown in **D**.) Vertical connective tissue septa extend anteriorly from the deep surface of the extensor retinaculum to the bone or joint capsule and form six fibroosseous canals, the tendon sheath compartments of the extensor tendons (extensor tendon compartments).
Note also the dorsal tubercle, which redirects the tendon of insertion of the extensor pollicis longus to the thumb (see also **D**).

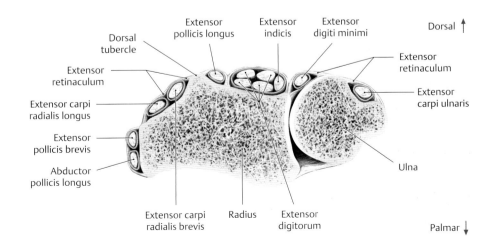

Dorsal tubercle

Extensor pollicis longus

Extensor indicis

Extensor digiti minimi

Dorsal ↑

Extensor retinaculum

Extensor retinaculum

Extensor carpi radialis longus

Extensor carpi ulnaris

Extensor pollicis brevis

Abductor pollicis longus

Ulna

Extensor carpi radialis brevis

Radius

Extensor digitorum

Palmar ↓

16.9 The Dorsal Digital Expansion

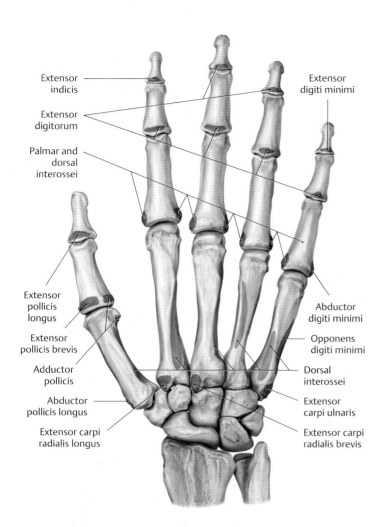

A Origins and insertions of the dorsal muscles of the right hand
The origins and insertions of the muscles are indicated by color shading
(red = origin, blue = insertion).

B Extensor tendons and intertendinous connections on the dorsum of the right hand
The tendons of insertion of the extensor digitorum are interlinked by variable oblique bands called *intertendinous connections*. The most proximal of the intertendinous connections are those extending between the index and middle fingers. No such connection is present on the tendon of the extensor indicis. The extensor digitorum inserts by a variable number of tendons. Generally, all of the fingers have at least two extensor tendon elements. In addition, the *index finger* and *little finger* have their own extensor muscles (extensor indicis and extensor digiti minimi) whose tendons always run on the ulnar side of the tendons of the common extensor digitorum. Because the index finger and little finger have their own extensors, they can more easily be moved independently of the other fingers.

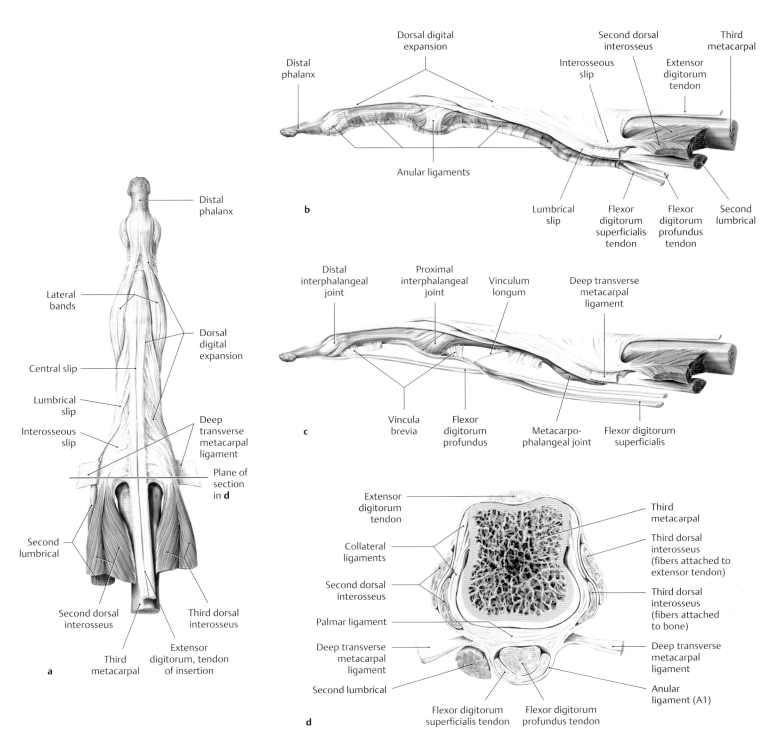

C Dorsal digital expansion

Dorsal digital expansion of the middle finger of the right hand (after Schmidt and Lanz).

a Posterior view.
b Radial view.
c After opening the common tendon sheath of the flexor digitorum superficialis and profundus muscles.
d Cross section at the level of the metacarpal head.

The dorsal digital expansion is more than an aponeurosis that incorporates slips from the extensor digitorum, lumbrical, and interosseous tendons. It is a complex system of interwoven fiber bands, joined by loose connective tissue to the periosteum of the phalanges. The dorsal digital expansion consists of a *central slip* and *lateral bands*, each of which has a *lateral part* and a *medial part*. The lateral part of the expansion receives slips from the tendons of the lumbrical and interosseous muscles (see **a**). This complex arrangement makes it possible for the long digital flexors and the short hand muscles to act on all three of the finger joints.

347

16.10 The Intrinsic Muscles of the Hand: Superficial Layer

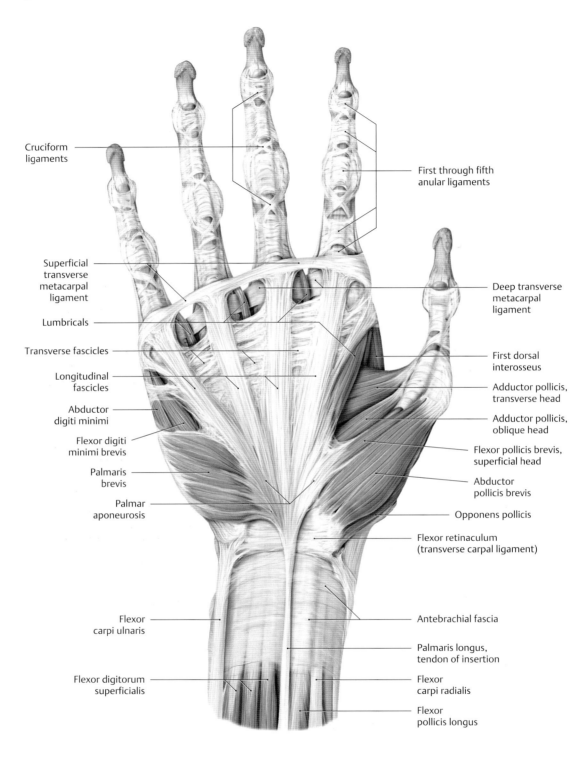

Cruciform ligaments

First through fifth anular ligaments

Superficial transverse metacarpal ligament

Deep transverse metacarpal ligament

Lumbricals

Transverse fascicles

First dorsal interosseus

Longitudinal fascicles

Adductor pollicis, transverse head

Abductor digiti minimi

Adductor pollicis, oblique head

Flexor digiti minimi brevis

Flexor pollicis brevis, superficial head

Palmaris brevis

Abductor pollicis brevis

Palmar aponeurosis

Opponens pollicis

Flexor retinaculum (transverse carpal ligament)

Flexor carpi ulnaris

Antebrachial fascia

Palmaris longus, tendon of insertion

Flexor digitorum superficialis

Flexor carpi radialis

Flexor pollicis longus

A The palmar aponeurosis and Dupuytren's contracture
Right hand, anterior view. The muscular fascia of the palm is thickened by firm connective tissue to form the *palmar aponeurosis*, which separates the palm from the subcutaneous fat to protect the soft tissues. It is composed mainly of longitudinal fiber bundles (*longitudinal fascicles*), which give it a fan-shaped arrangement. The longitudinal fascicles are held together by transverse fiber bundles (*transverse fascicles*) at the level of the metacarpal bones and by the superficial transverse metacarpal ligament at the level of the metacarpophalangeal joints. Two muscles, the palmaris brevis and palmaris longus, keep the palmar aponeurosis tense and prevent it from contracting, especially when the hand is clenched into a fist. Gradual atrophy or contracture of the palmar

aponeurosis leads to progressive shortening of the palmar fascia that chiefly affects the little finger and ring finger (*Dupuytren's contracture*). Over a period of years, the contracture may become so severe that the fingers assume a fixed flexed position with the fingertips touching the palm; this seriously compromises the grasping ability of the hand. The causes of Dupuytren's contracture are poorly understood, but it is a relatively common condition that is most prevalent in men over 40 years of age and is associated with chronic liver disease (e.g., cirrhosis). Treatment generally consists of complete surgical removal of the palmar aponeurosis.

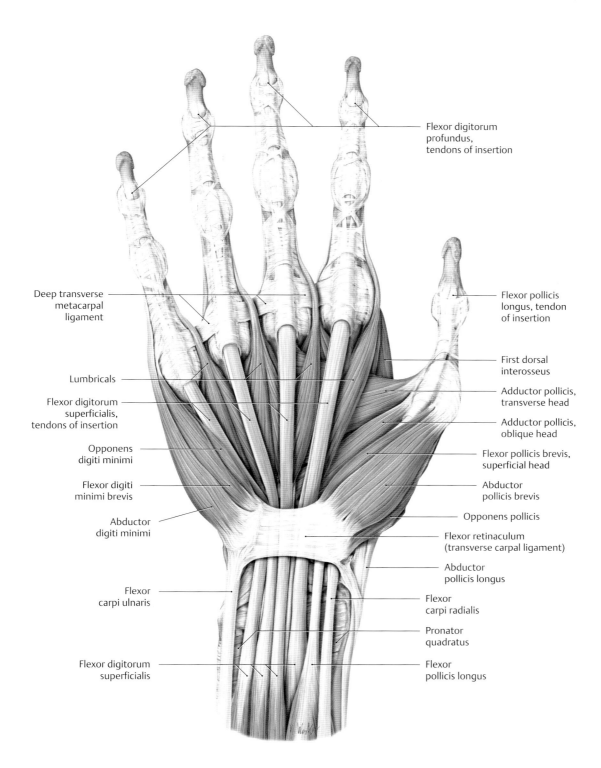

Flexor digitorum profundus, tendons of insertion

Deep transverse metacarpal ligament

Lumbricals

Flexor digitorum superficialis, tendons of insertion

Opponens digiti minimi

Flexor digiti minimi brevis

Abductor digiti minimi

Flexor carpi ulnaris

Flexor digitorum superficialis

Flexor pollicis longus, tendon of insertion

First dorsal interosseus

Adductor pollicis, transverse head

Adductor pollicis, oblique head

Flexor pollicis brevis, superficial head

Abductor pollicis brevis

Opponens pollicis

Flexor retinaculum (transverse carpal ligament)

Abductor pollicis longus

Flexor carpi radialis

Pronator quadratus

Flexor pollicis longus

B Superficial layer of the muscles of the right hand after removal of the palmar aponeurosis
Anterior view. The palmar aponeurosis, antebrachial (forearm) fascia, and palmaris brevis and longus muscles have been removed, along with the palmar and carpal tendon sheaths.

349

16.11 The Intrinsic Muscles of the Hand: Middle Layer

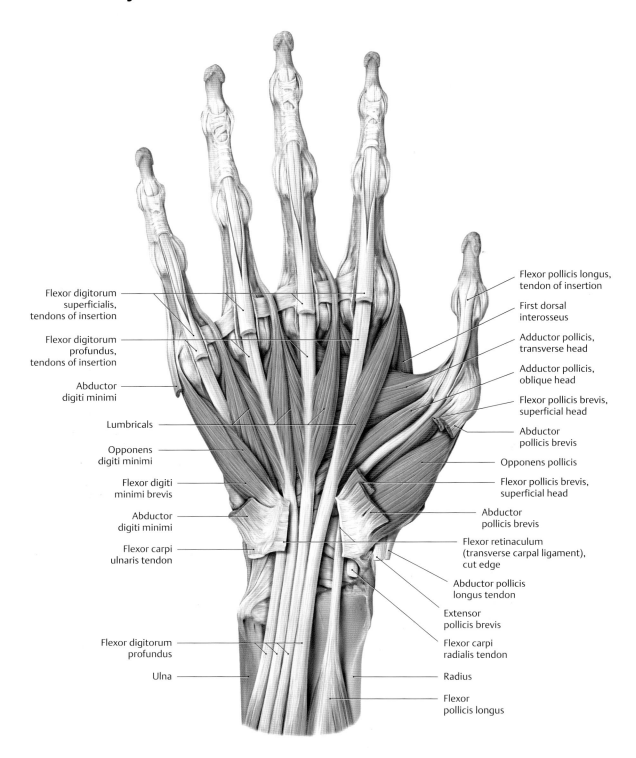

Flexor digitorum superficialis, tendons of insertion

Flexor digitorum profundus, tendons of insertion

Abductor digiti minimi

Lumbricals

Opponens digiti minimi

Flexor digiti minimi brevis

Abductor digiti minimi

Flexor carpi ulnaris tendon

Flexor digitorum profundus

Ulna

Flexor pollicis longus, tendon of insertion

First dorsal interosseus

Adductor pollicis, transverse head

Adductor pollicis, oblique head

Flexor pollicis brevis, superficial head

Abductor pollicis brevis

Opponens pollicis

Flexor pollicis brevis, superficial head

Abductor pollicis brevis

Flexor retinaculum (transverse carpal ligament), cut edge

Abductor pollicis longus tendon

Extensor pollicis brevis

Flexor carpi radialis tendon

Radius

Flexor pollicis longus

A Middle layer of the muscles of the right hand
Anterior view. The flexor digitorum superficialis muscle has been removed, and its four tendons of insertion have been divided at the level of the metacarpophalangeal joints. The first through third anular ligaments have been cut open to reveal the flexor tendons on the fin- gers. The flexor retinaculum (transverse carpal ligament) has been par- tially removed to open the carpal tunnel. Of the thenar muscles, por- tions of the abductor pollicis brevis and flexor pollicis brevis (superficial head) have been removed. Part of the abductor digiti minimi has been resected on the hypothenar side.

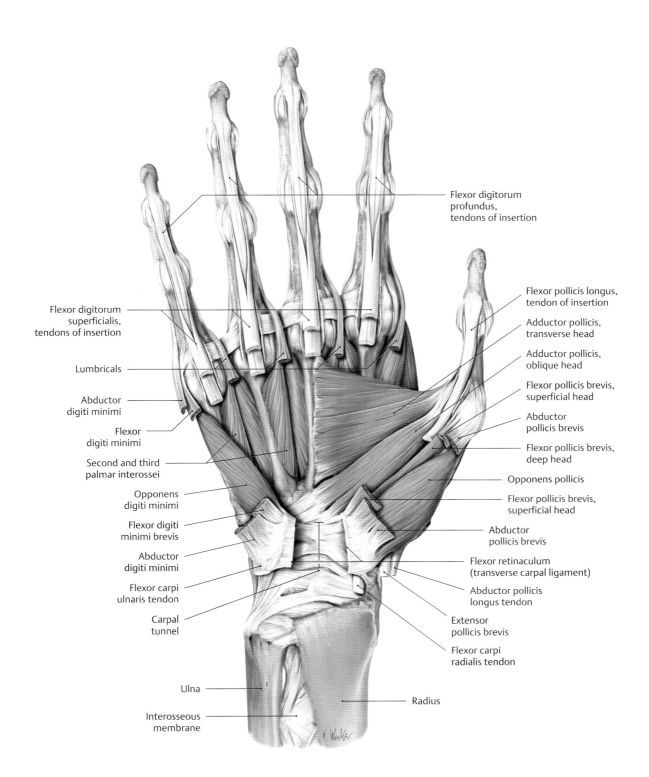

Flexor digitorum profundus, tendons of insertion

Flexor digitorum superficialis, tendons of insertion

Lumbricals

Abductor digiti minimi

Flexor digiti minimi

Second and third palmar interossei

Opponens digiti minimi

Flexor digiti minimi brevis

Abductor digiti minimi

Flexor carpi ulnaris tendon

Carpal tunnel

Ulna

Interosseous membrane

Flexor pollicis longus, tendon of insertion

Adductor pollicis, transverse head

Adductor pollicis, oblique head

Flexor pollicis brevis, superficial head

Abductor pollicis brevis

Flexor pollicis brevis, deep head

Opponens pollicis

Flexor pollicis brevis, superficial head

Abductor pollicis brevis

Flexor retinaculum (transverse carpal ligament)

Abductor pollicis longus tendon

Extensor pollicis brevis

Flexor carpi radialis tendon

Radius

B Middle layer of the muscles of the right hand
Anterior view. The flexor digitorum profundus muscle has been removed, and its four tendons of insertion and the lumbricals arising from them have been divided. The flexor pollicis longus and flexor digiti minimi muscles have also been removed.

16.12 The Intrinsic Muscles of the Hand: Deep Layer

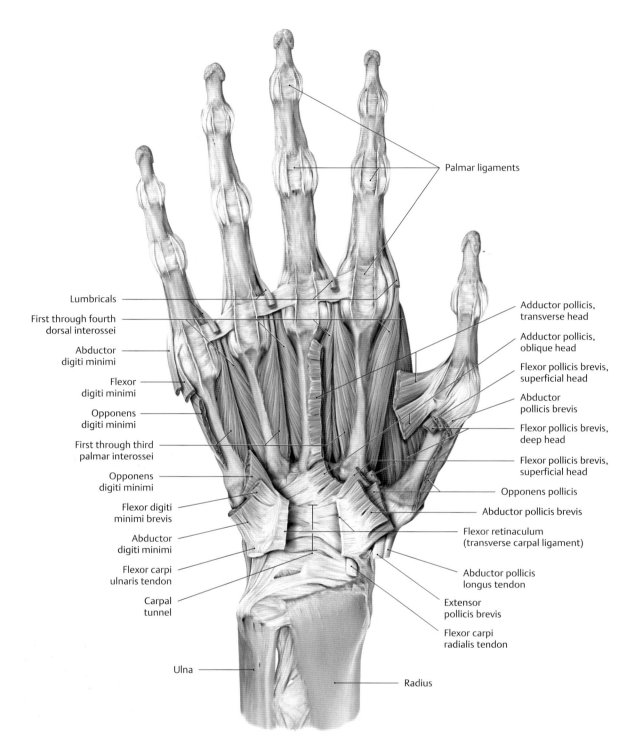

Palmar ligaments

Lumbricals

First through fourth dorsal interossei

Abductor digiti minimi

Flexor digiti minimi

Opponens digiti minimi

First through third palmar interossei

Opponens digiti minimi

Flexor digiti minimi brevis

Abductor digiti minimi

Flexor carpi ulnaris tendon

Carpal tunnel

Ulna

Adductor pollicis, transverse head

Adductor pollicis, oblique head

Flexor pollicis brevis, superficial head

Abductor pollicis brevis

Flexor pollicis brevis, deep head

Flexor pollicis brevis, superficial head

Opponens pollicis

Abductor pollicis brevis

Flexor retinaculum (transverse carpal ligament)

Abductor pollicis longus tendon

Extensor pollicis brevis

Flexor carpi radialis tendon

Radius

A Deep layer of the muscles of the right hand
Anterior view. The tendons of insertion, tendon sheaths, and anular ligaments of the long digital flexors have been completely removed. *Note* the exposed palmar ligaments, which combine with the tendon sheaths to form a trough that directs the long flexor tendons (see p. 291).

The first dorsal interosseus and first palmar interosseus muscles have been almost completely exposed by removal of the adductor pollicis. Both the opponens pollicis and the opponens digiti minimi have been partially removed.

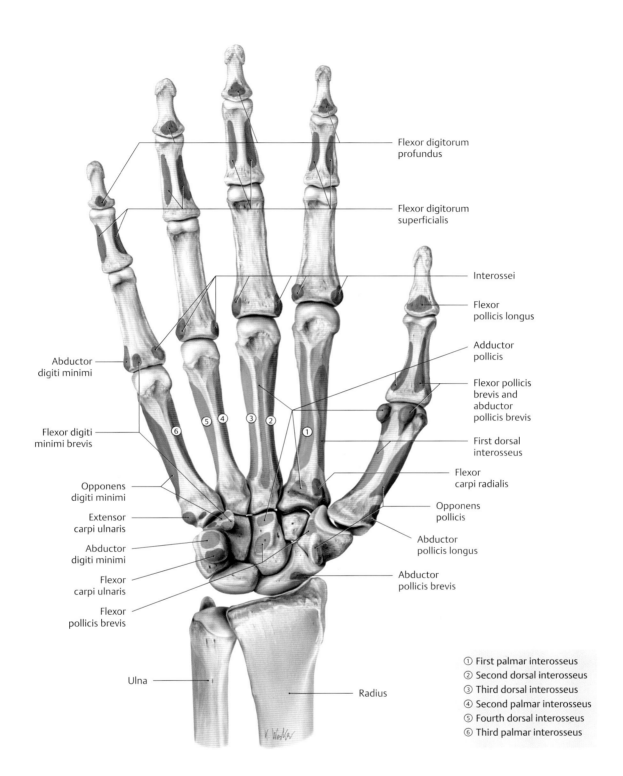

Flexor digitorum profundus

Flexor digitorum superficialis

Interossei

Flexor pollicis longus

Adductor pollicis

Flexor pollicis brevis and abductor pollicis brevis

First dorsal interosseus

Flexor carpi radialis

Opponens pollicis

Abductor pollicis longus

Abductor pollicis brevis

Abductor digiti minimi

Flexor digiti minimi brevis

Opponens digiti minimi

Extensor carpi ulnaris

Abductor digiti minimi

Flexor carpi ulnaris

Flexor pollicis brevis

Ulna

Radius

① First palmar interosseus
② Second dorsal interosseus
③ Third dorsal interosseus
④ Second palmar interosseus
⑤ Fourth dorsal interosseus
⑥ Third palmar interosseus

B Origins and insertions of the palmar muscles of the right hand
The origins and insertions of the muscles are indicated by color shading
(red = origin, blue = insertion).

17.1 The Arteries

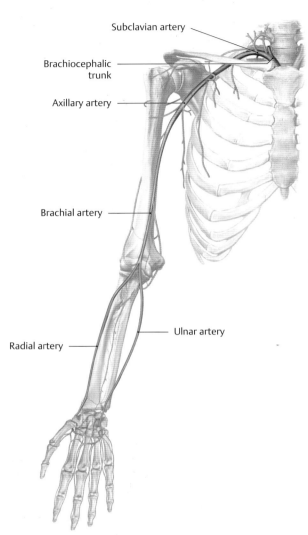

Subclavian artery

Brachiocephalic trunk

Axillary artery

Brachial artery

Ulnar artery

Radial artery

A Course of the different segments of the arteries supplying the shoulder and arm

Subclavian artery: The right subclavian artery arises from the brachiocephalic trunk (as shown here), and the left arises directly from the aortic arch. The vessel runs over the first rib between the anterior and middle scalene (interscalene space, scalene interval) and continues as the axillary artery (see below) on reaching the lateral border of the rib. Unlike the other arteries pictured here, the subclavian artery supplies blood not only to the upper limb (i.e., the shoulder girdle and arm) but also to

- a portion of the neck,
- the cerebral circulation, and
- the anterior chest wall.

Axillary artery: The continuation of the subclavian, the axillary artery runs from the lateral border of the first rib to the inferior border of the teres major muscle.

Brachial artery: The brachial artery is the continuation of the axillary artery. It ends at the elbow joint by dividing into the radial and ulnar arteries.

Radial artery: The radial artery runs distally on the radial side of the forearm from the division of the brachial artery, passing between the brachioradialis and flexor carpi radialis muscles on its way to the wrist. It terminates in the deep palmar arch.

Ulnar artery: This second division of the brachial artery runs below the pronator teres on the ulnar side of the forearm, under cover of the flexor carpi ulnaris, to the superficial palmar arch.

B Overview of the arteries of the shoulder and arm
The arteries of the shoulder and arm vary considerably in their origins and branching patterns (the principal variants are reviewed in Chapter 5, Neurovascular Systems: Topographical Anatomy). The branches are listed below in the order in which they arise from the parent vessels.

Branches of the subclavian artery
- Vertebral artery
- Internal thoracic artery (internal mammary artery)
- Thyrocervical trunk
  - Inferior thyroid artery
  - Ascending cervical artery
  - Suprascapular artery
  - Transverse cervical artery
- Costocervical trunk
  - Deep cervical artery
  - Supreme intercostal artery

Branches of the axillary artery
- Superior thoracic artery
- Thoracoacromial artery
  - Acromial branch
  - Clavicular branch
  - Deltoid branch
  - Pectoral branch
- Lateral thoracic artery
- Subscapular artery
  - Thoracodorsal artery
  - Circumflex scapular artery
- Anterior circumflex humeral artery
- Posterior circumflex humeral artery

Branches of the brachial artery
- Deep artery of the arm (deep brachial artery)
  - Medial collateral artery
  - Radial collateral artery
- Superior ulnar collateral artery (arterial network of the elbow)
- Inferior ulnar collateral artery (arterial network of the elbow)

Branches of the radial artery
- Radial recurrent artery (arterial network of the elbow)
- Palmar carpal branch (palmar carpal network)
- Superficial palmar branch (superficial palmar arch)
- Dorsal carpal branch (dorsal carpal network)
  - Dorsal metacarpal arteries
  - Dorsal digital arteries
- Princeps pollicis artery
- Radialis indicis artery
- Deep palmar arch
  - Palmar metacarpal arteries
  - Perforating branches

Branches of the ulnar artery
- Ulnar recurrent artery (arterial network of the elbow)
- Common interosseous artery
  - Posterior interosseous artery
  - Recurrent interosseous artery
  - Anterior interosseous artery
- Palmar carpal branch (palmar carpal network)
- Dorsal carpal branch (dorsal carpal network)
- Deep palmar branch (deep palmar arch)
- Superficial palmar arch
  - Common palmar digital arteries
  - Proper palmar digital arteries

C Arteries of the right upper limb
Anterior view with the forearm supinated. For clarity, some of the arteries listed in **B** are not illustrated.

D Arteries of the right hand
Posterior view.

E Main arterial branches in the right forearm (perforating branches)
a From the radial artery and ulnar artery (forearm supinated, anterior view).
b From the posterior interosseous artery (forearm pronated, posterior view).

Fasciocutaneous flaps with an excellent vascular pedicle can be harvested from the thin skin of the forearm. Composed of skin, subcutaneous tissue, and fascia, these flaps are supplied by branches of the major arteries and their accompanying veins. The skin flaps carry this vascular supply with them when they are transferred to the recipient site.

17.2 The Veins

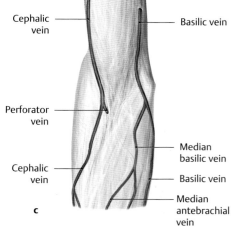

A Cutaneous veins and cutaneous nerves of the right elbow

Anterior view. The subcutaneous veins of the elbow are excellent sites for administering intravenous injections and drawing blood owing to their size and accessibility and the relatively thin skin in that region. But given their close relationship to the cutaneous nerves, as illustrated by the proximity of the basilic vein to the medial antebrachial cutaneous nerve, injections into these veins may cause severe transient pain, as in cases where an accidental "paravascular" injection irritates the surrounding connective tissue. "Rolling veins" refers to a condition in which the subcutaneous veins are exceptionally mobile within the subcutaneous fat. In approximately 3% of cases the ulnar artery may pass over the surface of the flexor muscles (superficial ulnar artery, see also p. 395). An unintended intra-*arterial* injection can have devastating consequences with certain medications. This complication can be avoided by palpating the vessel and confirming arterial-type pulsations before giving the injection and always drawing a small amount of blood back into the syringe (dark red = venous blood, bright red = arterial blood) before depressing the plunger.

B Cubital fossa of the right arm: variable course of the subcutaneous veins

a M-shaped venous pattern above the median antebrachial vein.

b Presence of an accessory cephalic vein from the venous plexuses on the extensor side of the forearm.

c Absence of the median cubital vein.

All of the illustrated variants are common.

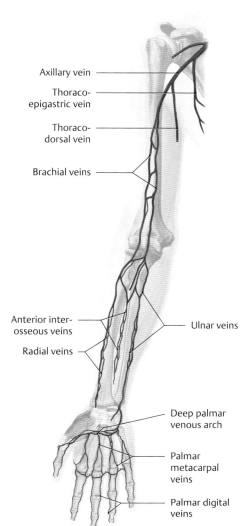

Axillary vein

Thoraco-
epigastric vein

Thoraco-
dorsal vein

Brachial veins

Anterior inter-
osseous veins

Radial veins

Ulnar veins

Deep palmar
venous arch

Palmar
metacarpal
veins

Palmar digital
veins

C Deep veins of the right upper limb
Anterior view.

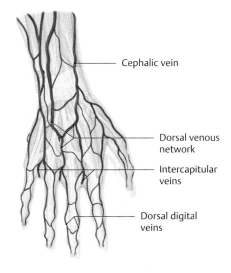

Cephalic vein

Dorsal venous
network

Intercapitular
veins

Dorsal digital
veins

E Superficial veins of the dorsum of the right hand

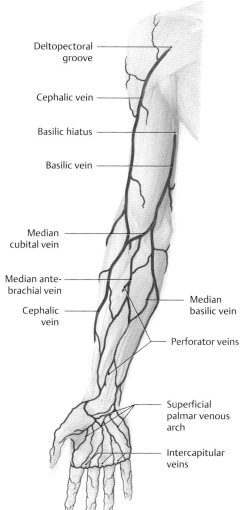

Deltopectoral
groove

Cephalic vein

Basilic hiatus

Basilic vein

Median
cubital vein

Median ante-
brachial vein

Cephalic
vein

Median
basilic vein

Perforator veins

Superficial
palmar venous
arch

Intercapitular
veins

D Superficial veins of the right upper limb
Anterior view. The main longitudinal trunks of the subcutaneous venous network of the arm are the median antebrachial vein, the basilic vein, and the cephalic vein.

Median antebrachial vein: This vein, unlike the cephalic and basilic, receives blood mainly from the cutaneous veins on the dorsum of the hand, draining the *flexor side of the forearm*. The *variable* median antebrachial vein opens into the corresponding longitudinal veins at the elbow, usually by way of the median cephalic vein and median basilic vein (see p. 379).

Basilic vein: This vein begins at the *elbow*, first ascending in the *epifascial* plane in the medial bicipital groove to the basilic hiatus, where it pierces the fascia in the middle of the arm. It terminates in a *subfascial* plane at the ulnar brachial vein.

Cephalic vein: In the *arm* the cephalic vein first ascends on the lateral side of the biceps brachii, then enters a groove between the deltoid and pectoralis major muscles (the deltopectoral groove). It finally opens into the axillary vein in the clavipectoral triangle (see p. 380).

F Overview of the main superficial and deep veins of the upper limb
Numerous connections exist between the deep and superficial veins of the arm—the perforator veins. Valves are incorporated into the veins at regular intervals, increasing the efficiency of venous return (see p. 65).

Deep veins of the upper limb
- Subclavian vein
- Axillary vein
- Brachial veins
- Ulnar veins
- Radial veins
- Anterior interosseous veins
- Posterior interosseous veins
- Deep palmar venous arch
- Palmar metacarpal veins

Superficial veins of the upper limb
- Cephalic vein
- Accessory cephalic vein
- Basilic vein
- Median cubital vein
- Median antebrachial vein
- Median cephalic vein
- Median basilic vein
- Dorsal venous network of the hand
- Superficial palmar venous arch

17.3 The Lymphatic Vessels and Lymph Nodes

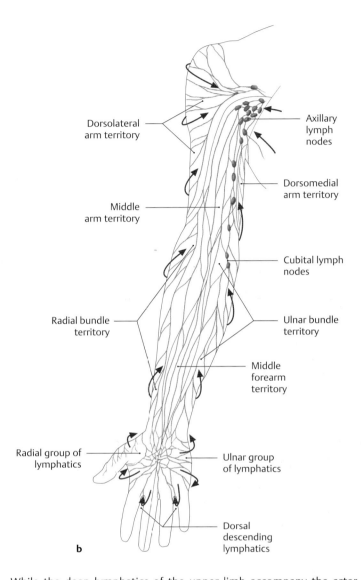

A Lymph vessels of the upper limb (after Schmidt and Lanz)
a Posterior view, **b** anterior view. The lymph vessels (lymphatics) in the upper limb are of two types:

- Superficial (epifascial) lymphatics
- Deep lymphatics

While the deep lymphatics of the upper limb accompany the arteries and deep veins, the superficial lymphatics lie in the subcutaneous tissue. In the forearm, they are most closely related to the cephalic and basilic veins. Numerous anastomoses exist between the deep and superficial systems. The arrows in the diagrams indicate the main directions of lymphatic drainage. Inflammations and infections of the hand generally incite a painful swelling of the axillary lymph nodes. When the lymph vessels are also involved, they are visible as red streaks beneath the skin (lymphangitis).

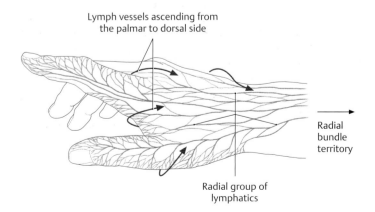

B Lymphatic drainage of the thumb, index finger, and dorsum of the hand (after Schmidt and Lanz)
The thumb, index finger, and part of the middle finger are drained by a radial group of lymph vessels that pass directly to the axillary lymph nodes. The other fingers are drained by an ulnar group of lymphatics (not shown here) that end at the cubital lymph nodes.

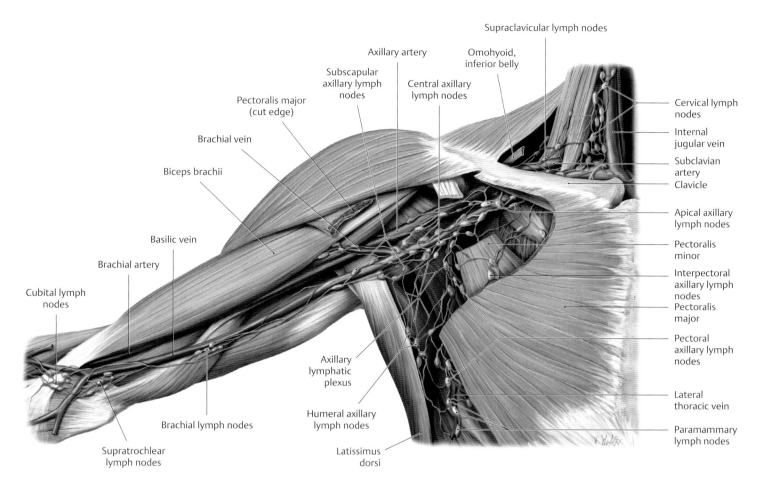

C Regional lymph nodes of the right upper limb

Anterior view. The lymph nodes of the axilla (*axillary lymph nodes*) are important collecting stations for the arm, shoulder girdle, and anterior chest wall. The 30 to 60 lymph nodes of the axilla are divided into several groups or levels, numbered I to III (see **E**), which are interconnected by lymph vessels. Taken together, the lymphatics in this region form an *axillary lymphatic plexus* lying within the fatty tissue. Lymphatic drainage from the axilla is collected in the subclavian trunk (not shown here). On the right side, the lymph is conveyed by the right jugular trunk and right bronchomediastinal trunk to the right lymphatic duct, which opens into the junction of the right subclavian and internal jugular veins (see p. 194).

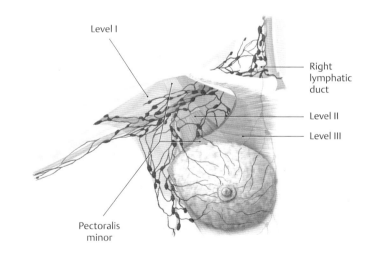

E Classification of axillary lymph nodes by level

The axillary lymph nodes have major clinical importance in breast cancer. A malignant breast tumor will metastasize (seed tumor cells) to the axillary nodes as it grows. As a guide for surgical removal, the axillary lymph nodes can be segregated into groups arranged in three levels, based on their relationship to the pectoralis minor muscle.

- Level I: all the lymph nodes lateral to the pectoralis minor.
- Level II: all the lymph nodes along the pectoralis minor.
- Level III: all the lymph nodes medial to the pectoralis minor (see p. 300).

D The axillary lymph nodes, grouped by levels

(after Henne-Bruns, Dürig, and Kremer)

Level I: lower axillary group

(lateral to pectoralis minor)

- Pectoral axillary lymph nodes
- Subscapular axillary lymph nodes
- Humeral axillary lymph nodes
- Paramammary lymph nodes

Level II: middle axillary group

(along the pectoralis minor)

- Interpectoral axillary lymph nodes
- Central axillary lymph nodes

Level III: upper, infraclavicular group

(medial to pectoralis minor)

- Apical axillary lymph nodes

17.4 The Brachial Plexus: Structure

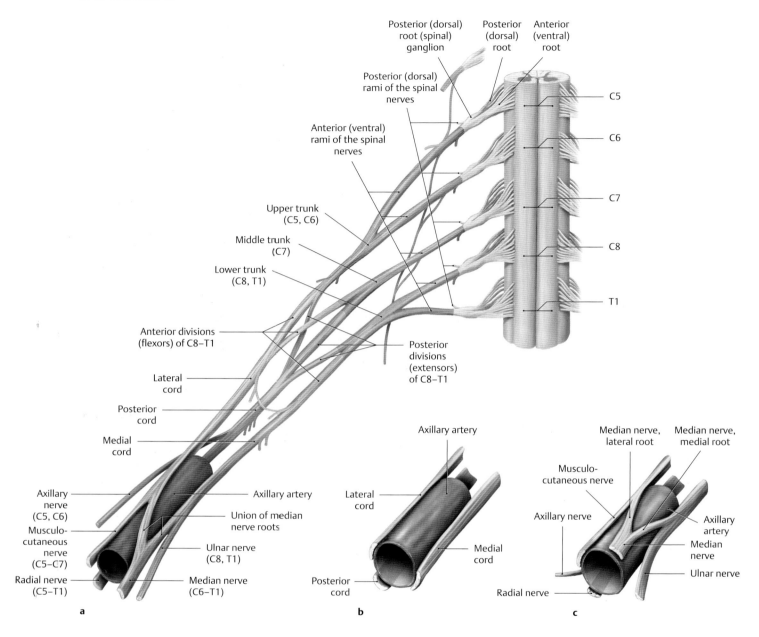

A Schematic representation of the structure of the brachial plexus

a Names and sequence of the various components of the brachial plexus.

b Relationship of the lateral, medial, and posterior cords of the brachial plexus to the axillary artery.

c Subdivision of the brachial plexus cords into their main branches.

B Number and location of the main components of the brachial plexus

Components	Number	Location
1. Plexus roots (anterior rami of the spinal nerves from cord segments C5–T1)	5	Between anterior and middle scalene (interscalene space)
2. The primary trunks: upper, middle, and lower	3	Lateral to the interscalene space and above the clavicle
3. The three anterior and three posterior divisions	6	Posterior to the clavicle
4. The lateral, medial, and posterior cords	3	In the axilla, posterior to the pectoralis minor

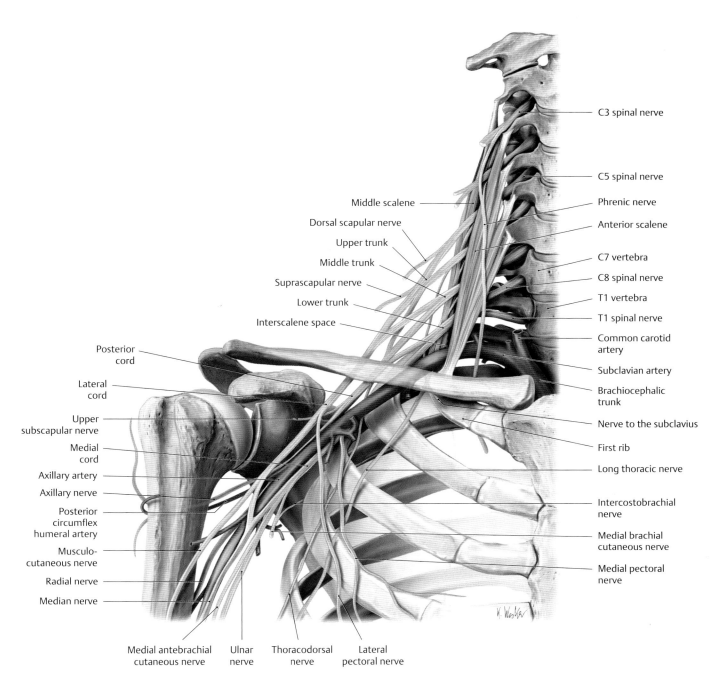

C Course of the brachial plexus and its relation to the thorax after passing through the interscalene space
Right side, anterior view.

D Spinal cord segments and nerves of the brachial plexus

Brachial plexus trunks and associated spinal cord segments
- Upper trunk C5 + C6
- Middle trunk C7
- Lower trunk C8 + T1

Brachial plexus cords and associated spinal cord segments
- Lateral cord C5–C7
- Medial cord C8–T1
- Posterior cord C5–T1

Nerves of the supraclavicular part of the brachial plexus (direct branches from the anterior rami or plexus trunks)
- Dorsal scapular nerve
- Long thoracic nerve
- Suprascapular nerve
- Nerve to the subclavius

Nerves of the infraclavicular part of the brachial plexus (short and long branches from the plexus cords)
- Lateral cord
  - Musculocutaneous nerve
  - Lateral pectoral nerve
  - Median nerve (lateral root)
- Medial cord
  - Median nerve (medial root)
  - Ulnar nerve
  - Medial pectoral nerve
  - Medial brachial cutaneous nerve
  - Medial antebrachial cutaneous nerve
- Posterior cord
  - Radial nerve
  - Axillary nerve
  - Upper subscapular nerve
  - Lower subscapular nerve
  - Thoracodorsal nerve

17.5 The Brachial Plexus: Supraclavicular Part

A Supraclavicular part of the brachial plexus
The supraclavicular part of the brachial plexus includes all nerves that arise directly from the plexus roots (anterior rami of the spinal nerves) or from the plexus trunks in the lateral cervical triangle between the anterior and middle scalene muscles. The different nerves of the supraclavicular plexus are predisposed to paralysis and/or compression in varying degrees based on their location and course (see **B–D**).

Nerve	Segment	Innervated muscle
Dorsal scapular nerve	C4, C5	• Levator scapulae • Rhomboid major • Rhomboid minor
Suprascapular nerve	C4–C6	• Supraspinatus • Infraspinatus
Long thoracic nerve	C5–C7	• Serratus anterior
Nerve to the subclavius	C5, C6	• Subclavius

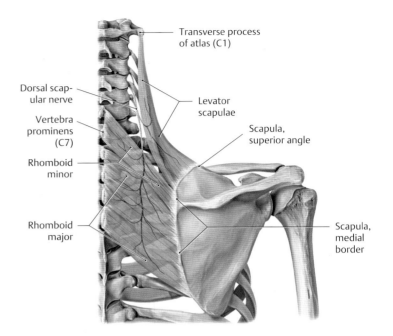

B The dorsal scapular nerve
Isolated paralysis of the dorsal scapular nerve is extremely rare owing to the protected location of the nerve between the deep nuchal muscles, the levator scapulae, and the rhomboids.

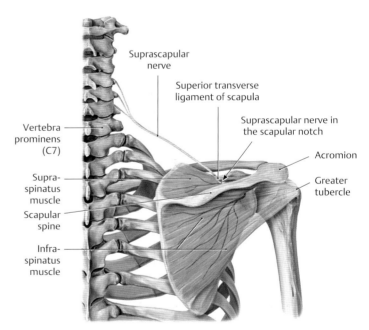

C The long thoracic nerve and nerve to the subclavius
Its long, superficial course on the serratus anterior along the lateral chest wall makes the long thoracic nerve susceptible to mechanical injury. The prolonged wearing of a heavy backpack is a common mechanism for this type of lesion. In iatrogenic cases, the nerve may be damaged by an axillary lymphadenectomy performed for a metastatic breast tumor. Clinically, loss of the serratus anterior muscle causes the medial scapular border to become elevated from the chest wall. This "winging" of the scapula is most conspicuous when the arm is raised forward, and generally the arm cannot be elevated past 90°.

D The suprascapular nerve
Injuries and chronic compression of the suprascapular nerve are uncommon conditions that lead to atrophy of the supraspinatus and infraspinatus muscles with weakness of arm abduction (especially during the initial phase owing to the "starter" function of the supraspinatus) and external rotation of the arm. Besides an isolated injury, the nerve may become compressed in the fibro-osseous canal between the scapular notch and the superior transverse scapular ligament (which is occasionally ossified to form a bony canal). The resulting symptoms are known collectively as "scapular notch syndrome" (see p. 243).

E Brachial plexus compression syndrome based on narrow anatomic passages in the shoulder region

In its course from the intervertebral foramina to the nerves of the upper limb, the brachial plexus must negotiate several narrow passages in which it may become compressed by surrounding structures. There are also extrinsic factors, such as carrying heavy loads, that may exert direct pressure on the brachial plexus. Several types of compression syndrome are distinguished:

1. Scalene syndrome or cervical rib syndrome:
   neurovascular compression in the interscalene space caused by a cervical rib or ligamentous structure (see **F**)

2. Costoclavicular syndrome:
   narrowing of the space between the first rib and clavicle (see **G**)

3. Hyperabduction syndrome:
   compression of the brachial plexus by the pectoralis minor muscle and coracoid process when the upper arm is raised above the head (see **H**)

4. Chronic heavy load on the shoulder girdle (e.g., "backpack paralysis")

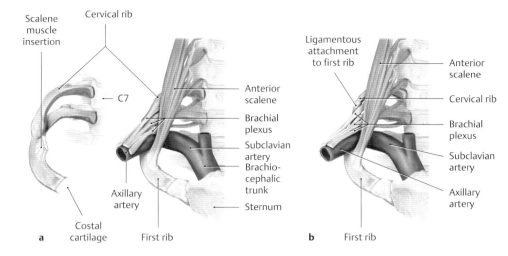

F Scalene syndrome due to narrowing of the interscalene space by a cervical rib

In approximately 1% of the population, cervical ribs may narrow the interscalene space bounded by the anterior and middle scalene muscles and the first rib. In this condition the trunks of the brachial plexus that pass through the interscalene space along with the subclavian artery are compressed from behind and below, placing varying degrees of tension on the neurovascular bundle. If there is no bony contact between a short cervical rib and the first rib (**b**), that site is often occupied by a ligamentous structure that can also cause neurovascular compression. The main clinical manifestations are pain radiating down the arm, chiefly to the ulnar side of the hand, and circulatory impairment caused by mechanical irritation of the periarterial sympathetic plexus of the subclavian artery.

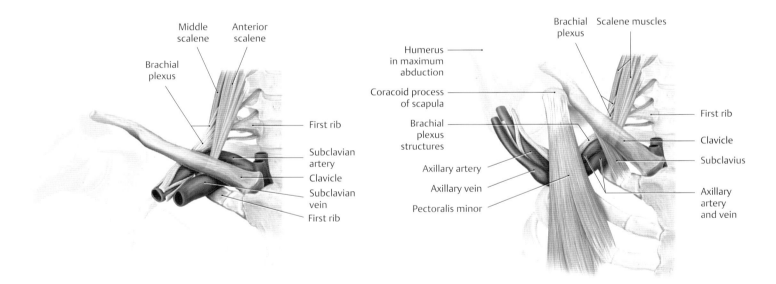

G Costoclavicular syndrome due to compression of the neurovascular bundle between the first rib and clavicle

Narrowing of the costoclavicular space is a rare condition that is most common in persons with drooping shoulders, a flat back, retracted shoulders (from carrying heavy loads), a deformed first rib, or a previous clavicular fracture. Any narrowing of the costoclavicular space can be aggravated by lowering and retracting the shoulder girdle. The complaints are similar to those in scalene syndrome and may be accompanied by signs of venous stasis caused by impaired return through the subclavian vein.

H Hyperabduction syndrome due to compression of the neurovascular bundle below the pectoralis minor and coracoid process

This rare syndrome is caused by neurovascular compression beneath the tendon of the pectoralis minor under the coracoid process. It is precipitated by maximum abduction or elevation of the arm on the affected side. A simple clinical test consists of pulling the arm upward and backward and holding it there. In normal cases, a definite radial artery pulse should still be palpable after 1 to 2 minutes, and the patient should not complain of radiating pain.

17.6 Infraclavicular Part of the Brachial Plexus: Overview and Short Branches

A Infraclavicular part of the brachial plexus
The infraclavicular part of the brachial plexus includes all the nerves that leave the plexus at the level of the plexus cords—the *short branches*—and those that continue down the arm as terminal branches of the individual plexus cords—the *long branches*. These nerves are reviewed below, beginning with the short branches.

Nerve	Segment	Innervated muscle	Cutaneous branches
Part I: Short branches			
• Upper and lower subscapular nerves	C5, C6	• Subscapularis • Teres major (upper only)	—
• Thoracodorsal nerve	C6–C8	• Latissimus dorsi	—
• Medial and lateral pectoral nerves	C5–T1	• Pectoralis major • Pectoralis minor	—
• Medial brachial cutaneous nerve	T1	—	• Medial brachial cutaneous nerve
• Medial antebrachial cutaneous nerve	C8, T1	—	• Medial antebrachial cutaneous nerve
• Intercostobrachial nerves*	T2, T3	—	• Lateral cutaneous branches
Part II: Long branches			
• Musculocutaneous nerve (see p. 366)	C5–C7	• Coracobrachialis • Biceps brachii • Brachialis	• Lateral antebrachial cutaneous nerve
• Axillary nerve (see p. 366)	C5, C6	• Deltoid • Teres minor	• Superior lateral brachial cutaneous nerve
• Radial nerve (see p. 368)	C5–T1	• Brachialis (contribution) • Triceps brachii • Anconeus • Supinator • Brachioradialis • Extensor carpi radialis longus • Extensor carpi radialis brevis • Extensor digitorum • Extensor digiti minimi • Extensor carpi ulnaris • Extensor pollicis longus • Extensor pollicis brevis • Extensor indicis • Abductor pollicis longus	• Inferior lateral brachial cutaneous nerve • Posterior brachial cutaneous nerve • Posterior antebrachial cutaneous nerve • Superficial branch of radial nerve
• Median nerve (see p. 372)	C6–T1	• Pronator teres • Pronator quadratus • Palmaris longus • Flexor carpi radialis • Flexor pollicis longus • Flexor digitorum profundus (half) • Flexor digitorum superficialis • Abductor pollicis brevis • Opponens pollicis • Flexor pollicis brevis (superficial head) • First and second lumbricals	• Palmar branch of median nerve • Common and proper palmar digital nerves
• Ulnar nerve (see p. 370)	C8, T1	• Flexor carpi ulnaris • Flexor digitorum profundus (half) • Palmaris brevis • Flexor digiti minimi • Abductor digiti minimi • Opponens digiti minimi • Adductor pollicis • Flexor pollicis brevis (deep head) • Palmar and dorsal interosseous muscles • Third and fourth lumbricals	• Palmar branch of ulnar nerve • Dorsal branch of ulnar nerve • Dorsal digital nerves • Common and proper palmar digital nerves

* These are the cutaneous branches of the intercostal nerves 2 and 3, which accompany the medial brachial cutaneous nerve.

B Sensory distribution of the medial brachial cutaneous nerve and medial antebrachial cutaneous nerve of the right arm
a Anterior view, **b** posterior view.

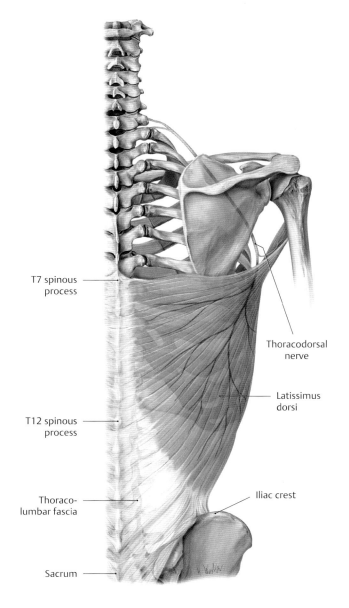

T7 spinous process

Thoracodorsal nerve

T12 spinous process

Latissimus dorsi

Thoraco-lumbar fascia

Iliac crest

Sacrum

C The thoracodorsal nerve
Right side, posterior view.

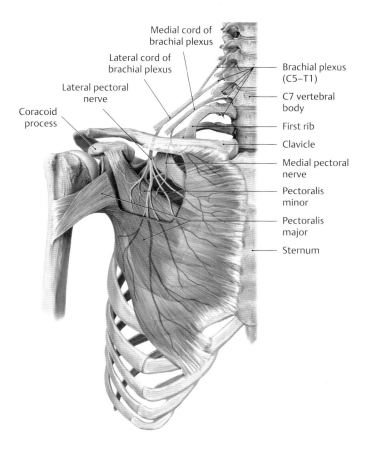

Medial cord of brachial plexus

Lateral cord of brachial plexus

Lateral pectoral nerve

Coracoid process

Brachial plexus (C5–T1)

C7 vertebral body

First rib

Clavicle

Medial pectoral nerve

Pectoralis minor

Pectoralis major

Sternum

D The medial and lateral pectoral nerves
Right side, anterior view.

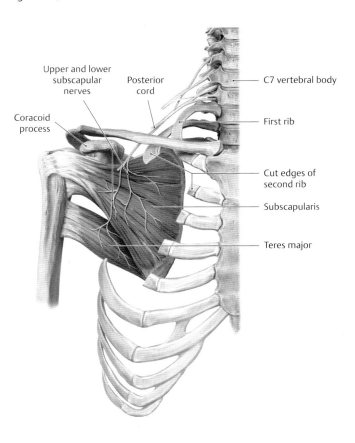

Upper and lower subscapular nerves

Posterior cord

Coracoid process

C7 vertebral body

First rib

Cut edges of second rib

Subscapularis

Teres major

F The upper and lower subscapular nerves
Right side, anterior view. The ribs have been partially removed.

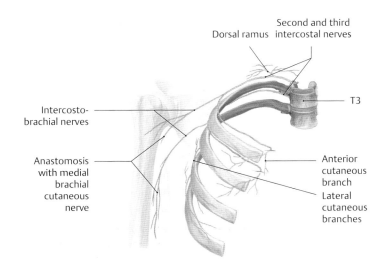

Second and third intercostal nerves

Dorsal ramus

Intercosto-brachial nerves

Anastomosis with medial brachial cutaneous nerve

T3

Anterior cutaneous branch

Lateral cutaneous branches

E Origin and cutaneous distribution of the intercostobrachial nerves of the right arm
Anterior view.

17.7 Infraclavicular Part of the Brachial Plexus: The Musculocutaneous Nerve and Axillary Nerve

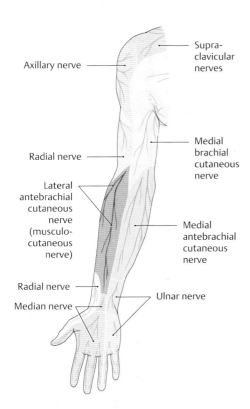

A Sensory distribution of the lateral antebrachial cutaneous nerve
Anterior view.

B Sensory distribution of the lateral antebrachial cutaneous nerve
Posterior view.

C Course of the musculocutaneous nerve after leaving the lateral cord of the brachial plexus
Right upper limb, anterior view. The musculocutaneous nerve leaves the lateral cord of the brachial plexus as a mixed nerve (one with motor and sensory branches) at the level of the lateral border of the pectoralis minor (not shown here) and runs a short course before piercing the coracobrachialis. It then runs between the biceps brachii and brachialis muscles to the elbow, where its terminal sensory branch supplies the skin on the radial side of the forearm.

D The musculocutaneous nerve (C 5–C 7)

Motor branches
• Muscular branches
– Coracobrachialis
– Biceps brachii
– Brachialis

Sensory branches
• Lateral antebrachial cutaneous nerve
• Articular branches (anterior part of the joint capsule of the elbow)

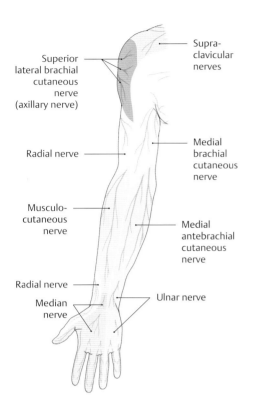

E Sensory distribution of the superior lateral brachial cutaneous nerve
Anterior view.

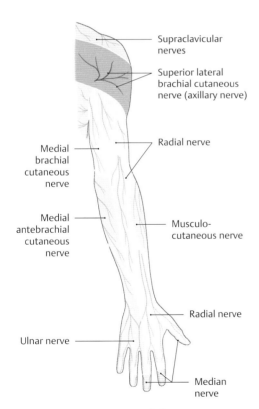

F Sensory distribution of the superior lateral brachial cutaneous nerve
Posterior view.

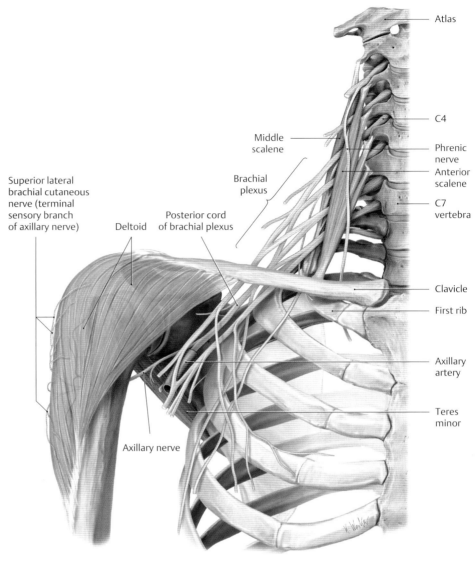

G Course of the axillary nerve after leaving the posterior cord of the brachial plexus

Right upper limb, anterior view. The axillary nerve leaves the posterior cord of the brachial plexus as a mixed nerve and runs backward through the deep part of the axilla, passing directly below the shoulder joint. It courses through the quadrangular space of the axilla (with the posterior circumflex humeral artery) and along the surgical neck to the posterior side of the proximal humerus. Its terminal sensory branch supplies the skin over the deltoid muscle. Isolated *axillary nerve palsy* may occur following an anteroinferior shoulder dislocation (or a traumatic reduction attempt), a humeral fracture at the level of the surgical neck, or prolonged pressure from an improperly adjusted crutch in the axilla.

H The axillary nerve (C 5 and C 6)

Motor branches

- Muscular branches
  - Deltoid
  - Teres minor

Sensory branch

- Superior lateral brachial cutaneous nerve

367

17.8 Infraclavicular Part of the Brachial Plexus: The Radial Nerve

A The radial nerve (C5–T1)

Motor branches

- Muscular branches (from the radial nerve)
  - Brachialis (contribution)
  - Triceps brachii
  - Anconeus
  - Brachioradialis
  - Extensor carpi radialis longus
  - Extensor carpi radialis brevis
- Deep branch (terminal branch: posterior interosseous nerve)
  - Supinator
  - Extensor digitorum
  - Extensor digiti minimi
  - Extensor carpi ulnaris
  - Extensor pollicis longus
  - Extensor pollicis brevis
  - Extensor indicis
  - Abductor pollicis longus

Sensory branches

- Articular branches (from the radial nerve)
  - Capsule of the shoulder joint
- Articular branches (from the posterior interosseous nerve)
  - Joint capsule of the wrist and the four radial metacarpophalangeal joints
- Posterior brachial cutaneous nerve
- Inferior lateral brachial cutaneous nerve
- Posterior antebrachial cutaneous nerve
- Superficial branches
  - Dorsal digital nerves
  - Ulnar communicating branch

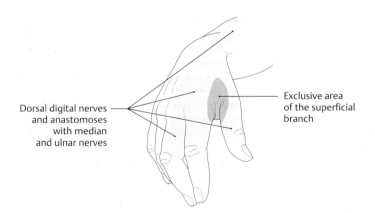

Dorsal digital nerves and anastomoses with median and ulnar nerves

Exclusive area of the superficial branch

C Wrist drop due to proximal and midlevel radial nerve lesions

When the radial nerve is damaged, the patient can no longer actively extend the hand at the wrist, and *wrist drop* (drop hand) is said to be present. Besides the dropped position of the wrist, clinical examination reveals areas of sensory loss on the radial surface of the dorsum and on the extensor surface of the thumb, index finger, and the radial half of the middle finger extending to the proximal interphalangeal joint. The sensory deficits are often confined to the area of the hand that receives sensory innervation exclusively from the radial nerve (the interosseous space between the thumb and index finger).

B Traumatic lesions and compression syndromes involving the radial nerve

The radial nerve may be damaged anywhere in its course as a result of injury or chronic compression. The clinical features depend critically on the *site of the lesion*. As a general rule, the more proximal the site of the lesion, the greater the number of extensor muscles that are affected. The characteristic feature of a proximal ("high") radial nerve lesion is *wrist drop* (see **C**), in which the patient is unable to extend the wrist or the metacarpophalangeal joints. Lesions at some sites may additionally cause sensory disturbances (pain, paresthesia, numbness), particularly in the exclusive sensory territory of the superficial branch on the radial side of the dorsum (first interosseous space between the thumb and index finger).

Proximal radial nerve lesion

- Chronic pressure in the axilla (e.g., due to prolonged crutch use).
  Clinical features: typical dropped wrist with loss of the triceps brachii (and sensory disturbances).
- Traumatic lesion due to a humeral shaft fracture at the level of the radial groove (spiral canal).
  Clinical features: usually a typical dropped wrist *without involvement of the triceps brachii*, since the muscular branches that supply the triceps brachii leave the radial nerve just before it enters the radial groove (sensory disturbances are present, however).
- Chronic compression of the radial nerve against the bony floor of the radial groove (e.g., during sleep or due to improper positioning of the patient during general anesthesia, exuberant callus formation after a fracture, or a tendon expansion from the lateral head of the triceps brachii). "Park bench palsy" is a common form caused by draping the arm over the back of a park bench.
  Clinical features: dropped wrist *without involvement of the triceps brachii.* Sensory disturbances are present. The prognosis is usually favorable, and the palsy should resolve in a few days.

Midlevel radial nerve lesion

- Chronic compression of the radial nerve in its passage through the lateral intermuscular septum and in the radial tunnel (e.g., by bridging vessels and connective-tissue septa).
  Clinical features: dropped wrist with sensory disturbances.

Distal radial nerve lesion

- Compression of the deep branch of the radial nerve at its entry into the supinator canal by a sharp-edged tendon of the superficial part of the supinator muscle: supinator syndrome or distal radial nerve compression syndrome.
  Clinical features: no typical wrist drop and no sensory disturbances involving the hand (before entering the supinator canal, the deep branch gives off the purely sensory superficial branch and muscular branches for the supinator, brachioradialis, and extensor carpi radialis longus and brevis). There are palsies involving the extensor pollicis brevis and longus, abductor pollicis longus, extensor digitorum, extensor indicis, and extensor carpi ulnaris.
- Trauma to the deep radial nerve branch caused by a fracture or dislocation of the radius.
  Clinical features: no wrist drop and no sensory disturbances.

Phrenic nerve

Anterior scalene

Posterior cord of brachial plexus

Axillary artery

Radial nerve

Posterior brachial cutaneous nerve

Radial nerve in radial groove

Inferior lateral brachial cutaneous nerve

Triceps brachii

Radial tunnel

Medial epicondyle

Brachialis

Deep branch of radial nerve in supinator canal

Posterior antebrachial cutaneous nerve

Supinator

Brachioradialis

Posterior interosseous nerve

Superficial branch of radial nerve

Radialis muscle group

Abductor pollicis longus

Extensor digitorum

Extensor pollicis brevis

Extensor pollicis longus

Dorsal digital nerves

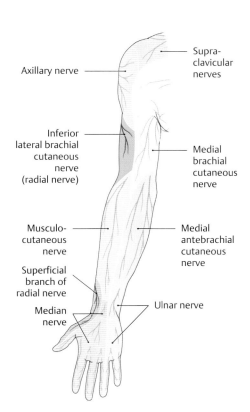

Axillary nerve

Supra-clavicular nerves

Inferior lateral brachial cutaneous nerve (radial nerve)

Medial brachial cutaneous nerve

Musculo-cutaneous nerve

Medial antebrachial cutaneous nerve

Superficial branch of radial nerve

Median nerve

Ulnar nerve

D Sensory distribution of the radial nerve
Anterior view.

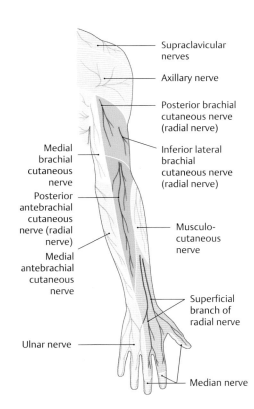

Supraclavicular nerves

Axillary nerve

Posterior brachial cutaneous nerve (radial nerve)

Inferior lateral brachial cutaneous nerve (radial nerve)

Medial brachial cutaneous nerve

Posterior antebrachial cutaneous nerve (radial nerve)

Medial antebrachial cutaneous nerve

Musculo-cutaneous nerve

Superficial branch of radial nerve

Ulnar nerve

Median nerve

E Sensory distribution of the radial nerve
Posterior view.

F Course of the radial nerve after leaving the posterior cord of the brachial plexus

Right upper limb, anterior view with the forearm pronated. The radial nerve is the direct continuation of the posterior cord of the brachial plexus. It winds around the back of the humerus in the radial groove, accompanied by the deep artery of the arm. After piercing the lateral intermuscular septum (not shown here) approximately 10 cm proximal to the radial epicondyle of the humerus, the radial nerve runs distally between the brachioradialis and brachialis muscles (*radial tunnel*, see p. 392) to the elbow, where it divides into a deep branch and a superficial branch. The deep branch passes between the superficial and deep parts of the supinator muscle (*supinator canal*) and continues to the wrist as the posterior (antebrachial) interosseous nerve. The superficial branch accompanies the radial artery down the forearm along the brachioradialis, passes to the extensor side between the radius and brachioradialis in the lower third of the forearm, and terminates as a main sensory branch on the radial dorsum of the hand and the dorsal margins of the radial 2½ digits (the thumb, index finger, and radial half of the middle finger).

369

17.9 Infraclavicular Part of the Brachial Plexus: The Ulnar Nerve

A The ulnar nerve (C8, T1)

Motor branches

- Muscular branches (directly from the ulnar half)
  - Flexor carpi ulnaris
  - Flexor digitorum profundus (ulnar half)
- Muscular branch (from the superficial ulnar nerve branch)
  - Palmaris brevis
- Muscular branches (from the deep ulnar nerve branch)
  - Abductor digiti minimi
  - Flexor digiti minimi
  - Opponens digiti minimi
  - Third and fourth lumbricals
  - Palmar and dorsal interosseous muscles
  - Adductor pollicis
  - Flexor pollicis brevis (deep head)

Sensory branches

- Articular branches
  - Capsule of the elbow joint and of the carpal and metacarpophalangeal joints
- Dorsal branch of the ulnar nerve (terminal branches: dorsal digital nerves)
- Palmar branch of the ulnar nerve
- Proper palmar digital nerve (from the superficial branch)
- Common palmar digital nerve (from the superficial branch; terminal branches: proper palmar digital nerves)

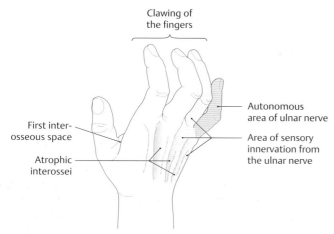

Clawing of the fingers

First interosseous space

Atrophic interossei

Autonomous area of ulnar nerve

Area of sensory innervation from the ulnar nerve

C Claw hand due to an ulnar nerve lesion

Besides the typical clawlike appearance of the hand, atrophy of the interossei leads to hollowing of the interosseous spaces in the metacarpus. Sensory abnormalities are frequently confined to the little finger (exclusive sensory territory of the ulnar nerve).

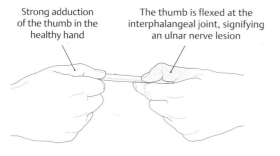

Strong adduction of the thumb in the healthy hand

The thumb is flexed at the interphalangeal joint, signifying an ulnar nerve lesion

B Traumatic lesions and compression syndromes involving the ulnar nerve

Ulnar nerve palsy is the *most common peripheral nerve paralysis*. The characteristic feature of an ulnar nerve lesion is a *"claw hand"* deformity (see **C**), in which *loss of the interosseous muscles* causes the fingers to be hyperextended at the metacarpophalangeal joints and slightly flexed at the proximal and distal interphalangeal joints. The deformity is least pronounced in the index and middle fingers because the first and second lumbrical muscles, which are innervated by the median nerve, can partially compensate for the clawing of those fingers. The thumb is markedly hyperextended due to the loss of the adductor pollicis and the dominance of the extensor pollicis longus and abductor pollicis. The interossei muscles atrophy in 2 to 3 months; this is most conspicuous in the first interosseous space and is accompanied by hypothenar atrophy. Sensory disturbances affect the ulnar portion of the hand, the ulnar half of the ring finger, and the entire little finger.

Proximal ulnar nerve lesion

- Traumatic lesions, usually occurring at the elbow joint due to the exposed position of the nerve in the ulnar groove (e.g., pressure from resting on the arm), displacement of the nerve from its groove, or articular injuries due to fractures.
- Chronic pressure on the nerve in the ulnar groove due to degenerative or inflammatory changes in the elbow joint, or chronic traction on the nerve caused by repetitive flexion and extension at the elbow joint (sulcus ulnaris syndrome).
- Possible compression between the tendons of origin of the flexor carpi ulnaris (cubital tunnel syndrome).
  Clinical features: claw hand and sensory disturbances.

Midlevel ulnar nerve lesion

- Traumatic lesions at the wrist (e.g., lacerations).
- Chronic compression of the nerve in the ulnar tunnel, a fibro-osseous canal between the palmar carpal ligament, pisiform bone, and flexor retinaculum (ulnar tunnel syndrome, see p. 405).
  Clinical features: claw hand and sensory disturbances that spare the hypothenar region (palmar branch is intact).

Distal ulnar nerve lesion

- Compression of the deep branch of the ulnar nerve in the palm due to chronic pressure (e.g., from an air hammer or other tools).
  Clinical features: claw hand with no sensory disturbances (superficial branch is intact).

D Positive "Froment sign" in the left hand

A positive Froment sign indicates palsy of the adductor pollicis muscle. When the patient is told to hold a piece of paper firmly between the thumb and index finger, he or she must use the flexor pollicis longus, which is innervated by the *median nerve*, rather than the paralyzed adductor pollicis, which is innervated by the *ulnar nerve*. Flexing the thumb at the interphalangeal joint signifies a positive test.

E Sensory distribution of the ulnar nerve
Anterior view.

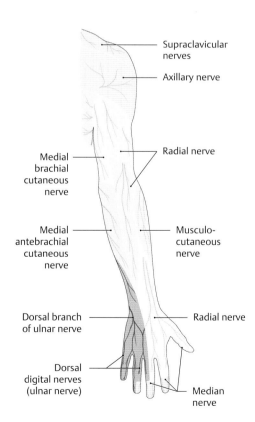

F Sensory distribution of the ulnar nerve
Posterior view.

G Course of the ulnar nerve from the brachial plexus

Right upper limb, anterior view. The ulnar nerve leaves the axilla as the continuation of the medial cord of the brachial plexus, initially descending in the medial bicipital groove. Halfway down the arm it crosses to the extensor side, piercing the medial intermuscular septum (see p. 386). It reaches the elbow joint between the septum and the medial head of the triceps and crosses over the joint on the medial side below the medial epicondyle, embedded in the bony ulnar groove. The nerve then passes to the flexor side of the forearm between the two heads of the flexor carpi ulnaris and runs beneath that muscle to the wrist. In the hand, the ulnar nerve runs on the flexor retinaculum radial to the pisiform bone, passing through the ulnar tunnel (see p. 405) to the palmar surface, where it divides into a superficial branch and a deep motor branch.

371

17.10 Infraclavicular Part of the Brachial Plexus: The Median Nerve

A The median nerve (C6–T1)

Motor branches

- Muscular branches (directly from the median nerve)
  - Pronator teres
  - Flexor carpi radialis
  - Palmaris longus
  - Flexor digitorum superficialis
- Muscular branches (from the anterior antebrachial interosseous nerve)
  - Pronator quadratus
  - Flexor pollicis longus
  - Flexor digitorum profundus (radial half)
- Thenar muscular branch ("thenar branch")
  - Abductor pollicis brevis
  - Flexor pollicis brevis (superficial head)
  - Opponens pollicis
- Muscular branches (from the common palmar digital nerves)
  - First and second lumbricals

Sensory branches

- Articular branches
  - Capsules of the elbow joint and wrist joints
- Palmar branch of median nerve (thenar eminence)
- Communicating branch to ulnar nerve
- Common palmar digital nerves
- Proper palmar digital nerves (fingers)

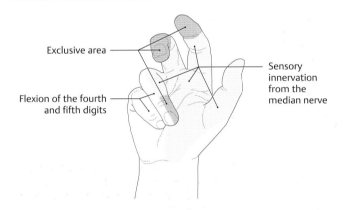

C "Hand of benediction" following a proximal median nerve lesion

When patients try to make a fist, they can flex only the ulnar fingers. This is the "hand of benediction" deformity. There may be associated sensory disturbances, particularly in the autonomous area of the nerve (tips of the radial 3½ digits).

In a healthy hand, the thumb can be abducted to fully grasp a cylindrical object

With a proximal median nerve lesion, the thumb cannot be fully abducted

B Traumatic lesions and compression syndromes involving the median nerve

Median nerve lesions in the arm caused by an acute injury or chronic pressure are among the most common peripheral nerve lesions. The clinical manifestations depend on the *site of the lesion*. The two main categories are proximal and distal nerve lesions, as illustrated by the *pronator teres syndrome* and the *carpal tunnel syndrome*. The hallmark of a proximal median nerve lesion is the "*hand of benediction*," which occurs when the patient tries to clench the hand into a fist (loss of the long digital flexors except for the part of the flexor digitorum profundus supplied by the ulnar nerve). This contrasts with distal median nerve lesions, which present selectively with thenar atrophy and sensory disturbances, as in carpal tunnel syndrome.

Proximal median nerve lesion

- Traumatic injury caused by a fracture or dislocation of the elbow joint.
- Chronic pressure injury from an anomalous supracondylar process connected to the medial epicondyle by a ligament ("Struthers' ligament," see p. 393), pressure from a tight bicipital aponeurosis, or a *pronator teres syndrome* in which the nerve is squeezed between the two heads of the pronator teres.
  Clinical features: Typical "hand of benediction" when fist closure is attempted, with incomplete pronation, loss of thumb opposition, impaired grasping ability, atrophy of the thenar muscles, and sensory disturbances affecting the radial part of the palm and radial 3½ digits (also autonomic trophic disturbances, such as decreased sweat secretion and increased cutaneous blood flow). The patient also has a positive "*bottle sign*" in which the fingers and thumb cannot fully close around a cylindrical object due to weakness of the abductor pollicis brevis.

Distal median nerve lesion

- The superficial location of the nerve in the distal forearm makes it vulnerable to cuts and lacerations (e.g., in attempted suicide).
- Chronic compression of the median nerve in the carpal tunnel (most common compression syndrome affecting the median nerve: carpal tunnel syndrome). Compression or entrapment of the nerve within the carpal tunnel can have various causes, such as fractures and dislocations of the carpal bones, inflammatory changes in the tendon sheaths, muscle variants (e.g., lumbricals passing through the carpal tunnel), and connective = tissue proliferation due to endocrine hormonal changes (diabetes mellitus, pregnancy, menopause).
  Clinical features: oath hand is not present. Initial signs consist of sensory disturbances (paresthesias and dysesthesias), chiefly affecting the tips of the index and middle fingers and thumb due to increased carpal tunnel pressure resulting from prolonged flexion or extension of the wrist during sleep ("brachialgia paraesthetica nocturna"). Chronic or severe damage leads to motor deficits involving the thenar muscles (thenar atrophy) with preservation of thenar sensation (intact palmar branch of the median nerve) and a positive bottle sign (see **D**). ·

D Positive "bottle sign" in the right hand

When proximal and distal median nerve lesions are present, the thumb and fingers cannot completely encircle a cylindrical vessel with the affected hand due to weakness or loss of the abductor pollicis brevis.

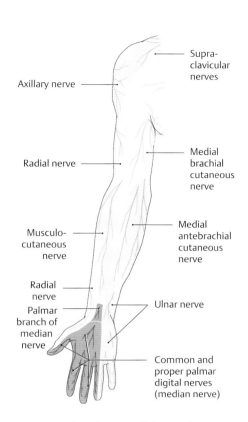

E Sensory distribution of the median nerve.
Anterior view.

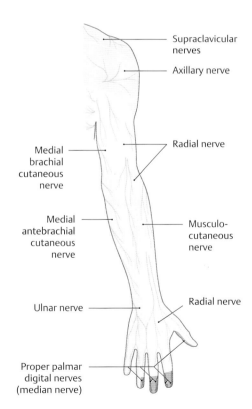

F Sensory distribution of the median nerve
Posterior view.

G Course of the median nerve after the union of its medial and lateral roots from the medial and lateral cords of the brachial plexus

Right upper limb, anterior view. Distal to the union of its brachial plexus roots, the median nerve runs in the medial bicipital groove above the brachial artery to the elbow and passes under the bicipital aponeurosis and between the two heads (humeral and ulnar) of the pronator teres to the forearm. After giving off the anterior antebrachial interosseous nerve distal to the pronator teres, the median nerve runs between the flexor digitorum superficialis and profundus to the wrist and passes beneath the flexor retinaculum (transverse carpal ligament) in the carpal tunnel to the palm of the hand, where it divides into its terminal branches (a motor branch for the thenar muscles and sensory branches for the skin on the palmar side of the radial 3½ digits).

18.1 Surface Anatomy and Superficial Nerves and Vessels: Anterior View

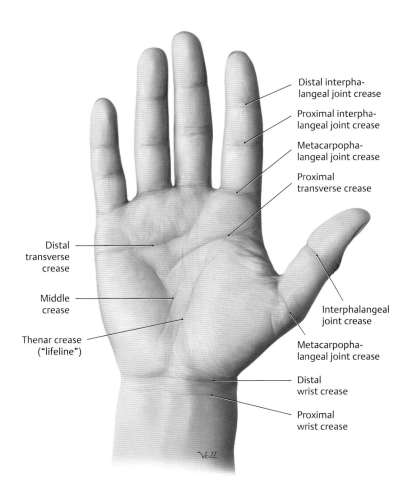

A Surface anatomy of the right upper limb
Anterior view. The palpable bony landmarks of the upper limb are reviewed on p. 239.

B Hand lines and flexion creases on the right palm with the wrist in slight flexion (after Schmidt and Lanz)
The *proximal wrist crease*, located approximately one finger width from the palm, coincides with the distal epiphyseal lines of the radius and ulna. The *distal wrist crease* usually overlies the midcarpal joint.

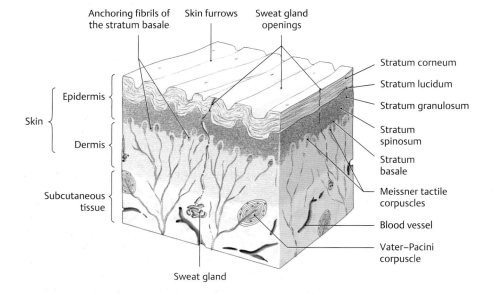

C Schematic structure of the ridged skin on the palm of the hand
The smooth, thin skin of the forearm gives way to the thicker, ridged skin on the palm of the hand. The papillary ridges are particularly high on the palmar skin of the fingers and, at 0.1 to 0.4 mm, are distinctly visible. The ridge pattern (dermatoglyphs) found on the bulbs of the fingers is unique for each individual. The tactile sensitivity of the fingertips is closely linked to the spatial distribution of tactile corpuscles and free nerve endings (e.g., 75–80 Vater–Pacini corpuscles per finger and approximately 100 free nerve endings per square millimeter).

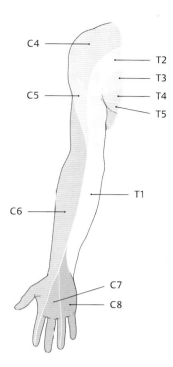

E Radicular (segmental) cutaneous innervation pattern (dermatomes) in the right upper limb
Anterior view. With the outgrowth of the upper limb during development, the sensory cutaneous segments become elongated in varying degrees to form narrow bands. In the process, segments C5–C7 become separated from the body wall.

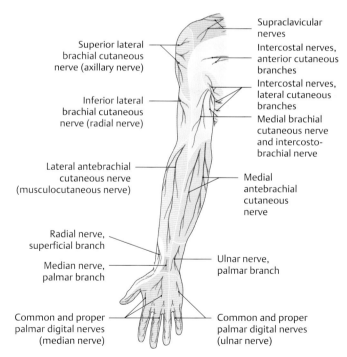

D Superficial cutaneous veins and nerves of the right upper limb
Anterior view. The arrangement of cutaneous veins about the elbow can vary considerably (see p. 356). This dissection does not show the cutaneous arteries that perforate the antebrachial fascia (particularly those arising from the radial artery, see also p. 355).

F Pattern of peripheral sensory cutaneous innervation in the right upper limb
Anterior view. The territories supplied by the peripheral cutaneous nerves (cutaneous branches) correspond to the areas of cutaneous nerve branching in the subcutaneous connective tissue that are demonstrable by dissection. The area served exclusively by a single nerve and thus rendered completely anesthetic by a lesion is much smaller because the individual sensory territories overlap extensively. *Note:* The sensory loss following damage to a *peripheral nerve* shows a completely different pattern than that of a damaged *nerve root*.

18.2 Surface Anatomy and Superficial Nerves and Vessels: Posterior View

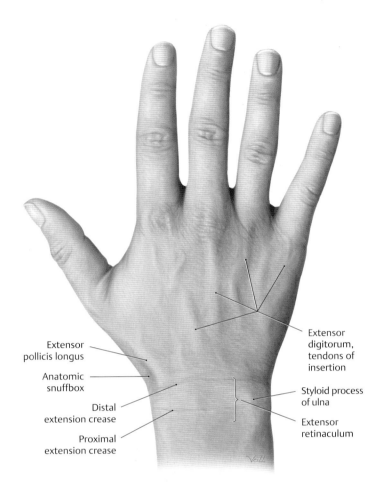

A Surface anatomy of the right upper limb
Posterior view. The palpable bony landmarks of the upper limb are reviewed on p. 239.

B Extension creases on the dorsum of the right hand (after Schmidt and Lanz)
In contrast to the palm, the dorsal surfaces of the hand and fingers bear indistinct extension creases that deepen with maximum dorsiflexion of the hand. The most proximal crease overlies the styloid process of the ulna, while the most distal crease approximately overlies the distal margin of the extensor retinaculum. Unlike the hairless ridged skin of the palm, the dorsum of the hand is covered by smooth, thin, hair-bearing skin.

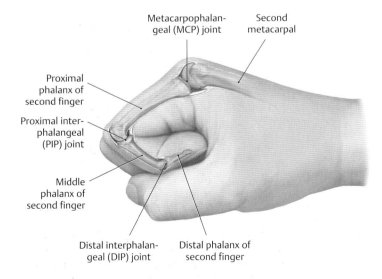

C Location of the MCP, PIP, and DIP joint spaces
Right hand closed into a fist, radial view.

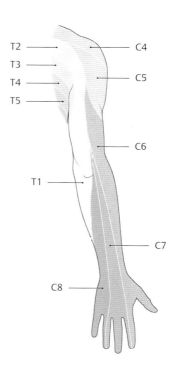

E Radicular (segmental) cutaneous innervation pattern (dermatomes) in the right upper limb
Posterior view. With the outgrowth of the limb during development, the sensory cutaneous segments become elongated in varying degrees to form narrow bands. As this occurs, segments C5–C7 become separated from the body wall.

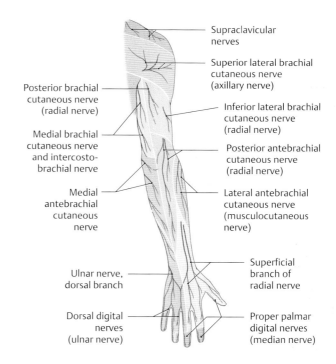

D Superficial cutaneous veins (subcutaneous veins) and cutaneous nerves of the right upper limb
Posterior view. The epifascial veins of the dorsum of the hand (dorsal venous network) display a highly variable branching pattern. Generally, the epifascial veins are clearly visible beneath the skin, receiving tributaries that include perforating veins from the palmar side of the hand. The cephalic vein on the radial side of the hand provides for most of the dorsal venous drainage, while the basilic vein provides for a lesser degree on the ulnar side. This dissection does not show the main branches of the posterior interosseous artery that perforate the antebrachial fascia on the back of the forearm (see also p. 355).

F Peripheral sensory cutaneous innervation pattern in the right upper limb
Posterior view. The color-coded areas that are supplied by the peripheral cutaneous nerves (cutaneous branches) correspond to the areas of cutaneous nerve branching in the subcutaneous connective tissue that are demonstrable by dissection. The areas of exclusive non-overlapping innervation of a specific nerve is much smaller.
Note that the sensory loss following damage to a *peripheral nerve* shows a completely different pattern from that caused by damage to a *nerve root* (see **E**).

377

18.3 The Shoulder Region: Anterior View

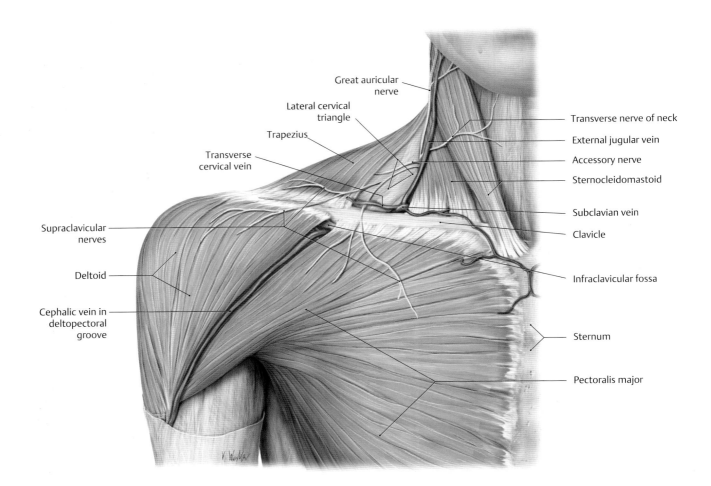

A Superficial veins and nerves of the right shoulder and neck region

Anterior view. The skin, platysma, muscle fasciae, and superficial layer of the cervical fascia have been removed in this dissection to demonstrate the branches of the cervical plexus (e.g., the great auricular nerve) and the superficial veins of the lateral and anterior neck. The *external jugular vein* and *anterior jugular vein* (not shown) are visible through the skin when the patient is lying supine and the veins are well filled. When *right-sided heart failure* is present, these veins may be engorged due to the damming back of venous blood and may be visible even when the patient is sitting upright. The *cephalic vein* crosses the shoulder in the groove between the pectoralis major and deltoid muscles (*deltopectoral groove*) and empties into the axillary vein. This site of entry into the axillary vein, and thus into the deep veins, is visible and palpable on the skin as the infraclavicular fossa. At the level of the lateral border of the first rib, the axillary vein becomes the subclavian vein.

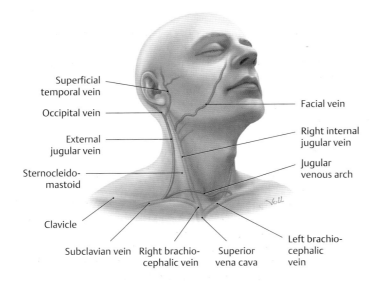

B Relationship of major superficial and deep veins in the neck to the sternocleidomastoid muscle

Anterior view. The internal jugular vein runs almost straight downward from the jugular foramen and unites with the subclavian vein just lateral to the sternoclavicular joint to form the brachiocephalic vein. When its course is projected onto the side of the neck, it follows a line drawn from the earlobe to the medial end of the clavicle. The *internal* jugular vein is crossed obliquely in its lower third by the sternocleidomastoid muscle, while the *external* jugular vein runs obliquely downward on the muscle and opens into the subclavian vein.

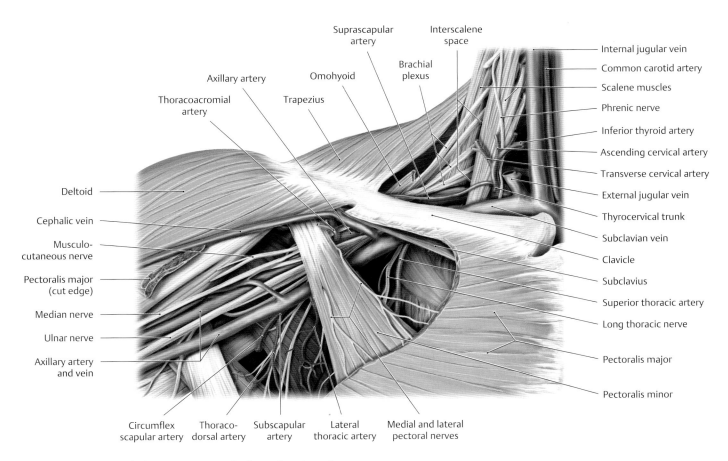

C Course of the right subclavian artery in the lateral neck region
Anterior view. The sternocleidomastoid and omohyoid muscles and all layers of the cervical fasciae have been removed to demonstrate the deep lateral cervical triangle and the passage of the subclavian artery and brachial plexus through the space between the anterior and middle scalene muscles (interscalene space). At the level of the first rib the subclavian artery becomes the axillary artery, which enters the axilla posterior to the tendon of insertion of the pectoralis minor.

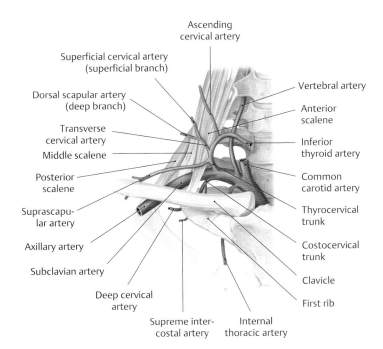

D Origin and branches of the right subclavian artery
Anterior view.

E Branches of the subclavian artery: normal anatomy and variants (after Lippert and Pabst)
a Normally (30% of cases), the subclavian artery gives off the following branches:
  • Thyrocervical trunk with the inferior thyroid artery, suprascapular artery, and transverse cervical artery
  • Vertebral artery
  • Internal thoracic artery
  • Costocervical trunk
b–e Variants:
b The transverse cervical artery arises toparately from the subclavian artery (30%).
c The internal thoracic artery arises from the thyrocervical trunk (10%).
d The thyrocervical trunk is made up of the inferior thyroid artery, suprascapular artery, and internal thoracic artery (8%).
e The subclavian artery gives off two main branches:
  1. One with the inferior thyroid and transverse cervical arteries.
  2. One with the internal thoracic and suprascapular arteries (4%).

379

18.4 The Axilla: Anterior Wall

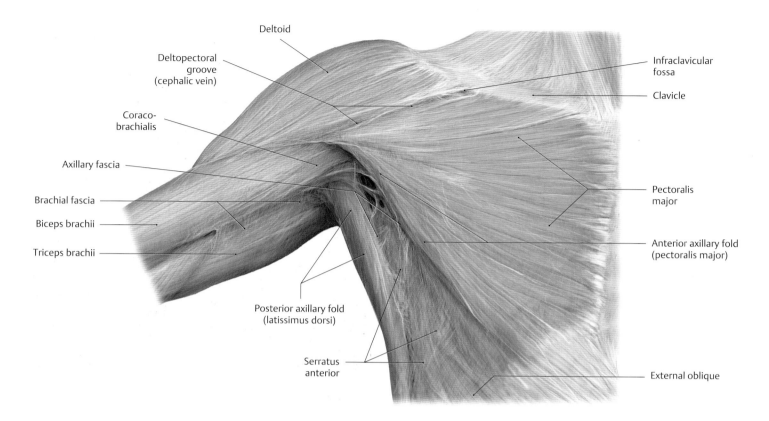

A The walls and fasciae of the right axilla

Anterior view. With the arm abducted, the axilla (axillary fossa) resembles a four-sided pyramid whose apex is approximately at the center of the clavicle and whose base is represented by the axillary *fascia*. The walls of the axilla are formed by various muscles and their fasciae:

Anterior wall: The anterior wall of the axilla consists of the pectoralis major and minor and the clavipectoral fascia (the pectoralis minor is not shown here; see **C** and **D**).

Posterior wall: This consists of the subscapularis, teres major (not shown here, see p. 305), and latissimus dorsi.

Lateral wall: This is narrow and formed by the intertubercular groove of the humerus.

Medial wall: This is formed by the lateral thoracic wall (ribs 1–4 and associated intercostal muscles) and the serratus anterior.

B The clavipectoral triangle and clavipectoral fascia

Right shoulder, anterior view. The clavicular part of the pectoralis major has been removed. In the clavipectoral triangle bounded by the deltoid, pectoralis major, and clavicle, the cephalic vein runs upward in the deltopectoral groove, pierces the clavipectoral fascia, and drains into the axillary vein at the level of the infraclavicular fossa.

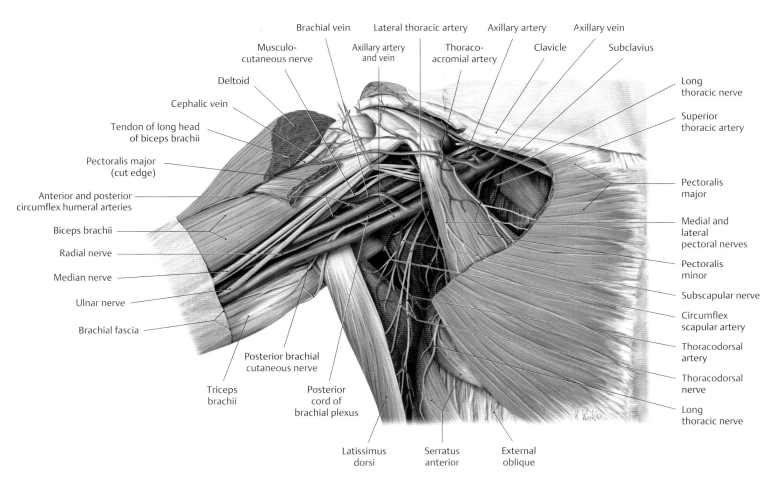

Brachial vein   Lateral thoracic artery   Axillary artery   Axillary vein

Musculo-
cutaneous nerve

Axillary artery
and vein

Thoraco-
acromial artery

Clavicle   Subclavius

Deltoid

Cephalic vein

Long
thoracic nerve

Superior
thoracic artery

Tendon of long head
of biceps brachii

Pectoralis major
(cut edge)

Pectoralis
major

Anterior and posterior
circumflex humeral arteries

Medial and
lateral
pectoral nerves

Biceps brachii

Radial nerve

Pectoralis
minor

Median nerve

Subscapular nerve

Ulnar nerve

Circumflex
scapular artery

Brachial fascia

Thoracodorsal
artery

Posterior brachial
cutaneous nerve

Thoracodorsal
nerve

Triceps
brachii

Posterior
cord of
brachial plexus

Long
thoracic nerve

Latissimus
dorsi

Serratus
anterior

External
oblique

**C The axilla after removal of the pectoralis major and clavipec-
toral fascia**

Right shoulder, anterior view. The axillary artery runs approximately 2
cm below the coracoid process and posterior to the pectoralis minor.

It relates laterally to the lateral cord of the brachial plexus and medially
to the medial cord (both are retracted slightly upward in the drawing).
The posterior cord of the brachial plexus, which runs behind the axillary artery, is just visible.

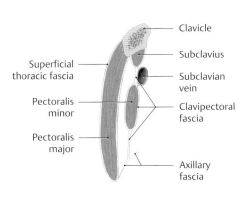

Clavicle

Subclavius

Superficial
thoracic fascia

Subclavian
vein

Pectoralis
minor

Clavipectoral
fascia

Pectoralis
major

Axillary
fascia

**D Location of the superficial and deep
thoracic fasciae**

Sagittal section through the anterior wall of
the right axilla. The clavipectoral fascia, known
also as the "deep" thoracic fascia, encloses
the pectoralis minor and subclavius muscles
and covers the subclavian vein while being
fused to its wall. The fascia is made tense by
the pectoralis minor. The clavipectoral fascia exerts traction on the vein wall that can
keep its lumen patent, thus facilitating venous
return to the superior vena cava.

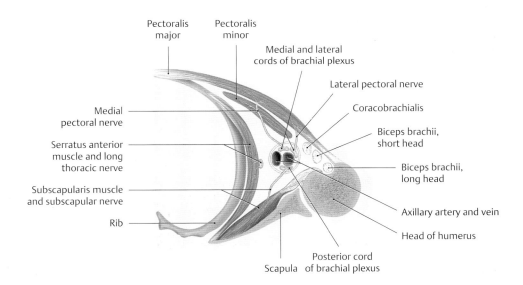

Pectoralis
major

Pectoralis
minor

Medial and lateral
cords of brachial plexus

Lateral pectoral nerve

Medial
pectoral nerve

Coracobrachialis

Serratus anterior
muscle and long
thoracic nerve

Biceps brachii,
short head

Subscapularis muscle
and subscapular nerve

Biceps brachii,
long head

Rib

Axillary artery and vein

Head of humerus

Scapula

Posterior cord
of brachial plexus

**E Schematic transverse section through
the right axilla**

Superior view. The three muscular walls and
the bony lateral wall of the axilla are clearly
delineated in this view. Neurovascular struc-

tures (axillary artery and vein plus the medial,
lateral, and posterior cords of the brachial
plexus) traverse the axilla, invested by a
fibrous sheath and embedded in the axillary
fat.

18.5 The Axilla: Posterior Wall

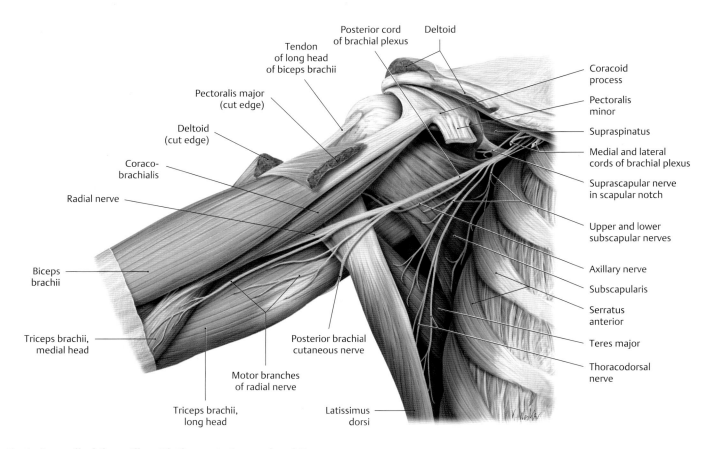

A Posterior wall of the axilla with the posterior cord and its branches

Right shoulder, anterior view. The medial and lateral cords of the brachial plexus and the axillary vessels have been removed to demonstrate the course of the *posterior* cord and its branches in the posterior axilla.

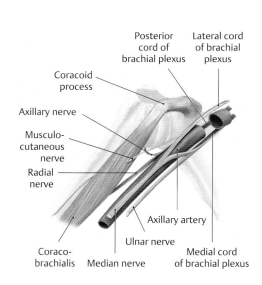

B Relationship of the medial, lateral, and posterior cords of the brachial plexus to the axillary artery

Note that the musculocutaneous nerve passes through the coracobrachialis, which aids in locating the nerve. Very rarely, this nerve may be compressed as it pierces the muscle.

C Origin and branches of the axillary artery

Right shoulder, anterior view.

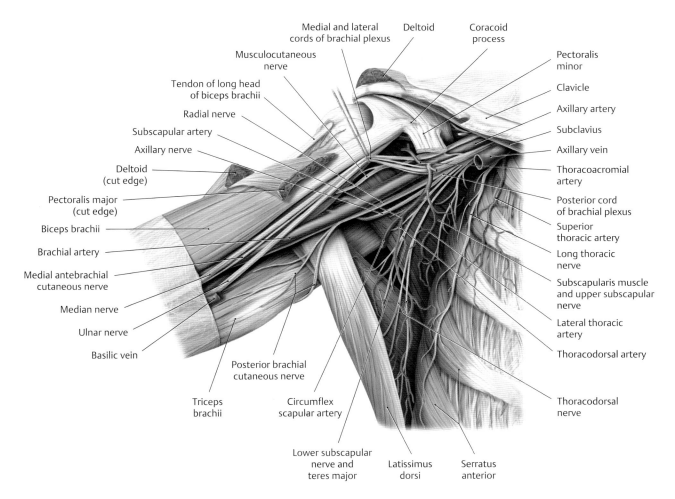

Medial and lateral cords of brachial plexus

Musculocutaneous nerve

Tendon of long head of biceps brachii

Radial nerve

Subscapular artery

Axillary nerve

Deltoid (cut edge)

Pectoralis major (cut edge)

Biceps brachii

Brachial artery

Medial antebrachial cutaneous nerve

Median nerve

Ulnar nerve

Basilic vein

Posterior brachial cutaneous nerve

Triceps brachii

Circumflex scapular artery

Lower subscapular nerve and teres major

Latissimus dorsi

Serratus anterior

Deltoid

Coracoid process

Pectoralis minor

Clavicle

Axillary artery

Subclavius

Axillary vein

Thoracoacromial artery

Posterior cord of brachial plexus

Superior thoracic artery

Long thoracic nerve

Subscapularis muscle and upper subscapular nerve

Lateral thoracic artery

Thoracodorsal artery

Thoracodorsal nerve

D Axilla with the entire anterior wall removed
Right shoulder, anterior view. The axillary vein has been removed, and the medial and lateral cords of the brachial plexus have been retracted upward to show more clearly the location and course of the posterior cord and its terminal branches, the radial nerve and axillary nerve.

Note the superficial course of the long thoracic nerve on the serratus anterior.

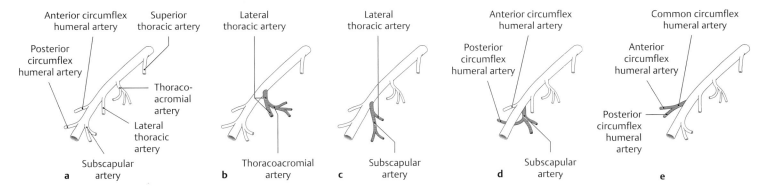

E Branches of the axillary artery: normal anatomy and variants
(after Lippert and Pabst)

a Normally (40% of cases), the axillary artery gives off the following branches:
Superior thoracic artery, thoracoacromial artery, lateral thoracic artery, subscapular artery, anterior circumflex humeral artery, and posterior circumflex humeral artery.

b–e Variants:
b The thoracoacromial artery arises from the lateral thoracic artery (10% of cases).

c Common origin of the lateral thoracic artery and subscapular artery (10% of cases).

d The posterior circumflex humeral artery arises from the subscapular artery (20% of cases).

e Common origin of the anterior and posterior circumflex humeral arteries (20% of cases). The common segment formed by both arteries is termed the common circumflex humeral artery.

18.6 Conduction Anesthesia of the Brachial Plexus: Principle, Pathways, and Administering the Block

A Principle of peripheral conduction anesthesia

Peripheral conduction anesthesia is a regional anesthetic technique that blocks conduction of action potentials. The area under anesthesia is thus distal to the puncture site. It is possible to anesthetize both individual peripheral nerves and the entire plexus.

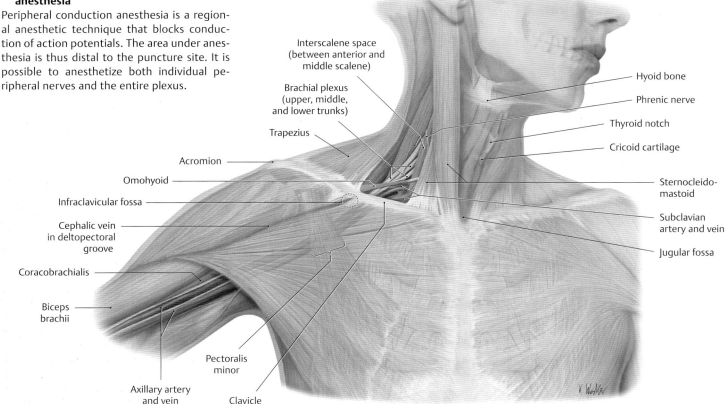

B Topography of the brachial plexus and anatomic landmarks

The brachial plexus is responsible for the motor and sensory nerve supply of the upper limbs. It is formed from the anterior rami of the spinal nerves C5–T1 (see p. 360). In the course of the plexus, first the trunks are formed, followed by the divisions, and then the cords. The trunks are located at the level of the interscalene space. The divisions are above and behind the clav icle. The cords run infraclavicular and start cranial or lateral to the axillary artery and at the level of the axilla, posterior (posterior cord), lateral (lateral cord), and medial (medial cord) to the axillary artery.

Note the important anatomic landmarks for the individual pathways: sternocleidomastoid, cricoid cartilage, thyroid, anterior and middle scalenes (interscalene space), clavicle, acromion, jugular fossa, infraclavicular fossa (Mohrenheim's fossa), coracobrachialis, and axillary artery. In addition, it is recommended to memorize the topographic anatomy in relation to the following structures, which could potentially get damaged: phrenic nerve, recurrent laryngeal nerve, cervical or thoracic and cervical sympathetic ganglia (e.g., stellate ganglion), vertebral artery, cervical epidural and subarachnoid space, and pleural dome.

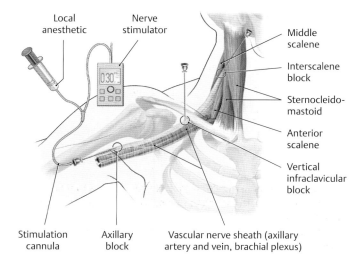

C Brachial plexus sheath and electrical nerve stimulation

From passage through the interscalene space to the axillary region, the entire brachial plexus, together with the accompanying axillary artery and vein, is enclosed by a connective-tissue sheath. Within this sheath, local anesthetic can dissipate more or less evenly, anesthetizing all nerves in this area. In order to target and effectively block one particular nerve, electrical nerve stimulation is performed. A stimulation cannula, only the tip of which is not isolated, emits a defined current pulse. This current pulse can trigger action potentials at the respective motor axons (for more details about the possible responses, see E). With correct positioning of the cannula, ensuing injection of 1 to 2 mL of a suitable local anesthetic should lead to immediate suppression of muscle function (extinction phenomenon).

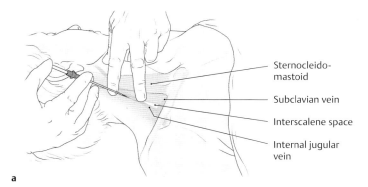

Sternocleidomastoid

Subclavian vein

Interscalene space

Internal jugular vein

a

D Clinically important pathways for brachial plexus block

In order to avoid mechanical lesions, usually the use of an electrical nerve stimulation device (see **C**) and atraumatic needles is recommended. Among common contraindications for all procedures mentioned here are infections of the puncture site and manifest coagulation disorders. Among more specific contraindications are contralateral phrenic nerve paresis and contralateral recurrent nerve paresis.

a Interscalene approach according to Meier: Allows for the most proximal brachial plexus block and thus procedures involving the neck and shoulder. Anatomic landmark is the posterior edge of the sternocleidomastoid at the level of the thyroid notch 2 cm above the cricoid cartilage. Puncture is made from the cranial direction down toward the interscalene space with the needle at 30° to the skin.

b Vertical-infraclavicular block according to Kilka, Geiger, and Mehrkens: Advantage over the axillary block (see below): in addition to blocking the cords, it safely blocks the musculocutaneous nerve. The anatomic landmarks are the anterior edge of the acromion and the center of the jugular fossa. The midpoint of the connecting line between those two points marks the puncture site and the lower edge of the clavicle. For better orientation, the index finger is placed in infraclavicular fossa (Mohrenheim's fossa). Puncture is made from medial of the index finger and strictly vertical to the exam table cover. A medial direction of puncture and puncturing too deep is to be avoided in any case due to the risk of pneumothorax.

c Axillary brachial plexus anesthesia: Most established, technically easiest, and least risky pathway to the brachial plexus. Among the indications are all procedures involving the hand, forearm, and distal upper arm. Anatomic landmark is the axillary artery medial to the coracobrachialis, which is usually easily palpable. Use two fingers to palpate the gap between the axillary artery and coracobrachialis, which is located directly distal to the anterior axillary fold (lateral edge of the pectoralis major). The puncture is made in this gap with the needle being held at a 30 to 45° angle parallel to the artery. After penetrating the vessel nerve sheath, which is felt as a sturdy, elastic resistance, the needle is lowered and advanced tangentially in the proximal direction all the way. By using a nerve stimulation device, the position of the tip of the needle can be optimized. "Problematic nerves" (= those difficult to anesthetize) include the radial nerve, which runs behind the axillary artery, and the musculocutaneous nerve, which has left the vessel nerve sheath significantly more proximal.

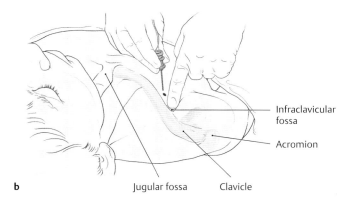

Infraclavicular fossa

Acromion

b Jugular fossa Clavicle

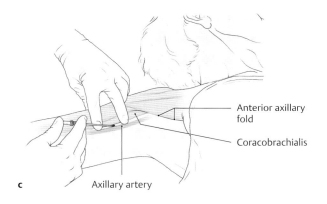

Anterior axillary fold

Coracobrachialis

c Axillary artery

a **b** **c** **d**

E Motor response of individual nerves of the upper limbs following electrical nerve stimulation

a Radial nerve: elbow joint extension (triceps brachii), extension and radial abduction of the wrist, supination of forearm, and finger extension.

b Musculocutaneous nerve: elbow joint flexion (biceps brachii).

c Ulnar nerve: ulnar flexion of the wrist, flexion of the metacarpophalangeal joints II–V.

d Median nerve: flexion and pronation of the wrist, flexion of the phalanges, including the thumb.

18.7 The Anterior Brachial Region

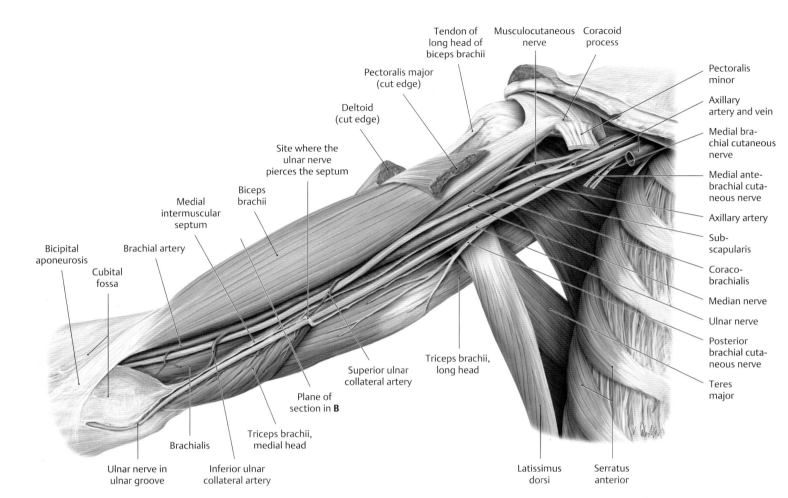

A Main neurovascular tract of the arm: the medial bicipital groove

The right arm has been abducted and slightly rotated externally and is viewed from the anterior view. The deltoid, pectoralis major, and pectoralis minor muscles have been removed. The medial bicipital groove is a subcutaneous longitudinal groove on the medial side of the arm that is bounded deeply by the biceps brachii and brachialis muscles and the medial intermuscular septum of the arm. It marks the location of the main neurovascular tract of the arm extending from the axilla to the cubital fossa. The *most superficial* structure of the tract is the *medial antebrachial cutaneous nerve*, which leaves the medial bicipital groove at the basilic hiatus in company with the basilic vein (see p. 375). The *most medial* structure is the *ulnar nerve*, which initially courses on the medial intermuscular septum. In the lower third of the arm, the ulnar nerve pierces the intermuscular septum and passes to the back of the septum, entering the ulnar groove on the medial epicondyle of the humerus. The *deep part of the medial bicipital groove* transmits the principal artery of the arm, the *brachial artery*, which extends from the axilla to the elbow accompanied by the *median nerve*.

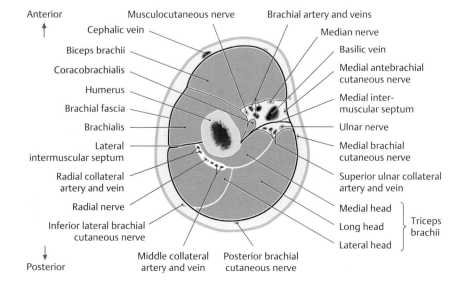

B Cross section through the middle third of the right arm

Distal view.

Note for orientation that the basilic hiatus (where the basilic vein perforates the deep fascia medial to the biceps) is distal to (below) the level of this section. Thus, the basilic vein and medial antebrachial cutaneous nerve are subfascial. The ulnar nerve and ulnar collateral artery have left the medial bicipital groove and have pierced the medial intermuscular septum, and thus lie posterior to it, in this section. Proximal to (above) this level, the artery deep of the arm (deep brachial artery) has split into its two terminal branches, the radial collateral and middle collateral arteries, which are seen here posterior to the humerus.

386

Deltoid branch Acromial branch

Axillary artery

Posterior circumflex humeral artery

Anterior circumflex humeral artery

Subscapular artery

Deep artery of arm

Brachial artery

Radial collateral artery

Middle collateral artery

Radial re-current artery

Radial artery

Posterior inter-osseous artery

Anterior inter-osseous artery

Thoraco-acromial artery

Pectoral branches

Lateral thoracic artery

Circumflex scapular artery

Teres major

Thoracodorsal artery

Superior ulnar collateral artery

Inferior ulnar collateral artery

Medial epicondyle of humerus

Ulnar recurrent artery

Common inter-osseous artery

Ulnar artery

C Course of the brachial artery in the arm

Right arm, anterior view. The brachial artery arises from the axillary artery at the level of the teres major and descends in the medial bicipital groove to the elbow. There it divides into the radial artery and ulnar artery. On its way down the arm, it gives off branches to the arm muscles as well as the deep artery of the arm, which runs on the extensor side of the arm and divides distal to the radial groove into the middle collateral artery (to the medial head of the triceps brachii) and the radial collateral artery (to the arterial network of the elbow). The brachial artery supplies the arterial network of the elbow through the superior and inferior ulnar collateral arteries. It is significant clinically that the brachial artery can be ligated distal to the origin of the profunda brachii with little risk (e.g., to control heavy posttraumatic bleeding) because the arterial network of the elbow (see **C**, p. 393) can establish an adequate collateral circulation. The biceps brachii is a useful landmark for locating the brachial artery, whose pulse is palpable all along the ulnar border of that muscle.

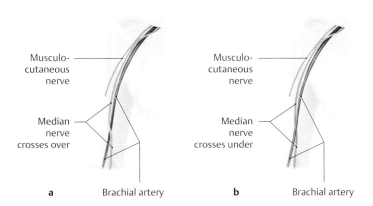

Musculo-cutaneous nerve

Median nerve crosses over

a   Brachial artery

Musculo-cutaneous nerve

Median nerve crosses under

b   Brachial artery

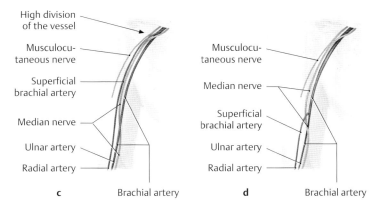

High division of the vessel

Musculocu-taneous nerve

Superficial brachial artery

Median nerve

Ulnar artery

Radial artery

c   Brachial artery

Musculocu-taneous nerve

Median nerve

Superficial brachial artery

Ulnar artery

Radial artery

d   Brachial artery

D Course of the brachial artery in the arm:
normal anatomy and variants (after von Lanz and Wachsmuth)
Right shoulder, anterior view.

a Usually (74% of cases) the median nerve *crosses over* the brachial artery in the lower third of the arm.

b–d Variants:

b The median nerve *crosses under* the brachial artery (very rare, 1% of cases).

c, d The brachial artery divides into a *superficial* brachial artery and a brachial artery while still in the arm ("high division" pattern, 25% of cases). Both of these arteries may be well developed and may flank the union of the median nerve roots and the median nerve itself. In this case the radial artery arises from the superficial brachial artery ("high origin of the radial artery"), while the ulnar artery is the continuation of the brachial artery (see p. 395).

18.8 The Shoulder Region: Posterior and Superior Views

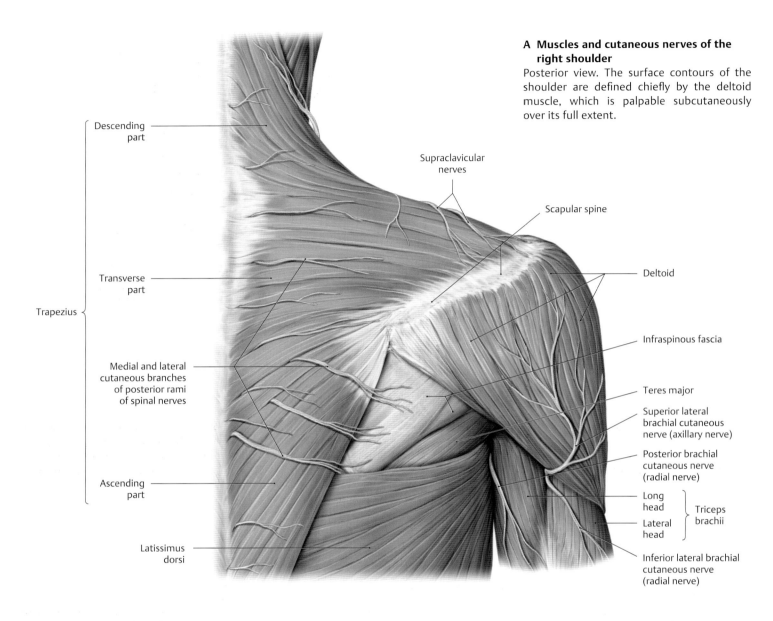

Trapezius
- Descending part
- Transverse part
- Medial and lateral cutaneous branches of posterior rami of spinal nerves
- Ascending part

Latissimus dorsi

Supraclavicular nerves

Scapular spine

Deltoid

Infraspinous fascia

Teres major

Superior lateral brachial cutaneous nerve (axillary nerve)

Posterior brachial cutaneous nerve (radial nerve)

Triceps brachii
- Long head
- Lateral head

Inferior lateral brachial cutaneous nerve (radial nerve)

A Muscles and cutaneous nerves of the right shoulder

Posterior view. The surface contours of the shoulder are defined chiefly by the deltoid muscle, which is palpable subcutaneously over its full extent.

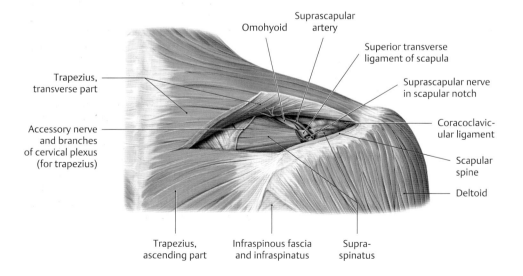

Trapezius, transverse part

Accessory nerve and branches of cervical plexus (for trapezius)

Omohyoid

Suprascapular artery

Superior transverse ligament of scapula

Suprascapular nerve in scapular notch

Coracoclavicular ligament

Scapular spine

Deltoid

Trapezius, ascending part

Infraspinous fascia and infraspinatus

Supraspinatus

B Suprascapular region of the right shoulder from the posterior view

A flap from the transverse part of the trapezius muscle has been raised to reveal the suprascapular region, and the central portion of the supraspinatus has been removed.

Note the course of the suprascapular nerve in its fibro-osseous canal *below* the superior transverse ligament of the scapula in the scapular notch. Compression of this nerve in its canal, especially on extreme external rotation of the shoulder, can lead to paralysis of the supra- and infraspinatus muscles (*scapular notch syndrome*). Ossification of the superior transverse ligament of the scapula creates a scapular foramen that can also cause suprascapular nerve compression (see p. 243).

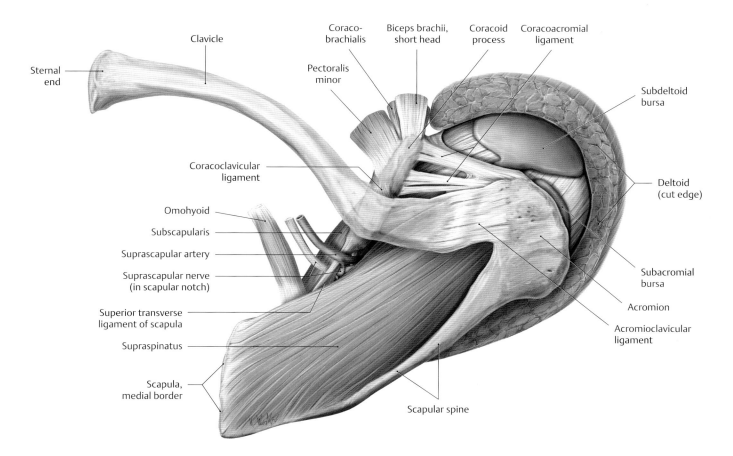

Sternal end — Clavicle
Coraco-brachialis
Biceps brachii, short head
Coracoid process
Coracoacromial ligament
Pectoralis minor
Subdeltoid bursa
Coracoclavicular ligament
Deltoid (cut edge)
Omohyoid
Subscapularis
Suprascapular artery
Suprascapular nerve (in scapular notch)
Subacromial bursa
Superior transverse ligament of scapula
Supraspinatus
Acromion
Acromioclavicular ligament
Scapula, medial border
Supraspinatus
Scapular spine

C Suprascapular region of the right shoulder, viewed from above
The trapezius and deltoid muscles have been removed to demonstrate the *supraspinatus*, which originates in the supraspinous fossa and passes laterally beneath the subacromial bursa in the subacromial space to insert on the greater tubercle. The suprascapular artery and nerve run along the anterior border of the supraspinatus at the level of the superior transverse ligament of the scapula, just lateral to the omohyoid insertion—the artery above the ligament and the nerve below it (see **B** and **D**).

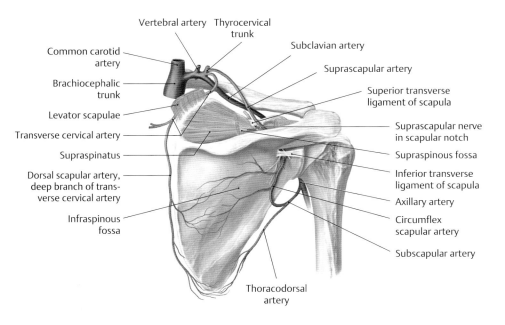

Vertebral artery   Thyrocervical trunk
Subclavian artery
Common carotid artery
Suprascapular artery
Brachiocephalic trunk
Superior transverse ligament of scapula
Levator scapulae
Transverse cervical artery
Suprascapular nerve in scapular notch
Supraspinatus
Supraspinous fossa
Dorsal scapular artery, deep branch of transverse cervical artery
Inferior transverse ligament of scapula
Axillary artery
Infraspinous fossa
Circumflex scapular artery
Subscapular artery
Thoracodorsal artery

D Scapular arcade
Right scapula, posterior view. The suprascapular artery arises from the thyrocervical trunk and passes *over* the *superior* transverse ligament of the scapula to enter the supraspinous fossa. From there it runs past the neck of the scapula, passing *under* the *inferior* transverse ligament of the scapula (often absent), and enters the infraspinous fossa, where it communicates with the circumflex scapular artery (from the subscapular artery) and the deep branch (dorsal scapular artery) of the transverse cervical artery.

Note the anastomosis between the suprascapular artery and the circumflex scapular artery (*scapular arcade*). It is important clinically because it can provide a collateral circulation in response to ligation or occlusion of the axillary artery (see also p. 390).

389

18.9 The Posterior Brachial Region

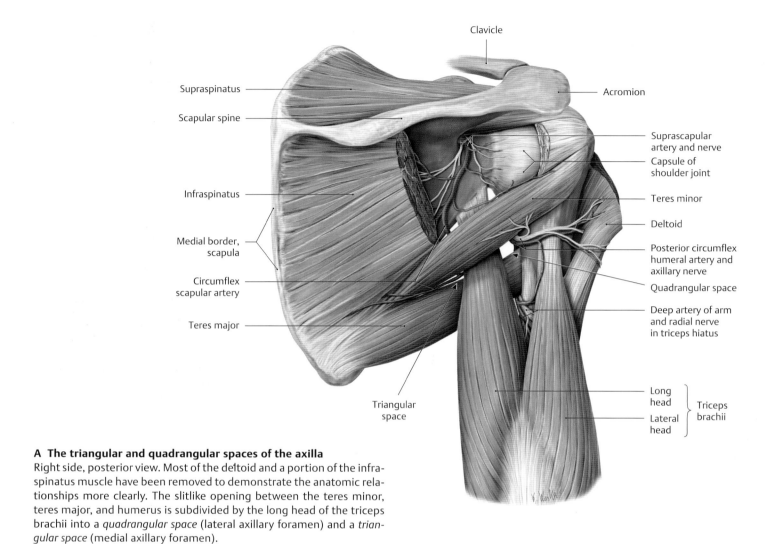

A The triangular and quadrangular spaces of the axilla
Right side, posterior view. Most of the deltoid and a portion of the infraspinatus muscle have been removed to demonstrate the anatomic relationships more clearly. The slitlike opening between the teres minor, teres major, and humerus is subdivided by the long head of the triceps brachii into a *quadrangular space* (lateral axillary foramen) and a *triangular space* (medial axillary foramen).

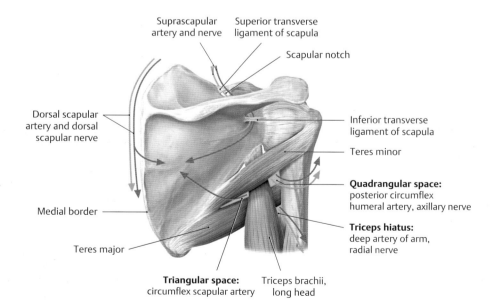

B Neurovascular tracts associated with the scapula
Right side, posterior view. The triangular and quadrangular spaces of the axilla and the triceps hiatus provide important passageways that transmit neurovascular structures from the anterior to the posterior scapular region.

Passageways	Structures transmitted
• Triangular space	Circumflex scapular artery
• Quadrangular space	Posterior circumflex humeral artery and axillary nerve
• Triceps hiatus	Deep artery of arm and radial nerve

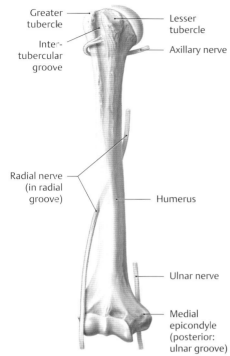

E Nerves that are closely related to the humerus
Right humerus, anterior view.

C Course of the radial nerve in the radial groove

Right shoulder and upper arm, posterior view. The lateral head of the triceps brachii has been divided to show how the radial nerve spirals around the humerus. The dissection shows the bony radial groove between the origins of the medial and lateral heads of the triceps brachii. At the distal end of the groove, the radial nerve passes through the lateral intermuscular septum to the front of the humerus and continues in the radial tunnel to the cubital fossa (not shown here; see also p. 392).

Note that the radial nerve branches for the triceps brachii arise proximal to the radial groove. Thus, the triceps brachii may still be functional after a humeral shaft fracture at the level of the radial groove, even though the radial nerve has been damaged, because the muscular branches to the triceps arise proximal to the site of the lesion.

F Branches of the brachial artery: normal anatomy and variants (after von Lanz and Wachsmuth)

a Typically (77% of cases), the deep artery of the arm and the posterior circumflex humeral artery arise from the brachial artery.

b, c Variants:
b The deep artery of the arm arises from the posterior circumflex humeral artery (7%).
c As in **b**, but the posterior circumflex humeral artery runs through the triceps hiatus rather than the quadrangular space (16%).

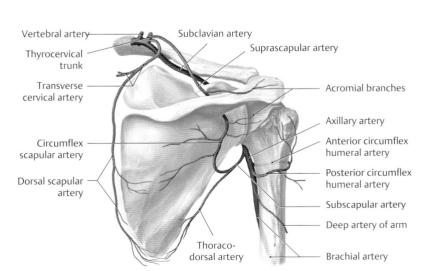

D Arterial supply to the scapular region
Right shoulder, posterior view.

18.10 The Elbow (Cubital Region)

Skin, subcutaneous tissue, and superficial fascia

Medial antebrachial cutaneous nerve

Cephalic vein

Biceps brachii

Brachial vein and artery, median nerve

Brachialis

Brachioradialis

Lateral ante-brachial cutaneous nerve (musculocutaneous nerve)

Tendon of biceps brachii

Perforator vein

Radial artery

Extensor carpi radialis longus

Cephalic vein

Median antebrachial vein

Basilic vein

Biceps brachii fascia

Triceps brachii

Inferior ulnar collateral artery

Superior ulnar collateral artery, ulnar nerve

Medial epicondyle

Pronator teres

Flexor carpi radialis

Palmaris longus

Bicipital aponeurosis

Flexor carpi ulnaris

A Cubital fossa after removal of the fasciae and epifascial neurovascular structures
Right arm, anterior view. The *median nerve* and the *musculocutaneous nerve* with its main branches are clearly visible (variants in the course of the median nerve are shown in **D**). The brachioradialis muscle must be retracted (as in **B**) before the radial nerve can be seen.

Skin, subcutaneous tissue, and superficial fascia

Medial antebrachial cutaneous nerve

Cephalic vein

Brachialis

Radial tunnel

Musculocutaneous nerve

Brachioradialis

Radial nerve {
Muscular branches

Deep branch

Superficial branch
}

Biceps brachii tendon

Radial recurrent artery

Ulnar artery

Radial artery

Supinator

Pronator teres

Basilic vein

Biceps brachii

Brachial artery

Triceps brachii

Median nerve

Superior ulnar collateral artery, ulnar nerve

Medial epicondyle

Median nerve

Pronator teres, humeral head

Pronator teres, ulnar head

Flexor carpi radialis

Palmaris longus

Flexor carpi ulnaris

B Deep dissection of the cubital fossa
Right arm, anterior view. The distal muscle belly of the biceps brachii has been removed, and the muscles of the radialis group (brachioradialis, extensor carpi radialis longus, and extensor carpi radialis brevis) have been pulled aside to better demonstrate the course of the *radial nerve*. After passing through the radial tunnel, the nerve gives off its sensory superficial branch and its muscular branches to the muscles of the radialis group before entering the supinator (see p. 393). Portions of the pronator teres have been retracted medially to demonstrate the course of the median nerve between the two heads of that muscle.

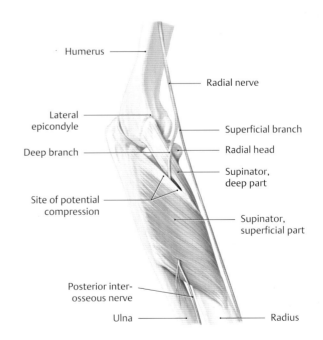

C Arterial anastomoses around the elbow joint: the arterial network of the elbow

Right arm, anterior view. The arterial anastomoses in the elbow region form a vascular network that is fed by several arteries:

- The middle collateral artery and radial collateral artery from the deep artery of the arm (communicate with the radial artery via the radial recurrent artery and interosseous recurrent artery)
- The superior ulnar collateral artery and inferior ulnar collateral artery from the brachial artery (communicate with the ulnar artery via the ulnar recurrent artery)

Because of this arterial network, the brachial artery can be ligated distal to the origin of the deep artery of the arm without compromising the blood supply to the elbow region.

D Relationship of the median nerve to the pronator teres: normal anatomy and variants (after von Lanz and Wachsmuth)

Right arm, anterior view.

a In the great majority of cases (95%) the median nerve runs between the two heads of the pronator teres.

b, c Variants:

b The median nerve pierces the humeral head of the pronator teres (2% of cases).

c The median nerve runs on the bone beneath the ulnar head of the pronator teres (3% of cases).

E Supracondylar process of the humerus

Distal humerus, right arm, anterior view. The *supracondylar process* is an unusual anomaly (0.7% of the population), a bony outgrowth above the medial epicondyle (see p. 214). When present, it can serve as an attachment for a connective tissue band referred to as Struthers' ligament, which ends on the medial epicondyle. The resulting fibro-osseous *supracondylar canal* can entrap and compress the brachial artery and median nerve.

F Relationship of the radial nerve to the supinator

Right elbow region, radial view. Just proximal to the supinator muscle, the radial nerve divides into its deep motor branch and superficial sensory branch. This arrangement can lead to entrapment and compression of the deep motor branch, with resulting selective palsy of the extensor muscles (and abductor pollicis longus) served by this nerve.

393

18.11 The Anterior Forearm Region

Median nerve

Biceps brachii

Brachialis

Biceps brachii tendon

Radial artery

Brachio-radialis

Extensor carpi radialis longus

Extensor carpi radialis brevis

Flexor carpi radialis

Abductor pollicis longus

Radial artery

Flexor pollicis longus

Thenar muscles

Palmar aponeurosis

Inferior ulnar collateral artery

Superior ulnar collateral artery, ulnar nerve

Medial epicondyle

Brachial artery

Pronator teres

Flexor carpi radialis

Bicipital aponeurosis

Palmaris longus

Flexor carpi ulnaris

Flexor digitorum superficialis

Ulnar artery

Median nerve

Ulnar nerve

Hypothenar muscles

A Right forearm, anterior view, superficial layer

The fasciae and superficial neurovascular structures have been removed. Most of the forearm's neurovascular structures are obscured in this view. (The superficial veins are shown in **D**, p. 375.)

Median nerve

Biceps brachii

Brachialis

Brachio-radialis

Radial nerve, superficial branch

Biceps brachii tendon

Common inter-osseous artery

Posterior inter-osseous artery

Anterior inter-osseous artery

Pronator teres

Flexor digitorum superficialis, radial head

Radial artery

Flexor pollicis longus

Abductor pollicis longus

Median nerve

Pronator quadratus

Flexor carpi radialis

Thenar muscles

Palmar branch of median nerve

Superior ulnar collateral artery, ulnar nerve

Inferior ulnar collateral artery

Medial epicondyle

Pronator teres, humeral head

Flexor carpi radialis

Palmaris longus

Pronator teres, ulnar head

Flexor digitorum superficialis, humeroulnar head

Flexor carpi ulnaris

Ulnar artery

Ulnar nerve

Flexor digitorum profundus

Flexor digitorum superficialis tendons

Flexor retinaculum

Hypothenar muscles

B Right forearm, anterior view, deep layer

The pronator teres, flexor digitorum superficialis, palmaris longus, and flexor carpi radialis have been partially removed to demonstrate the median nerve, the superficial branch of the radial nerve, and the radial and ulnar arteries (variants in the course of the arteries are shown in **D**).

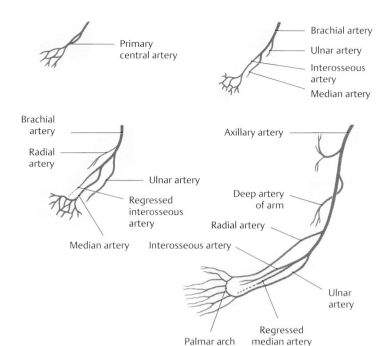

C Development of the arteries of the upper limb (after Stark)

The vascular system in the embryonic arm does not develop directly into the mature anatomy but undergoes several basic changes. The early limb bud is supplied by a central vascular trunk that develops distally into the *common interosseous artery*. As development proceeds, a second longitudinal trunk, called the *median artery*, is formed parallel to the median nerve. That vessel provides most of the blood supply to the forearm and hand, while the interosseous artery regresses. Finally, the initially small muscular branches enlarge on the ulnar and radial sides to form the *ulnar artery* and the *radial artery*, which replace the median artery in primates and assume its functions. The interosseous artery remains the principal vessel of the arm in nonmammals, while the median artery is the dominant vessel in lower mammals. The interosseous and median arteries may persist in humans as well-developed atavistic anomalies (see **D**), providing most of the blood supply to the palm of the hand.

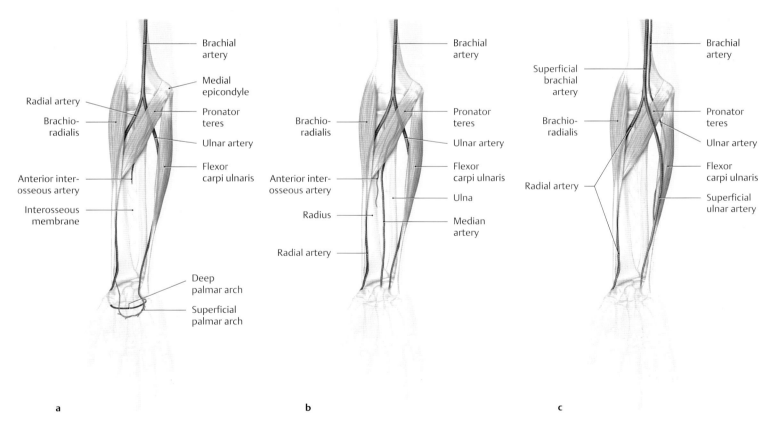

D Arteries of the forearm: normal anatomy and variants
(after Lippert and Pabst)
Right forearm, anterior view.

a Typical arterial anatomy in the forearm (84% of cases).

b, c Variants:

b A persistent median artery is present, often arising from the ulnar artery distal to the origin of the common interosseous artery (8% of cases).

c Accessory superficial arteries are present in the forearm (superficial antebrachial arteries, 8% of cases), such as a superficial ulnar artery arising from a superficial brachial artery, which runs over the surface of the flexor muscles and may unite distally with the ulnar artery. The presence of this vessel is a potential hazard during intravenous injections in the cubital area (see p. 356). Accessory superficial arteries most commonly develop in cases where the brachial artery divides in the arm into a superficial brachial artery (which becomes the radial artery in the forearm) and a brachial artery (which becomes the ulnar artery in the forearm; see "high division" pattern, p. 387).

18.12 The Posterior Forearm Region and the Dorsum of the Hand

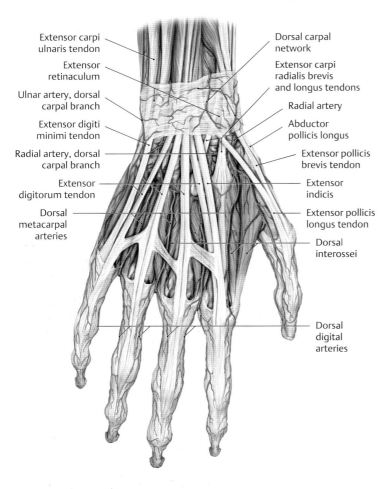

Labels (left figure):
- Extensor carpi ulnaris tendon
- Extensor retinaculum
- Ulnar artery, dorsal carpal branch
- Extensor digiti minimi tendon
- Radial artery, dorsal carpal branch
- Extensor digitorum tendon
- Dorsal metacarpal arteries
- Dorsal carpal network
- Extensor carpi radialis brevis and longus tendons
- Radial artery
- Abductor pollicis longus
- Extensor pollicis brevis tendon
- Extensor indicis
- Extensor pollicis longus tendon
- Dorsal interossei
- Dorsal digital arteries

Labels (right figure):
- Triceps brachii, lateral head
- Olecranon
- Anconeus
- Extensor carpi ulnaris
- Interosseous recurrent artery
- Passage through interosseous membrane
- Posterior interosseous artery
- Extensor carpi ulnaris
- Site where anterior interosseous artery pierces membrane
- Extensor indicis
- Interosseous membrane
- Ulnar artery, dorsal carpal branch
- Extensor retinaculum
- Radial artery, dorsal carpal branch
- Extensor carpi radialis brevis tendon
- Radial collateral artery
- Brachioradialis
- Arterial network of elbow and lateral epicondyle
- Supinator
- Extensor digitorum
- Extensor carpi radialis brevis and longus
- Extensor pollicis longus
- Abductor pollicis longus
- Extensor pollicis brevis
- Extensor carpi radialis longus tendon
- Radial artery
- Extensor pollicis longus tendon

A Arteries of the dorsum of the hand and the extensor sides of the fingers in the right hand

The skin, subcutaneous tissue, and dorsal fascia of the hand have been removed to demonstrate the dorsal arteries (for clarity, the veins and nerves have also been removed). The dorsum of the hand receives most of its blood supply from the radial artery, while the ulnar artery contributes only one small vessel (the dorsal carpal branch). The perforating branches, however, create numerous connections between the palmar and dorsal arteries of the hand. In the fingers, these connections are provided by lateral anastomoses between the dorsal digital arteries and the proper palmar digital arteries (not seen here).

B Deep dissection of the arteries on the extensor side of the forearm and the dorsum of the hand in the right arm

In the elbow region the anconeus muscle has been released from its origin and reflected to the side. The triceps brachii has also been released from its origin at a more proximal level. On the extensor side of the forearm, the extensor carpi ulnaris and extensor digitorum have been partially resected.

Note how the posterior interosseous artery pierces the interosseous membrane just below the lower border of the supinator and enters the extensor compartment of the forearm. In the distal forearm, parts of the extensor pollicis longus and extensor indicis have been removed to demonstrate the site where the anterior interosseous artery pierces the interosseous membrane to reach the back of the forearm. Both arteries are important sources of blood to the extensor compartment.

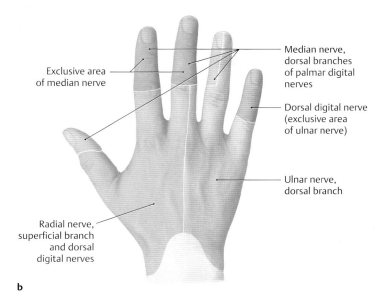

C Nerve supply to the dorsum of the hand

Right hand, posterior view.

a The cutaneous nerves on the dorsum of the hand. *Note* that the index and middle fingers and the radial part of the ring finger are supplied by different nerves in their proximal and distal portions.

- *Distal:* by the dorsal branches of the palmar digital nerves from the *median nerve*.
- *Proximal:* by the dorsal digital nerves from the *radial nerve* (to about the proximal interphalangeal joints of the index and middle fingers) and from the *ulnar nerve* (also to the level of the proximal interphalangeal joints of the middle and ring fingers).

b Exclusive and overlapping areas of sensory innervation on the dorsum of the hand, for ulnar, median, and radial nerves. In lighter shading, areas are indicated that receive sensory innervation mostly from the corresponding nerve. Because the sensory distribution of each nerve in actuality overlaps extensively with the adjacent sensory territories of the other nerves, an isolated nerve lesion does not render its entire territory anesthetic. Instead, extensive or complete loss of sensation is restricted to areas where there is little or no overlap, depicted in heavier shading.

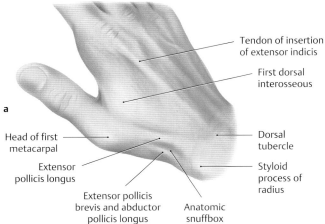

D Boundaries of the anatomic snuffbox

a Surface anatomy of the dorsum of the right hand, posterolateral view.

b Muscles and tendons of the dorsum of the right hand, radial view. The three-sided "anatomic snuffbox" is bounded on the palmar side by the tendons of insertion of the abductor pollicis longus and extensor pollicis brevis and dorsally by the tendon of insertion of the extensor pollicis longus. The floor is formed mostly by the scaphoid and trapezium carpal bones. Fractures of the scaphoid bone are thus often associated with deep tenderness in the snuffbox. The snuffbox is bounded proximally by the extensor retinaculum.

Note that the radial artery runs deep in the snuffbox between the trapezium and scaphoid, providing a landmark for dissection.

397

18.13 The Palm of the Hand: Epifascial Nerves and Vessels

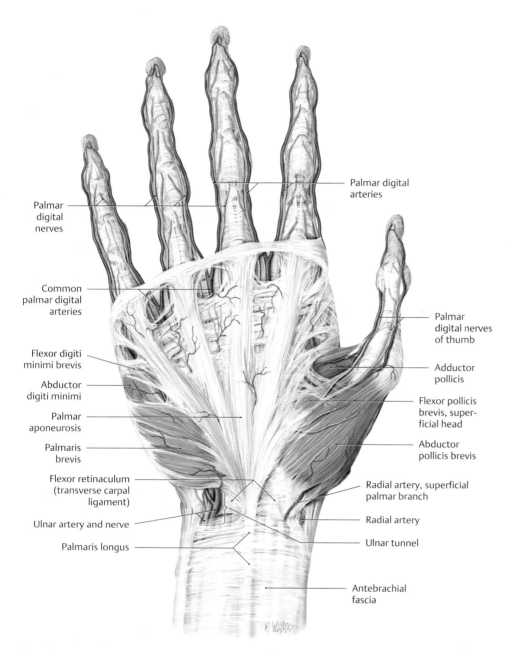

Palmar digital arteries

Palmar digital nerves

Common palmar digital arteries

Flexor digiti minimi brevis

Abductor digiti minimi

Palmar aponeurosis

Palmaris brevis

Flexor retinaculum (transverse carpal ligament)

Ulnar artery and nerve

Palmaris longus

Palmar digital nerves of thumb

Adductor pollicis

Flexor pollicis brevis, superficial head

Abductor pollicis brevis

Radial artery, superficial palmar branch

Radial artery

Ulnar tunnel

Antebrachial fascia

A Superficial arteries and nerves of the palm

Right hand, anterior view. All of the fasciae except the palmar aponeurosis have been removed to demonstrate the superficial neurovascular structures of the palm. The palmar carpal ligament has also been removed to demonstrate the neurovascular structures that pass through the ulnar tunnel (the ulnar artery and nerve; see p. 405).

Note the superficial palmar branch of the radial artery, which is highly variable in its course. In the case shown, it runs between the origins of the abductor and flexor pollicis brevis to the palm of the hand. In approximately 30% of cases it combines with the ulnar artery to form the superficial palmar arch (not shown here; see also p. 400).

Palmar digital nerve with dorsal branch

Metacarpophalangeal joint

Dorsal digital artery

Dorsal digital nerve

Common palmar digital artery

Proper palmar digital artery

Proper palmar digital nerve

B Nerves and vessels of the right middle finger

Lateral view. The arteries of the palm are anterior to the nerves, but they are dorsal to the nerves in the fingers (generally crossing at the level of the metacarpophalangeal joint). The lateral and distal dorsal surfaces of the fingers are supplied by branches of the proper palmar digital nerves (from the median nerve).

C Nerve supply to the palm of the hand
Right hand, anterior view.

a–c Innervation patterns in the palm of the hand (after Schmidt and Lanz). The sensory innervation pattern is marked by the presence of connecting branches between the median nerve and ulnar nerve. The following innervation patterns are most frequently encountered:
a Most commonly (46% of cases) the median nerve and ulnar nerve are interconnected by an ulnar communicating branch.

b Variant 1 (20% of cases): The median nerve and ulnar nerve are cross-connected by an ulnar communicating branch and a median communicating branch.
c Variant 2 (20% of cases): There are no communicating branches between the median and ulnar nerves.
d **Exclusive and overlapping areas of sensory innervation of the hand, palmar view.** Non-overlapping areas of exclusive innervation are indicated by darker shading. Compare with the dorsal aspect (**C**, p. 397).

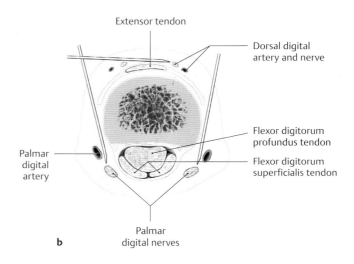

D The Oberst nerve block
Right hand, posterior view. This type of local anesthesia is clinically useful for injuries of the fingers, specifically for wounds that require suturing.

a The injection sites are located in the interdigital folds.
b After the dorsal nerve branches have been numbed, the needle is advanced on both the radial and ulnar sides toward the palmar nerves, and a subcutaneous bolus of 1 to 2 mL of local anesthetic is injected at each site.

E Blood supply to the flexor tendons of the finger within the tendon sheath
(after Lundborg)
Right middle finger, lateral view. The flexor tendons are supplied within their sheath by branches of the palmar digital arteries that are transmitted to the tendons through the mesotendons (vinculum longum and vinculum breve).

399

18.14 The Palm of the Hand: Vascular Supply

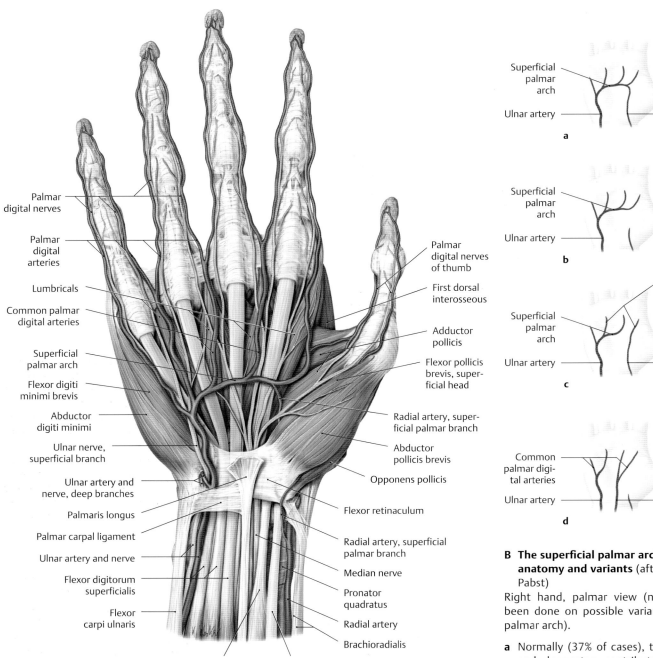

Labels (clockwise from left):
- Palmar digital nerves
- Palmar digital arteries
- Lumbricals
- Common palmar digital arteries
- Superficial palmar arch
- Flexor digiti minimi brevis
- Abductor digiti minimi
- Ulnar nerve, superficial branch
- Ulnar artery and nerve, deep branches
- Palmaris longus
- Palmar carpal ligament
- Ulnar artery and nerve
- Flexor digitorum superficialis
- Flexor carpi ulnaris
- Flexor pollicis longus
- Flexor carpi radialis
- Palmar digital nerves of thumb
- First dorsal interosseous
- Adductor pollicis
- Flexor pollicis brevis, superficial head
- Radial artery, superficial palmar branch
- Abductor pollicis brevis
- Opponens pollicis
- Flexor retinaculum
- Radial artery, superficial palmar branch
- Median nerve
- Pronator quadratus
- Radial artery
- Brachioradialis

A The superficial palmar arch and its branches
Right hand, anterior (palmar) view. The palmar aponeurosis and other fasciae have been removed to demonstrate the *superficial palmar arch* (variants are shown in **B**).

B The superficial palmar arch: normal anatomy and variants (after Lippert and Pabst)
Right hand, palmar view (no studies have been done on possible variants of the *deep* palmar arch).

a Normally (37% of cases), the radial artery and ulnar artery contribute equally to the superficial palmar arch.

b–d Variants:

b The palmar arch arises entirely from the ulnar artery (37% of cases).

c All of the common palmar digital arteries arise from the ulnar artery except for the first, which arises from the radial artery (13%).

d The ulnar artery and a median artery give off the common palmar digital arteries (very rare).

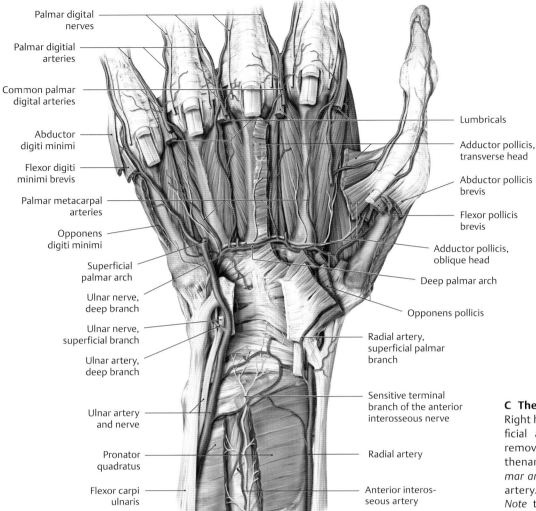

Palmar digital nerves

Palmar digitial arteries

Common palmar digital arteries

Abductor digiti minimi

Flexor digiti minimi brevis

Palmar metacarpal arteries

Opponens digiti minimi

Superficial palmar arch

Ulnar nerve, deep branch

Ulnar nerve, superficial branch

Ulnar artery, deep branch

Ulnar artery and nerve

Pronator quadratus

Flexor carpi ulnaris

Lumbricals

Adductor pollicis, transverse head

Abductor pollicis brevis

Flexor pollicis brevis

Adductor pollicis, oblique head

Deep palmar arch

Opponens pollicis

Radial artery, superficial palmar branch

Sensitive terminal branch of the anterior interosseous nerve

Radial artery

Anterior interosseous artery

C The deep palmar arch and its branches

Right hand, anterior (palmar) view. The superficial and deep flexor tendons have been removed along with the thenar and hypothenar muscles to demonstrate the *deep palmar arch* as the terminal branch of the radial artery.

Note the end branch of the anterior interosseous antebrachial nerve, which extends between the interosseous membrane and pronator quadratus distally and supplies sensory innervation to the capsule of the wrists.

Palmar digital arteries

Common palmar digital arteries

Superficial palmar arch

Palmar carpal branches to the palmar carpal network

Interosseous membrane

Ulnar artery

Common interosseous artery

Proper palmar digital arteries

Perforating branches

Deep palmar arch

Anterior interosseous artery

Radial artery

Posterior interosseous artery

Interosseous recurrent artery

a

Dorsal digital arteries

Perforating branches

Dorsal metacarpal arteries

Ulnar artery, dorsal carpal branch

Posterior interosseous artery

Dorsal carpal artery

Radial artery

Dorsal carpal network

b

D Arterial anastomoses in the hand

The ulnar artery and radial artery are interconnected by the superficial and deep palmar arch, the perforating branches, and the dorsal carpal network.

Palmar

Palmar digital artery

Superficial palmar arch

Deep palmar arch

Palmar carpal network

Radial artery

Dorsal

Dorsal digital artery

Dorsal metacarpal artery

Palmar metacarpal artery

Perforating branch

Dorsal carpal artery

Dorsal carpal network

Posterior interosseous artery

c

a Right hand, anterior (palmar) view.
b Right hand, posterior (dorsal) view.
c Right middle finger, lateral view.

401

18.15 The Carpal Tunnel

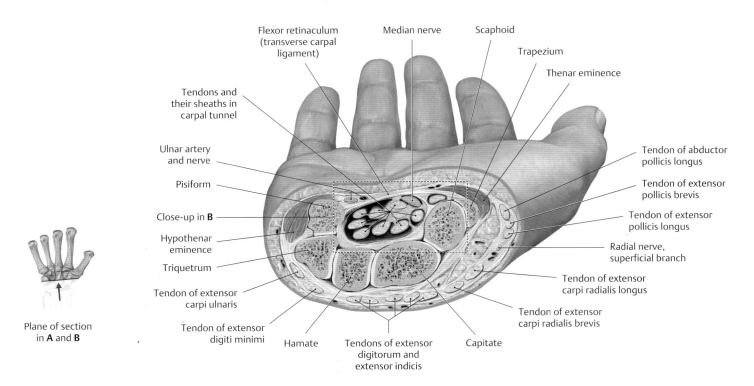

Flexor retinaculum (transverse carpal ligament)

Median nerve

Scaphoid

Trapezium

Thenar eminence

Tendons and their sheaths in carpal tunnel

Ulnar artery and nerve

Pisiform

Close-up in **B**

Hypothenar eminence

Triquetrum

Tendon of extensor carpi ulnaris

Tendon of extensor digiti minimi

Hamate

Tendons of extensor digitorum and extensor indicis

Capitate

Tendon of abductor pollicis longus

Tendon of extensor pollicis brevis

Tendon of extensor pollicis longus

Radial nerve, superficial branch

Tendon of extensor carpi radialis longus

Tendon of extensor carpi radialis brevis

Plane of section in **A** and **B**

A Cross section through the right wrist (see also **B**)
Distal view. The *carpal tunnel* is a fibro-osseous canal (see p. 288) through which pass the median nerve and the tendons of insertion of the flexor digitorum superficialis, and flexor digitorum profundus, flexor pollicis longus. Its dorsal boundary is formed by the carpal sulcus on the anterior surface of the carpal bones, and its palmar boundary is the flexor retinaculum (also known clinically as the transverse carpal ligament). The ulnar artery and ulnar nerve pass through the *ulnar tunnel* on the palmar side of the flexor retinaculum (see p. 405).

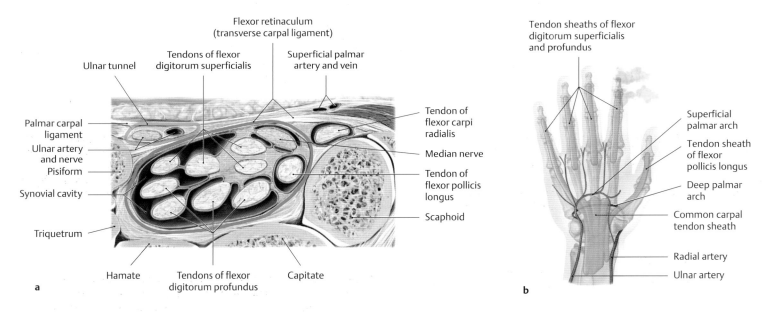

Flexor retinaculum (transverse carpal ligament)

Tendons of flexor digitorum superficialis

Superficial palmar artery and vein

Ulnar tunnel

Palmar carpal ligament

Ulnar artery and nerve

Pisiform

Synovial cavity

Triquetrum

Hamate

Tendons of flexor digitorum profundus

Capitate

Tendon of flexor carpi radialis

Median nerve

Tendon of flexor pollicis longus

Scaphoid

Tendon sheaths of flexor digitorum superficialis and profundus

Superficial palmar arch

Tendon sheath of flexor pollicis longus

Deep palmar arch

Common carpal tendon sheath

Radial artery

Ulnar artery

a

b

B Relationship of the palmar arches to the carpal and digital tendon sheaths (after Schmidt and Lanz)
a Tendon sheaths in the carpal tunnel (detail from **A**). The long flexor tendons pass through the carpal tunnel, encased in their palmar tendon sheaths. The tendons of the flexor digitorum superficialis and profundus are contained in their own ulnar synovial sheath. Radial to this sheath is the tendon of the flexor pollicis longus. The common mesotendon of all the digital flexor tendons is attached to the radial and palmar walls of the carpal tunnel. The median nerve generally occupies a separate space just deep to the flexor retinaculum (the variable course of the tendon sheaths is described on p. 344).
b Relationship of the carpal and digital tendon sheaths to the palmar arches.

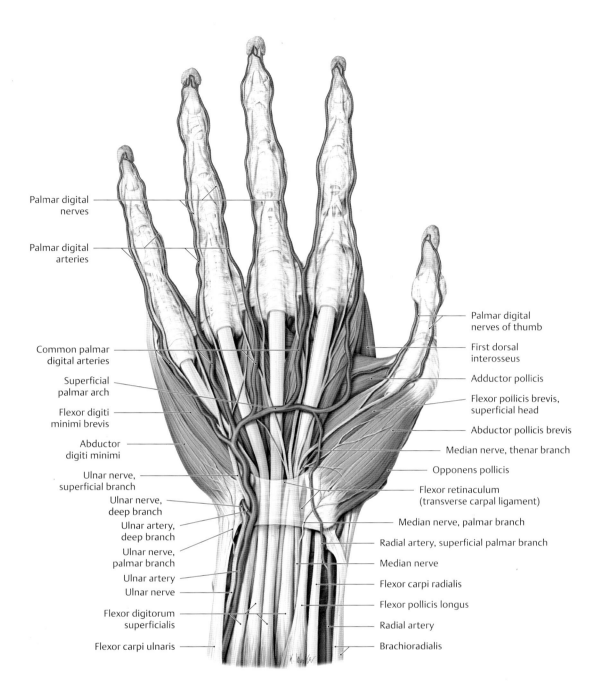

Palmar digital nerves

Palmar digital arteries

Common palmar digital arteries

Superficial palmar arch

Flexor digiti minimi brevis

Abductor digiti minimi

Ulnar nerve, superficial branch

Ulnar nerve, deep branch

Ulnar artery, deep branch

Ulnar nerve, palmar branch

Ulnar artery

Ulnar nerve

Flexor digitorum superficialis

Flexor carpi ulnaris

Palmar digital nerves of thumb

First dorsal interosseus

Adductor pollicis

Flexor pollicis brevis, superficial head

Abductor pollicis brevis

Median nerve, thenar branch

Opponens pollicis

Flexor retinaculum (transverse carpal ligament)

Median nerve, palmar branch

Radial artery, superficial palmar branch

Median nerve

Flexor carpi radialis

Flexor pollicis longus

Radial artery

Brachioradialis

C View into the carpal tunnel of the right hand
Anterior (palmar) view. The flexor retinaculum is transparent to reveal the contents of the carpal tunnel. The ulnar tunnel has been opened to expose the ulnar artery and nerve.
Note the superficial course of the median nerve in the carpal tunnel and the origin of its thenar (motor) branch just distal to the flexor retinacu-

lum (variants are shown in **D**). During surgical division of the flexor retinaculum for carpal tunnel syndrome, the hand surgeon must be aware of its variable course to avoid cutting the thenar branch.
The superficial palmar branch of the radial artery runs on the flexor retinaculum in the case shown here, but frequently it passes through the thenar muscles (see p. 320).

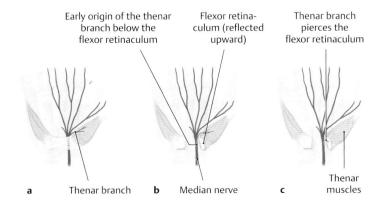

Early origin of the thenar branch below the flexor retinaculum

Flexor retinaculum (reflected upward)

Thenar branch pierces the flexor retinaculum

a   Thenar branch   b   Median nerve   c

Thenar muscles

D Origin of the thenar (motor) branch of the median nerve: normal anatomy and variants (after Schmidt and Lanz)
a   Normally (46 % of cases) the median nerve gives off its thenar branch distal to the flexor retinaculum (transverse carpal ligament).

b, c Variants:
b   The thenar branch has a subligamentatous origin and course (31 % of cases).
c   The thenar branch pierces the flexor retinaculum (transverse carpal ligament; approximately 23 % of all cases), making it vulnerable during surgical division of the retinaculum.

403

18.16 The Ulnar Tunnel and Anterior Carpal Region

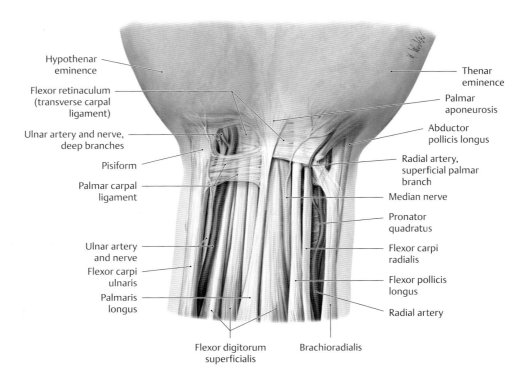

Hypothenar eminence

Flexor retinaculum (transverse carpal ligament)

Ulnar artery and nerve, deep branches

Pisiform

Palmar carpal ligament

Ulnar artery and nerve

Flexor carpi ulnaris

Palmaris longus

Flexor digitorum superficialis

Thenar eminence

Palmar aponeurosis

Abductor pollicis longus

Radial artery, superficial palmar branch

Median nerve

Pronator quadratus

Flexor carpi radialis

Flexor pollicis longus

Radial artery

Brachioradialis

A Superficial structures of the anterior carpal region
Right hand, anterior view. The skin and antebrachial fascia have been removed to demonstrate the superficial structures of the anterior carpal region, which is bounded distally by the flexor retinaculum (transverse carpal ligament). The tendons of insertion of the flexor carpi ulnaris, palmaris longus, and flexor carpi radialis in particular are clearly visible and palpable beneath the skin, especially when the fist is tightly clenched and the wrist is in slight flexion (see **B**). The tendon of the flexor carpi radialis is a useful landmark for locating the *radial artery pulse*. The flexor carpi ulnaris tendon is palpable proximally over the pisiform bone.
Note: Due to their superficial course, the median and ulnar nerves and the radial and ulnar arteries are particularly susceptible to injury from lacerations of the wrist.

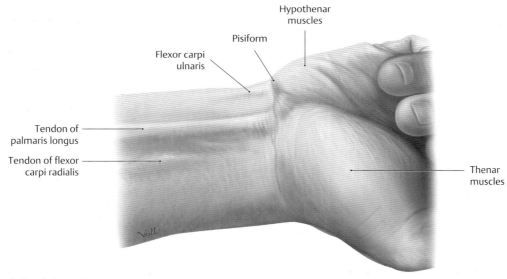

Hypothenar muscles

Pisiform

Flexor carpi ulnaris

Tendon of palmaris longus

Tendon of flexor carpi radialis

Thenar muscles

B Surface anatomy of the right wrist
Anterior view.

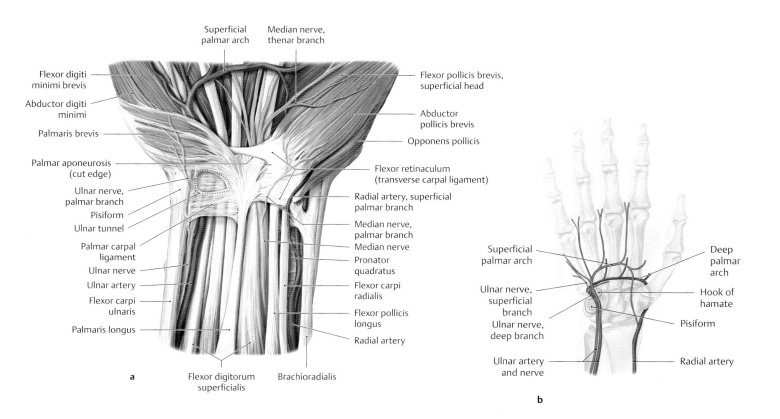

Superficial palmar arch

Median nerve, thenar branch

Flexor digiti minimi brevis

Abductor digiti minimi

Palmaris brevis

Palmar aponeurosis (cut edge)

Ulnar nerve, palmar branch

Pisiform

Ulnar tunnel

Palmar carpal ligament

Ulnar nerve

Ulnar artery

Flexor carpi ulnaris

Palmaris longus

Flexor pollicis brevis, superficial head

Abductor pollicis brevis

Opponens pollicis

Flexor retinaculum (transverse carpal ligament)

Radial artery, superficial palmar branch

Median nerve, palmar branch

Median nerve

Pronator quadratus

Flexor carpi radialis

Flexor pollicis longus

Radial artery

a Flexor digitorum superficialis Brachioradialis

Superficial palmar arch

Deep palmar arch

Ulnar nerve, superficial branch

Ulnar nerve, deep branch

Hook of hamate

Pisiform

Ulnar artery and nerve

Radial artery

b

C Course of the ulnar artery and nerve in the ulnar tunnel and deep palm
Right hand, anterior view.

a The palmar aponeurosis and antebrachial fascia have been removed to demonstrate the course of the ulnar artery and nerve through the ulnar tunnel.

b Bony landmarks within the ulnar tunnel. The pisiform bone on the ulnar side of the wrist and the hook of the hamate bone, which lies more distally and radially, provide the bony landmarks between which the ulnar artery and nerve pass through the ulnar tunnel.

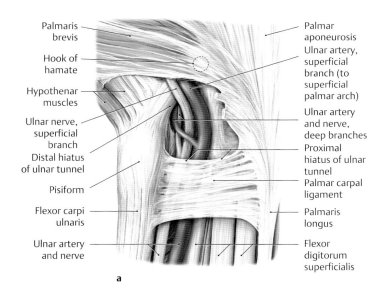

Palmaris brevis

Hook of hamate

Hypothenar muscles

Ulnar nerve, superficial branch

Distal hiatus of ulnar tunnel

Pisiform

Flexor carpi ulnaris

Ulnar artery and nerve

Palmar aponeurosis

Ulnar artery, superficial branch (to superficial palmar arch)

Ulnar artery and nerve, deep branches

Proximal hiatus of ulnar tunnel

Palmar carpal ligament

Palmaris longus

Flexor digitorum superficialis

a

Palmaris brevis

Abductor digiti minimi and flexor digiti minimi

Pisohamate ligament

Pisiform

Tendon of flexor carpi ulnaris

Tendon of flexor digitorum superficialis

Palmar aponeurosis

Hook of hamate

Distal hiatus of ulnar tunnel

Flexor retinaculum

Proximal hiatus of ulnar tunnel

Palmar carpal ligament

Tendon of palmaris longus

b

D Apertures and walls of the ulnar tunnel with (a) and without (b) the nerves and vessels (after Schmidt and Lanz)
Right hand, anterior view. The *palmar* roof of the ulnar tunnel is formed by skin and subcutaneous fat, the palmar carpal ligament (proximal), and the palmaris brevis muscle (distal). The ulnar tunnel is bounded *dorsally* by the flexor retinaculum (transverse carpal ligament) and the pisohamate ligament. The *entrance* to the tunnel begins at the level of the pisiform bone below the palmar carpal ligament (proximal hiatus).

The *outlet* is at the level of the hook of the hamate, marked by a taut, transverse, crescent-shaped tendinous arch between the pisiform and the hook of the hamate (distal hiatus), the latter giving attachment to the flexor digiti minimi. The *deep branches* of the ulnar artery and nerve reach the central compartment of the palm on the pisohamate ligament, passing deep to the tendinous arch. The *superficial branches* of the artery and nerve run distally above the tendinous arch, passing deep to the palmaris brevis.

405

The Lower Limb

19.1 The Lower Limb: General Aspects

A Unique features and specialized function of the human lower limb

The evolution of the lower limb into a mechanism specifically adapted for bipedal locomotion, along with the specialization of the upper limb for visually guided manipulation, is a distinctive feature of the anatomy of the human primate. The uniquely human conformation of shapes and proportions is the end result of a process that rearranged the primate center of gravity and the positions of internal organs, dramatically altering the form and biomechanics of the trunk to produce a progressively more efficient bipedal gait. Other primates have the capacity to assume an erect body posture and to walk upright, but only for short periods and at a much greater relative expenditure of energy. The habitual upright gait of humans has been achieved through a series of anatomic adaptations of the musculoskeletal system. The most critical of these adaptations occurred in the vertebral column and pelvis. The design of the human vertebral column differs markedly from that of other primates: the simple "arch and cord" construction of the chimpanzee spine has been abandoned in favor of the human double-S-shaped curve, which allows the human axial skeleton to act as a shock-absorbing spring (see p. 103), while shifting the entire weight of the trunk over the load-bearing surface of the feet. This shift to an upright posture has imposed the full weight of the abdominal viscera upon the pelvis. Concomitantly, the iliac wings of the pelvis have spread farther apart, and the sacrum has broadened, to generate a structure in humans that is now specialized for bearing the load of the viscera. The efficiency of upright gait has been improved further by stabilization of the pelvis and secure anchoring to the spine via the sacrum. The unique proportions of the human lower limb provide a dramatic demonstration of the extent of this specialization. Because their function is more exclusively directed toward support and locomotion, the legs are exceptionally long and powerful in humans. While the leg length is 111% of trunk length in orangutans and 128% in chimpanzees, it measures 171% of trunk length in humans. The specialization of the human lower limb for bipedal gait is also reflected in the substantial changes in function of certain muscles, particularly the gluteal muscles, the knee-joint extensors, and the muscles of the calf.

B Overview of the skeleton of the lower limb

a Right lower limb, anterior view.
b Right lower limb, posterior view (the foot is in maximum plantar flexion in both views).

As in the upper limb, the skeleton of the lower limb consists of a limb girdle and the attached free limb.

- The pelvic girdle in adults is formed by the paired hip bones (ossa coxae, innominate bones). They differ from the shoulder girdle in that they are firmly integrated into the axial skeleton through the sacroiliac joints (see p. 142). The two hip bones combine with the sacrum and pubic symphysis to form the *pelvic ring* (see p. 413).
- The free limb consists of the thigh (femur), the leg (tibia and fibula), and the foot. It is connected to the pelvic girdle by the hip joint.

a Interphalangeal joints of the foot

b

C Palpable bony prominences of the right lower limb

a Anterior view, **b** posterior view.

Almost all the skeletal elements of the lower limb have bony prominences, margins, or surfaces (e.g., the medial tibial surface) that can be palpated through the skin and soft tissues. The only exceptions are structures that are largely covered by muscle, such as the hip joint, the neck and shaft of the femur, and large portions of the fibular shaft. Several standard anatomic landmarks have been defined in the lower limb for use in measur-

ing the length of the leg and certain skeletal elements. They are the anterior superior iliac spine, the greater trochanter of the femur, the medial joint space of the knee (superior margin of the medial tibial condyle), and the medial malleolus. The clinical evaluation of leg length discrepancy is important because "true" shortening of the leg (a disparity of anatomic leg lengths), as well as functional leg shortening (e.g., due to muscle contractures), can lead to *pelvic tilt* and scoliotic deformity of the spine (see p. 133).

D Leg length measurement in the standing position

Leg length discrepancy can be measured with reasonable accuracy in the standing patient by placing wooden blocks of known thickness (0.5 cm, 1 cm, 2 cm) beneath the foot of the shorter leg until the pelvis is horizontal. Horizontal position is confirmed when noting that both iliac crests are at the same level when palpated from behind and the anal fissure is vertical. If the pelvis cannot be leveled by placing blocks under the apparently shorter limb, then a "functional" leg length discrepancy is present rather than a "true" discrepancy. Most cases of this kind are caused by a fixed pelvic tilt secondary to a hip joint contracture or scoliosis. The measured leg lengths in these cases may actually be equal, and the pelvic tilt only mimics a length discrepancy.

409

19.2   The Anatomic and Mechanical Axes of the Lower Limb

a Center of rotation of the femoral head (hip joint)

Mechanical axis (Mikulicz line)

Anatomic axis of the femur

81°

174°

93°

Intercondylar eminence of the tibial plateau (knee joint)

Knee baseline

Ankle mortise

Talocrural joint

b Gluteus maximus (superior part)

Iliotibial tract

Biceps femoris

c Sartorius

Semi-tendinosus

Gracilis

Mechanical axis

A   The mechanical axis of the leg (the Mikulicz line)
a Normal mechanical axis, anterior view.
b Mechanical axis in genu varum, posterior view.
c Mechanical axis in genu valgum, posterior view.

In an individual with normal axial alignment, the large joints of the lower limb (the hip, knee, and ankle) lie on a straight line that represents the mechanical longitudinal axis of the leg (the *Mikulicz line*). This mechanical axis extends from the center of rotation of the femoral head through the intercondylar eminence of the tibial plateau and down through the center of the ankle *mortise* (the pocket created by the fibula and tibia for the talus in the ankle joint, from Arabic, *murtazz*, fastened). While the mechanical axis and anatomic axis coincide in the *tibial shaft*, the anatomic and mechanical axes of the *femoral shaft* diverge at a 6° angle. Thus, the longitudinal anatomic axes of the femur

and tibia do not lie on a straight line but form a laterally open angle of 174° at the level of the knee joint in the coronal plane (the *femorotibial angle*). In genu varum (**b**) the center of the knee joint is lateral to the mechanical axis, and in genu valgum (**c**) it is medial to the mechanical axis. Both conditions impose abnormal, unbalanced loads on the joints (see **B**) that gradually cause degenerative changes to develop in the bone and cartilage (osteoarthritis of the knee) accompanied by stretching of the associated joint capsule, ligaments, and muscles. In genu varum (**b**), for example, the medial joint complex of the knee is subjected to abnormal pressure, while the lateral joint structures (e.g., the lateral collateral ligament), iliotibial tract, and biceps femoris muscle are subjected to abnormal tension. Genu varum also places greater stress on the lateral border of the foot, resulting in a fallen pedal arch.

a   **b**

B   Position of the mechanical axes with the feet slightly apart and together
Anterior view.

a In upright stance with the feet placed slightly apart, the mechanical axis runs almost vertically through the center of the three large joints.
b The legs are generally considered "straight" if, when the feet are together, the opposing medial malleoli and knees are touching. Accordingly, the intercondylar distance and the intermalleolar distance between the legs provide an index for the measurement of genu varum and genu valgum. When this stance is attempted, an intercondylar distance greater than 3 cm or an intermalleolar distance greater than 5 cm is considered abnormal (see **C**).

a   Intercondylar distance   b   Intermalleolar distance   c

C The normal leg axes at different ages
a Infant, **b** small child, **c** school-age child.
Up to about 20° of genu varum is considered normal during the first year of life. Up to about 10° of genu valgum is also considered normal through 2 years of age. By the time the child enters school, the legs are essentially straight as a result of musculoskeletal growth.

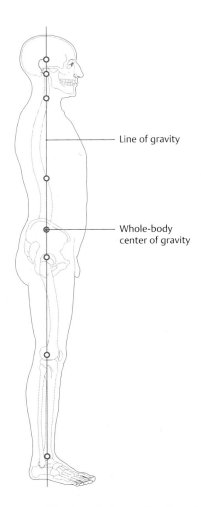

Line of gravity

Whole-body
center of gravity

D Normal anatomic position in relation to the line of gravity
Right lateral view. The *line of gravity* runs vertically from the whole-body center of gravity to the ground. In normal upright humans, it intersects the external auditory canal, the dens of the axis (dental process C 2), the inflection points between the normal curves in the vertebral column (between the cervical and thoracic curves, and thoracic and lumbar curves), the whole-body center of gravity, and the hip, knee, and ankle joints. Chronic deviation of any reference point from this line imposes abnormal stresses on different clusters of musculoskeletal elements.

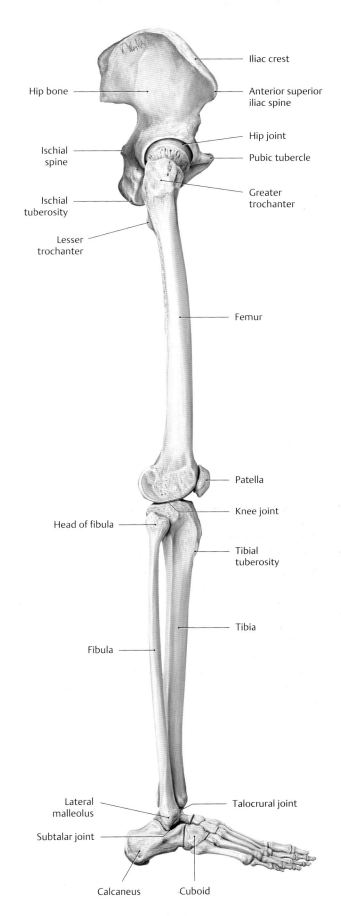

Iliac crest
Hip bone
Anterior superior
iliac spine
Hip joint
Ischial
spine
Pubic tubercle
Greater
trochanter
Ischial
tuberosity
Lesser
trochanter
Femur
Patella
Knee joint
Head of fibula
Tibial
tuberosity
Tibia
Fibula
Lateral
malleolus
Talocrural joint
Subtalar joint
Calcaneus
Cuboid

E Skeleton of the right lower limb
Right lateral view.

411

19.3 The Bones of the Pelvic Girdle

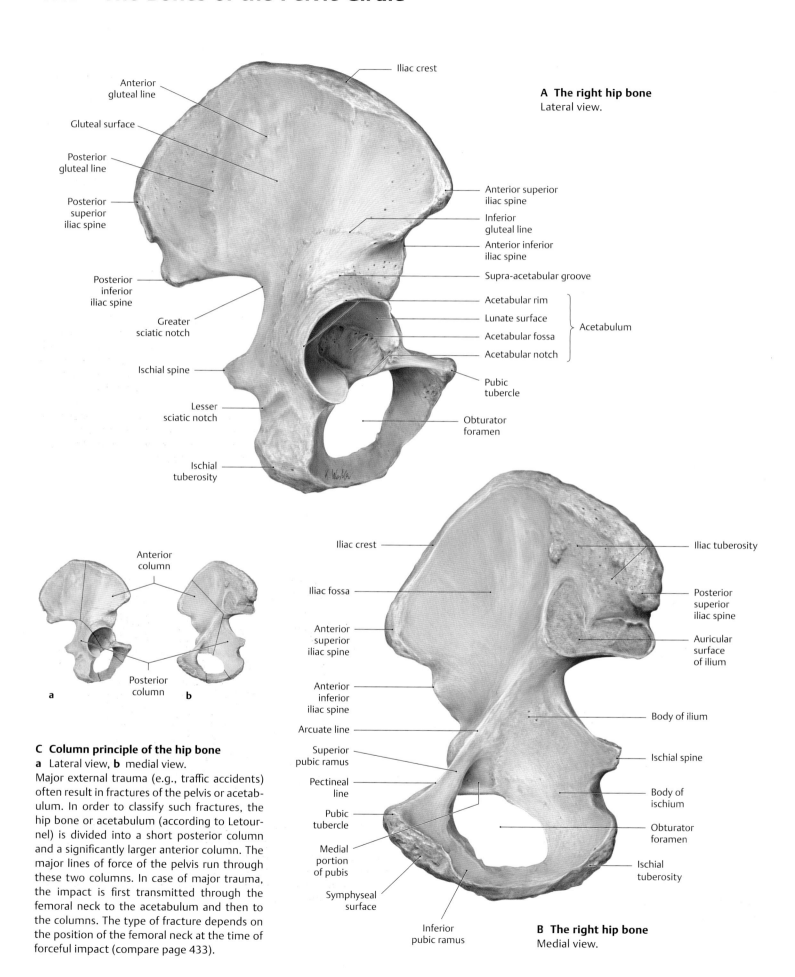

A The right hip bone
Lateral view.

Iliac crest

Anterior gluteal line

Gluteal surface

Posterior gluteal line

Posterior superior iliac spine

Posterior inferior iliac spine

Greater sciatic notch

Ischial spine

Lesser sciatic notch

Ischial tuberosity

Anterior superior iliac spine

Inferior gluteal line

Anterior inferior iliac spine

Supra-acetabular groove

Acetabular rim

Lunate surface

Acetabular fossa

Acetabular notch

Acetabulum

Pubic tubercle

Obturator foramen

C Column principle of the hip bone
a Lateral view, **b** medial view.

Anterior column

Posterior column

a

b

Major external trauma (e.g., traffic accidents) often result in fractures of the pelvis or acetabulum. In order to classify such fractures, the hip bone or acetabulum (according to Letournel) is divided into a short posterior column and a significantly larger anterior column. The major lines of force of the pelvis run through these two columns. In case of major trauma, the impact is first transmitted through the femoral neck to the acetabulum and then to the columns. The type of fracture depends on the position of the femoral neck at the time of forceful impact (compare page 433).

Iliac crest

Iliac fossa

Anterior superior iliac spine

Anterior inferior iliac spine

Arcuate line

Superior pubic ramus

Pectineal line

Pubic tubercle

Medial portion of pubis

Symphyseal surface

Inferior pubic ramus

Iliac tuberosity

Posterior superior iliac spine

Auricular surface of ilium

Body of ilium

Ischial spine

Body of ischium

Obturator foramen

Ischial tuberosity

B The right hip bone
Medial view.

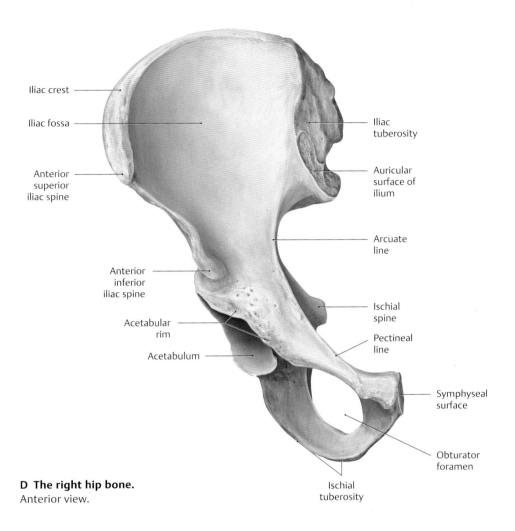

Iliac crest

Iliac fossa

Anterior superior iliac spine

Anterior inferior iliac spine

Acetabular rim

Acetabulum

Iliac tuberosity

Auricular surface of ilium

Arcuate line

Ischial spine

Pectineal line

Symphyseal surface

Obturator foramen

Ischial tuberosity

D The right hip bone.
Anterior view.

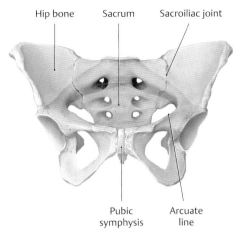

Hip bone   Sacrum   Sacroiliac joint

Pubic symphysis   Arcuate line

E The pelvic girdle and pelvic ring
Anterior view. The paired hip bones that make up the pelvic girdle are connected to each other at the cartilaginous pubic symphysis and to the sacrum at the sacroiliac joints (see p. 142). This creates a stable ring, the bony pelvic ring (shaded in red), that permits very little motion. This stability throughout the pelvic ring is an important prerequisite for the transfer of trunk loads to the lower limb necessary for normal gait.

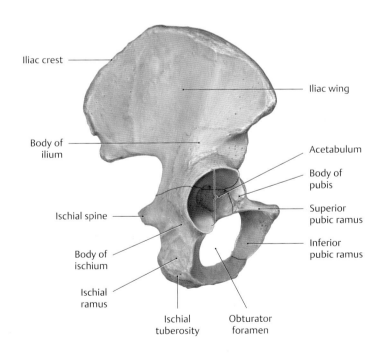

Iliac crest

Iliac wing

Body of ilium

Acetabulum

Body of pubis

Superior pubic ramus

Inferior pubic ramus

Ischial spine

Body of ischium

Ischial ramus

Ischial tuberosity

Obturator foramen

F The triradiate cartilage of a right hip bone: the junction of the ilium, ischium, and pubis.
Lateral view.

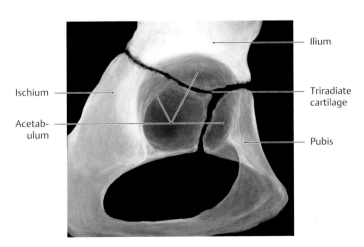

Ilium

Ischium

Acetabulum

Triradiate cartilage

Pubis

G Schematic radiograph of the right acetabulum of a child
Lateral view (lateral projection). The bony elements of the hip bone come together in the acetabulum, with the ilium and ischium each comprising two fifths of the acetabulum and the pubis one fifth. Definitive fusion of the Y-shaped growth plate (triradiate cartilage) occurs between the 14th and 16th years of life.

19.4 The Femur: Importance of the Femoral Neck Angle

A The right femur
Anterior view.

B The right femur
Posterior view.

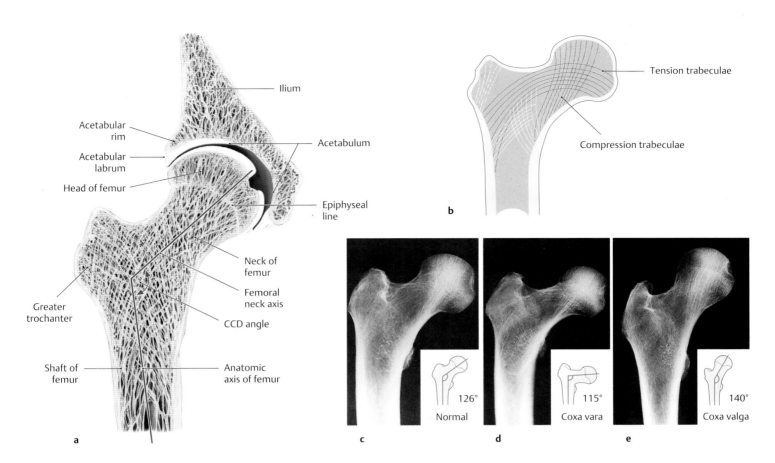

a

b

c   **d**   **e**

C The arrangement and prominence of tension trabeculae and compression trabeculae as a function of the femoral neck angle
Right femur, anterior view.

a Coronal section through the right hip joint at the level of the fovea on the femoral head. The angle between the longitudinal axis of the femoral neck and the axis of the femoral shaft is called the femoral neck angle or CCD angle (centrum-collum-diaphysis angle). This angle normally measures approximately 126° in adults and 150° in newborns. It decreases continually during growth due to the constant bone remodeling that occurs in response to the changing stress patterns across the hip.

b The trabecular pattern associated with a normal femoral neck angle.
c–e Radiographs in the sagittal projection.
c Normal femoral neck angle with a normal bending load.
d A *decreased* femoral neck angle (coxa vara) leads to a greater bending load with higher tensile stresses, thereby stimulating the formation of more tension trabeculae.
e An *increased* femoral neck angle (coxa valga) leads to a greater pressure load with higher compressive stresses, stimulating the formation of more compression trabeculae.

a   **b**

a   **b**

D Compressive and tensile stresses in a bone model
a An *axial* (centered) weight placed atop a Plexiglas model of a pillar creates a uniform pressure load that is evenly distributed over the cross section of the pillar and whose sum is equal to the applied weight.
b A *nonaxial* (eccentric) weight placed on an overhang creates a bending load that generates both tensile and compressive stresses in the pillar.

E The principle of the tension band (after Pauwels)
a The bending load acting on an I-beam model can be reduced by placing a high-tensile-strength member (chain) on the side opposite the bending force. This added member transforms the bending load into a pure compressive load.
b In the leg, the fascia lata on the lateral side of the thigh is thickened to form the iliotibial tract (see p. 479). By functioning as a tension band, the iliotibial tract reduces the bending loads on the proximal femur.

415

19.5 The Femoral Head and Deformities of the Femoral Neck

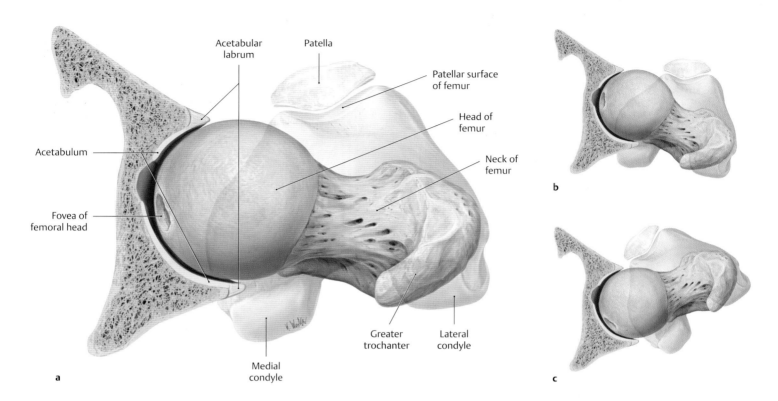

Acetabular labrum

Patella

Patellar surface of femur

Head of femur

Neck of femur

Acetabulum

Fovea of femoral head

b

Greater trochanter

Lateral condyle

Medial condyle

a

c

A The right femur

Proximal view. For clarity, the acetabulum has been sectioned in the horizontal plane. The distal end of the femur (with patella) has been added in light shading.

a Hip joint with centered femoral head, **b** hip joint externally rotated, **c** hip joint internally rotated.

Note the orientation of the acetabulum, which is angled forward by approximately 17°. This anterior angle affects the stability and "seating" of the femoral head in the hip joint (see p. 427). With the femoral head centered in the acetabulum and the femur slightly medially rotated (**a**), the distal femur and thus the knee joint point slightly inward (physiologic internal rotation of the knee). The position of the foot is additionally influenced by the external rotation of the tibia (see p. 421) (see **D**).

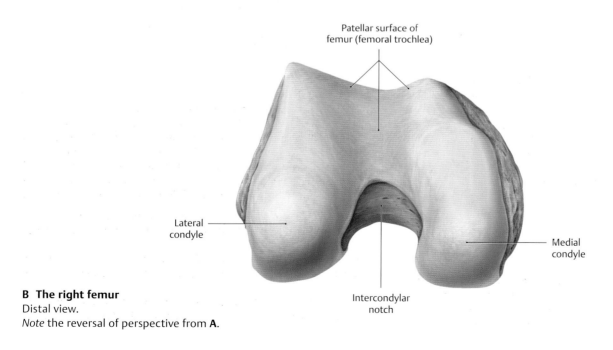

Patellar surface of femur (femoral trochlea)

Lateral condyle

Medial condyle

Intercondylar notch

B The right femur

Distal view.

Note the reversal of perspective from **A**.

C The right femur.
Medial view.
Note the transverse condylar axis and the femoral neck axis. When the axes are superimposed, the two lines intersect each other at a 12° angle in adults (anteversion angle, see also **D** and **A**). This angle is considerably larger at birth, measuring 30° to 40°, but decreases to the normal adult value by the end of the 2nd decade.

D Rotational deformities of the femoral neck
Right hip joint, superior view. Increased or decreased torsion of the femoral shaft results in torsion angles of varying size. When the hip is centered, this leads to increased internal or external rotation of the leg with a corresponding change in gait (a "toeing-in" or "toeing-out" gait). When the condylar axis is taken as the reference point, femoral torsion may be described as normal (**a**), increased (**b**), or decreased (**c**).

a A normal anteversion angle of approximately 12° with the foot directed forward (taking into account tibial torsion of 23°, see p. 421).
b An increased anteversion angle (*coxa anteverta*) typically leads to a toeing-in gait accompanied by a pronounced limitation of external rotation.
c The femoral neck is retroverted (points backward in relation to the condylar axis). The result is *coxa retroverta* with a toeing-out gait.

19.6 The Patella

A Location of the patella

Right knee joint, lateral view. The red line indicates the plane of section in **C**.

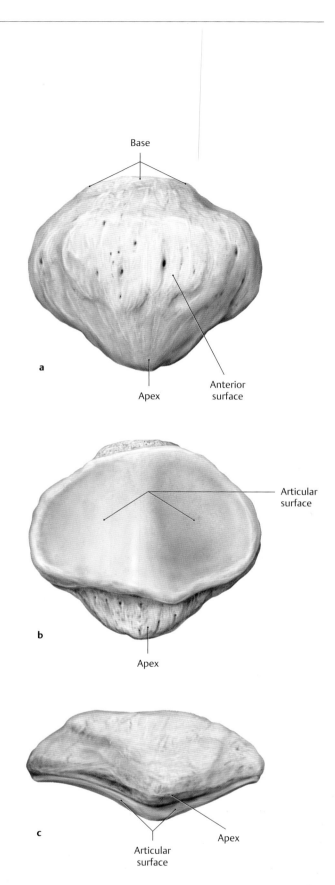

B Right patella

a Anterior view, **b** posterior view, **c** distal view.

Note that the *apex* of the patella points downward.

C Cross section through the femoropatellar joint

Right knee, distal view. The level of the cross section is shown in **A**. The femoropatellar joint is the site where the patellar surface of the femur, often called the femoral trochlea (by analogy with the distal humerus), articulates with the posterior articular surface of the patella. The patella is a sesamoid bone (the largest sesamoid) embedded in the quadriceps tendon. The patella is well centered when the ridge on the undersurface of the patella is seated within the groove of the femoral trochlea. The main functional role of the patella is to lengthen the effective lever arm of the quadriceps femoris muscle (the only extensor muscle of the knee), thereby reducing the force required to extend the knee joint (see also p. 482).

D Bipartite patella

Because the patella develops from multiple ossification centers, the failure of an ossification center to fuse results in a two-part (bipartite) patella. The upper lateral quadrant of the patella is most commonly affected. A fracture should always be considered in the radiographic differential diagnosis of a bipartite patella.

E The evaluation of patellar shape

Diagrams of tangential radiographs of the patella ("sunrise" view: supine position, knee flexed 60°, caudocranial beam directed parallel to the posterior patellar surface). Each diagram shows the relation of the patella to the femoral trochlea in a horizontal plane through the right knee joint. The posterior articular surface of the patella bears a vertical ridge dividing it into a lateral facet and a medial facet. Generally, the lateral facet is slightly concave, while the medial facet is slightly convex. The angle between the lateral and medial facets, called the patellar facet angle, is normally 130° ± 10°. Wiberg, Baumgart, and Ficat devised the following scheme for the classification of patellar shape based on the facet angle:

a Patella with medial and lateral facets of approximately equal size and a facet angle within the normal range.
b Most common patellar shape with a slightly smaller medial facet.
c A distinctly smaller medial facet ("medial hypoplasia").
d Patellar dysplasia with a very steep medial facet ("hunter's hat" configuration).

Besides the various patellar shapes, the patellar surface of the femur (the femoral trochlea) has a variable morphology (described in the Hepp classification system). Developmental dysplasias of the patella and femoral trochlea lead to patellar instability marked by recurrent lateral or medial subluxation or dislocation of the patella.

19.7 The Tibia and Fibula

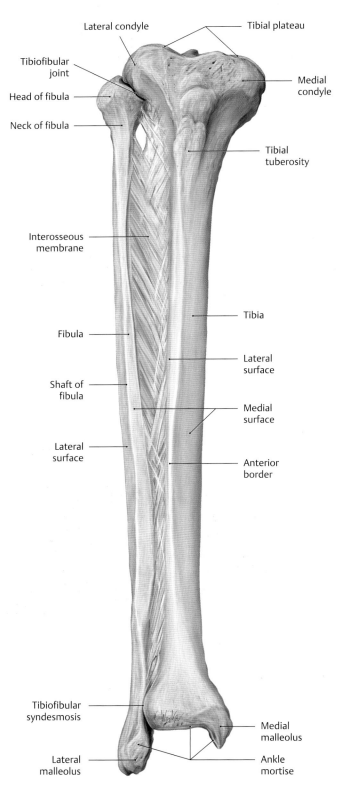

Lateral condyle

Tibial plateau

Tibiofibular joint

Head of fibula

Neck of fibula

Medial condyle

Tibial tuberosity

Interosseous membrane

Fibula

Tibia

Lateral surface

Shaft of fibula

Medial surface

Lateral surface

Anterior border

Tibiofibular syndesmosis

Medial malleolus

Lateral malleolus

Ankle mortise

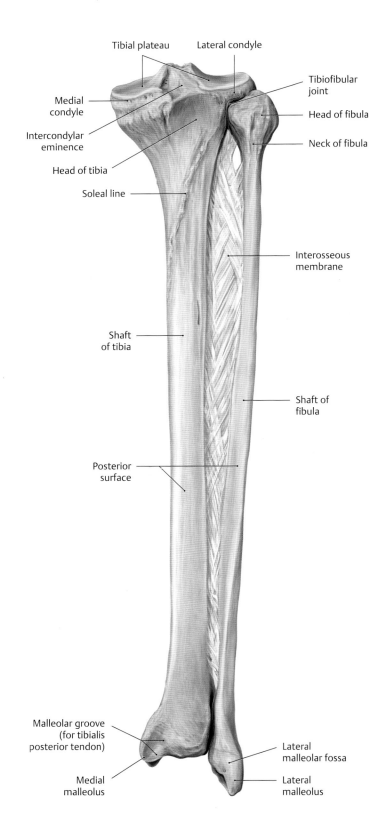

Tibial plateau

Lateral condyle

Medial condyle

Tibiofibular joint

Intercondylar eminence

Head of fibula

Head of tibia

Neck of fibula

Soleal line

Interosseous membrane

Shaft of tibia

Shaft of fibula

Posterior surface

Malleolar groove (for tibialis posterior tendon)

Lateral malleolar fossa

Medial malleolus

Lateral malleolus

A The tibia, fibula, and crural interosseous membrane

Right leg, anterior view. The tibia and fibula articulate at two joints that allow only very limited motion (rotation). Proximally, near the knee, is the synovial tibiofibular joint; distally, at the ankle, is the tibiofibular *syndesmosis* (fibrous joint with bony elements united by ligaments). The crural interosseous membrane (see also **F**) is a sheet of tough connective tissue that serves as an origin for several muscles in the leg. Additionally, it acts with the tibiofibular syndesmosis to stabilize the ankle mortise.

B The tibia, fibula, and crural interosseous membrane

Right leg, posterior view.

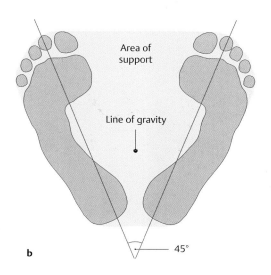

C Normal orientation of the tibia and its role in stability
When the transverse axes of the upper tibia (tibial plateau) and lower tibia (ankle mortise) are superimposed, they form an angle of approximately 23°; i.e., the transverse axis of the ankle joint is rotated 23° laterally relative to the transverse axis of the tibial plateau (*normal tibial*

orientation, **a**). As a result of this, the longitudinal anatomic axis of the foot does not lie in the sagittal plane, and the toes point outward when the upper tibia is directed forward (**b**). This significantly improves the stability of bipedal stance by placing the line of gravity close to the center of the area of support (see p. 411).

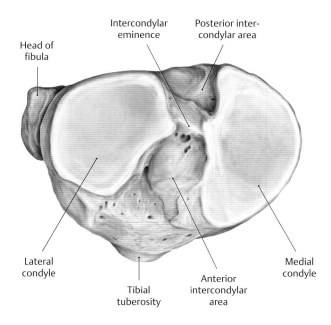

D The right tibial plateau
Proximal view.

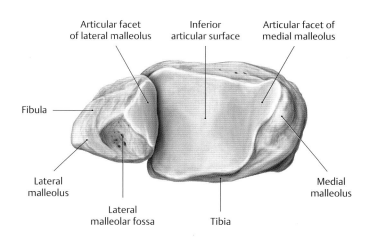

E The right ankle mortise
Distal view.

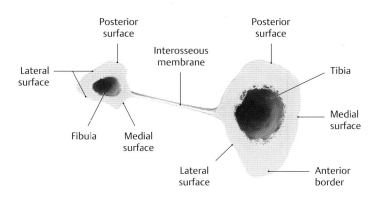

F Cross section through the middle third of the right leg
Proximal view.

19.8 The Bones of the Foot from the Dorsal and Plantar Views

Distal phalanx of great toe

Head

Proximal phalanx of great toe — Shaft

Base

Head

First meta-tarsal

Shaft

Base

Medial cuneiform

Intermediate cuneiform

Navicular

Head of talus

Talus — Neck of talus

Body of talus

Calcaneal tuberosity

Distal phalanx of little toe

Middle phalanx of little toe

Proximal phalanx of little toe

Lateral cuneiform

Tuberosity of fifth metatarsal

Cuboid

Calcaneus

A The bones of the right foot
Dorsal view.

Antetarsus (phalanges)

Metatarsus (metatarsal bones)

Tarsus (tarsal bones)

C Anatomic subdivisions of the pedal skeleton

Right foot, dorsal view. In the nomenclature of *descriptive* anatomy, the skeletal elements of the foot are subdivided into three adjoining segments:

• The tarsus, composed of seven bones
• The metatarsus, composed of five bones
• The antetarsus, composed of 14 phalanges

Compare this diagram with the *functional* subdivisions in **D**.

B The right talus and calcaneus
Dorsal view. The two tarsal bones have been separated at the subtalar joint to demonstrate their articular surfaces.

Navicular articular surface

Superior facet of trochlea of talus

Medial malleolar facet

Medial tubercle

Posterior process of talus — Groove for flexor hallucis longus tendon

Lateral tubercle

Lateral malleolar facet

Anterior talar articular surface

Articular surface for cuboid

Tarsal sinus

Sulcus calcanei

Posterior talar articular surface

Sustentac-ulum tali

Middle talar articular surface

Calcaneal body

D Functional subdivisions of the pedal skeleton

Right foot, dorsal view. The skeleton of the foot is often subdivided as follows based on functional and clinical criteria:

- The hindfoot (calcaneus and talus)
- The midfoot (cuboid, navicular, and cuneiforms)
- The forefoot (the metatarsals and phalanges)

Forefoot

Midfoot

Hindfoot

Distal phalanx of little toe

Middle phalanx of little toe

Proximal phalanx of little toe

Fifth metatarsal

Tuberosity of fifth metatarsal

Groove for fibularis longus tendon

Tuberosity of cuboid

Cuboid

Calcaneus

Distal phalanx of great toe

Proximal phalanx of great toe

Sesamoids

First metatarsal

Medial cuneiform

Intermediate cuneiform

Lateral cuneiform

Navicular

Head of talus

Neck of talus

Body of talus

Sustentaculum tali

Posterior process of talus (medial tubercle)

E The bones of the right foot
Plantar view.

Groove for flexor hallucis longus tendon

Medial process of calcaneal tuberosity

Lateral process of calcaneal tuberosity

Calcaneal tuberosity

Articular surface for cuboid

Tarsal sinus

Anterior facet for calcaneus

Navicular articular surface

Middle facet for calcaneus

Sulcus tali

Posterior facet for calcaneus

Medial tubercle

Groove for flexor hallucis longus tendon

Lateral tubercle

F The right talus and calcaneus
Plantar view. The two tarsal bones have been separated at the subtalar joint to demonstrate their articular surfaces.

423

19.9 The Bones of the Foot from the Lateral and Medial Views; Accessory Tarsal Bones

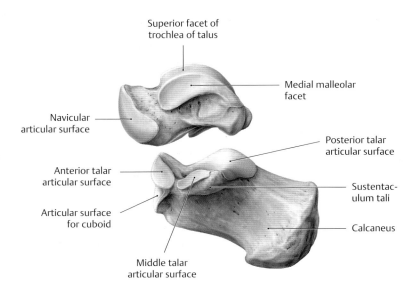

A The right talus and calcaneus
Medial view. The two tarsal bones have been separated at the subtalar joint to demonstrate their articular surfaces.

C Sustentaculum tali ("supports talus")

- The sustentaculum tali is a bony protuberance of the medial calcaneus.
- It is palpable approximately 1.5 cm below the tip of the medial malleolus.
- It supports the talus on its balcony-like protrusion.
- It marks the end of the tarsal canal, which divides the two chambers of the lower ankle joint (see p. 459).
- It serves as a support for the tendon of the flexor hallucis longus (thereby supporting the calcaneus in upright position, see p. 466).
- It has a longitudinal groove for the flexor digitorum longus (see p. 466).
- Two ligaments insert at the sustentaculum tali: the spring ligament and part of the deltoid ligament (see p. 460).
- It is a common location for fractures associated with snowboarding.

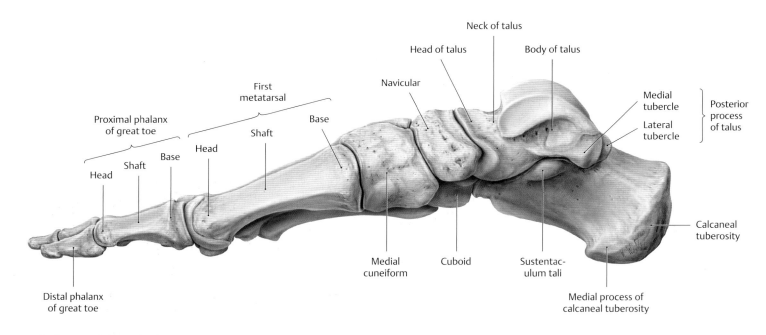

B The bones of the right foot
Medial view.

C The right talus and calcaneus

Lateral view. The two tarsal bones have been separated at the subtalar joint to demonstrate their articular surfaces.

E Accessory tarsal bones

Right foot, dorsal view. A number of accessory (inconstant) ossicles are sometimes found in the foot. While they rarely cause complaints, they do require differentiation from fractures. A clinically important accessory bone is the external tibial bone, which can be a source of discomfort when tight shoes are worn.

D The bones of the right foot

Lateral view.

19.10 The Hip Joint: Articulating Bones

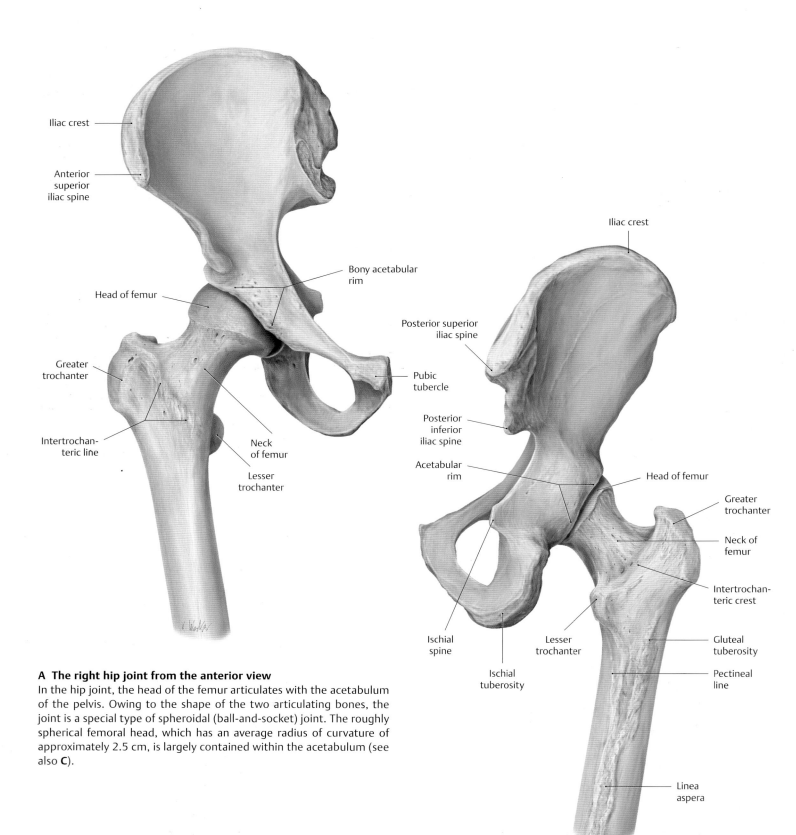

Iliac crest

Anterior superior iliac spine

Head of femur

Greater trochanter

Intertrochan-teric line

Bony acetabular rim

Neck of femur

Lesser trochanter

Iliac crest

Posterior superior iliac spine

Pubic tubercle

Posterior inferior iliac spine

Acetabular rim

Head of femur

Greater trochanter

Neck of femur

Intertrochan-teric crest

Ischial spine

Lesser trochanter

Gluteal tuberosity

Ischial tuberosity

Pectineal line

Linea aspera

A The right hip joint from the anterior view
In the hip joint, the head of the femur articulates with the acetabulum of the pelvis. Owing to the shape of the two articulating bones, the joint is a special type of spheroidal (ball-and-socket) joint. The roughly spherical femoral head, which has an average radius of curvature of approximately 2.5 cm, is largely contained within the acetabulum (see also **C**).

B The right hip joint from the posterior view

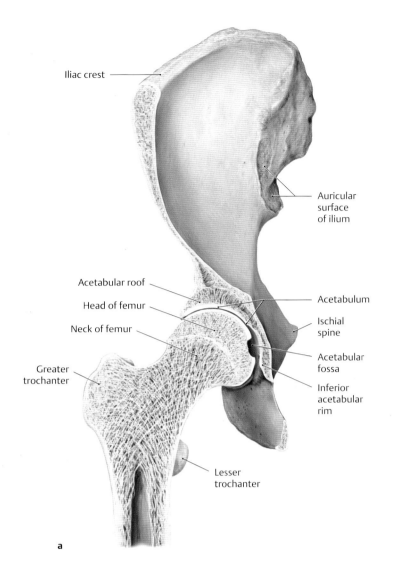

Iliac crest

Auricular surface of ilium

Acetabular roof

Head of femur

Neck of femur

Acetabulum

Ischial spine

Acetabular fossa

Inferior acetabular rim

Greater trochanter

Lesser trochanter

a

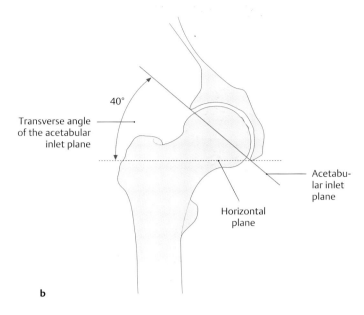

40°

Transverse angle of the acetabular inlet plane

Acetabular inlet plane

Horizontal plane

b

C Transverse angle of the acetabular inlet plane in the adult

Right hip joint, anterior view. Coronal section at the level of the acetabular fossa. The acetabular inlet plane, or bony acetabular rim, faces inferolaterally (*transverse angle*) and also anteroinferiorly (*sagittal angle*; see **D**). The inferolateral tilt of the acetabulum can be determined by drawing a line from the superior acetabular rim to the inferior acetabular rim (lowest point of the acetabular notch) and measuring the angle between that line and the true horizontal. This transverse angle normally measures approximately 51° at birth, 45° at 10 years of age, and 40° in adults (after Ullmann and Sharp). The value of the transverse angle affects several parameters, including the degree of lateral coverage of the femoral head by the acetabulum (the *center-edge angle* of Wiberg, see p. 439).

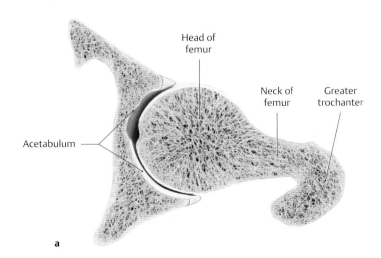

Head of femur

Neck of femur

Greater trochanter

Acetabulum

a

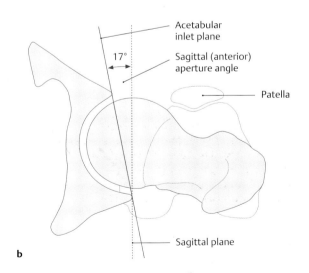

Acetabular inlet plane

17°

Sagittal (anterior) aperture angle

Patella

Sagittal plane

b

D Sagittal angle of the acetabular inlet plane in the adult

Right hip joint, superior view. Horizontal section through the center of the femoral head.

The bony acetabular rim is angled anteroinferiorly relative to the sagittal plane (compare this with the horizontal plane in **C**). This aperture angle measures approximately 7° at birth and increases to 17° by adulthood (after Chassard and Lapine).

19.11 The Ligaments of the Hip Joint: Stabilization of the Femoral Head

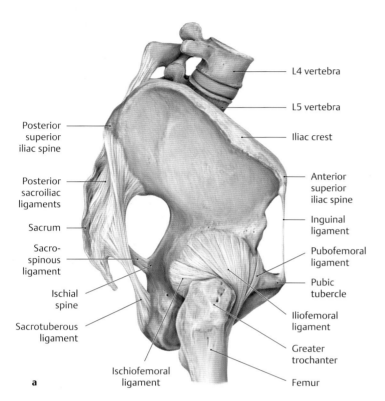

a

Posterior superior iliac spine
Posterior sacroiliac ligaments
Sacrum
Sacrospinous ligament
Ischial spine
Sacrotuberous ligament
Ischiofemoral ligament

L4 vertebra
L5 vertebra
Iliac crest
Anterior superior iliac spine
Inguinal ligament
Pubofemoral ligament
Pubic tubercle
Iliofemoral ligament
Greater trochanter
Femur

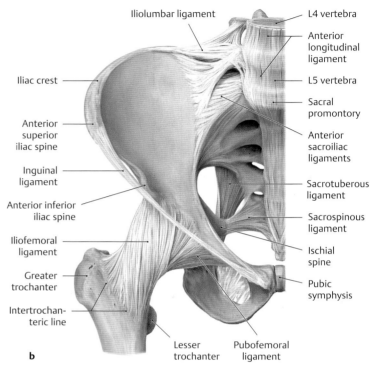

b

Iliolumbar ligament
Iliac crest
Anterior superior iliac spine
Inguinal ligament
Anterior inferior iliac spine
Iliofemoral ligament
Greater trochanter
Intertrochanteric line

L4 vertebra
Anterior longitudinal ligament
L5 vertebra
Sacral promontory
Anterior sacroiliac ligaments
Sacrotuberous ligament
Sacrospinous ligament
Ischial spine
Pubic symphysis
Lesser trochanter
Pubofemoral ligament

c

Iliolumbar ligament
L4 vertebra
L5 vertebra
Posterior sacroiliac ligaments
Ischial spine
Sacrospinous ligament
Sacrotuberous ligament
Ischiofemoral ligament
Ischial tuberosity

Iliac crest
Posterior superior iliac spine
Iliofemoral ligament
Greater trochanter
Intertrochanteric crest
Lesser trochanter

A The ligaments of the right hip joint

a Lateral view, **b** anterior view, **c** posterior view.
The strongest of the three ligaments, the iliofemoral ligament, arises from the anterior inferior iliac spine and fans out at the front of the hip, attaching along the intertrochanteric line (see **b**). With a tensile strength greater than 350 N, it is the most powerful ligament in the human body and provides an important constraint for the hip joint: it keeps the pelvis from tilting posteriorly in the upright stance, without the need for muscular effort. It also limits adduction of the extended limb (particularly the lateral elements of the ligament) and stabilizes the pelvis on the stance side during gait; i.e., it acts with the small gluteal muscles to keep the pelvis from tilting toward the swing side.

B The ligaments of the hip joint

- Iliofemoral ligament
- Pubofemoral ligament
- Ischiofemoral ligament
- Zona orbicularis (anular ligament)*
- Ligament of head of femur**

* Not visible externally, it encircles the femoral neck like a buttonhole (see p. 431, **C**).
** Has no mechanical function, but transmits vessels that supply the femoral head (see also p. 431).

a b

c d

C Actions of the ligaments as a function of joint position

a Right hip joint in extension, lateral view. The capsular ligaments of the hip joint (see facing page) form a ringlike collar that encircles the femoral neck. When the hip is extended, these ligaments become twisted upon themselves (as shown here), pushing the femoral head more firmly into the acetabulum (joint-stabilizing function of the ligaments).

b Right hip joint in flexion, lateral view. During flexion (anteversion), the ligament fibers are lax and press the femoral head less firmly into the acetabulum, allowing a greater degree of femoral mobility.

c, d The twisting mechanism of the capsular ligaments can be represented by a model consisting of two disks interconnected by parallel bands. The situation in **c** represents the position of the ligaments when the hip joint is extended. When one of the two disks rotates (blue arrow), the bands become twisted and draw the two disks closer together (red arrows). Panel **d** models the situation in the flexed hip. The ligaments are no longer twisted, so the distance between the two disks is increased (after Kapandji).

a b

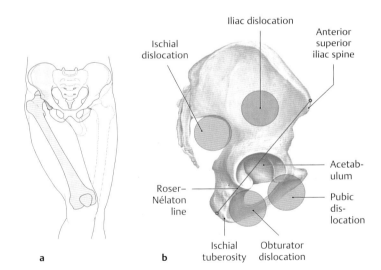

a b

D Weak spots in the capsule of the right hip joint

a Anterior view, **b** posterior view.

There are weak spots in the joint capsule (color-shaded areas) located between the ligaments that strengthen the fibrous membrane (see **A**). External trauma may cause the femoral head to dislocate from the acetabulum at these sites (see **E**).

The combination of great ligament strength and the close congruity of the femoral head in the acetabulum makes the hip joint very stable and dislocations relatively rare. The situation is different, however, following a hip replacement arthroplasty. The hip joint ligaments must be at least partially divided to implant the prosthesis, and the risk of dislocation is markedly increased.

E Traumatic dislocation of the hip

a It is most common for the femoral head to dislocate upward and backward from the acetabulum (iliac dislocation) between the iliofemoral ligament and ischiofemoral ligament. Typically, this is caused by a fall from a great height, a motor vehicle accident (front-end collision), etc. In this type of dislocation, the leg assumes a position of adduction and slight internal rotation.

b Lateral view. Position of the femoral head in various types of dislocation. The greater trochanter may be above or below the Roser–Nélaton line.

429

19.12 The Ligaments of the Hip Joint: Nutrition of the Femoral Head

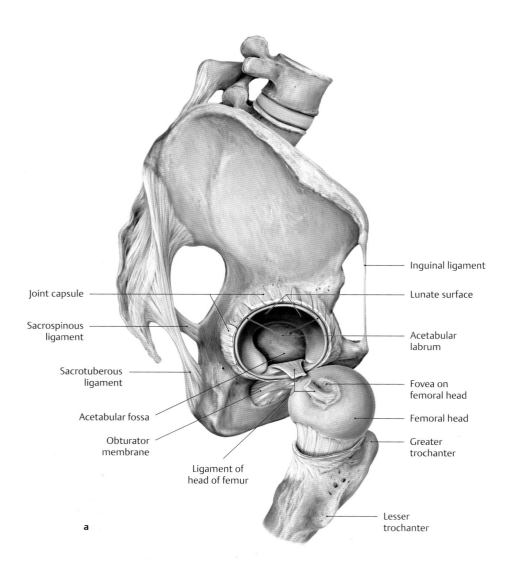

Joint capsule

Sacrospinous ligament

Sacrotuberous ligament

Acetabular fossa

Obturator membrane

Ligament of head of femur

Inguinal ligament

Lunate surface

Acetabular labrum

Fovea on femoral head

Femoral head

Greater trochanter

Lesser trochanter

a

A The ligaments of the right hip joint

a Lateral view. The joint capsule has been divided at the level of the acetabular labrum, and the femoral head has been dislocated to expose the divided ligament of the head of the femur. This ligament transmits important nutrient blood vessels for the femoral head.

b Anterior view. The fibrous membrane of the joint capsule has been removed at the level of the femoral neck to show the conformation of the synovial membrane. This membrane extends laterally from the acetabular rim, and about 1 cm proximal to the attachment of the fibrous membrane, it is reflected onto the femoral neck within the joint cavity. It continues up the femoral neck to the chondro-osseous junction of the femoral head (see also the coronal section in **C**).

c Posterior view.

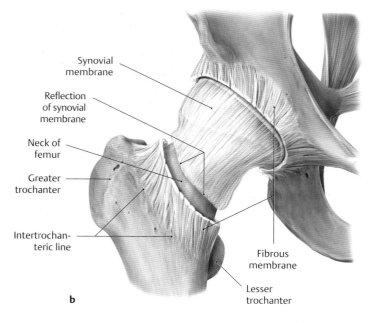

Synovial membrane

Reflection of synovial membrane

Neck of femur

Greater trochanter

Intertrochanteric line

Fibrous membrane

Lesser trochanter

b

Fibrous membrane

Synovial membrane

c

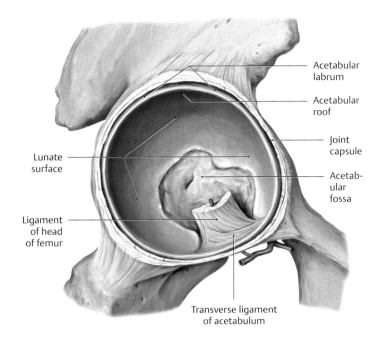

Labels (clockwise from top): Acetabular labrum · Acetabular roof · Joint capsule · Acetabular fossa · Transverse ligament of acetabulum · Ligament of head of femur · Lunate surface

B The acetabulum of the right hip joint with the femoral head removed

Lateral view. The cartilage-covered articular surface of the acetabulum is crescent-shaped (lunate surface) and is broadest and thickest over the acetabular roof. The lunate surface is bounded externally by the slightly protruding bony rim of the acetabulum, which is extended by a lip (the acetabular labrum) composed of tough connective tissue and fibrocartilage. The cartilaginous articular surface lines much of the acetabular fossa, which is occupied by loose, fibrofatty tissue and is bounded inferiorly by the transverse acetabular ligament in the area of the acetabular notch (not visible here). The ligament of the head of the femur, which has been sectioned in the drawing, transmits blood vessels that nourish the femoral head (see **C**).

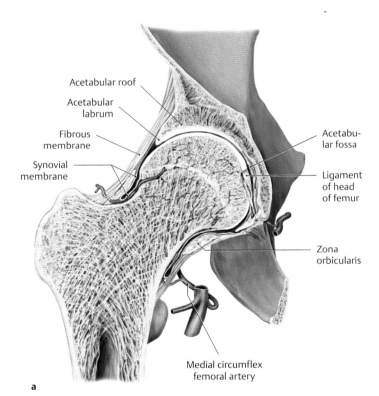

a

Labels (left): Acetabular roof · Acetabular labrum · Fibrous membrane · Synovial membrane · Ligament of head of femur · Medial circumflex femoral artery
Labels (right): Acetabular fossa · Ligament of head of femur · Zona orbicularis

Labels (b): Head of femur · Femoral neck vessels · Synovial membrane · Fibrous membrane · Ligament of head of femur · Medial circumflex femoral artery · Iliopsoas tendon · Deep artery of thigh · Lateral circumflex femoral artery · Lesser trochanter

b

C The blood supply to the femoral head

a Coronal section through the right hip joint, anterior view.
b Course of the femoral neck vessels in relation to the joint capsule (right femur, anterior view).

The femoral head derives its blood supply from the lateral and medial circumflex femoral arteries and the artery of the ligament of the head of the femur, which branches from the obturator artery (see p. 550). If the anastomoses between the vessels of the ligament of the head of the femur and the femoral neck vessels are absent or deficient due to the avulsion of blood vessels caused by a dislocation or femoral neck fracture, the bony tissue in the head of the femur may become necrotic (avascular necrosis of the femoral head).

431

19.13 Cross-sectional and X-Ray Anatomy of the Hip Joint. Typical Medical Condition of the Elderly: Femoral Neck Fractures

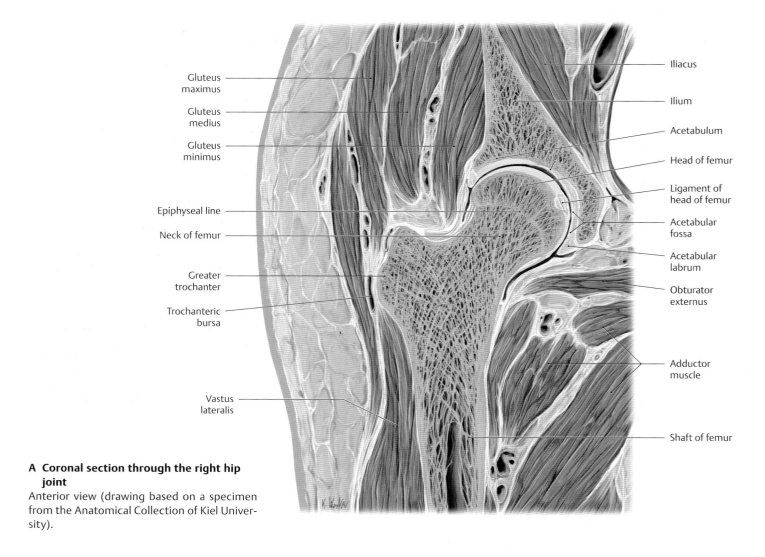

A Coronal section through the right hip joint

Anterior view (drawing based on a specimen from the Anatomical Collection of Kiel University).

B MRI of the hip region: coronal T1-weighted spin-echo (SE) image at the level of the acetabular fossa (from Vahlensieck M, Reiser M. MRT des Bewegungsapparates. 3rd ed. Stuttgart: Thieme; 2006).

C Classification of proximal femoral fractures

Among the femoral fractures close to the hip joint, the medial femoral fractures (see **F**) are typical injuries of the osteoporotic bones of the elderly. Often, the cause is minimal trauma, such as falling on the greater trochanter or the outstretched leg.

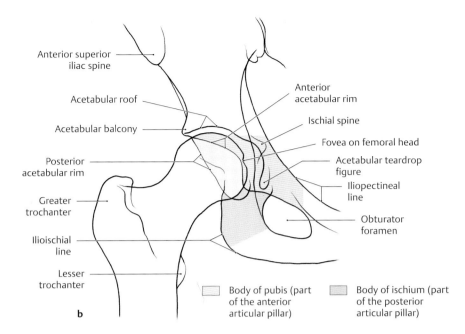

a   b

D X-ray of the hip joint and diagnostic reference levels in case of acetabular fractures

a X-ray of the hip joint in a sagittal beam path (section of a pelvis survey radiograph; from Möller TB, Reif E. Taschenatlas der Röntgenanatomie. 2nd ed. Stuttgart: Thieme; 1998); **b** reference lines important for diagnostic radiology, mainly X-rays of the hip socket.

The pelvis survey radiograph is supplemented only when needed (i.e., when it is not sufficent for making a diagnosis, e.g., in undisplaced femoral fractures) with the help of particular positioning (e.g., ala and obturator view in which the healthy or injured side, respectively, is lifted at 45°) or MRI (see **E**) or CT. The CT is required as soon as an acetabular fracture has been diagnosed.

Particular reference lines in the anteroposterior (AP) view of the pelvis are important for diagnosis or for therapeutic surgical procedures in cases of acetabular fractures: anterior and posterior socket rim, acetabular roof, Köhler's teardrop (equivalent to the depth of the acetabular fossa), and iliopectineal or ilioischial line.

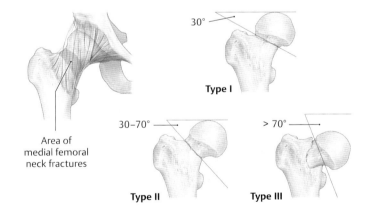

a   b

E Radiologic diagnosis of proximal femoral fractures (from Bohndorf K, Imhof H, Fischer W. Radiologische Diagnostik der Knochen und Gelenke. 2nd ed. Stuttgart: Thieme; 2006)

a Normal X-ray of a medial, undisplaced femoral fracture in a sagittal beam path; **b** MRI identifies fracture: T1-weighted coronal cross section of the same patient with fracture-related edema (red arrows).

Whereas diagnosing displaced factures usually is not a problem since they are visible in AP views of the hip (see **Da**), both undisplaced femoral fractures and stress fractures often appear in conventional X-rays only as slight abnormalities of the trabecular bone structure, so an MRI is needed to identify a fracture (because fracture-related edema can be identified through the lesser signals it emits).

F Medial femoral fractures (classification according to Pauwels)

Medial femoral fractures are much more common than lateral femoral fractures (95% of cases compared to 5% of cases). Medial femoral fractures are always intracapsular and due to common complications associated with them (e.g., ischemic femoral head necrosis, delayed fracture healing, and development of pseudarthrosis) are of particular clinical relevance. In particular, the damage to epiphyseal vessels as a result of intracapsular femoral head fractures leads to impaired blood flow to the femoral head. Medial femoral fractures are classified according to Pauwels by the inclination angle of the fracture line relative to the horizontal line (type I: 0–30°, type II: 30–70°, and type III: > 70°). The steeper the angle, meaning the steeper the course of the fracture line, the greater the risk of the femoral head sliding off and the greater the danger of pseudarthrosis.

433

19.14 Cross-sectional Anatomy of the Hip Joint: Sonographic Representation of Hip Joint Effusion

A Transverse section through the right hip joint
Superior view (drawing based on a specimen from the Anatomical Collection of Kiel University).

B MRI of the hip region: axial (transverse) T1-weighted SE image at the level of the femoral neck (from Vahlensieck and Reiser. MRT des Bewegungsapparates. 3rd ed. Stuttgart: Thieme; 2006).
The synovial bursae shown in **A** are not visible because in T1-weighted MRI, they always appear as low signal intensity and are barely distinguishable from muscles, which are also low signal intensity.
Note: With MRI, axial (transverse) cross sections are always inferior views.

Near transducer

Iliopectineal bursa

Iliopsoas

Gluteus medius

Proximal

Distal

Joint capsule

Hypoechoic area

b   Head of femur   **Away from transducer**   Neck of femur

a   Transducer

Effusion   Articular capsule

c   Head of femur   Neck of femur

Acetabular labrum   Iliopectineal bursa   Iliopsoas   Joint capsule   Gluteus medius

d   Acetabular fossa   Head of femur   Effusion   Neck of femur

C Diagostic ultrasonography of a longitudinal section of the hip: normal and showing hip joint effusion

a Position of the transducer from the front and in the longitudinal direction to the femoral neck; **b** sonogram of a normal finding (from Konermann W, Gruber G. Ultraschalldiagnostik der Bewegungsorgane. 2nd ed. Stuttgart: Thieme; 2006); **c** sonogram of hip joint effusion (from Niethard FU, Pfeil J. Orthopädie. 5th ed. Stuttgart: Thieme; 2005); **d** schematic view of the sonogram. Ultrasonography delivers real-time pictures. Structures at the top of the screen are close to the transducer; those at the bottom are farther away; those on the left side are proximal, those on the right side are distal.

In addition to the diagnostic ultrasound of the embryonic hip joint, the standardized diagnostic ultrasound of the hip joint is of great significance as it is cost-effective and quickly done. Just as in diagnostic x-rays, two almost perpendicular sectional planes (transverse and longitudinal relative to the femoral neck) are recorded. The sonographic examination of the hip joint is performed with the patient lying down. The hip and knee joints are in neutral position (**a**). The longitudinal section allows for a very good evaluation of the anterior parts of the articular capsule and the osseous and periarticular structures of the hip joint. The surface contours of the anterior margin, the crescent-shaped femoral head, and the femoral neck appear as echoic structures. The articular capsule runs parallel to the femoral head and neck and is generally separated from the femoral neck by a narrow low echoic area (**b**). Hip disorders, which are accompanied by increased intra-articular volume (e.g., effusion as part of synovialitis or bacterial coxitis), can be very well shown with the help of an anterior longitudinal section because the effusion appears as a capsular distention at the anterior side of the femoral neck (see **c**). A lateral difference of more than 2 mm between the healthy and affected area (between the articular capsule and the femoral neck) is viewed as significant and implies increased intra-articular volume.

Note: Diagnostic ultrasound helps to show periarticular fluid buildup, e.g., in the case of trochanteric bursitis (= above the greater trochanter).

19.15 The Movements and Biomechanics of the Hip Joint

a

12°

Lumbar lordosis

b

Posterior superior
iliac spine

Anterior superior
iliac spine

20°

c

Iliopsoas   Rectus femoris

Degree of
loss of
extension

0°

B Range of extension of the right hip joint determined with the Thomas maneuver

The Thomas maneuver is used to measure the range of hip extension while the patient lies supine on a hard surface.

a Starting position with a slight degree of anterior pelvic tilt (approximately 12°). In this position it cannot be determined whether or not there is a flexion contraction of the hip joint. This is because the patient can compensate for any limitation of extension by increasing lumbar lordosis (arching the lower back to hyperlordosis) and increasing the degree of anterior pelvic tilt.

b Pelvic tilt can be temporarily eliminated by drawing the opposite hip joint (in this case, the left hip) into a position of maximum flexion. If the right thigh remains flat on the table, the right hip joint will be in approximately 20° of extension (*normal extension*).

c If hip extension is limited (e.g., due to a shortened rectus femoris or iliopsoas muscle), and the opposite (left) hip is placed in maximum flexion, the femur of the affected leg will be raised from the table by an amount equal to the loss of extension. Increased lumbar lordosis is generally present when hip extension is limited and is easily detected clinically by palpating the lower back.

A The axes of motion in the hip joint

Right hip joint, anterior view. As a spheroidal joint, the hip has three principal axes of motion, all of which pass through the center of the femoral head (the rotational center of the hip) and are mutually perpendicular. Accordingly, the joint has three degrees of freedom, allowing movement in six principal directions:

1. Transverse axis: flexion and extension
2. Sagittal axis: abduction and adduction
3. Longitudinal axis: internal rotation and external rotation

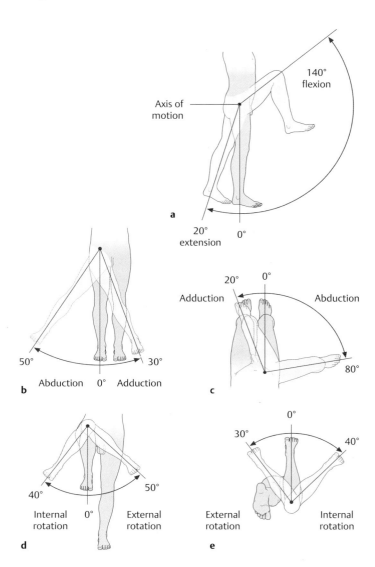

C Range of motion of the hip joint from the neutral (0°) position
(after Debrunner)

The range of motion of the hip joint is measured using the neutral zero method (see p. 50).

a Range of flexion/extension.
b Range of abduction/adduction with the hip extended.
c Range of abduction/adduction with the hip flexed 90°.
d Range of internal rotation/external rotation with the hip flexed 90°.
e Range of internal rotation/external rotation in the prone position with the hip extended (when measuring rotation, the examiner uses the leg, flexed 90°, as a pointer to determine the range of motion).

D Hip joint load depending on the femoral neck angle

Each illustration shows a one-legged stance, standing on the right leg, anterior view. **a** Normal femoral neck angle, around 126°, see p. 415 (the femoral neck angle is also known as the CCD angle—centrum-collum-diaphysis angle, with centrum standing for the center of the femoral head); **b** increased femoral neck angle (coxa valga); **c** decreased femoral neck angle (coxa vara).

The resultant force vector *R* determines the hip joint load when walking or standing on one leg. It is calculated using the partial body weight *K*, muscle force *M*, and length of the lever arms (see p. 51). With a normal CCD angle, the lever arm of the body weight is around 3 times more than the one of the muscle force, meaning in a one-legged stance, the hip joint load is 4 times (*R* = 4) larger than the body weight *K*. Since the lever arm of muscle force in coxa valga (coxa vara) decreases (increases), the hip joint load increases in coxa valga (*R* = 7) and decreases in coxa vara (*R* = 3). *S* is the partial-body center of gravity.

Note: Due to this relationship, surgically changing the femoral neck angle (osteotomy) influences the hip joint load.

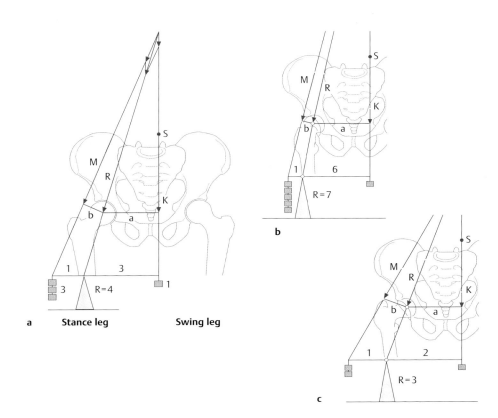

a **Stance leg** **Swing leg**

b

c

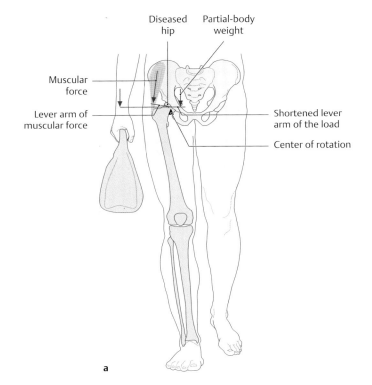

Muscular force

Lever arm of muscular force

Diseased hip

Partial-body weight

Shortened lever arm of the load

Center of rotation

a

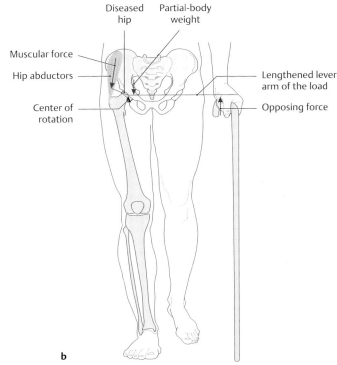

Diseased hip

Partial-body weight

Muscular force

Hip abductors

Center of rotation

Lengthened lever arm of the load

Opposing force

b

E Reducing the stresses on an osteoarthritic right hip

Anterior view. In patients with advanced osteoarthritis of the hip, various measures can be taken to alleviate the stresses, and thus the pain, on the affected side.

a Shift the partial-body center of gravity (see above) toward the affected side. One way to do this is by carrying a shopping bag *on the affected right side*, as shown here. This moves the partial-body center of gravity closer to the center of the femoral head, thereby *shortening* the lever arm of the load (in this case, the partial-body weight)

and also reducing the torque generated by the partial-body weight. The same effect is produced by adopting a *Duchenne limp*—an unconscious response in which the patient leans over the affected side with the upper body during the stance phase of gait (see also p. 536).

b Use a cane *on the unaffected (left) side*. While this *lengthens* the lever arm of the load (the partial-body weight), it also provides a force (the cane) that counteracts the body load at the end of that lever arm. This reduces the torque generated by the load (as in **a**).

19.16 The Development of the Hip Joint

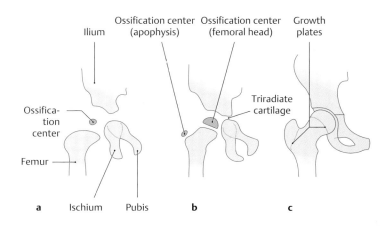

B Stages in the radiographic development of the hip joint
Schematic representations of AP radiographs taken at various stages in the development of the right hip joint. The ossification centers are indicated by dark shading.

a Ossification center
b

A Radiographic appearance of the right hip joint
Anteroposterior projection.

a Boy, 2 years of age (original film from the Department of Diagnostic Radiology, Schleswig-Holstein University Hospital, Kiel Campus, Prof. S. Müller-Hülsbeck, M.D.).
Note: The ossification center for the femoral head is already visible.
b Man 25 years of age (from Möller TB, Reif E. Taschenatlas der Röntgenanatomie. 2nd ed. Stuttgart: Thieme; 1998).

a The ossification center for the femoral head can be identified at 6 months of age.
b Ossification centers for the femoral head and greater trochanter are visible at 4 years of age.
c At 15 years of age, the growth plates have not yet fused.

The anatomic differentiation of all structures that comprise the hip joint is largely complete by the 12th week of development (crown–rump length 80 mm). Whereas ossification of the acetabulum begins between the 3rd and 6th months of fetal development, the ossification center for the capital femoral epiphysis (femoral head) does not appear until about 5 to 6 months after birth. The ossification center for the apophysis of the greater trochanter appears during the 4th year of life. Fusion of the growth plates takes place between 16 and 18 years of age in the proximal femur and at about 15 years of age in the triradiate cartilage.

a

 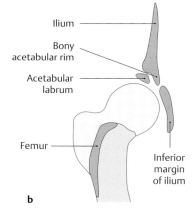

b

C Ultrasound evaluation of the infant hip (from Niethard FU, Pfeil J. Orthopädie. 5th ed. Stuttgart: Thieme; 2005).
a Normal hip joint in a 5-month-old child.
b Hip dislocation (type IV) in a 3-month-old child.

Ultrasonography is the most important imaging method for screening the infant hip, demonstrating potential morphological changes during the 1st year of life without exposure to ionizing radiation. The child is examined in the lateral decubitus position (on his or her side, other hip on the examination table) with the ultrasound transducer placed

longitudinally over the hip joint and perpendicular to the skin. The key landmark is the superior acetabular rim, i. e., the bony and cartilaginous roof of the acetabulum (see **D**). Infant hips are classified into four types based on their sonographic features:

- Type I   Normal hip
- Type II   Physiologically immature hip
- Type III Subluxated hip
- Type IV   Dislocated hip

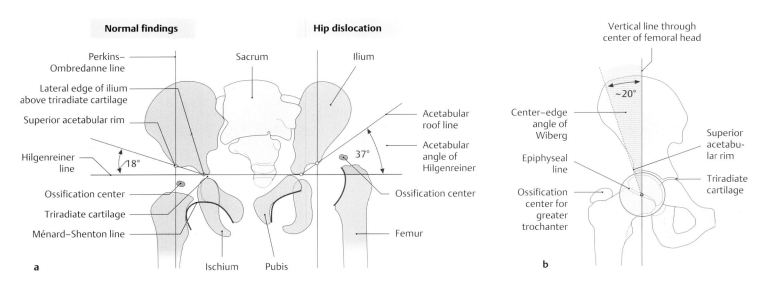

D Radiographic evaluation of the pediatric hip
Schematic representations of AP pelvic radiographs. Radiographic evaluation of the infant hip is feasible after 3 months of age, by which time there has been sufficient ossification of the joint. Both hips should always be imaged on the same radiograph.

a Normal findings (left half of figure) contrasted with findings in congenital hip dislocation (right half of figure) in a 2-year-old child. The following standard reference lines are used in the radiographic analysis of the infant hip:

- *Hilgenreiner line:* connects the inferolateral edge of the ilium above the triradiate cartilage on both sides.
- *Perkins–Ombredanne line:* drawn from the most lateral edge of the acetabular roof, perpendicular to the Hilgenreiner line.
- *Menard–Shenton line:* curved line drawn from the superior border of the obturator foramen along the medial border of the femoral neck.
- *Acetabular angle of Hilgenreiner (AC angle):* angle formed by the intersection of the Hilgenreiner line and a line connecting the

superior acetabular rim with the lowest part of the ilium at the triradiate cartilage (see p. 413). This angle measures approximately 35° at birth, approximately 25° at 1 year of age, and should be less than 10° by 15 years of age.

Typically, the acetabular angle of Hilgenreiner is increased on the affected (left) side, while the center–edge angle of Wiberg (see below) is decreased. Additionally, there is a discontinuity in the Menard–Shenton line, and the Perkins–Ombredanne line runs medial to the femoral shaft.

b Evaluation of lateral femoral head coverage based on the center–edge angle of Wiberg (drawing of a radiograph of the right hip in a 5-year-old child). The angle is formed by a vertical line through the center of the femoral head (within the future epiphyseal line) and a line drawn from the center of the femoral head to the superior acetabular rim. The center–edge angle should not be less than 10° between 1 and 4 years of age, and it should be in the range of 15 to 20° at 5 years of age.

E Clinical examination of congenital dysplasia and dislocation of the hip
Hip dysplasia is characterized by an abnormal development of the acetabulum (acetabular dysplasia) in which the steep, flattened acetabular roof provides insufficient coverage for the femoral head (see also **D**). The principal complication is dislocation of the hip, since the femoral head is poorly contained in the dysplastic acetabulum and may be displaced upward and backward as a result of muscular traction or external loads. The *etiology* of hip dysplasia and dislocation is related to endogenous factors (familial disposition, maternal hormone status), as well as exogenous factors.

The following *clinical signs* may direct attention to a dysplastic or dislocated hip:

- Instability of the hip joint: paucity of kicking activity or a positive Ortolani click caused by subluxation of the femoral head. The Ortolani test requires a very experienced examiner. While still considered part of the clinical examination, it is performed less often today owing to the availability of ultrasound.
- Leg shortening with asymmetry of the posterior leg folds and gluteal folds.
- Limitation of abduction due to increased reflex tension from the hip adductors.

439

19.17 The Knee Joint: Articulating Bones

Femur

Patella

Lateral epicondyle

Lateral femoral condyle

Lateral tibial condyle

Tibial plateau

Fibula

Tibia

Medial epicondyle

Medial femoral condyle

Medial tibial condyle

Tibial tuberosity

Popliteal surface

Intercondylar notch

Lateral epicondyle

Lateral femoral condyle

Intercondylar eminence

Tibiofibular joint

Head of fibula

Neck of fibula

Soleal line

Tibia

Shaft of fibula

a

b

A The right knee joint from the anterior view (a) and posterior view (b)

Three bones articulate at the knee joint: the femur, tibia, and patella. The femur and tibia form the *femorotibial joint*, while the femur and patella form the *femoropatellar joint*. Both joints are contained within a common capsule and have communicating articular cavities (see p. 450). Contrasting with the elbow joint, where the forearm bones articulate with the humerus, the fibula is *not* included in the knee joint. It forms a separate, rigid articulation with the tibia called the *tibiofibular joint*.

a   b

B The knee joint

Right knee joint: **a** anteroposterior projection, **b** lateral projection (original films from the Department of Diagnostic Radiology, Schleswig-Holstein University Hospital, Kiel Campus, Prof. S. Müller-Hülsbeck, M. D.).

There are three standard radiographic views of the knee that demonstrate the joint in three planes: anteroposterior, lateral, and tangential. The *anteroposterior (AP) view* is particularly useful for evaluating the width of the joint space and the contours of the tibial plateau. *Lateral views* are good for evaluating the shape of the femoral condyles and the height of the patella. The *tangential (sunrise) view* is used mainly for examining the femoropatellar joint and evaluating the position of the patella in the femoral trochlea (see **C**).

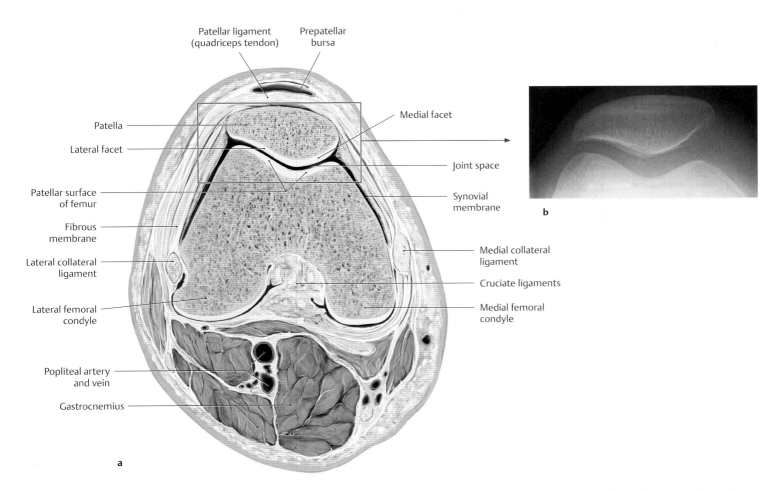

C The femoropatellar joint

a Transverse section at the level of the femoropatellar joint. Right knee joint in slight flexion, distal view (drawn from a specimen in the Anatomical Collection of Kiel University).

b Tangential radiographic view of the patella and femoral trochlea ("sunrise" view of the right knee joint in 60° flexion with the beam parallel to the posterior patellar surface). This view is excel-

lent for evaluating the articular surface of the patella and the femoral trochlea. The radiographic "joint space" appears particularly wide owing to the relatively thick articular cartilage in this region (articular cartilage is not visible on radiographs). (Original film from the Department of Diagnostic Radiology, Schleswig-Holstein University Hospital, Kiel Campus, Prof. S. Müller-Hülsbeck, M. D.).

19.18 The Ligaments of the Knee Joint: An Overview

A The capsule, ligaments, and periarticular bursae of the popliteal fossa

Right knee, posterior view. Besides the ligaments that reinforce the joint capsule (the oblique popliteal ligament and arcuate popliteal ligament), the capsule is strengthened posteriorly by the tendinous attachments of the muscles in the popliteal region. There are several sites where the joint cavity communicates with periarticular bursae—these include the subpopliteal recess, the semimembranosus bursa, and the medial subtendinous bursa of the gastrocnemius.

a

b

B Gastrocnemio-semimembranosus bursa ("Baker cyst") in the popliteal region

a Depiction of a Baker cyst in the right popliteal fossa. A painful swelling behind the knee may be caused by a cystic outpouching of the joint capsule ("synovial popliteal cyst"). This frequently results from a joint effusion (e.g., in rheumatoid arthritis) causing a rise of intra-articular pressure. A common *Baker cyst* is a cystic protrusion occurring in the medial part of the popliteal fossa between the semimembranosus tendon and the medial head of the gastrocnemius at the level of the posteromedial femoral condyle (gastrocnemio-semimembranosus bursa = communication between the semimembranosus bursa and the medial subtendinous bursa of the gastrocnemius).

b Axial MR image of a knee with a Baker cyst. The cystic mass in the popliteal fossa and its communication with the joint cavity appear as conspicuous areas of high signal intensity in the T2-weighted image (from Vahlensieck M, Reiser M. MRT des Bewegungsapparates. 3rd ed. Stuttgart: Thieme; 2006).

D Location of the cruciate ligaments and menisci in the knee joint

Anterior view of the right knee, in which the capsule and patella are shown in light shading. The cruciate ligaments are colored dark blue, the menisci red.

E Overview of the ligaments of the knee joint

Because its articulating bony surfaces are not closely apposed over a large area, the knee must rely upon a group of strong and extensive ligaments for stability. These ligaments of the knee joint can be segregated into two groups, extrinsic and intrinsic.

Extrinsic ligaments

• Anterior side
  – Patellar ligament
  – Medial longitudinal patellar retinaculum
  – Lateral longitudinal patellar retinaculum
  – Medial transverse patellar retinaculum
  – Lateral transverse patellar retinaculum
• Medial and lateral sides
  – Medial collateral ligament (tibial collateral ligament)
  – Lateral collateral ligament (fibular collateral ligament)
• Posterior side
  – Oblique popliteal ligament
  – Arcuate popliteal ligament

Intrinsic ligaments

– Anterior cruciate ligament
  – Posterior cruciate ligament
  – Transverse ligament of the knee
  – Posterior meniscofemoral ligament

C The anterior and lateral capsule and ligaments of the right knee joint

Anterior view. The capsule and ligaments at the front of the knee serve mainly to stabilize the patella. The key stabilizers for this purpose are the tendons of insertion of the rectus femoris and vastus medialis and lateralis, the longitudinal and transverse patellar retinacula, and, at a deeper level, the meniscopatellar ligaments.

19.19 The Knee Joint: The Cruciate and Collateral Ligaments

Patellar surface of femur

Anterior cruciform ligament

Transverse liga- ment of knee

Lateral meniscus

Lateral collateral ligament

Anterior ligament of fibular head

Fibula

Posterior cruciate ligament

Medial meniscus

Medial collateral ligament

Patellar ligament

Patella

Intercondylar notch

Lateral femoral condyle

Anterior cruciate ligament

Posterior meniscofemoral ligament

Lateral meniscus

Lateral collateral ligament

Posterior ligament of fibular head

Head of fibula

Interosseous membrane

Tibia

Medial femoral condyle

a

b

A The cruciate ligaments of the right knee joint

a Anterior view. The patellar ligament has been reflected downward with the attached patella.
b Posterior view.

The cruciate ligaments of the knee stretch between the anterior and posterior intercondylar areas of the tibia (not visible here; see p. 446) and the intercondylar notch of the femur.

- The anterior cruciate ligament runs from the anterior intercondylar area of the tibia to the medial surface of the lateral femoral condyle.

- The posterior cruciate ligament is thicker than the anterior ligament and runs approximately at right angles to it, passing from the posterior intercondylar area to the lateral surface of the medial femoral condyle.

The cruciate ligaments keep the articular surfaces of the femur and tibia in contact while stabilizing the knee joint primarily in the sagittal plane. Some portions of the cruciate ligaments are taut in every position of the joint (see p. 448).

Femur

Quadriceps femoris

Femoro-patellar joint

Patellar ligament

Medial surface of tibia

Medial epicondyle

Medial femoral condyle

Medial meniscus

Medial collateral ligament

Fibula

a

Quadriceps tendon

Lateral epicondyle

Lateral femoral condyle

Lateral collateral ligament

Posterior ligament of fibular head

Head of fibula

Fibula

Patella

Patellar surface of femur

Lateral meniscus

Patellar ligament

Anterior ligament of fibular head

Tibial tuberosity

b

B The collateral ligaments and patellar ligament of the right knee joint

a Medial view, **b** lateral view.

The knee joint has two collateral ligaments:

- The medial collateral ligament on the medial view of the knee.
- The lateral collateral ligament on the lateral view of the knee.

The *medial collateral ligament* (tibial collateral ligament) is the broader of the two ligaments. It runs obliquely downward and forward from the medial epicondyle of the femur to the medial surface of the upper tibia approximately 7 to 8 cm below the tibial plateau. The *lateral collateral ligament* (fibular collateral ligament) is a round cord that runs obliquely downward and backward from the lateral epicondyle of the femur to the head of the fibula. Both of the collateral ligaments are taut when the knee is in *extension* (see **A**). When the knee is in *flexion*, the radius of curvature is decreased, and the origins and insertions of the collateral ligaments move closer together, causing the ligaments to become lax. Both collateral ligaments stabilize the knee joint in the coronal plane. Thus, damage or rupture of these ligaments can be diagnosed by examining the mediolateral stability of the knee and the extent of medial and lateral opening of the joint space with manipulation.

Note the different relationship of each collateral ligament to the joint capsule and associated meniscus. The *medial* collateral ligament is firmly attached both to the capsule and the medial meniscus, whereas the *lateral* collateral ligament has no direct contact with the capsule or the lateral meniscus. As a result, the medial meniscus is less mobile than the lateral meniscus and is thus far more susceptible to injury (see also p. 447).

445

19.20 The Knee Joint: The Menisci

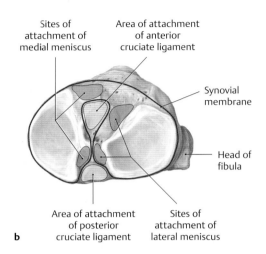

a

b

A The tibial plateau with the medial and lateral menisci and the sites of attachment of the menisci and cruciate ligaments

Right tibial plateau, proximal view with the cruciate and collateral ligaments divided and the femur removed.

a Shape and attachments of the menisci: The medial and lateral menisci are both crescent-shaped when viewed from above (L. *meniscus* = crescent). Their ends (the anterior and posterior horns) are attached by short ligaments to the bone of the anterior and posterior intercondylar areas of the tibia. The *lateral meniscus* forms almost a complete ring, while the *medial meniscus* has a more semicircular shape. On the whole, the medial meniscus is less mobile than the lateral meniscus because its points of attachment to the bone are spaced farther

apart (see **b**), and it is also firmly attached peripherally to the medial collateral ligament. The lateral meniscus, by contrast, has no attachment to the lateral collateral ligament (see **E**).

b Sites of attachment of the medial and lateral menisci and the cruciate ligaments: The red line indicates the tibial attachment of the synovial membrane, which covers the cruciate ligaments anteriorly and at the sides. The cruciate ligaments lie in the subsynovial connective tissue of the joint capsule and are covered posteriorly by the heavy fibrous membrane. Because the cruciate ligaments migrate forward into the knee joint during development, they are extracapsular but intra-articular in their location (see also p. 450), and they derive their blood supply from the popliteal fossa (middle genicular artery, see p. 561).

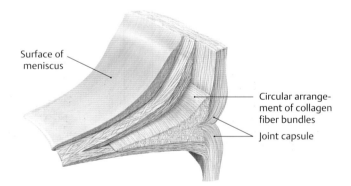

B Blood supply to the menisci

Schematic coronal section through the femorotibial joint. The fibrous portions of the menisci located adjacent to the capsule have a rich blood supply (the medial and lateral inferior articular arteries from the popliteal artery, see p. 561). But the more central portions of the menisci, composed of fibrocartilage, are avascular and are nourished entirely by the synovial fluid (arrows).

C Structure of the meniscus

The meniscus has a wedge-shaped cross section, the base of the wedge being directed toward the periphery and attached to the joint capsule. The surface facing the tibial plateau is flat, while the upper surface facing the femoral condyles is concave. The central, inner two thirds of the menisci are composed of fibrocartilage and the outer third of tough connective tissue. The bundles of collagen fibers in both the fibrocartilage and the connective tissue have a predominantly circular arrangement, reflecting the high tensile stresses that develop in the menisci. The ability of the meniscal tissue to move outward in response to loading is similar to that found in intervertebral disks (converting pressure to tensile forces) (after Petersen and Tillmann).

D Coronal section through the femorotibial joint

Right knee, anterior view. An essential task of the menisci is to increase the surface area available for load transfer across the knee joint. With their different curvatures, the menisci compensate for the mismatch in the articulating surfaces of the femur and tibia. They absorb approximately one third of the loads imposed on the knee, and they help to distribute the pressures more evenly within the femorotibial joint.

E Movements of the menisci during flexion of the knee

The drawings show a right knee joint from the lateral view in extension (**a**) and flexion (**b**) and the associated tibial plateau viewed from above in extension (**c**) and flexion (**d**).

Note that the medial meniscus, which is anchored more securely than the lateral meniscus, undergoes considerably less displacement during knee flexion.

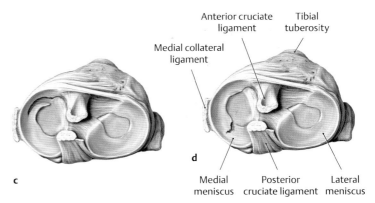

F Different patterns of meniscal tears

Right tibial plateau, proximal view.

a Peripheral tear.
b Bucket-handle tear.
c Longitudinal or flap tear of the anterior horn.
d Radial tear of the posterior horn.

The medial meniscus, being less mobile, is injured far more often than the lateral meniscus. Meniscal injuries most commonly result from sudden extension or rotational movements of the flexed knee (external and internal rotation) while the leg is fixed, as may occur while skiing or playing soccer. The resultant shearing forces can tear the substance of the meniscus or avulse it from its peripheral attachment. The cardinal feature of a fresh meniscal injury is a painful limitation of active and passive knee extension immediately after the trauma, while the patient favors the knee by keeping it slightly flexed. Degenerative changes in the menisci occur with aging and are exacerbated by excessive loads and angular deformities of the knee (genu varum or valgum, see p. 410).

19.21 The Movements of the Knee Joint

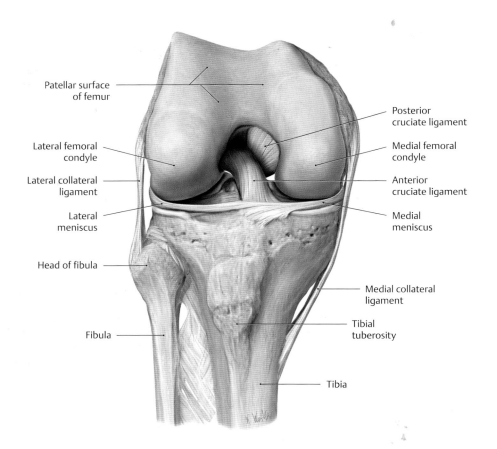

Patellar surface of femur

Lateral femoral condyle

Lateral collateral ligament

Lateral meniscus

Head of fibula

Fibula

Posterior cruciate ligament

Medial femoral condyle

Anterior cruciate ligament

Medial meniscus

Medial collateral ligament

Tibial tuberosity

Tibia

A The right knee joint in flexion
Anterior view with the joint capsule and patella removed.

a

b

c

C Behavior of the cruciate and collateral ligaments in flexion and extension
Right knee, anterior view. Ligament fibers that are taut are colored red.

a Extension.
b Flexion.
c Flexion and internal rotation.

While the collateral knee ligaments are taut *only in extension* (**a**), the cruciate ligaments, or at least portions of them, are taut *in every joint position*: the medial portions of both cruciate ligaments in extension (**a**), the lateral part of the anterior cruciate ligament and the entire posterior cruciate ligament in flexion (**b**), the medial part of the anterior ligament and the entire posterior ligament in flexion and internal rotation (**c**). The cruciate ligaments thus help stabilize the knee in any joint position.

a

b

B Condition after rupture of the anterior cruciate ligament
a Right knee joint in flexion, anterior view.
b Right knee joint in flexion, medial view.

The instability that results from a cruciate ligament rupture allows the tibia to be moved forward or backward like a drawer relative to the femur, depending on whether the anterior or posterior cruciate ligament has been torn ("anterior or posterior drawer sign," elicited with the Lachman test). A rupture of the anterior cruciate ligament, as shown in the diagram, is approximately 10 times more common than a rupture of the posterior ligament. The most common mechanism of injury is an internal rotation trauma with the leg fixed (see **D**). A lateral blow to the fully extended knee, with foot planted, tends to cause concomitant rupture of the anterior cruciate ligament and the medial collateral ligament, and tearing of the attached medial meniscus, referred to colloquially as the "unhappy triad."

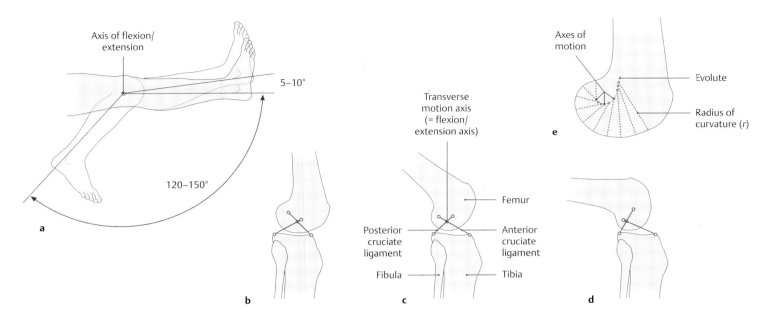

D Flexion and extension of the knee joint

Right knee joint, lateral view.

Flexion and extension of the knee joint take place about a transverse axis (**a**) that passes through the dynamic center of rotation in any joint position. That center is located at the point where both the collateral ligaments and the cruciate ligaments intersect (**b**). With increasing flexion of the knee (**c, d**), the dynamic flexion axis moves upward and backward along a curved line (the evolute, **e**). The momentary distance from that curve to the articular surface of the femur is equal to the changing radius of curvature (*r*) of the femoral condyle. The total range of motion, especially in flexion, depends on various parameters (soft-tissue restraints, active insufficiency or hamstring tightness, see p. 485).

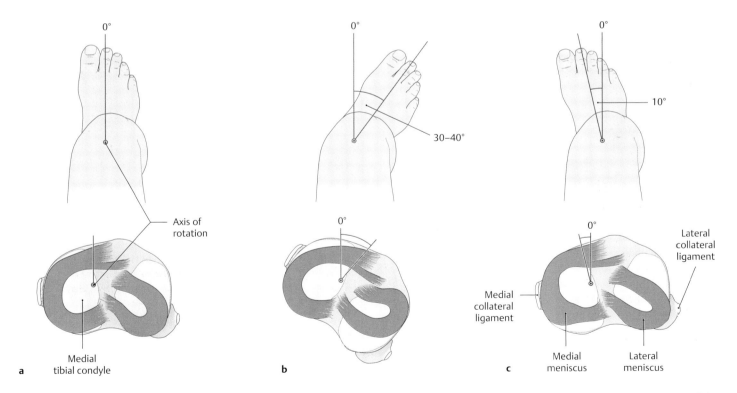

E Rotational movements of the tibia relative to the femur with the knee flexed 90°

Right knee joint, proximal view of the flexed knee and corresponding tibial plateau.

a Neutral (0°) position.
b External rotation.
c Internal rotation.

The axis of tibial rotation runs vertically through the medial part of the medial tibial condyle. Because the cruciate ligaments (not shown here) twist around each other during internal rotation, the range of internal rotation in the knee (approximately 10°) is considerably smaller than the range of external rotation (30–40°). As a result, the majority of cruciate ligament tears occur during internal rotation and involve the anterior cruciate ligament.

Note the different degrees of displacement of the lateral and medial menisci.

449

19.22 The Knee Joint: Capsule and Joint Cavity

Femur

Suprapatellar pouch

Synovial fold lying with anterior cruciate ligament

Lateral femoral condyle

Lateral collateral ligament

Lateral meniscus

Patellar surface of femur

Medial femoral condyle

Medial meniscus

Alar folds

Position of Hoffa's fat pad

Infrapatellar fat pad

Patella (articular surface)

Cut edge of joint capsule

Suprapatellar pouch

Fibula

Tibia

A The right knee with the joint capsule opened

The patella has been reflected downward. In the anterior meniscofemoral portion of the joint capsule, variable folds of the capsule project into the joint cavity (alar folds on both sides of the infrapatellar fat pad), increasing its capacity.

C Anterior femoral and tibial attachments of the joint capsule

Right knee joint, anterior view.

Quadriceps tendon

Suprapatellar pouch

Femur

Lateral collateral ligament

Subpopliteal recess

Fibula

Patella

Lateral meniscus

Patellar ligament

Infrapatellar bursa

Tibia

B Extent of the joint cavity

Right knee joint, lateral view. The joint cavity was demonstrated by injecting a liquid plastic into the knee joint and later removing the capsule after the plastic had cured.

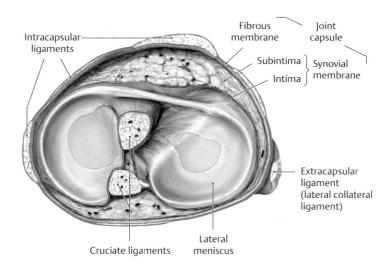

Intracapsular ligaments

Fibrous membrane

Joint capsule

Subintima

Intima

Synovial membrane

Extracapsular ligament (lateral collateral ligament)

Cruciate ligaments

Lateral meniscus

D Structure of the articular capsule

Right knee after removal of femur (articular capsule and ligaments severed), superior view.

Note: The cruciate ligaments run in the subintima of the synovial membrane and are thus intracapsular but extra-articular (compare p. 43). In contrast, the menisci are intra-articular because they are not covered by a synovial intima and have direct contact with synovial fluid.

Femur

Supra-
patellar
pouch

Quadri-
ceps
tendon

Patella

Prepatellar
bursa

Patellar
ligament

Infrapatellar
fat pad

Anterior inter-
condylar area

Infrapatellar
bursa

Tibia

Popliteal
artery and
vein

Anterior
cruciate
ligament

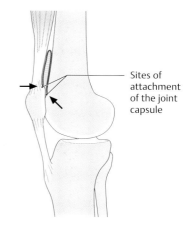

Sites of
attachment
of the joint
capsule

a

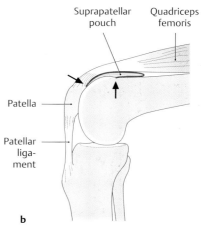

Suprapatellar
pouch

Quadriceps
femoris

Patella

Patellar
liga-
ment

b

c

E Mid-sagittal section through the right knee joint

Note the extent of the suprapatellar pouch (also called the suprapatellar *bursa*) and compare it with **F**. *Note* also the placement of the infrapatellar fat pad between the anterior intercondylar area and the deep surface of the patellar ligament. A fall onto the knee or chronic mechanical irritation due to frequent kneeling can cause pain and inflammation of the bursae about the patella: infrapatellar bursitis ("clergyman's knee") and prepatellar bursitis (drawn from a specimen in the Anatomical Collection of Kiel University).

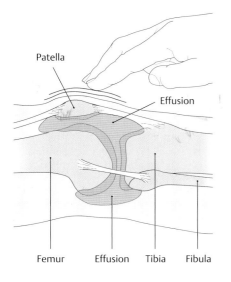

Patella

Effusion

Femur   Effusion   Tibia   Fibula

F The "ballottable patella sign" of knee effusion

When an effusion develops in the knee joint due to inflammatory changes or injury, various degrees of joint swelling may be seen. To differentiate an intra-articular effusion from swelling of the joint capsule itself, the leg is placed in a position of maximum extension. This will force the (potentially increased) intra-articular fluid out of the suprapatellar pouch and into the space between the patella and femur. The examiner then pushes the patella downward with the index finger. If there is excessive fluid in the joint, the patella will rebound when released, signifying a positive test.

G Unfolding of the suprapatellar pouch during flexion

Right knee joint, medial view.

a Neutral (0°) position.
b 80° of flexion.
c 130° of flexion.

The suprapatellar pouch extends proximally from the superior pole of the patella, turns back distally, and inserts at the chondro-osseous junction on the patellar surface of the femur. This redundant fold provides a reserve capacity when the knee is flexed, opening up completely past about 130° of flexion.

451

19.23 Cross-sectional Anatomy of the Knee

A Magnetic resonance imaging of the knee joint
(from Vahlensieck M, Reiser M. MRT des Bewegungsapparates. 3rd ed. Stuttgart: Thieme; 2006)

T1-weighted sagittal sequences at the level of the outer meniscus (**a**) and the cruciate ligaments (**b**).

The strength of MRI when evaluating joints includes the differentiated representation of the joint's internal structure, the capsular ligament apparatus, the surrounding soft tissue, and the subchondral bone. In addition to the T1-weighted images, which are primarily suited for anatomic orientation and tissue characterization, the T2-weighted pro-

ton-density fat saturation sequences (PDFS) play an important role in the diagnosis of joint damage because they are very sensitive to edematous changes (e.g., fractures) and allow for the high signal intensity of the hyaline articular cartilage (see **B**). (In MRI, fat emits a high signal, which, however, is often adverse and thus needs to be suppressed.)

Note: In sagittal cross sections, the posterior cruciate ligament is clearly visible in its entirety, even its archlike course from posterior to superior. In contrast, the anterior cruciate ligament is only visible in its entirety when the knee joint, as shown here, is externally rotated at 15 to 20°.

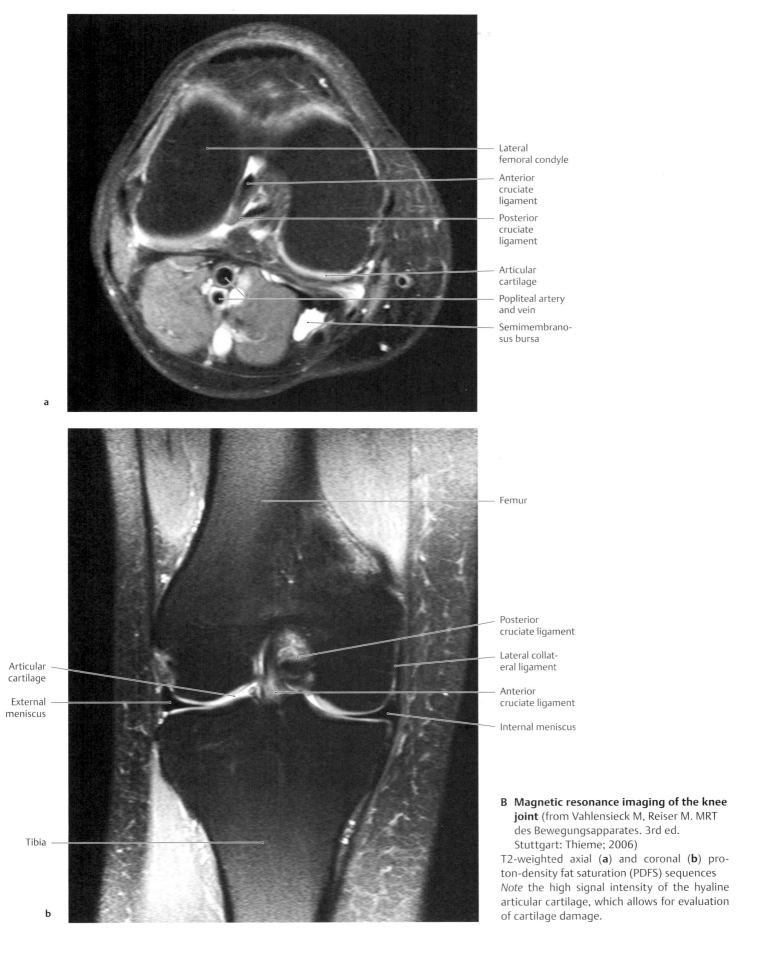

a

—— Lateral
femoral condyle

—— Anterior
cruciate
ligament

—— Posterior
cruciate
ligament

—— Articular
cartilage

—— Popliteal artery
and vein

—— Semimembrano-
sus bursa

—— Femur

Posterior
cruciate ligament

Lateral collat-
eral ligament

Anterior
cruciate ligament

Internal meniscus

Articular
cartilage

External
meniscus

Tibia

b

**B Magnetic resonance imaging of the knee
joint** (from Vahlensieck M, Reiser M. MRT
des Bewegungsapparates. 3rd ed.
Stuttgart: Thieme; 2006)
T2-weighted axial (**a**) and coronal (**b**) pro-
ton-density fat saturation (PDFS) sequences
Note the high signal intensity of the hyaline
articular cartilage, which allows for evaluation
of cartilage damage.

19.24 The Joints of the Foot: Overview of the Articulating Bones and Joints

a

A The articulating bones in different joints of the right foot

a Anterior view with the talocrural joint in plantar flexion.
b Posterior view with the foot in the neutral (0°) position.

b

B Overview of the joints in the foot

- Talocrural joint (ankle joint)
- Subtalar joint (talocalcaneal joint and talocalcaneonavicular joint)*
- Calcaneocuboid joint (between the calcaneus and cuboid bone)
- Talonavicular joint (between the talus and navicular bone)
- Transverse tarsal joint**
- Cuneonavicular joint (between the cuneiform and navicular bones)
- Intercuneiform joints (between the cuneiform bones)
- Cuneocuboid joint (between the lateral cuneiform and cuboid bones)
- Tarsometatarsal joints
- Intermetatarsal joints (between the bases of the metatarsal bones)
- Metatarsophalangeal joints
- Proximal interphalangeal joints
- Distal interphalangeal joints

* In the subtalar joint, the talus articulates with the calcaneus and the navicular bone to form two separate articulations: the talocalcaneal joint posteriorly and the talocalcaneonavicular joint anteriorly. Both are often referred to collectively as the "subtalar joint."

** Consists of the calcaneocuboid joint and talonavicular joint.

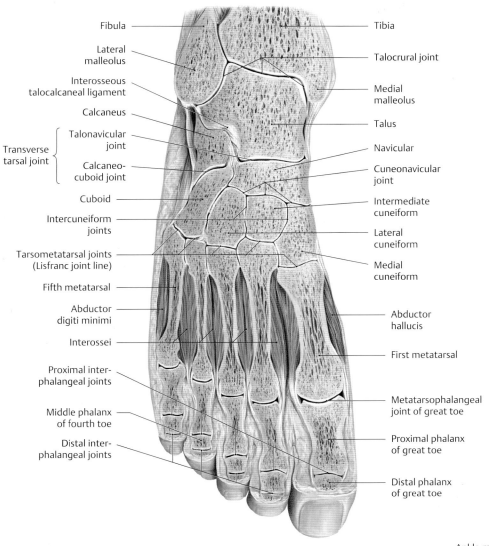

Fibula

Lateral malleolus

Interosseous talocalcaneal ligament

Calcaneus

Talonavicular joint

Calcaneo-cuboid joint

Transverse tarsal joint

Cuboid

Intercuneiform joints

Tarsometatarsal joints (Lisfranc joint line)

Fifth metatarsal

Abductor digiti minimi

Interossei

Proximal inter-phalangeal joints

Middle phalanx of fourth toe

Distal inter-phalangeal joints

Tibia

Talocrural joint

Medial malleolus

Talus

Navicular

Cuneonavicular joint

Intermediate cuneiform

Lateral cuneiform

Medial cuneiform

Abductor hallucis

First metatarsal

Metatarsophalangeal joint of great toe

Proximal phalanx of great toe

Distal phalanx of great toe

Plane of section

C Oblique transverse section through the foot

Right foot, superior view. The foot is plantar flexed at the talocrural (ankle) joint (drawn from a specimen in the Anatomical Collection of Kiel University).

Ankle mortise

Extensor hallucis

Extensor digitorum

Tibialis anterior

Tibia

Articular facet of lateral malleolus

Medial malleolus

Superior surface of talar dome

Tibialis posterior

Flexor digitorum longus

Flexor hallucis longus

Posterior tibial vessels

Abductor hallucis

Quadratus plantae

Tibiofibular syndesmosis

Fibula

Talocrural joint

Articular facet of medial malleolus

Lateral malleolus

Subtalar (talo-calcaneal) joint

Fibularis brevis

Fibularis longus

Calcaneus

Flexor digitorum brevis

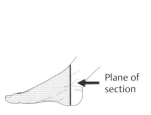

Plane of section

D Coronal section through the talocrural and subtalar joints

Right foot, proximal view. The talocrural joint is plantar flexed, and the subtalar joint is sectioned through its posterior compartment (drawn from a specimen in the Anatomical Collection of Kiel University).

19.25 The Joints of the Foot: Articular Surfaces

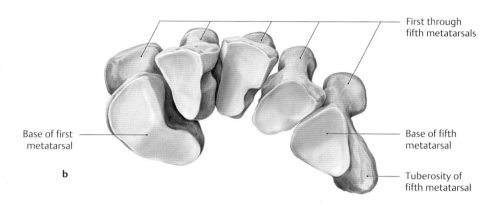

Base of first proximal phalanx

a

First through fifth metatarsals

Base of first metatarsal

Base of fifth metatarsal

Tuberosity of fifth metatarsal

b

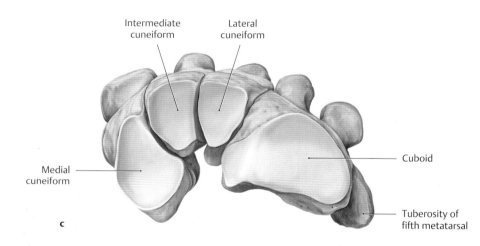

Intermediate cuneiform

Lateral cuneiform

Medial cuneiform

Cuboid

Tuberosity of fifth metatarsal

c

Navicular

Cuboid

d

A Proximal articular surfaces
Right foot, proximal view.

a Metatarsophalangeal joints: bases of the first through fifth proximal phalanges.
b Tarsometatarsal joints: bases of the first through fifth metatarsals.
c Cuneonavicular joint and calcaneocuboid joint: proximal articular surfaces of the medial, intermediate, and lateral cuneiform bones and the cuboid.
d Talonavicular joint and calcaneocuboid joint: proximal articular surfaces of the navicular and cuboid bones.

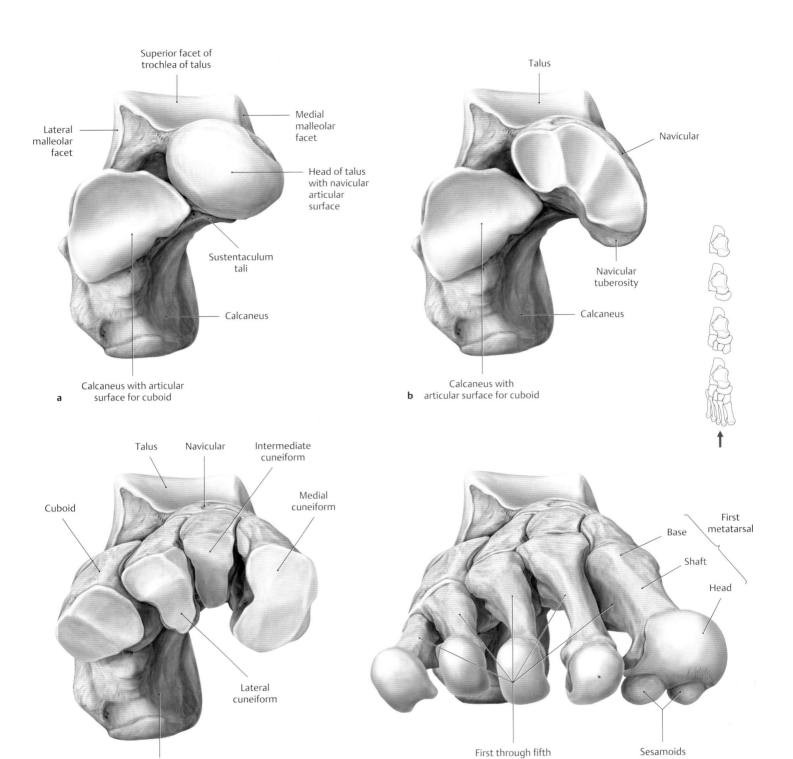

a

Superior facet of trochlea of talus

Lateral malleolar facet

Medial malleolar facet

Head of talus with navicular articular surface

Sustentaculum tali

Calcaneus

Calcaneus with articular surface for cuboid

b

Talus

Navicular

Navicular tuberosity

Calcaneus

Calcaneus with articular surface for cuboid

c

Talus

Navicular

Intermediate cuneiform

Medial cuneiform

Cuboid

Lateral cuneiform

Calcaneus

d

First metatarsal

Base

Shaft

Head

First through fifth metatarsals

Sesamoids

B Distal articular surfaces
Right foot, distal view.

a The talonavicular joint and calcaneocuboid joint: distal articular surfaces of the calcaneus and talus.
b The cuneonavicular joint and calcaneocuboid joint: distal articular surfaces of the navicular and calcaneus.

c The tarsometatarsal joints: distal articular surfaces of the medial, intermediate, and lateral cuneiform and the cuboid.
d Metatarsophalangeal joints: heads of the first through fifth metatarsals.

19.26 The Joints of the Foot: The Talocrural and Subtalar Joints

Tibia
Fibula
Lateral malleolus
Medial malleolus
Talus
Navicular

a Superior facet of trochlea of talus (anterior diameter)

Tibia
Fibula
Ankle mortise
Lateral malleolus
Calcaneus

b Sustentaculum tali   Superior facet of trochlea of talus (posterior diameter)

Head of talus
Neck of talus
Anterior diameter
Medial malleolar facet
Superior facet of trochlea of talus
Posterior diameter
Lateral malleolar facet

c Lateral tubercle

A The articulating skeletal elements of the talocrural joint
a Right foot, anterior view.
b Right foot, posterior view.
c Trochlea of the right talus, superior view.

The talocrural joint, called also the ankle joint, is formed by the distal ends of the tibia and fibula (the ankle mortise, see also **B**) articulating with the trochlea of the talus. This provides the talocrural joint with good bony and ligamentous stability and helps to stabilize the body in an erect posture. However, due to the shape of the talar trochlea (the anterior part, the superior surface, is approximately 5 to 6 mm broader

than the posterior part), the bony stability of the talocrural joint differs in flexion and extension. When the broader anterior part of the trochlea articulates with the ankle mortise in *dorsiflexion* (where the foot moves closer to the leg, as in squatting), the syndesmotic ligaments (see p. 460) are tightly stretched, and there is excellent bony stability. But when the narrower posterior part of the trochlea comes in contact with the ankle mortise in *plantar flexion* (e.g., standing on the toes), the talus no longer provides a high degree of bony stability within the ankle mortise.

Fibula
Inferior articular surface
Tibia
Lateral malleolus
Medial malleolus
Articular facet of lateral malleolus   Articular facet of medial malleolus

B The articular surfaces of the ankle mortise
Right foot, distal view.

Navicular articular surface
Navicular
Medial cuneiform
First metatarsal
Plantar aponeurosis   Long plantar ligament   Plantar calcaneo-navicular ligament

Tibia
Medial malleolus
Talus
Interosseous talocalcaneal ligament
Sustentaculum tali
Calcaneus

C Overview of an opened subtalar joint
Right foot, medial view. The interosseous talocalcaneal ligament has been divided, and the talus has been displaced upward to demonstrate the articular surfaces of the subtalar joint.

Note the course of the plantar calcaneonavicular ligament, which functions with the long plantar ligament and plantar aponeurosis to support the longitudinal arch of the foot (see also **D** and p. 467).

D Course of the plantar calcaneonavicular ligament

Right foot, plantar view. The plantar calcaneonavicular (spring) ligament stretches between the sustentaculum tali and the navicular. It completes the bony socket of the talocalcaneal joint from the plantar side.

Fifth meta-tarsal

Medial cuneiform

Navicular

Cuboid

Plantar calcaneonavicular ligament

Calcaneus

Sustentaculum tali

Talus

Medial cuneiform

Navicular

Plantar calcaneo-navicular ligament

Talus

Cuboid

Bifurcate ligament

Dorsal calcaneocuboid ligament

Anterior compartment

Posterior compartment

Subtalar joint

Calcaneus

Divided interosseous talocalcaneal ligament

E The articular surfaces of an opened subtalar joint

Right foot, dorsal view (after separation of the talus). In the subtalar joint, the talus articulates with the calcaneus and the navicular. It consists of two completely separate articulations:

- a posterior compartment (the talocalcaneal joint) and
- an anterior compartment (the talocalcaneonavicular joint).

The boundary between the two compartments is formed by the interosseous talocalcaneal ligament located in the tarsal canal (bony canal formed by the sulcus tali and sulcus calcanei; its entrance is the tarsal sinus). The plantar calcaneonavicular ligament, which has cartilage cells in its medial surface, loops like a tendon around the plantar head of the talus, which acts as a fulcrum. It stabilizes the position of the talus on the calcaneus and helps to support the apex of the longitudinal pedal arch (see p. 467). Overstretching of the plantar calcaneonavicular (spring) ligament due to flattening of the plantar vault promotes the development of flat foot.

459

19.27 **The Ligaments of the Foot**

A The ligaments of the right foot, medial view
The medial and lateral collateral ligaments, along with the syndesmotic ligaments (see **E**), are of major importance in stabilizing and guiding the subtalar joint, because portions of these ligaments are taut in every joint position and thus in every movement. The ligaments of the foot are classified by their location as belonging to the talocrural or subtalar joint, the metatarsus, the forefoot, or the sole of the foot.

B The ligaments of the right foot, lateral view
Sprains of the ankle joint and especially of its lateral ligaments (usually supination trauma = buckling of the ankle in a supinated position) are extremely common injuries. They often occur during plantar flexion of the foot, a position that provides less bony stability to the talocrural joint (see p. 458). Most of these injuries occur during sports and other leisure activities when the ankle gives way on uneven ground. Typically, the trauma will cause stretching or tearing of the anterior talofibular ligament, the calcaneofibular ligament, or both. If the leg is twisted violently while the foot is fixed, there may also be separation of the ankle mortise with disruption of the tibiofibular syndesmosis (see **D**).

a

b

C The ligaments of the right foot

a Anterior view (talocrural joint in plantar flexion).
b Posterior view (plantigrade foot position).

The anterior and posterior portions of the talocrural joint capsule have been removed to demonstrate more clearly the placement of the ligaments.

E The ligaments of the talocrural joint (the ligaments of the subtalar joint are reviewed on p. 459).

Lateral ligaments*
- Anterior talofibular ligament
- Posterior talofibular ligament
- Calcaneofibular ligament

Medial ligaments*
- Deltoid ligament
  - Anterior tibiotalar part
  - Posterior tibiotalar part
  - Tibionavicular part
  - Tibiocalcaneal part

Syndesmotic ligaments of the ankle mortise
- Anterior tibiofibular ligament
- Posterior tibiofibular ligament

*The medial and lateral ligaments are also termed the medial and lateral collateral ligaments.

a   b   c

D Weber fractures

A Weber fracture is an avulsion fracture of the lateral malleolus of the fibula. Weber fractures are classified as type A, B, or C depending on whether the fibula is fractured below, level with, or above the syndesmosis. The syndesmosis *may* be torn in a Weber type B fracture (as shown here), but it is *always* torn in a Weber type C fracture.

19.28 **The Movements of the Foot**

Axis of talocrural joint motion

Axis of subtalar joint motion

b

Axis of motion in the transverse tarsal and tarsometatarsal joints

a

c

Axis of talocrural joint motion

Axis of subtalar joint motion

d

A The principal axes of motion in the right foot
a Anterior view with the talocrural joint in plantar flexion.
b Posterior view in the functional position (see **B**).
c Isolated right forefoot, proximal view.
d Superior view.

The axes of articular motion in the foot are complex, and the descriptions of movements in the pedal joints are often inconsistent and confusing. The following axes of motion are important in clinical parlance and for the testing of joint motion (compare with the facing page):

- **Axis of talocrural joint motion (plantar flexion/dorsiflexion):** This axis runs almost transversely through the lateral and medial malleoli. It forms an approximately 82° angle with the tibial shaft axis in the frontal plane, and it forms a 10° angle with the frontal plane on the medial side (**a, d**).
- **Axis of subtalar joint motion (inversion/eversion):** This axis runs obliquely upward through the foot in a posterolateral-to-anteromedial direction, i.e., from the lateral calcaneus through the medial portion of the tarsal canal to the center of the navicular bone. It forms an approximately 30° angle with the horizontal plane and a 20° angle with the sagittal plane (**b, d**).
- **Axis of forefoot motion in the transverse tarsal joint and tarsometatarsal joints (pronation/supination):** This axis lies approximately in the sagittal plane, running from the calcaneus through the navicular and along the second ray (**a, c**).

B The functional position of the foot
Right foot, lateral view. In the neutral (0°) position, the skeleton of the foot is angled approximately 90° relative to the skeleton of the leg. This *plantigrade foot position* is termed the "functional position" and is an important basis for normal standing and walking.

Medial malleolus

Tibial axis

Lateral malleolus

Calcaneal axis

a

b

c

C Axis of the hindfoot
Distal right leg and hindfoot, posterior view.

a With normal axial alignment in the hindfoot, the tibial axis and calcaneal axis lie on a vertical line (pes rectus). The calcaneal axis bisects a line drawn between the two malleoli.
b Pes valgus: the foot is in an everted position.
c Pes varus: the foot is in an inverted position.

D Normal range of motion of the talocrural joint
Lateral view.

a Right foot on the ground (stance leg).
b Right foot off the ground (swing leg).

Starting from the neutral (0°) (plantigrade) position, the non-weight-bearing foot has an approximately 40 to 50° range of plantar flexion and an approximately 20 to 30° range of dorsiflexion (extension). When the foot is planted on the ground (in the stance phase of gait), the leg can be moved approximately 50° backward (plantar flexion) and 30° forward (dorsiflexion).

E Range of motion of the subtalar joint
Right foot, anterior view.

a Everted by 10°.
b Neutral (0°) position.
c Inverted by 20°.

Rotation of the calcaneus medially (inversion) and laterally (eversion) is measured from the neutral (0°) position. This is done clinically by holding the leg stationary and moving the calcaneus back and forth. Estimation of the range of inversion/eversion is based on the calcaneal axis.

F Range of pronation/supination of the transverse tarsal and tarsometatarsal joints.
Right foot, anterior view.

a Range of pronation of the forefoot: 20°.
b Range of supination of the forefoot: 40°.

Range of motion is tested with the hindfoot fixed. Pronation/supination of the forefoot is tested by rotating the forefoot outward relative to the hindfoot (raising the lateral border of the foot) or inward (raising the medial border of the foot).

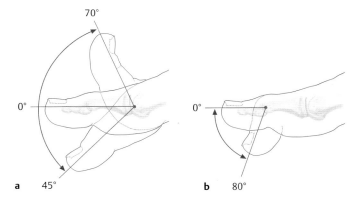

G Total range of motion of the forefoot and hindfoot
Right foot, anterior view.

a Eversion and pronation of the forefoot: 30°.
b Inversion and supination of the forefoot: 60°.

Because the movements in the joints are complex, and different joint movements are almost always mechanically coupled, the range of all joint movements can be assessed by holding the leg stationary and raising the entire foot in the medial and lateral directions.

H Range of motion of the joints of the great toe
Lateral view.

a Flexion/extension of the first metatarsophalangeal joint.
b Flexion of the first interphalangeal joint.

The toes, especially the great toe, can be passively extended to approximately 90°. This is an important prerequisite for walking, especially during the phase between heel take-off and toe strike.

19.29 Overview of the Plantar Vault and the Transverse Arch

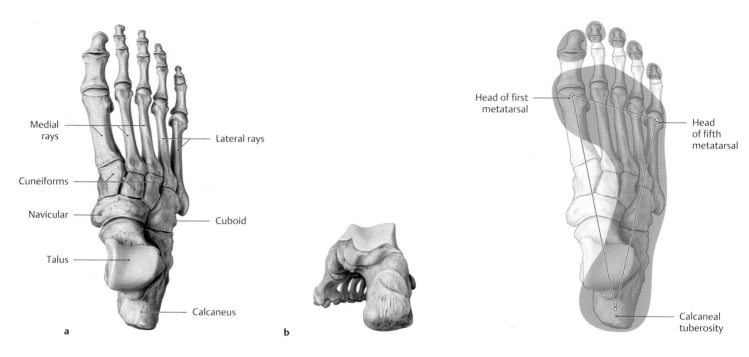

a

b

A The plantar vault
a Right foot, superior view.
b Right foot, posteromedial view.

From the perspective of structural engineering, the forces borne by the foot are distributed among two lateral (fibular) rays and three medial (tibial) rays. The lateral rays extend across the cuboid bone to the calcaneus, while the medial rays extend across the cuneiform and navicular bones to the talus. The arrangement of these rays—adjacent distally and overriding proximally—creates a lon-

gitudinal arch and a transverse arch in the sole of the foot. These plantar arches enable the foot to adapt optimally to uneven terrain, ensuring that the compressive forces can be transmitted under optimum mechanical conditions in any situation. The arches thus perform a kind of shock-absorber function, creating a springy flexibility that helps the foot absorb vertical loads. The deficient arches in a flatfoot or a splayfoot, for example, can lead to considerable pain during walking.

B The plantar architecture of the right foot
Superior view showing the bony points of support for the plantar vault and the associated footprint. The area that is outlined by interconnecting the bony supports (the calcaneal tuberosity and the heads of the first and fifth metatarsals) has the shape of a triangle. By contrast, the area of ground contact defined by the plantar soft tissues (the footprint or *podogram*) is considerably larger. The calluses typically found on the heel and the balls of the great and little toes confirm that these areas bear the brunt of the loads.

a

b

C Transfer of compressive stresses in the weight-bearing foot
Schematic sagittal section at the level of the first ray, medial view.

a During stance, the partial body weight on the talocrural joint is transferred across the talus to the forefoot and hindfoot.

b A schematic radiograph illustrates the parallel arrangement of the cancellous bony trabeculae. The pattern conforms to the compressive stresses (indicated by color shading) that result from the loads acting on the forefoot and hindfoot (**a**) (after Rauber and Kopsch).

Plantar ligaments

Base of first proximal phalanx

a Deep transverse metatarsal ligament

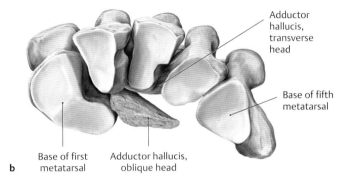

Adductor hallucis, transverse head

Base of fifth metatarsal

Base of first metatarsal

Adductor hallucis, oblique head

b

Deep transverse metatarsal ligament

Proximal phalanx of great toe

Metatarso-phalangeal joint of great toe

Adductor hallucis, transverse head

Plantar ligaments

First metatarsal

Adductor hallucis, oblique head

Medial cuneiform

Cuboid

Tibialis posterior

Fibularis longus

Medial malleolus

Sustentac-ulum tali

Calcaneus

Talus

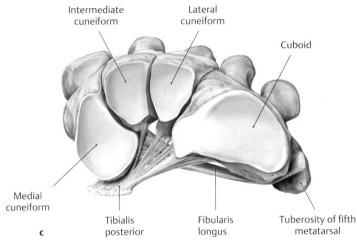

Intermediate cuneiform

Lateral cuneiform

Cuboid

Medial cuneiform

Tibialis posterior

Fibularis longus

Tuberosity of fifth metatarsal

c

D Active and passive stabilizers of the transverse arch, plantar view

Right foot. Both active and passive stabilizing structures maintain the curvature of the transverse pedal arch. The passive stabilizers are ligaments, and the active stabilizers are muscles. In the foot, ligamentous structures are usually able to maintain the pedal arches without assistance from the muscles. But when the loads on the foot are increased, as during walking or running on uneven ground, active muscular forces are recruited to give additional support.

E Active and passive stabilizers of the transverse arch, proximal view

Right foot.

a Arch stabilizers in the forefoot (anterior arch). The deep transverse metatarsal ligament stabilizes the anterior arch at the level of the metatarsal heads. The arch of the forefoot thus relies entirely on *passive* stabilizers, while the arches of the metatarsus and tarsus (**b, c**) have only *active* stabilizers.

b Stabilizers of the metatarsal arch. The transverse head of the adductor hallucis is the primary muscular stabilizer of the metatarsal arch.

c The principal arch-supporting muscle in the tarsal region is the fibularis longus. After winding around the cuboid, its tendon of insertion runs from the lateral border of the foot and across the sole to the medial cuneiform bone and the base of the first metatarsal. Another active stabilizer in this region is the tibialis posterior, whose tendon of insertion gives off expansions to the cuneiform bones. Like the fibularis longus, its oblique course enables it to support the longitudinal arch in addition to its transverse component.

19.30 The Longitudinal Arch of the Foot

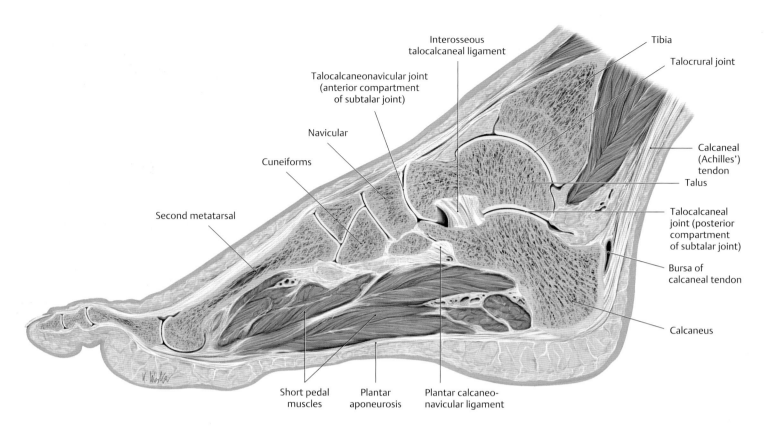

Interosseous talocalcaneal ligament

Talocalcaneonavicular joint (anterior compartment of subtalar joint)

Navicular

Cuneiforms

Second metatarsal

Tibia

Talocrural joint

Calcaneal (Achilles') tendon

Talus

Talocalcaneal joint (posterior compartment of subtalar joint)

Bursa of calcaneal tendon

Calcaneus

Short pedal muscles

Plantar aponeurosis

Plantar calcaneo-navicular ligament

A Active stabilizers of the longitudinal arch

Sagittal section at the level of the second ray of the right foot, medial view. The second ray (consisting of the second toe, second metatarsal, intermediate cuneiform, navicular, and calcaneus) forms the highest arch within the overall longitudinal plantar arch, its height diminishing laterally. The main active stabilizers of the longitudinal arch are the *short muscles of the foot*: abductor hallucis, flexor hallucis brevis, flexor digitorum brevis, quadratus plantae, and abductor digiti minimi (drawn from a specimen in the Anatomical Collection of Kiel University).

Navicular   Talus

Medial cuneiform

Flexor hallucis longus

Flexor digitorum longus

Medial malleolus

Medial tubercle

Plantar aponeurosis

Long plantar ligament

Plantar calcaneonavicular ligament

Sustentaculum tali

B Passive stabilizers of the longitudinal arch

Right foot, medial view. The main passive stabilizers of the longitudinal arch are the plantar aponeurosis, the long plantar ligament, and the plantar calcaneonavicular (spring) ligament. The plantar aponeurosis is particularly important owing to its long lever arm, while the plantar calcaneonavicular ligament is the weakest component (shortest dis-

tance from the apex of the longitudinal arch). The *tendons of insertion of the long flexors* of the foot (flexor hallucis longus and flexor digitorum longus) also help to prevent sagging of the longitudinal arch. The flexor hallucis longus, which runs beneath the sustentaculum tali, is particularly effective in tightening the longitudinal arch like the chord of an arc.

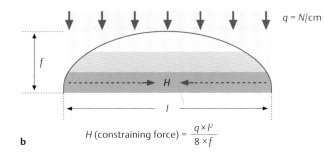

a Plantar calcaneonavicular ligament

Plantar aponeurosis — Long plantar ligament

$q = N/cm$

H (constraining force) $= \dfrac{q \times l^2}{8 \times f}$

D Footprints (podograms) of right feet (after Rauber and Kopsch)
a Normal plantar arches (pes rectus).
b Increased height of the longitudinal arch (pes cavus).
c Loss of the transverse arch (splayfoot = pes transversoplanus).
d Loss of the longitudinal arch (flatfoot = pes planus).

Foot deformities—deviations from a normal, healthy foot shape—may be congenital, or acquired through paralysis or trauma. Structural abnormalities caused by chronic loads imposed on the foot by the body weight are referred to specifically as *static deformities*.

C Support of the longitudinal arch
a Ligamentous support of the longitudinal arch (right foot, medial view).
b Calculating the constraining force (*H*) needed to maintain the arch (after Rauber and Kopsch).

Comparing the longitudinal arch of the foot to a theoretical parabolic arch, we see that a constraining force (*H*) must be applied to maintain the arch curvature. The magnitude of this force depends on the load (*q*), the chord length of the arch (*l*), and the height of the arch (*f*). As a result, the structures that are most effective in maintaining the pedal arch are those closest to the ground, since the long lever arm of those structures requires the least expenditure of force. The formula also dictates that the constraining force must increase as the distance *l* between the points of support increases, or as the arch becomes flatter (smaller *f*).

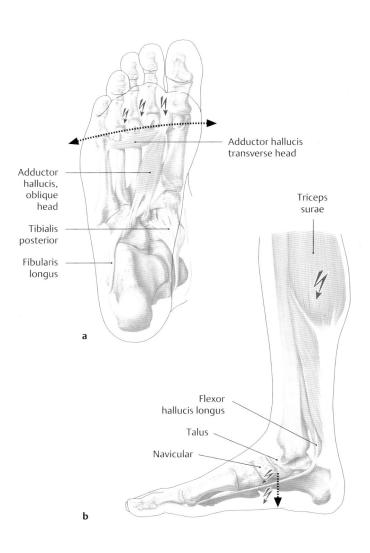

Adductor hallucis transverse head

Adductor hallucis, oblique head

Triceps surae

Tibialis posterior

Fibularis longus

a

E Location of pain associated with splayfoot and flatfoot (after Loeweneck)
a Right splayfoot viewed from the plantar aspect. The collapse of the transverse arch results in a broadened forefoot (arrows) with greater pressure acting on the heads of the second through fourth metatarsals and the associated metatarsophalangeal joints. Typically, very painful calluses will form between the balls of the great and little toes in this situation.
b Right flatfoot viewed from the medial aspect. With collapse of the longitudinal arch, marked by downward displacement of the talus and navicular (arrow), weight bearing often incites a diffuse foot pain that is most intense in the area of the stretched calcaneonavicular (spring) ligament. Calf pain may also develop as a result of sustained, increased tension on the calf muscles (and the pedal muscles as well, which must compensate for the deficient passive stabilizers).

Flexor hallucis longus

Talus

Navicular

b

467

19.31 The Sesamoid Bones and Deformities of the Toes

A Cross section through the head of the first metatarsal at the level of the sesamoids

Great toe of right foot, proximal view. The plane of section is indicated in **B**. The lateral and medial sesamoids are hemispheric bones, each presenting a slightly convex dorsal articular surface that articulates with the grooved plantar articular surfaces on the head of the first metatarsal. Sesamoids protect the tendons from excessive friction. They are important functionally for their ability to lengthen the effective lever arm of the muscle, so that muscular forces can be applied more efficiently. The development of sesamoids can be interpreted as a functional adaptation to the presence of pressure tendons.

B The sesamoids of the great toe

Right foot, posteromedial view. The tendon of the flexor hallucis longus runs between the two sesamoids. The box around the sesamoids indicates the plane of section shown in **A**.

C The articular surfaces of the sesamoids

Right foot, dorsal view with the first metatarsal removed.

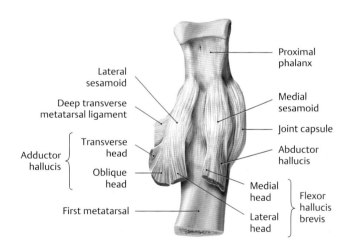

D The capsule and ligaments of the sesamoids and muscular attachments

First metatarsophalangeal joint of the right foot, plantar view. Both sesamoids are attached to the joint capsule and to the collateral ligaments of the metatarsophalangeal joint. They are embedded in the tendons of insertion of the following muscles:

- Medial sesamoid – Abductor hallucis
  – Medial head of flexor hallucis brevis

- Lateral sesamoid – Lateral head of flexor hallucis brevis
  – Transverse head of adductor hallucis
  – Oblique head of adductor hallucis

a

b

E Change in the first intermetatarsal angle and first metatarsophalangeal angle in hallux valgus

Right foot, superior view.

a Skeleton of a normal right foot.
b Lateral deviation of the first ray with subluxation of the metatarsophalangeal joint in hallux valgus.

In a normal foot, the *first intermetatarsal angle* (angle between the longitudinal axes of the first and second metatarsals) should not exceed 8°. The *first metatarsophalangeal angle* (angle between the longitudinal axes of the proximal phalanx of the great toe and the first metatarsal) should be less than 20°. In hallux valgus and also in splayfoot, which generally precedes it, both the intermetatarsal angle and metatarsophalangeal angle are significantly increased.

G Etiology of hallux valgus

Hallux valgus usually develops secondary to splayfoot. When a broadened forefoot is forced into a narrow, pointed shoe, the outer toes are crowded against the middle toes. This results in the pressure points and pain that are typical of hallux valgus and predominantly affect the medial side of the head of the first metatarsal, with chronic irritation of the first metatarsophalangeal joint and the overlying bursa (bursitis), in addition to reactive bone changes (exostosis). The middle toes are squeezed together anteriorly and become clawed (hammer toes, claw toes) (after Debrunner).

F Pathogenic mechanism of hallux valgus

Right forefoot, superior view. As the first metatarsal deviates medially and the great toe deviates laterally, a muscular imbalance develops marked by a change in the direction of tendon pull, which perpetuates and exacerbates the deformity. Most notably, the abductor hallucis moves laterally with the medial sesamoid, causing it to become an *adductor*. Meanwhile, the long flexor and extensor tendons move laterally, reinforcing the lateral angulation at the first metatarsophalangeal joint.

H Claw toes and hammer toes

Toe deformities are a very common associated feature of hallux valgus and splayfoot. When the foot is placed into a tight shoe with a high heel, it tends to slide forward and downward, and the resulting pressure leads to a typical cramped deformity with degenerative changes in the toe joints and painful callus formation. The claw toe deformity is characterized by marked hyperextensibility of the metatarsophalangeal joint with flexion of the proximal and distal interphalangeal joints. With hammer toes, there is less pronounced dorsiflexion of the metatarsophalangeal joint.

469

19.32 X-Ray and Cross-sectional Anatomy of the Foot

A X-ray anatomy of the foot
a Upper ankle joint in anterior-posterior beam path, **b** rearfoot in lateral beam path, **c** forefoot in dorsal plantar beam path (from Möller TB, Reif E. Taschenatlas der Röntgenanatomie. 2nd ed. Stuttgart: Thieme; 1998).

The conventional X-ray is still the basis for medical imaging of the foot. It provides the highest spatial resolution and a good overview of the overall shape of the foot.

a

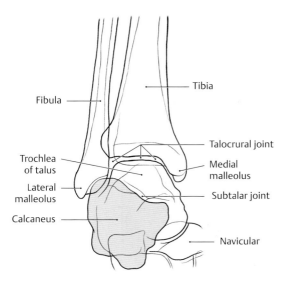

- Tibia
- Fibula
- Talocrural joint
- Trochlea of talus
- Medial malleolus
- Lateral malleolus
- Subtalar joint
- Calcaneus
- Navicular

b

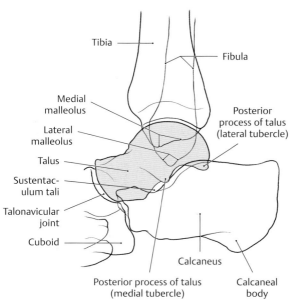

- Tibia
- Fibula
- Medial malleolus
- Posterior process of talus (lateral tubercle)
- Lateral malleolus
- Talus
- Sustentaculum tali
- Talonavicular joint
- Cuboid
- Calcaneus
- Posterior process of talus (medial tubercle)
- Calcaneal body

c

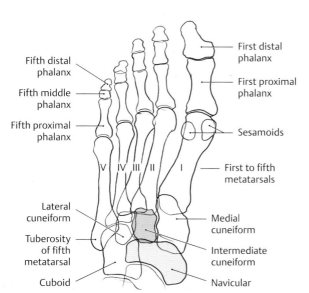

- Fifth distal phalanx
- First distal phalanx
- Fifth middle phalanx
- First proximal phalanx
- Fifth proximal phalanx
- Sesamoids
- V IV III II   I
- First to fifth metatarsals
- Lateral cuneiform
- Medial cuneiform
- Tuberosity of fifth metatarsal
- Intermediate cuneiform
- Cuboid
- Navicular

B Magnetic resonance imaging of the right foot (from Vahlensieck M, Reiser M. MRT des Bewegungsapparates. 3rd ed. Stuttgart: Thieme; 2006) T1-weighted **a** sagittal, **b** coronal, and **c** axial (transverse) sequences.

Lateral malleolus
Fibularis longus tendon
Fibularis brevis tendon
Small saphenous vein
Abductor digiti minimi
Calcaneus
Lateral cuneiform
Fourth metatarsal
Cuboid

a

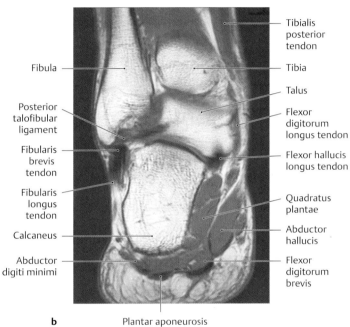

Tibialis posterior tendon
Tibia
Talus
Flexor digitorum longus tendon
Flexor hallucis longus tendon
Quadratus plantae
Abductor hallucis
Flexor digitorum brevis
Fibula
Posterior talofibular ligament
Fibularis brevis tendon
Fibularis longus tendon
Calcaneus
Abductor digiti minimi
Plantar aponeurosis

b

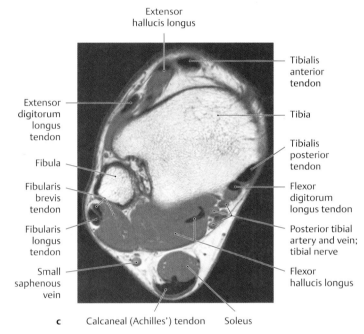

Extensor hallucis longus
Tibialis anterior tendon
Tibia
Tibialis posterior tendon
Flexor digitorum longus tendon
Posterior tibial artery and vein; tibial nerve
Flexor hallucis longus
Extensor digitorum longus tendon
Fibula
Fibularis brevis tendon
Fibularis longus tendon
Small saphenous vein
Calcaneal (Achilles') tendon
Soleus

c

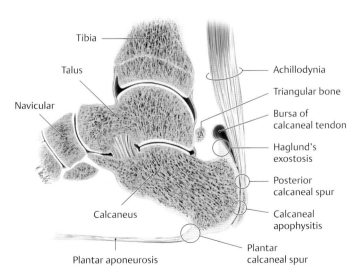

Tibia
Talus
Navicular
Calcaneus
Plantar aponeurosis
Achillodynia
Triangular bone
Bursa of calcaneal tendon
Haglund's exostosis
Posterior calcaneal spur
Calcaneal apophysitis
Plantar calcaneal spur

C Anatomic localization of clinically important disorders of the heel region

Heel pain is a very common symptom in patients of doctors specializing in foot surgery. In addition to the physical examination, only a few medical imaging techniques are necessary to make a diagnosis and treat-

ment plan. Aside from typical bone diseases (osteoporosis and tumors), the following causes for heel pain need to be considered:

- Plantar heel spur: osseous exostosis at the calcaneal insertion of the plantar aponeurosis (often as a result of chronic plantar fascitis).
- Calcaneal apophysitis: defect in the bony apophysis of the calcaneal tuberosity during growth; pain results from overload of the cartilaginous growth plate.
- Posterior heel spur: prominent exostosis at the insertion on the calcaneus of the calcaneal (Achilles') tendon (insertional tendinopathy of the chondral apophyseal enthesis).
- Haglund's exostosis: proximally located dorsal calcaneal tuberosity (benign cartilaginous growth); pain results from inflammation of the adjacent bursa (bursa of the calcaneal tendon).
- Triangular bone: accessory bone of the foot at the posterior talus.
- Achillodynia: painful peridentinitis of the calcaneal (Achilles') tendon; symptoms include hyperthermia, swelling, and impaired function.

19.33 **Human Gait**

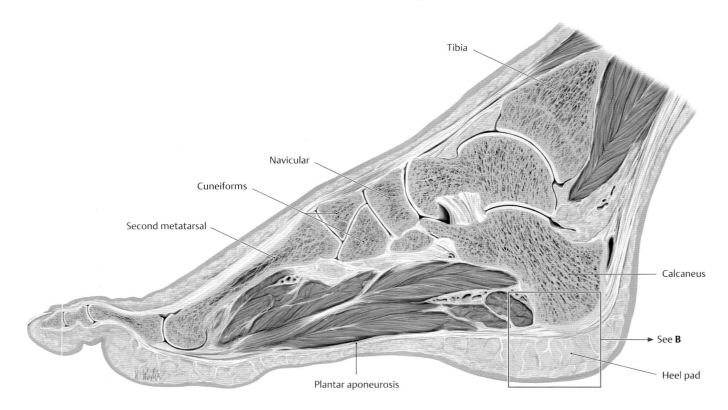

A The pressure chamber system in the sole of the foot
Sagittal section through the right foot at the level of the second ray, medial view (see detail in **B**).

During walking and particularly in the stance phase, large compressive forces are exerted on the heel pad and on the balls of the great and little toes. To distribute these concentrated forces more evenly over a larger area, the sole of the foot is covered by a layer of subcutane- ous connective tissue up to 2 cm thick. As a functional adaptation to these demands, the tissue has a "pressure chamber" construction that acts as a shock absorber while also enhancing the mechanical stability of the sole. Without this pressure chamber construction, the loads on the foot would generate very high, localized stresses that would result in pressure necrosis (drawn from a specimen in the Anatomical Collection of Kiel University).

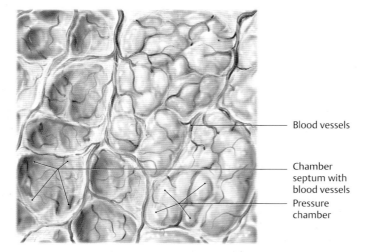

B The plantar pressure chambers
Detail from **A**.

Each of the pressure chambers contains an internal fibrofatty tissue covered externally by tough connective tissue made up of collagen fibers. These fibrous septa are firmly attached between the plantar aponeurosis and plantar skin and are supplied by an extensive network of blood vessels that further stabilize the walls of the pressure chambers (see close-up in **C**).

C Structure of the pressure chambers
Detail from **B**.

The fatty tissue has been removed from the chambers on the left side of the drawing to demonstrate the blood vessels that permeate the septa. (The sole of the foot is one of the most highly vascularized regions of the body surface.)

a

Step width
(track width)

Stance phase
(60%)

Swing phase
(40%)

0%
(heel strike)

60%
(toe-off)

100%
of gait cycle
(heel strike)

Stance phase

Longitudinal axis
of the foot

Step length

b

D Movements of the leg during one gait cycle

During normal walking, each leg functions alternately as the stance leg and swing leg. The stance phase begins when the heel contacts the ground (heel strike) and ends when the toes push off from the ground (toe-off). This phase makes up 60% of the gait cycle. The swing phase begins with the toe-off and ends with the heel strike. It makes up 40% of the gait cycle (100% of gait cycle = the period between two heel strikes of the same foot).

In the neutral position, the longitudinal axis of the foot relative to the line of direction shows an external rotation of 7°. This slight external rotation of the foot occurs also during walking.

E Step width (a) and step length (b)

The step width (track width) is evaluated from behind. Generally, it is narrower than the distance between the two hip joints. The step length (evaluated from the side) equals approximately 2 to 3 foot lengths.

The track width and step length define the area of support and thus play a critical role in stability. This is particularly important in hemiplegic patients, for example, in whom impaired proprioception can lead to instabilities of gait and stance.

473

20.1 The Muscles of the Lower Limb: Classification

In most mammals, the upper and lower limbs share many functions and have analogous functional groups of muscles. In humans, however, the specializations of the upper limb for manipulation and the lower limb for ambulation have imposed radically different requirements upon their respective muscle groups. For instance, the shoulder girdle has considerable freedom of motion on the trunk and is acted upon by an array of muscles, but the pelvic ring is firmly fixed to the vertebral column and changes position very little relative to the trunk, and has no comparable muscles to move it. In contrast, the hip and gluteal muscles have evolved into massive and powerful movers and stabilizers of the femur, counteracting the loads imposed by support of the whole body weight on two limbs and maintaining balance and stability during bipedal locomotion; these muscles are, in aggregate, larger than their counterparts that act upon the humerus, with a significantly different arrangement and orientation.

As with the upper limb (see p. 296), the muscles of the lower limb can be classified on the basis of origin, topography, function, and innervation. Each such classification system has advantages and disadvantages, so several schemes are presented here. Segregation of muscles that act at the hip into specific functional groups is valid only for a particular joint position, because the axis of motion changes relative to the muscles as the joint is dynamically reoriented, causing abductors to become adductors, for example. Muscles surrounding the hip can be categorized topographically into an inner and outer group, relative to the pelvic girdle (see **A**). Muscles acting on the knee and foot can be grouped logically in an arrangement that uses both functional and topographical criteria, because these muscles tend to be clustered by functional groups into discrete compartments and act in a consistent way on joints with restricted ranges of motion. As with the upper limb, it is also instructive to categorize the lower limb's muscles by the pattern of their innervation (see **E**), a pattern that reveals the underlying logic of different clinical syndromes involving nerve damage.

A The hip and gluteal muscles

Inner hip muscles
- Psoas major
- Psoas minor
- Iliacus

} Act in unison as the "iliopsoas"

Outer hip muscles
- Gluteus maximus
- Gluteus medius
- Gluteus minimus
- Tensor fasciae latae
- Piriformis
- Obturator internus
- Gemelli
- Quadratus femoris

Muscles of the adductor group*
- Obturator externus
- Pectineus
- Adductor longus
- Adductor brevis
- Adductor magnus
- Adductor minimus
- Gracilis

* For functional reasons, the muscles of the adductor group, all of which are located on the medial side of the thigh, are classified as hip muscles because they act mainly on the hip joint.

B The thigh muscles

Anterior thigh muscles
- Sartorius
- Quadriceps femoris
  - Rectus femoris
  - Vastus medialis
  - Vastus lateralis
  - Vastus intermedius
  - (Articularis genus, the "fifth head" of quadriceps femoris, see p. 482)

Posterior thigh muscles
- Biceps femoris
- Semimembranosus
- Semitendinosus

} The hamstrings

C The leg muscles

Anterior compartment
- Tibialis anterior
- Extensor digitorum longus
- Extensor hallucis longus
- Fibularis tertius

Lateral compartment
- Fibularis longus
- Fibularis brevis

Posterior compartment
Superficial part
- Triceps surae
  - Soleus
  - Gastrocnemius (medial and lateral heads)
- Plantaris

Deep part
- Tibialis posterior
- Flexor digitorum longus
- Flexor hallucis longus
- Popliteus

D The short muscles of the foot

Dorsal muscles
- Extensor digitorum brevis
- Extensor hallucis brevis

Plantar muscles
Medial compartment
- Abductor hallucis
- Flexor hallucis brevis (medial and lateral heads)

Lateral compartment
- Abductor digiti minimi
- Flexor digiti minimi brevis
- Opponens digiti minimi

Central compartment
- Flexor digitorum brevis
- Adductor hallucis (transverse and oblique heads)
- Quadratus plantae
- First through fourth lumbricals
- First through third plantar interossei
- First through fourth dorsal interossei

E Classification of muscles based on their motor innervation
All the muscles of the lower limb are supplied by branches of the lumbar plexus (T12–L4) and the sacral plexus (L5–S3). They may be supplied by short, direct branches or by long nerves emanating from the corresponding plexus (see p. 530). See also **F**.

Nerve or plexus	Muscles supplied
Lumbar plexus	
Direct branches (muscular branches) (L1–L3)	Psoas major and minor
Nerves of the lower limb arising from the lumbar plexus	
Femoral nerve (L2–L4)	Iliacus, pectineus; sartorius, quadriceps femoris
Obturator nerve (L2–L4)	Obturator externus, pectineus, adductor longus, adductor brevis, adductor magnus (deep part), adductor minimus, gracilis
Sacral plexus	
Direct branches (muscular branches) (L5–S2)	Piriformis, obturator internus, gemelli, quadratus femoris
Nerves of the lower limb arising from the sacral plexus	
Superior gluteal nerve (L4–S1)	Tensor fasciae latae, gluteus medius and minimus
Inferior gluteal nerve (L5–S2)	Gluteus maximus
Sciatic nerve (L4–S3) (see **F**)	Adductor magnus (superficial part, tibial part), biceps femoris (long head, tibial part), biceps femoris (short head, fibular part), semimembranosus (tibial part), semitendinosus (tibial part)
• Common fibular* nerve (L4–S2)	
– Deep fibular nerve	Tibialis anterior, extensor digitorum longus and brevis, fibularis tertius, extensor hallucis longus and brevis
– Superficial fibular nerve	Fibularis longus and brevis
• Tibial nerve (L4–S3)	Popliteus, triceps surae, plantaris, tibialis posterior, flexor digitorum longus, flexor hallucis longus
– Medial plantar nerve	Abductor hallucis, flexor hallucis brevis (medial head), flexor digitorum brevis, first lumbrical
– Lateral plantar nerve	Flexor hallucis brevis (lateral head), adductor hallucis, abductor digiti minimi, flexor digiti minimi brevis, opponens digiti minimi, quadratus plantae, second to fourth lumbricals, first through third plantar interossei, first through fourth dorsal interossei

* The common fibular nerve and its divisions are also referred to as "peroneal nerves."

Sacral plexus
- Superior gluteal nerve
- Inferior gluteal nerve
- Sciatic nerve
- Tibial nerve
- Common fibular nerve
- Superficial fibular nerve
- Deep fibular nerve
- Tibial nerve
- Medial plantar nerve
- Lateral plantar nerve

Lumbar plexus
- Obturator nerve
- Femoral nerve

F The branches of the lumbosacral plexus that innervate the muscles of the lower limb
Right leg, lateral view. The anterior rami of the lumbar and sacral nerves, with contributions from the subcostal nerve and coccygeal nerve (not shown here), combine to form the lumbosacral plexus. While the branches arising from the lumbar plexus run *anterior to* the hip joint and mainly supply the muscles on the anterior and medial views of the thigh, the branches from the sacral plexus run *behind* the hip joint to supply the posterior thigh muscles and all the muscles of the leg and foot. The grossly visible division of the sciatic nerve into its two terminal branches (the tibial nerve and common fibular nerve) is generally located just above the knee joint, as pictured here (*low division*). But the nerve fibers that make up the two terminal branches become organized into bundles at a much more proximal level, where they already appear as separate nerve branches within their common fibrous sheath. In the *high division* pattern, the nerve divides into its terminal branches while still in the lesser pelvis (see p. 553).

20.2 The Hip and Gluteal Muscles: The Inner Hip Muscles

A Schematic of the inner hip muscles

Iliopsoas

Origin:
- ① Psoas major (superficial layer): lateral surfaces of the T12 vertebral body, the L1–L4 vertebral bodies, and the associated intervertebral disks
- ① Psoas major (deep layer): costal processes of the L1–L5 vertebrae
- ② Iliacus: the iliac fossa

Insertion: Common insertion on the lesser trochanter of the femur as the iliopsoas ③ (psoas minor inserts into the iliopectineal arch, not depicted; see **B**)

Action:
- Hip joint: flexion and external rotation
- Lumbar spine: unilateral contraction (with the femur fixed) bends the trunk laterally to the same side, bilateral contraction raises the trunk from the supine position

Innervation: Femoral nerve (iliacus) and direct branches from the lumbar plexus (psoas) (L1–L3)

Properties and clinical aspects of the iliopsoas muscle

The iliopsoas is classified as a hip flexor, along with the rectus femoris, sartorius, and tensor fasciae latae. It is the most powerful flexor, its long vertical travel making it an important muscle for standing, walking, and running. As a typical postural muscle with a preponderance of slow-twitch red (type I) fibers, however, the iliopsoas is inherently susceptible to pathological shortening (particularly in older patients with a sedentary lifestyle or chronic immobilization conditions) and requires regular stretching to maintain normal tone (see pp. 56 and 499). Shortening (contracture) of the hip flexors leads to

- increased anterior pelvic tilt,
- increased lumbar lordosis, and
- limitation of hip extension.

Unilateral shortening of the iliopsoas, in which the ilium on the affected side is tilted forward, can be diagnosed with the Thomas maneuver (see p. 436). This condition leads to pelvic torsion, in which the pelvis becomes twisted upon itself. This mainly alters the function of the sacroiliac joints but also compromises the intervertebral joints and the lumbosacral junction (increased lordosis of the lumbar spine with degenerative changes in the vertebral bodies, see p. 130). Patients with *bilateral* iliopsoas weakness or paralysis are unable to raise the trunk from the supine position, despite intact abdominal muscles, without using their arms and are greatly limited in their ability to walk and climb stairs without assistance.

Twelfth rib

Psoas minor

Psoas major

L5 vertebra

Promontory

Iliac crest

Iliacus

Anterior superior iliac spine

Sacrotuberous ligament

Inguinal ligament

Iliopsoas

Sacrospinous ligament

Greater trochanter

Inter-trochanteric line

Lesser trochanter

Iliopectineal arch

Ischial spine

Pubic symphysis

Pubic tubercle

B The inner hip muscles
Anterior view.
Note: In the lower extremity, the directional terms "posterior" and "anterior" are better used than "dorsal" and "ventral"; for background, see rotation of the extremities on p. 21.

The psoas major unites with the iliacus at the level of the inguinal ligament to form a conjoined muscle, the iliopsoas. Approximately 50% of the population also has a psoas minor muscle (as shown here), which arises from the T12 and L1 vertebrae and inserts into the iliopectineal arch (iliac fascia).

20.3 The Hip and Gluteal Muscles: The Outer Hip Muscles

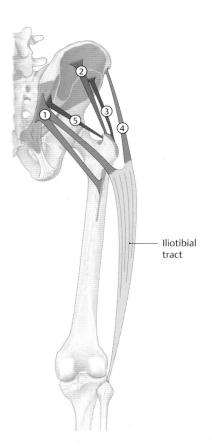

Iliotibial tract

A Schematic of the vertically oriented outer hip muscles

① **Gluteus maximus**

Origin:	Lateral part of the dorsal surface of the sacrum, posterior part of the gluteal surface of the ilium (behind the posterior gluteal line), also from the thoracolumbar fascia and sacrotuberous ligament
Insertion:	• Upper fibers: iliotibial tract • Lower fibers: gluteal tuberosity
Action:	• Entire muscle: extends and externally rotates the hip, stabilizes the hip in both the sagittal and coronal planes • Upper fibers: abduction • Lower fibers: adduction
Innervation:	Inferior gluteal nerve (L5–S2)

② **Gluteus medius**

Origin:	Gluteal surface of the ilium (below the iliac crest between the anterior and posterior gluteal line)
Insertion:	Lateral surface of the greater trochanter of the femur
Action:	• Entire muscle: abducts the hip, stabilizes the pelvis in the coronal plane • Anterior part: flexion and internal rotation • Posterior part: extension and external rotation
Innervation:	Superior gluteal nerve (L4–S1)

③ **Gluteus minimus**

Origin:	Gluteal surface of the ilium (below the origin of gluteus medius)
Insertion:	Anterolateral surface of the greater trochanter of the femur
Action:	• Entire muscle: abducts the hip, stabilizes the pelvis in the coronal plane • Anterior part: flexion and internal rotation • Posterior part: extension and external rotation
Innervation:	Superior gluteal nerve (L4–S1)

④ **Tensor fasciae latae**

Origin:	Anterior superior iliac spine
Insertion:	Iliotibial tract
Action:	• Tenses the fascia lata • Abduction, flexion, and internal rotation of the hip joint
Innervation:	Superior gluteal nerve (L4–S1)

⑤ **Piriformis**

Origin:	Pelvic surface of the sacrum
Insertion:	Apex of the greater trochanter of the femur
Action:	• External rotation, abduction, and extension of the hip joint • Stabilizes the hip joint
Innervation:	Direct branches from the sacral plexus (S1, S2)

B Schematic of the horizontally oriented outer hip muscles

① **Obturator internus**

Origin:	Inner surface of the obturator membrane and its bony boundaries
Insertion:	Medial surface of the greater trochanter
Action:	External rotation, adduction, and extension of the hip joint (also active in abduction, depending on the position of the joint)
Innervation:	Direct branches from the sacral plexus (L5, S1)

② **Gemelli**

Origin:	• Gemellus superior: ischial spine • Gemellus inferior: ischial tuberosity
Insertion:	Jointly with obturator internus tendon (medial surface, greater trochanter)
Action:	External rotation, adduction, and extension of the hip joint (also active in abduction, depending on the position of the joint)
Innervation:	Direct branches from the sacral plexus (L5, S1)

③ **Quadratus femoris**

Origin:	Lateral border of the ischial tuberosity
Insertion:	Intertrochanteric crest of the femur
Action:	External rotation and adduction of the hip joint
Innervation:	Direct branches from the sacral plexus (L5, S1)

a

b

C The outer hip muscles: superficial layer
Right side, posterior view.
Note the position of the gluteus maximus muscle in relation to the axis of hip abduction and adduction. While the fibers of the gluteus maximus that run *above* the axis and insert on the tibia via the iliotibial tract are active in abducting the hip joint, the muscle fibers that run *below* the axis are active in adduction.

D The outer hip muscles: deep layer
Right side, posterior view.

a With the gluteus maximus removed.
b With the gluteus medius removed.

If there is weakness or paralysis of the small gluteal muscles (gluteus medius and minimus), the pelvis can no longer be stabilized in the coronal plane and will tilt toward the unaffected side (positive Trendelenburg sign, see also p. 536).

20.4 The Hip and Gluteal Muscles: The Adductor Group

A Schematic of the adductors

① **Obturator externus**

Origin:	Outer surface of the obturator membrane and its bony boundaries
Insertion:	Trochanteric fossa of the femur
Action:	• Adduction and external rotation of the hip joint
	• Stabilizes the pelvis in the sagittal plane
Innervation:	Obturator nerve (L3, L4)

② **Pectineus**

Origin:	Pecten pubis
Insertion:	Pectineal line and the proximal linea aspera of the femur
Action:	• Adduction, external rotation, and slight flexion of the hip joint
	• Stabilizes the pelvis in the coronal and sagittal planes
Innervation:	Femoral nerve, obturator nerve (L2, L3)

③ **Adductor longus**

Origin:	Superior pubic ramus and anterior side of the symphysis
Insertion:	Linea aspera: medial lip in the middle third of the femur
Action:	• Adduction and flexion (up to 70°) of the hip joint (extends the hip past 80° of flexion)
	• Stabilizes the pelvis in the coronal and sagittal planes
Innervation:	Obturator nerve (L2–L4)

④ **Adductor brevis**

Origin:	Inferior pubic ramus
Insertion:	Linea aspera: medial lip in the upper third of the femur
Action:	• Adduction and flexion (up to 70°) of the hip joint (extends the hip past 80° of flexion)
	• Stabilizes the pelvis in the coronal and sagittal planes
Innervation	Obturator nerve (L2, L3)

⑤ **Adductor magnus**

Origin:	Inferior pubic ramus, ischial ramus, and ischial tuberosity
Insertion:	• Deep part ("fleshy insertion"): medial lip of linea aspera
	• Superficial part ("tendinous insertion"): adductor tubercle of femur
Actions	• Adduction, extension, and slight flexion of the hip joint (the tendinous insertion is also active in internal rotation)
	• Stabilizes the pelvis in the coronal and sagittal planes
Innervation:	• Deep part: obturator nerve (L2–L4)
	• Superficial part: tibial nerve (L4)

⑥ **Adductor minimus (upper division of adductor magnus)**

Origin:	Inferior pubic ramus
Insertion:	Medial lip of the linea aspera
Action:	Adduction, external rotation, and slight flexion of the hip joint
Innervation:	Obturator nerve (L2–L4)

⑦ **Gracilis**

Origin:	Inferior pubic ramus below the pubic symphysis
Insertion:	Medial border of the tibial tuberosity (along with the tendons of sartorius and semitendinosus)
Action:	• Hip joint: adduction and flexion
	• Knee joint: flexion and internal rotation
Innervation:	Obturator nerve (L2, L3)

Axis of flexion/extension

Adductor brevis

Linea aspera

Adductor longus

B Reversal of muscle actions, illustrated for the adductor brevis and longus

Right hip joint, lateral view. The femur in 80° of flexion is shown in lighter shading. In addition to their primary action as adductors, both muscles may be active in flexion and extension, depending on the joint position.

• They assist in flexion from the neutral (0°) position to approximately 70°.

• Their actions reverse past approximately 80° of flexion, and they become active in extension.

The flexor components of both muscles are transformed into extensor components as soon as their insertion (the linea aspera) moves higher than their origin (the inferior or superior pubic ramus).

Promontory

Iliac crest

Anterior superior
iliac spine

Anterior inferior
iliac spine

Superior
pubic ramus

Obturator
externus

Adductor
minimus

Pectineus

Femur

Greater
trochanter

Lesser
trochanter

Pectineus

Adductor
brevis

Adductor
longus

Gracilis

Adductor
magnus

Adductor
hiatus

Adductor
magnus,
tendinous
part

Medial
epicondyle

Patella

Gracilis tendon
of insertion

Tibial
tuberosity

Fibula

Tibia

**C The adductors (obturator externus; pectineus; adductors
longus, brevis, magnus, and minimus; and gracilis)**
Anterior view. A portion of the adductors, pectineus, and gracilis muscles on the left side have been removed just past their origins to demonstrate the course of the obturator externus more clearly.

Note: Unilateral shortening of the adductors leads to functional leg
shortening on the affected side.

481

20.5 The Anterior Thigh Muscles: The Extensor Group

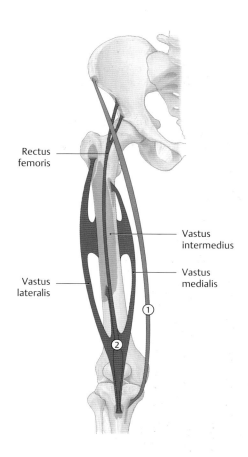

Rectus femoris

Vastus intermedius

Vastus medialis

Vastus lateralis

A Schematic of the extensors

① **Sartorius**

Origin: Anterior superior iliac spine
Insertion: Medial to the tibial tuberosity (together with gracilis and semitendinosus)
Action:
- Hip joint: flexion, abduction, and external rotation
- Knee joint: flexion and internal rotation
Innervation: Femoral nerve (L2, L3)

② **Quadriceps femoris**

Origin:
- Rectus femoris: anterior inferior iliac spine (straight head), acetabular roof of the hip joint (reflected head)
- Vastus medialis: medial lip of the linea aspera, distal part of the intertrochanteric line
- Vastus lateralis: lateral lip of the linea aspera, lateral surface of the greater trochanter
- Vastus intermedius: anterior side of the femoral shaft
- Articularis genus (distal fibers of the vastus intermedius): anterior side of the femoral shaft at the level of the suprapatellar recess

Insertion:
- On the tibial tuberosity via the patellar ligament (entire muscle)
- Both sides of the tibial tuberosity on the medial and lateral condyles via the medial and lateral longitudinal patellar retinacula (vastus medialis and lateralis)
- The suprapatellar recess of the knee joint capsule (articularis genus)

Action:
- Hip joint: flexion (rectus femoris)
- Knee joint: extension (all parts), prevents entrapment of the capsule (articularis genus)

Innervation: Femoral nerve (L2–L4)

B Deficient stabilization of the knee joint due to weakness or paralysis of quadriceps femoris
Right lower limb, lateral view.

a When the quadriceps femoris is intact and the knee is in slight flexion, the line of gravity falls *behind* the transverse axis of knee motion. As the only extensor muscle of the knee joint, the quadriceps femoris keeps the body from tipping backward and ensures stability.
b With weakness or paralysis of the quadriceps femoris, the knee joint can no longer be actively extended. In order to stand upright, the patient must hyperextend the knee so that the line of gravity, and thus the whole-body center of gravity, is shifted forward, in front of the knee, to utilize gravity as the extending force. The joint is stabilized in this situation by the posterior capsule and ligaments of the knee.

Line of gravity

a

b

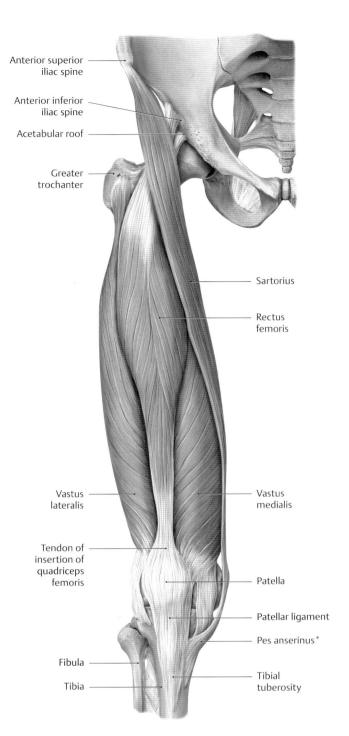

Anterior superior iliac spine

Anterior inferior iliac spine

Acetabular roof

Greater trochanter

Sartorius

Rectus femoris

Vastus lateralis

Vastus medialis

Tendon of insertion of quadriceps femoris

Patella

Patellar ligament

Pes anserinus*

Fibula

Tibia

Tibial tuberosity

Sartorius

Greater trochanter

Intertrochanteric line

Lesser trochanter

Rectus femoris, reflected head

Rectus femoris, straight head

Vastus intermedius

Vastus lateralis

Vastus medialis

Quadriceps femoris

Rectus femoris

Sartorius

Lateral longitudinal patellar retinaculum

Medial longitudinal patellar retinaculum

C The extensors (quadriceps femoris and sartorius)
Right side, anterior view. As its name implies, the quadriceps femoris is basically a four-headed muscle consisting of the rectus femoris and the vastus medialis, lateralis, and intermedius (the vastus intermedius, covered here by the rectus femoris, is visible in **D**). It may also be considered as having a fifth head, the articularis genus. The latter is composed of distal fibers of the vastus intermedius and so does not constitute a separate muscle. But because its fibers insert in the suprapatellar recess (not shown), unlike the other four parts, which all attach to the patellar ligament, the articularis genus is often regarded as the fifth head of the quadriceps femoris.
Note: The only biarticular part of the quadriceps femoris is the rectus femoris, which acts on both the hip and knee joints.

* The pes anserinus is the common tendinous expansion for the gracilis, sartorius, and semitendinosus.

D The extensors (deep portion of the quadriceps femoris)
Right side, anterior view. The sartorius and rectus femoris have been removed to their origins and insertions.
The area of origin of the rectus femoris is intimately related to the anterior aspect of the capsule of the hip joint, a relation with functional and clinical consequences. Pathological swelling of the joint capsule can cause pain that induces reflex reactions when the rectus is used for knee flexion; such reflex reactions are the basis of a useful test. With the patient lying prone, the examiner flexes the patient's knee. This causes passive stretching of the rectus femoris and adds significant pressure to a hip joint capsule already distended by effusion. The patient reflexively "escapes" the painful stimulus by raising the buttock, a positive "rectus sign."

483

20.6 The Posterior Thigh Muscles: The Flexor Group

A Schematic of the flexors

① **Biceps femoris**

Origin:	• Long head: ischial tuberosity, sacrotuberous ligament (common head with semitendinosus)
	• Short head: lateral lip of the linea aspera in the middle third of the femur
Insertion:	Head of fibula
Action:	• Hip joint (long head): adduction, extends the hip, stabilizes the pelvis in the sagittal plane
	• Knee joint (entire muscle): flexion and external rotation
Innervation:	• Tibial nerve, L5–S2 (long head)
	• Common fibular nerve, L5–S2 (short head)

② **Semimembranosus**

Origin:	Ischial tuberosity
Insertion:	Medial tibial condyle, oblique popliteal ligament, popliteus fascia
Action:	• Hip joint: adduction, extends the hip, stabilizes the pelvis in the sagittal plane
	• Knee joint: flexion and internal rotation
Innervation:	Tibial nerve (L5–S2)

③ **Semitendinosus**

Origin:	Ischial tuberosity and sacrotuberous ligament (common head with long head of biceps femoris)
Insertion:	Medial to the tibial tuberosity in the pes anserinus (along with the tendons of gracilis and sartorius)
Action:	• Hip joint: adduction, extends the hip, stabilizes the pelvis in the sagittal plane
	• Knee joint: flexion and internal rotation
Innervation:	Tibial nerve (L5–S2)

④ **Popliteus**

Origin:	Lateral femoral condyle, posterior horn of the lateral meniscus
Insertion:	Posterior tibial surface (above the origin of soleus)
Action:	Flexes and unlocks the knee by internally rotating the femur on the fixed head of the tibia 5°
Innervation:	Tibial nerve (L4–S1)

B Passive and active muscle insufficiency illustrated for ischiocrural muscles

a The ischiocrural hamstring muscles extend from the ischium over the hip joint and knee joint to the lower leg.

b Passive muscle insufficiency (lack of muscle length): With the knee outstretched, the ischiocrural muscles do not stretch enough to allow for maximal bending of the hip joint.

c Active muscle insufficiency (lack of muscle strength): With hip extended, the ischiocrural muscles cannot shorten enough to allow for maximal bending of the knee joint (see also muscle and soft tissue suspension, p. 50).

a

b

C The flexors (the hamstrings and popliteus)

Right side, posterior view.

a The *hamstrings* are the posterior thigh muscles that arise from the ischium and insert on the leg: biceps femoris, semimembrano-

sus, and semitendinosus. All but the short head of the biceps femoris are "biarticular," spanning both the hip and knee joints.

b A portion of the long head of the biceps femoris has been removed to display the short head and its origin from the lateral lip of the linea aspera.

20.7 The Leg Muscles: The Anterior and Lateral Compartments (Extensor and Fibularis Group)

A Schematic of the anterior compartment

B Schematic of the lateral compartment

① **Tibialis anterior**

Origin: Upper two thirds of the lateral surface of the tibia, the crural interosseous membrane, and the highest part of the superficial crural fascia

Insertion: Medial and plantar surface of the medial cuneiform, the medial base of the first metatarsal

Action:
- Talocrural joint: dorsiflexion
- Subtalar joint: inversion (supination)

Innervation: Deep fibular nerve (L4, L5)

② **Extensor digitorum longus**

Origin: Lateral tibial condyle, head of the fibula, medial surface of the fibula, and the crural interosseous membrane

Insertion: By four slips to the dorsal aponeuroses of the second through fifth toes and the bases of the distal phalanges of the second through fifth toes

Action:
- Talocrural joint: dorsiflexion
- Subtalar joint: eversion (pronation)
- Extends the metatarsophalangeal and interphalangeal joints of the second through fifth toes

Innervation: Deep fibular nerve (L4, L5)

③ **Extensor hallucis longus**

Origin: Middle third of the medial surface of the fibula, the crural interosseous membrane

Insertion: Dorsal aponeurosis of the great toe and the base of its distal phalanx

Action:
- Talocrural joint: dorsiflexion
- Subtalar joint: active in both eversion and inversion (pronation/supination), depending on the initial position of the foot
- Extends the metatarsophalangeal and interphalangeal joints of the great toe

Innervation: Deep fibular nerve (L4, L5)

④ **Fibularis tertius (part of extensor digitorum longus) (see also pp. 510 and 514)**

Origin: Anterior border of the distal fibula

Insertion: Base of the fifth metatarsal

Action:
- Talocrural joint: dorsiflexion
- Subtalar joint: eversion (pronation)

Innervation: Deep fibular nerve (L5, S1)

① **Fibularis longus**

Origin: Head of the fibula, proximal two thirds of the lateral surface of the fibula (arising partly from the intermuscular septa)

Insertion: Plantar side of the medial cuneiform, base of the first metatarsal

Action:
- Talocrural joint: plantar flexion
- Subtalar joint: eversion (pronation)
- Supports the transverse arch of the foot

Innervation: Superficial fibular nerve (L5, S1)

② **Fibularis brevis**

Origin: Distal half of the lateral surface of the fibula, intermuscular septa

Insertion: Tuberosity at the base of the fifth metatarsal (with an occasional division to the dorsal aponeurosis of the fifth toe)

Action:
- Talocrural joint: plantar flexion
- Subtalar joint: eversion (pronation)

Innervation: Superficial fibular nerve (L5, S1)

Femur

Lateral
epicondyle

Patella

Medial
epicondyle

Lateral
tibial
condyle

Medial
tibial
condyle

Head of
fibula

Tibial
tuberosity

Shaft of tibia

Tibialis
anterior

Extensor
digitorum
longus

Extensor
hallucis
longus

Lateral
malleolus

Medial
malleolus

Tendons of
extensor
digitorum
longus

Tendon of
extensor
hallucis
longus

First through fifth
distal phalanges

Femur

Patella

Head of
fibula

Lateral
tibial
condyle

Lateral tibial
surface

Interosseous
membrane

Fibularis
longus

Fibularis
brevis

Lateral
malleolus

Calcaneus

Cuboid

Tendon of
fibularis
longus

Tendon of
insertion of
fibularis brevis

Tuberosity
of fifth
metatarsal

First metatarsal

Medial
cuneiform

Cuboid

Tendon of
insertion of
fibularis longus

**E Course of the fibularis longus tendon on
the sole of the foot**
Right foot, plantar view.

**C The anterior compartment
(tibialis anterior, extensor digitorum
longus, and extensor hallucis longus)**
Right leg, anterior view.

**D The lateral compartment
(fibularis longus and brevis)**
Right leg, lateral view.

487

20.8 The Leg Muscles: The Posterior Compartment (Superficial Flexor Group)

① Triceps surae

Origin:	• Soleus: posterior surface of the head and neck of the fibula; attached to the soleal line of the tibia via a tendinous arch
	• Gastrocnemius, medial head: medial epicondyle of the femur
	• Gastrocnemius, lateral head: lateral epicondyle of the femur
Insertion:	The calcaneal tuberosity via the calcaneal (Achilles') tendon
Action:	• Talocrural joint: plantar flexion
	• Knee joint: flexion (gastrocnemius)
Innervation:	Tibial nerve (S1, S2)

② Plantaris

Origin:	Lateral epicondyle proximal to the lateral head of gastrocnemius
Insertion:	The calcaneal tuberosity via the calcaneal (Achilles') tendon
Action:	Negligible due to its small cross section; may act to prevent compression of the posterior leg musculature during knee flexion
Innervation:	Tibial nerve (S1, S2)

A Schematic of the superficial flexors

B Rupture of the calcaneal (Achilles') tendon

Right leg, posterior view. The calcaneal (Achilles') tendon is the common tendon of insertion of the muscles that comprise the triceps surae (the soleus and both heads of the gastrocnemius). The tendon has an average length of 20 to 25 cm, a mean cross-sectional area of approximately 70 to 80 mm², and a breaking strength of 60 to 100 N/mm². A healthy tendon can thus bear a load of nearly 1 ton. It is very unlikely, then, that the calcaneal tendon will rupture unless it has been subjected to chronic excessive loads (in high jumpers, for example). Repetitive microtrauma can compromise the blood supply to the tendon, causing it to degenerate and gradually lose its strength. This is particularly damaging in the area where the tendon already has the least blood flow: approximately 2 to 6 cm proximal to its insertion on the calcaneal tuberosity. This is the most common site of a degenerative calcaneal tendon rupture, which is eventually precipitated by a trivial injury. The rupture is accompanied by a whiplike snapping sound. Afterward the patient loses active plantar flexion and has only residual flexion from the deep flexor muscles (see also pp. 510–514).

— Triceps surae

— Calcaneal (Achilles') tendon

— Rupture site

— Calcaneal tuberosity

Femur

Lateral femoral epicondyle

Medial femoral epicondyle

Plantaris

Gastroc-nemius, lateral head

Gastroc-nemius, medial head

Triceps surae

Soleus

Plantaris tendon

Medial malleolus

Talus

Navicular

First metatarsal

Calcaneal (Achilles') tendon

Lateral malleolus

Calcaneal tuberosity

a

Gastrocnemius, medial head

Plantaris

Gastrocnemius, lateral head

Medial tibial condyle

Head of fibula

Tendinous arch of soleus

Plantaris tendon

Soleus

Gastrocnemius, medial head

Triceps surae

Gastrocnemius, lateral head

Talocrural joint

Calcaneal (Achilles') tendon

Talus

Subtalar joint

Calcaneus

b

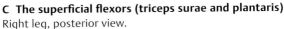

C The superficial flexors (triceps surae and plantaris)
Right leg, posterior view.

a The three heads of the triceps surae are clearly distinguishable: the medial and lateral heads of the gastrocnemius and the soleus. The plantaris, which arises proximal to the lateral head of the gastrocnemius, is often viewed as the fourth head of the triceps surae.

b Portions of the lateral and medial heads of the gastrocnemius have been removed to expose the soleus and the plantaris with its long, narrow tendon of insertion.

489

20.9 The Leg Muscles: The Posterior Compartment (Deep Flexor Group)

A Schematic of the deep flexors

Crural chiasm

Plantar chiasm

① **Tibialis posterior**

Origin:	Crural interosseous membrane and the adjacent borders of the tibia and fibula
Insertion:	Tuberosity of the navicular; medial, intermediate, and lateral cuneiforms; bases of the second through fourth metatarsals
Action:	• Talocrural joint: plantar flexion
	• Subtalar joint: inversion (supination)
	• Supports the longitudinal and transverse arches of the foot
Innervation:	Tibial nerve (L4, L5)

② **Flexor digitorum longus**

Origin:	Middle third of the posterior surface of the tibia
Insertion:	Bases of the second through fifth distal phalanges
Action:	• Talocrural joint: plantar flexion
	• Subtalar joint: inversion (supination)
	• Metatarsophalangeal and interphalangeal joints of the second through fifth toes: plantar flexion
Innervation:	Tibial nerve (L5–S2)

③ **Flexor hallucis longus**

Origin:	Distal two thirds of the posterior surface of the fibula, adjacent crural interosseous membrane
Insertion:	Base of the distal phalanx of the great toe
Action:	• Talocrural joint: plantar flexion
	• Subtalar joint: inversion (supination)
	• Metatarsophalangeal and interphalangeal joints of the great toe: plantar flexion
	• Supports the medial longitudinal arch of the foot
Innervation:	Tibial nerve (L5–S2)

④ **Popliteus**

Origin:	Lateral femoral condyle, posterior horn of lateral meniscus
Insertion:	Posterior tibial surface (above) the origin of the soleus
Action:	Flexes and unlocks the knee by internally rotating the femur on the fixed tibia 5°
Innervation:	Tibial nerve (L4–S1)

Tibialis posterior

Tibia

Calcaneal tuberosity

Calcaneus

Talus

Tendons of insertion of tibialis posterior

Medial cuneiform

Interosseous membrane

Fibula

Lateral malleolus

Cuboid

Tuberosity of cuboid

Tuberosity of fifth metatarsal

First through fifth meta-tarsals

B Insertion of the tibialis posterior
Right foot in plantar flexion, plantar view. With its fan-shaped insertion, the tibialis posterior assists in stabilizing both the longitudinal and transverse arches of the foot.

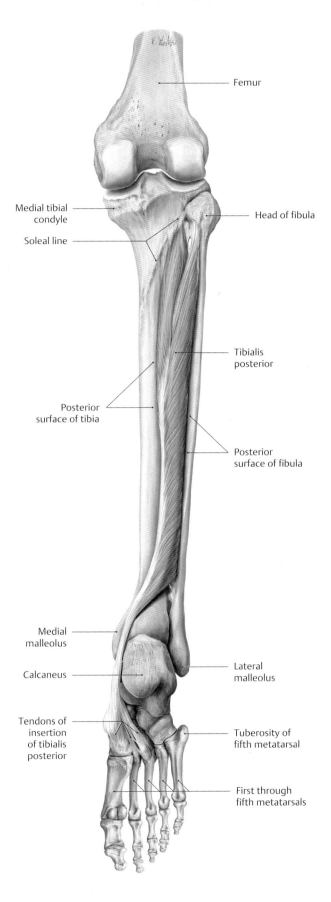

Femur

Medial tibial
condyle

Head
of fibula

Popliteus

Medial tibial
condyle

Head of fibula

Soleal line

Tibialis
posterior

Tibialis
posterior

Flexor
digitorum
longus

Posterior
surface of tibia

Flexor
hallucis
longus

Posterior
surface of fibula

Medial
malleolus

Calcaneal
tuberosity

Medial
malleolus

Lateral
malleolus

Calcaneus

Lateral
malleolus

Tibialis
posterior
tendon

Tendons of
insertion
of tibialis
posterior

Tuberosity of
fifth metatarsal

Flexor
hallucis
longus
tendon

Flexor
digitorum
longus
tendons

First through
fifth metatarsals

**C The deep flexors (tibialis posterior, flexor digitorum longus,
and flexor hallucis longus)**
Right leg with the foot in plantar flexion, posterior view.

D The tibialis posterior
Right leg with the flexor digitorum longus and flexor hallucis longus
removed. Foot in plantar flexion, posterior view.

20.10 The Short Muscles of the Foot: Dorsum, and Medial and Lateral Compartments of the Plantar Surface

A Dorsal view

① **Extensor digitorum brevis**

Origin: Dorsal surface of the calcaneus
Insertion: Dorsal aponeurosis of the second through fourth toes, bases of the middle phalanges of these toes
Action: Extension of the metatarsophalangeal and proximal interphalangeal joints of the second through fourth toes
Innervation: Deep fibular nerve (L5, S1)

② **Extensor hallucis brevis**

Origin: Dorsal surface of the calcaneus
Insertion: Dorsal aponeurosis of the great toe, base of the proximal phalanx of the great toe
Action: Extension of the metatarsophalangeal joint of the great toe
Innervation: Deep fibular nerve (L5, S1)

① **Abductor hallucis**

Origin: Medial process of the calcaneal tuberosity, plantar aponeurosis, flexor retinaculum
Insertion: Base of the proximal phalanx of the great toe via the medial sesamoid
Action: First metatarsophalangeal joint: flexion and medial abduction of the great toe; supports the longitudinal arch
Innervation: Medial plantar nerve (S1, S2)

② **Flexor hallucis brevis**

Origin: Cuboid, lateral cuneiform
Insertion: • Medial head: base of the proximal phalanx of the great toe via the medial sesamoid
• Lateral head: base of the proximal phalanx of the great toe via the lateral sesamoid
Action: Flexes the first metatarsophalangeal joint, supports the longitudinal arch
Innervation: Medial plantar nerve (S1, S2)

③ **Adductor hallucis** (for clarity, the adductor hallucis is depicted here, although it is located in the central compartment)

Origin: • Oblique head: bases of the second through fourth metatarsals, cuboid, lateral cuneiform
• Transverse head: metatarsophalangeal joints of the third through fifth toes, deep transverse metatarsal ligament
Insertion: Base of the first proximal phalanx by a common tendon via the lateral sesamoid
Action: Flexes the first metatarsophalangeal joint, adducts the great toe; transverse head supports the transverse arch, oblique head supports the longitudinal arch
Innervation: Lateral plantar nerve (S2, S3)

④ **Abductor digiti minimi**

Origin: Lateral process and inferior surface of the calcaneal tuberosity, plantar aponeurosis
Insertion: Base of the proximal phalanx of the little toe, tuberosity of the fifth metatarsal
Action: Flexes the metatarsophalangeal joint of the little toe, abducts the little toe, supports the longitudinal arch
Innervation: Lateral plantar nerve (S1–S3)

⑤ **Flexor digiti minimi brevis**

Origin: Base of the fifth metatarsal, long plantar ligament
Insertion: Base of the proximal phalanx of the little toe
Action: Flexes the metatarsophalangeal joint of the little toe
Innervation: Lateral plantar nerve (S2, S3)

⑥ **Opponens digiti minimi (often included with flexor digiti minimi brevis)**

Origin: Long plantar ligament, plantar tendon sheath of the fibularis longus
Insertion: Fifth metatarsal
Action: Pulls the fifth metatarsal slightly in the plantar and medial direction
Innervation: Lateral plantar nerve (S2, S3)

B Plantar view of the medial and lateral compartments

Tendons of
insertion of extensor
digitorum brevis

Fifth distal
phalanx

Fifth middle
phalanx

Fifth proximal
phalanx

First through
fifth meta-
tarsals

Tendon of
insertion of
extensor
hallucis brevis

Extensor
hallucis
brevis

Medial
cuneiform

Extensor
digitorum
brevis

Intermediate
cuneiform

Tuberosity
of fifth
metatarsal

Navicular

Talus

Trochlea of talus

Calcaneus

**C The dorsal muscles of the foot (extensor digitorum brevis and
extensor hallucis brevis)**
Right foot, dorsal view.

Metatarso-
phalangeal
joint capsules

Medial
sesamoid

Lateral
sesamoid

Adductor
hallucis, trans-
verse head

Flexor hallucis
brevis, medial
head

Flexor digiti
minimi brevis

Flexor hallucis
brevis, lateral
head

Opponens
digiti minimi

Adductor
hallucis,
oblique head

Tuberosity
of fifth
metatarsal

Tendon of
insertion of
fibularis
longus

Abductor
digiti minimi

Long plantar
ligament

Abductor
hallucis

Lateral process

Medial process

Calcaneal
tuberosity

**D The plantar muscles of the medial and lateral compartments
(abductor hallucis, adductor hallucis,* flexor hallucis brevis,
abductor digiti minimi, flexor digiti minimi brevis, and
opponens digiti minimi)**
Right foot, plantar view.

* The adductor hallucis is considered part of the central compartment
(see p. 494).

493

20.11 The Short Muscles of the Foot: Central Compartment of the Plantar Surface

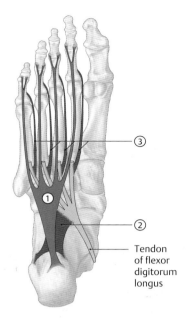

A Plantar view of flexor digitorum brevis, quadratus plantae, and lumbricals

Tendon of flexor digitorum longus

① **Flexor digitorum brevis**

Origin: Medial tubercle of the calcaneal tuberosity, plantar aponeurosis
Insertion: The sides of the middle phalanges of the second through fifth toes
Action: • Flexes the metatarsophalangeal and proximal interphalangeal joints of the second through fifth toes
               • Supports the longitudinal arch of the foot
Innervation: Medial plantar nerve (S1, S2)

② **Quadratus plantae**

Origin: Medial and plantar borders on the plantar side of the calcaneal tuberosity
Insertion: Lateral border of the flexor digitorum longus tendon
Action: Redirects and augments the pull of the flexor digitorum longus
Innervation: Lateral plantar nerve (S1–S3)

③ **First through fourth lumbricals**

Origin: Medial borders of the flexor digitorum longus tendons
Insertion: Dorsal aponeuroses of the second through fifth toes
Action: • Flexes the metatarsophalangeal joints of the second through fifth toes
               • Extension of the interphalangeal joints of the second through fifth toes
               • Moves the toes closer together (adducts the second through fifth toes toward the great toe)
Innervation: • First lumbrical: medial plantar nerve (S2, S3)
               • Second through fourth lumbricals: lateral plantar nerve (S2, S3)

B Plantar view of plantar and dorsal interossei

④ **First through third plantar interossei**

Origin: Medial border of the third through fifth metatarsals
Insertion: Medial base of the proximal phalanx of the third through fifth toes
Action: • Flexes the metatarsophalangeal joints of the third through fifth toes
               • Extension of the interphalangeal joints of the third through fifth toes
               • Moves the toes closer together (adducts the third through fifth toes toward the second toe)
Innervation: Lateral plantar nerve (S2, S3)

⑤ **First through fourth dorsal interossei**

Origin: By two heads from opposing sides of the first through fifth metatarsals
Insertion: • First interosseus: medial base of the second proximal phalanx, dorsal aponeurosis of the second toe
               • Second through fourth interossei: lateral base of the second through fourth proximal phalanges, dorsal aponeurosis of the second through fourth toes
Action: • Flexes the metatarsophalangeal joints of the second through fourth toes
               • Extension of the interphalangeal joints of the second through fourth toes
               • Spreads the toes apart (abducts the third and fourth toes from the second toe)
Innervation: Lateral plantar nerve (S2, S3)

* The adductor hallucis, though part of the central compartment, is not pictured here (see p. 493).

First metatarsal

Third plantar interosseus

Medial cuneiform

Flexor digitorum brevis

Tendon of fibularis longus

Quadratus plantae

Tendon of flexor digitorum longus

Calcaneal tuberosity

a

Tendons of insertion of flexor digitorum longus

First dorsal interosseus

First through fourth lumbricals

Third plantar interosseus

Tendon of fibularis longus

Quadratus plantae

Flexor digitorum longus

Sustentaculum tali

Flexor digitorum brevis

Posterior process of talus

b

C The plantar muscles of the central compartment
Right foot, plantar view.

a Flexor digitorum brevis, quadratus plantae, the first through fourth lumbricals (always numbered in the medial-to-lateral or tibial-to-fibular direction), the first through third plantar interossei, and the first through fourth dorsal interossei (for clarity, the adductor hallucis, though part of the central compartment, is not shown; see p. 493).

b Flexor digitorum brevis has been removed to its origin to display more clearly the insertion of quadratus plantae on the lateral margin of the flexor digitorum longus tendon.

Note: The "movable origins" of the first through fourth lumbricals form the medial borders of the flexor digitorum longus tendons. When the flexor digitorum longus contracts and therefore shortens, the origins of the lumbricals move proximally. This "prestretching" of the lumbricals improves their ability to contract, enabling them to develop greater force.

495

20.12 Overview of Muscle Functions: Hip Joint

A Movements of the hip joint

Type of movement	Range of motion	Muscle	Innervation	Nerve segment
Flexion	120–140°	• Iliopsoas (psoas major and iliacus)	• Direct branches from lumbar plexus and femoral nerve	• L1–L3
		• Rectus femoris	• Femoral nerve	• L2–L4
		• Tensor fasciae latae	• Superior gluteal nerve	• L4–S1
		• Sartorius	• Femoral nerve	• L2, L3
		• Pectineus	• Femoral nerve, obturator nerve	• L2, L3
		• Adductor longus	• Obturator nerve	• L2–L4
		• Adductor brevis	• Obturator nerve	• L2, L3
		• Gracilis	• Obturator nerve	• L2, L3
		• Gluteus medius and minimus, anterior parts	• Superior gluteal nerve	• L4–S1
Extension	20°	• Gluteus maximus	• Inferior gluteal nerve	• L5–S2
		• Semitendinosus	• Tibial nerve	• L5–S2
		• Semimembranosus	• Tibial nerve	• L5–S2
		• Biceps femoris, long head	• Tibial nerve	• L5–S2
		• Gluteus medius and minimus (posterior parts)	• Superior gluteal nerve	• L4–S1
		• Adductor magnus	• Obturator nerve	• L2–L4
			• Tibial nerve	• L4
		• Piriformis	• Direct branches from sacral plexus	• S1, S2
		• Obturator internus	• Direct branches from sacral plexus	• L5, S1
Abduction	50–80°	• Gluteus medius	• Superior gluteal nerve	• L4–S1
		• Tensor fasciae latae	• Superior gluteal nerve	• L4–S1
		• Gluteus maximus (upper fibers)	• Inferior gluteal nerve	• L5–S2
		• Gluteus minimus	• Superior gluteal nerve	• L4–S1
		• Piriformis	• Direct branches from sacral plexus	• S1, S2
		• Sartorius	• Femoral nerve	• L2, L3
		• Piriformis	• Direct branches from sacral plexus	• L5–S2
Adduction	20–30°	• Adductor magnus	• Obturator nerve	• L2–L4
			• Tibial nerve	• L4
		• Adductor longus	• Obturator nerve	• L2–L4
		• Adductor brevis	• Obturator nerve	• L2, L3
		• Gluteus maximus (lower fibers)	• Inferior gluteal nerve	• L5–S2
		• Pectineus	• Femoral nerve, obturator nerve	• L2, L3
		• Gracilis	• Obturator nerve	• L2, L3
		• Semitendinosus	• Tibial nerve	• L5–S2
		• Semimembranosus	• Tibial nerve	• L5–S2
		• Biceps femoris, long head	• Tibial nerve	• L5–S2
		• Quadratus femoris	• Direct branches from sacral plexus	• L5, S1
		• Obturator internus	• Direct branches from sacral plexus	• L5, S1
		• Obturator externus	• Obturator nerve	• L3, L4
Internal rotation	40°	• Gluteus medius and minimus (anterior parts)	• Superior gluteal nerve	• L4–S1
		• Tensor fasciae latae	• Superior gluteal nerve	• L4–S1
		• Adductor magnus (tendinoas insertion)	• Tibial nerve	• L4
External rotation	30–50°	• Gluteus maximus	• Inferior gluteal nerve	• L5–S2
		• Obturator internus	• Direct branches from sacral plexus	• L5, S1
		• Quadratus femoris	• Direct branches from sacral plexus	• L5, S1
		• Obturator externus	• Obturator nerve	• L3, L4
		• Gluteus medius and minimus (posterior parts)	• Superior gluteal nerve	• L4–S1
		• Adductor magnus	• Obturator nerve	• L2–L4
			• Tibial nerve	• L4
		• Adductor longus	• Obturator nerve	• L2–L4
		• Adductor brevis	• Obturator nerve	• L2, L3
		• Pectineus	• Femoral nerve, obturator nerve	• L2, L3
		• Sartorius	• Femoral nerve	• L2, L3
		• Iliopsoas (psoas major and iliacus)	• Direct branches from lumbar plexus and femoral nerve	• L1–L3

a Flexion

b Extension

c Abduction

d Adduction

e Internal rotation

f External rotation

B Movements of the hip joint

a Flexors

c Abductors

g Internal rotators

b Extensors

d Side-by-side comparison of adductors

C Functional muscle testing of the hip joint

In order to test the strength of each muscle, the patient is asked to resist (push back against) the examiner. The force generated by the muscle action is measured using a scale from 0 to 5.

e Adductors in side-lying position with strength unimpaired

f External rotators

D Clinical symptoms of hip muscle shortening and weakness

Muscles	Symptoms of muscle shortening	Symptoms of muscle weakness
Flexors	Shortened hip flexors lead to the pelvis tilting forward with increased lumbar lordosis and impaired hip extension range. One-sided shortening leads to pelvic torsion with ensuing functional impairment mainly in the sacroiliac joint of the affected side.	Activities such as climbing stairs, walking uphill, shifting from supine position to sitting position, or moving the upper body forward when sitting up are considerably impaired with weak flexors. When walking, instead of hip joint flexion, the leg is moved forward by circumduction or through movements of the pelvis.
Extensors	Contractions of the gluteus maximus are rare. Shortened ischiocrural muscles lead to a characteristic posture with increased hip extension and flexion of the lumbar spine.	A lack of stability in stance phase is due to weak hip joint extensors. It is compensated for through shifting of the upper body (to achieve support from the iliofemoral ligament).
Abductors	Shortened abductors lead to pelvic shift in the frontal plane and functional leg elongation of the affected side. The body compensates for leg length discrepancy through increased flexion of the knee joint.	Due to the lack of muscular support, the pelvis cannot be kept in place in stance phase. It drops to the healthy side (positive Trendelenburg sign). In case of slight weakness, the upper body shifts to the affected side, thus preventing the pelvis from dropping (Duchenne sign).
Adductors	Shortened adductors also lead to pelvic shift in the frontal plane and functional leg elongation of the affected side.	Generally, weakness becomes noticeable during extreme movements, e.g., horse riding, skiing (e.g., rider cannot keep himself on horse).
Internal rotators	The hip joint can no longer rotate externally to the full extent, so sitting cross-legged is no longer possible.	Leads to a significant predominance of external rotation (= change of gait pattern: forward section of foot increasingly points outward when walking).
External rotators	The one-sided pull at the sacrum, especially with shortening of the short external rotators, leads to functional impairment of the sacroiliac joint of the affected side.	Increased internal rotation of the affected leg (forward section of foot increasingly points inward when walking).

20.13 Overview of Muscle Functions: Knee Joint

A Movements of the knee joint

Type of movement	Range of motion	Muscle	Innervation	Nerve segment
Flexion	120–150°	• Semimembranosus • Semitendinosus • Biceps femoris, long head • Biceps femoris, short head • Gracilis • Sartorius • Gastrocnemius, medial and lateral heads • Popliteus • Plantaris	• Tibial nerve • Tibial nerve • Tibial nerve • Common fibular nerve • Obturator nerve • Femoral nerve • Tibial nerve • Tibial nerve • Tibial nerve	• L5–S2 • L5–S2 • L5–S2 • L5–S2 • L2, L3 • L2, L3 • S1, S2 • L4–S1 • S1, S2
Extension	5–10°	• Quadriceps femoris – Rectus femoris – Vastus lateralis – Vastus medialis – Vastus intermedius	• Femoral nerve	• L2–L4
Internal rotation	10°	• Semimembranosus • Semitendinosus • Gracilis • Sartorius • Popliteus	• Tibial nerve • Tibial nerve • Obturator nerve • Femoral nerve • Tibial nerve	• L5–S2 • L5–S2 • L2, L3 • L2, L3 • L4–S1
External rotation	30–40°	• Biceps femoris, long head • Biceps femoris, short head	• Tibial nerve • Common fibular nerve	• L5–S2 • L5–S2

c Internal rotation with the knee joint flexed

a Flexion

b Extension

B Movements of the knee joint

d External rotation with the knee joint extended

C Clinical symptoms of knee muscle shortening and weakness

Muscles	Symptoms of muscle shortening	Symptoms of muscle weakness
Flexors	Impaired knee extension with bent hip or impaired hip flexion with hip out-stretched. Shortened flexors, especially the ischiocrural (hamstring) muscles on both sides, lead to straightening of the pelvis and flattening of the lumbar spine. If the shortening affects only one side, the differing pull causes pelvic tilt and functional disorder of the sacroiliac joint.	Weakness of the ischiocrural muscles makes itself felt in both the knee and the hip joint. When standing, the result is increased pelvic tilt forward with simultaneous knee hyperextension. The clinical symptoms are similar to those of extensor weakness.
Extensors	In the case of muscle shortening, the rectus femoris is most commonly affected since it is the only part of the quadriceps femoris that crosses two joints. The result is impaired knee flexion or impaired hip extension with increased lumbar lordosis.	In case of muscle weakness, essential functions are significantly impaired, e.g., climbing stairs, walking uphill, standing up, and sitting down. Compensation occurs through shifting the center of gravity forward via knee hyperextension (genu recurvatum): "Gravity turns into stretching force."
Internal rotators		Increased external rotation of the lower leg
External rotators		Increased internal rotation of the lower leg

a Flexors

b Extensors

D Functional muscle testing of the knee joint

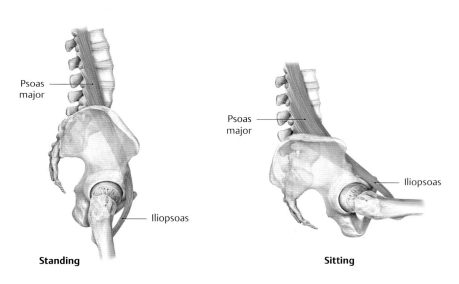

Psoas major

Psoas major

Iliopsoas

Iliopsoas

Standing

Sitting

Ischiocrural muscles

Quadriceps femoris

E Muscular dysbalance

Iliacus not shown. Special testing of every joint includes not only movement tests (neutral zero method, see p. 50) but also functional tests. The primary goal is not to test a muscle's force and ability to stretch but to detect muscular imbalances and coordination impairment. If there is an imbalance between a muscle and its antagonist, it is called a muscular dysbalance. What is commonly meant by this is an imbalance between tonic and phasic muscles.

Tonic muscles primarily consist of slow-twitch muscle fibers and in case of disorders tend to shorten (see p. 56). **Phasic muscles** consist of fast-twitch fibers and tend to weaken (atrophy) in case of disorders. Those disorders are the result of the insufficient adaptation of the musculoskeletal system to the civilized way of life, which includes prolonged sitting, inactivity, habitual movements, and abnormal postures in daily life and at work. Increased variety of motion and better quality of motion are easy ways to counteract the lack of stimuli to muscles.

Examples of the development of muscular dysbalances:
- Prolonged sitting leads to increased structural shortening of the iliopsoas muscles (these muscles reach their original length in standing position) and significant weakening of the hip extensors (mainly the gluteus maximus and ischiocrural muscles) and thus indirectly leads to increased susceptibility to disorders of the hyperlordotic lumbar spine.
- High heels lead to increased load on the quadriceps femoris with corresponding increased tonus; the ischiocrural muscles, as antagonists, however, shorten due to the constant lack of stimuli.

20.14 Overview of Muscle Functions: Ankle Joints

A Movements of the upper and lower ankle joint and the transverse tarsal joint

Type of movement	Range of motion	Muscle	Innervation	Nerve segment
Plantar flexion	40–50°	• Triceps surae	• Tibial nerve	• S1, S2
		• Fibularis longus	• Superficial fibular nerve	• L4, L5
		• Fibularis brevis	• Superficial fibular nerve	• L4, L5
		• Flexor hallucis longus	• Tibial nerve	• L5–S2
		• Flexor digitorum longus	• Tibial nerve	• L5–S2
		• Tibialis posterior	• Tibial nerve	• L4, L5
		• Plantaris	• Tibial nerve	• S1, S2
Dorsiflexion	20–30°	• Tibialis anterior	• Deep fibular nerve	• L4, L5
		• Extensor digitorum longus	• Deep fibular nerve	• L4, L5
		• Extensor hallucis longus	• Deep fibular nerve	• L4, L5
Inversion and supination	60°	• Tibialis posterior	• Tibial nerve	• L4, L5
		• Flexor hallucis longus	• Tibial nerve	• L5–S2
		• Flexor digitorum longus	• Tibial nerve	• L5–S2
		• Tibialis anterior	• Deep fibular nerve	• L4, L5
		• (Extensor hallucis longus)	• Deep fibular nerve	• L4, L5
Eversion and pronation	30°	• Fibularis longus	• Superficial fibular nerve	• L5, S1
		• Fibularis brevis	• Superficial fibular nerve	• L5, S1
		• Extensor digitorum longus	• Deep fibular nerve	• L4, L5
		• (Extensor hallucis longus)	• Deep fibular nerve	• L4, L5

a Plantar flexion

b Dorsiflexion

c Lifting the medial border of the foot (inversion and supination)

d Lifting the lateral border of the foot (eversion and pronation)

B Movements of the upper and lower ankle joint and the transverse tarsal joint

C Location of tendons of the long muscles of the foot relative to the axes of the upper and lower ankle joint

Superior view of both axes of the upper and lower ankle joint. Depending on the course of the tendons, the muscles can plantar flex and dorsal extend while at the same time pronating (everting) and supinating (inverting).

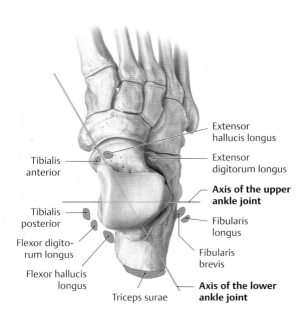

Tibialis anterior

Tibialis posterior

Flexor digitorum longus

Flexor hallucis longus

Triceps surae

Extensor hallucis longus

Extensor digitorum longus

Axis of the upper ankle joint

Fibularis longus

Fibularis brevis

Axis of the lower ankle joint

a Plantar flexors
(standing on the toes)

c Supinators

b Dorsiflexors

d Pronators

D Functional muscle testing of the ankle joint

E Clinical symptoms of muscle shortening and weakness of the upper and lower ankle joint

Muscles	Symptoms of muscle shortening	Symptoms of muscle weakness
Plantar flexors	Shortening of plantar flexors, mainly the triceps surae, leads to club foot (pes equinovarus). The resulting functional leg elongation when standing is compensated for by increased knee flexion. When walking, during swing phase, increased hip flexon is required in order to allow for the functionally longer leg to swing forward.	Tiptoe position is usually not possible, and jumping power is considerably impaired. Also common is development of talipes calcaneus (no rollover during walking). In stance phase, there is increased knee extension.
Dorsi-flexors	Shortening of dorsiflexors leads to impaired plantar flexion and impaired rollover during walking. Often development of club foot (no rollover during walking) develops.	The forward section of the foot cannot be sufficiently lifted during swing phase. To compensate for it, there is increased bending of the hip and knee. This characteristic gait pattern is also known as stork legs.
Supinators	Shortening leads to pes equinovarus. There is increased load on the lateral bottom of the foot during walking.	Weakened supinators result in valgus position (talipes valgus) with increased load on the inside edge of the foot.
Pronators	If the pronators (e.g., the fibularis muscles) are affected by shortening, the foot is plantar flexed and pronated (pes equinovalgus).	Weakened pronators often result in distortion of the upper and lower ankle joint (so-called supination trauma).

21.1 The Muscles of the Medial and Anterior Thigh, Hip, and Gluteal Region

Iliac crest

Iliacus

Anterior superior iliac spine

Psoas minor

Psoas major

Obturator internus

Pubic symphysis

Sartorius

Adductor longus

Rectus femoris

Vastus medialis

Patella

Patellar ligament

Pes anserinus (common tendon of insertion)

Tibialis anterior

L5 vertebral body

Promontory

Sacrum

Piriformis

Gluteus maximus

Adductor magnus

Semi-tendinosus

Gracilis

Semi-membranosus

Gastroc-nemius

Tibia

A The muscles of the thigh, hip, and gluteal region
Right side, medial view.

Iliac crest

Iliacus

Anterior superior iliac spine

Tensor fasciae latae

Iliopsoas

Rectus femoris

Iliotibial tract

Vastus lateralis

Head of fibula

Anterior longitudinal ligament

Promontory

Psoas major

Piriformis

Inguinal ligament

Pubic symphysis

Pectineus

Adductor longus

Sartorius

Gracilis

Adductor magnus

Vastus medialis

Patella

Patellar ligament

Pes anserinus

a

Sartorius

Rectus femoris

Vastus intermedius

Sartorius

Gracilis

Pes anserinus (common tendon of insertion)

Semi-tendinosus

b

B The muscles of the thigh, hip, and gluteal region
Right side, anterior view.
a The fascia lata of the thigh (see p. 545) has been removed as far as the lateral iliotibial tract.

b Portions of the sartorius and rectus femoris have also been removed.

503

21.2 The Muscles of the Anterior Thigh, Hip, and Gluteal Region: Origins and Insertions

A The muscles of the thigh, hip, and gluteal region
Right side, anterior view. The origins and insertions of the muscles are indicated by color shading (red = origin, blue = insertion).

a The iliopsoas and tensor fasciae latae have been partially removed. The sartorius, rectus femoris, vastus lateralis, and vastus medialis have been completely removed.

b The quadriceps femoris, iliopsoas, tensor fasciae latae, and pectineus have been completely removed. The midportion of the adductor longus has been removed.

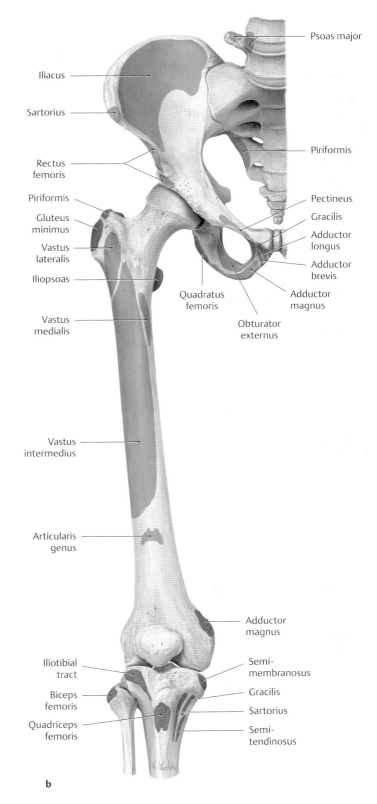

B The muscles of the thigh, hip, and gluteal region
Right side, anterior view. The origins and insertions of the muscles are indicated by color shading (red = origin, blue = insertion).

a All of the muscles have been removed except for adductor magnus and quadratus femoris.

b All of the muscles have been removed.

Note the adductor hiatus, through which the femoral artery and vein enter the popliteal fossa of the leg.

21.3 The Muscles of the Lateral and Posterior Thigh, Hip, and Gluteal Region

- L4 spinous process
- Iliac crest
- Posterior superior iliac spine
- Gluteus medius
- Anterior superior iliac spine
- Gluteus maximus
- Tensor fasciae latae
- Sartorius
- Rectus femoris
- Iliotibial tract
- Biceps femoris, long head
- Vastus lateralis
- Patella
- Patellar ligament
- Head of fibula
- Tibial tuberosity
- Fibularis longus
- Tibialis anterior
- Gastrocnemius

A The muscles of the thigh, hip, and gluteal region
Right side, lateral view. *Note* the tensor fasciae latae and gluteus maximus muscles, whose tendons of insertion strengthen land thicken the lateral part of the fascia lata. This thickened band, called *the iliotibial* tract because it runs between the *iliac* crest and the lateral side of the upper *tibia*, functions mechanically as a tension band to reduce the bending loads on the proximal femur (after Pauwels, see also p. 415).

L5 spinous
process

Iliac crest

Anterior
superior
iliac spine

Gluteus
medius

Tensor
fasciae latae

Gluteus
maximus

Greater
trochanter

Adductor
magnus

Iliotibial
tract

Semi-
tendinosus

Biceps femoris,
long head

Gracilis

Semi-
membranosus

Popliteal fossa

Plantaris

Gastrocnemius,
medial and
lateral heads

a

Gluteus
medius

Iliac crest

Anterior
superior
iliac spine

Gluteus
minimus

Tensor
fasciae latae

Piriformis

Gluteus
medius
(cut edge)

Quadratus
femoris

Gluteus
maximus

Adductor
magnus

Gluteus
maximus

Gemellus
superior

Gemellus
inferior

Obturator
internus

Sacro-
tuberous
ligament

Ischial
tuberosity

Iliotibial
tract

Semi-
tendinosus

Biceps
femoris,
long head

Gracilis

Semi-
membranosus

Plantaris

Pes anserinus

Gastrocnemius,
medial and
lateral heads

b

B The muscles of the thigh, hip, and gluteal region
Right side, posterior view.
a The fascia lata has been removed as far as the iliotibial tract (the portion over the buttock is called the gluteal fascia).

b The gluteus maximus and gluteus medius have been partially
removed.

21.4 The Muscles of the Posterior Thigh, Hip, and Gluteal Region: Origins and Insertions

A The muscles of the thigh, hip, and gluteal region
Right side, posterior view. The origins and insertions of the muscles are indicated by color shading (red = origin, blue = insertion).

a The semitendinosus and biceps femoris have been partially removed.

The gluteus maximus and medius have been completely removed.
b The hamstrings (semitendinosus, semimembranosus, and biceps femoris) and gluteus minimus have been completely removed.

a

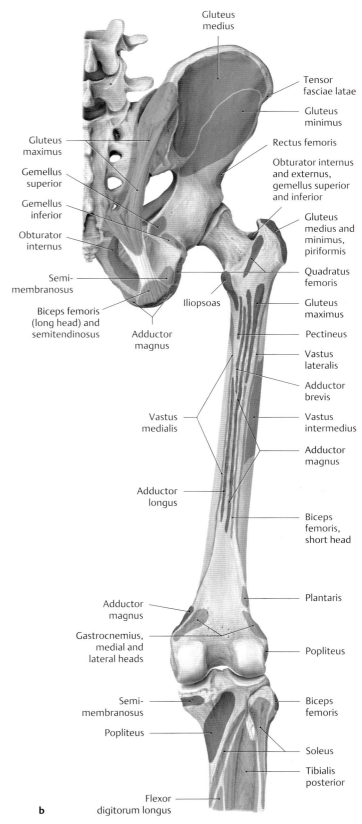

b

B The muscles of the thigh, hip, and gluteal region

Right side, posterior view. The origins and insertions of the muscles are indicated by color shading (red = origin, blue = insertion).

a All muscles have been removed except for the adductor brevis, adductor longus, gemellus superior and inferior, and obturator externus.

b All of the muscles have been removed.

21.5 The Muscles of the Lateral and Anterior Leg: Origins and Insertions

Biceps femoris, long head

Biceps femoris, short head

Head of fibula

Gastrocnemius, lateral head

Soleus

Triceps surae

Fibularis brevis

Lateral malleolus, fibula

Calcaneal (Achilles') tendon

Calcaneus

Rectus femoris

Vastus lateralis

Iliotibial tract

Patella

Patellar ligament

Lateral tibial condyle

Fibularis longus

Tibialis anterior

Extensor digitorum longus

Extensor hallucis longus

Extensor digitorum brevis

Fibularis tertius (variable)

Fibularis longus

Fibularis brevis

Extensor digitorum longus

a

Rectus femoris

Vastus lateralis

Iliotibial tract

Patellar ligament

Tibial tuberosity

Fibularis longus

Extensor digitorum longus

Fibularis tertius (variable)

b

Gracilis

Sartorius

Vastus medialis

Patella

Pes anserinus (common tendon of insertion of sartorius, gracilis, and semitendinosus)

Gastrocnemius, medial head

Soleus

Tibia

Tibialis anterior

Extensor hallucis longus

Medial malleolus

Extensor hallucis brevis

Interossei

Extensor digitorum longus

Extensor hallucis longus

A The muscles of the right leg
a Lateral view, **b** anterior view.

a

b

B The muscles of the right leg

Anterior view. The origins and insertions of the muscles are indicated by color shading (red = origin, blue = insertion).

a The tibialis anterior and fibularis longus have been completely removed, as have the distal portions of the extensor digitorum longus tendons. The fibularis tertius is a division of the extensor digitorum longus.

b All of the muscles have been removed.

21.6 The Muscles of the Posterior Leg: Origins and Insertions

Gracilis

Semi-
tendinosus

Semi-
membranosus

Gastroc-
nemius,
medial head

Iliotibial
tract

Plantaris

Biceps
femoris

Gastroc-
nemius,
lateral head

Fibularis
longus

Soleus

Flexor
digitorum longus

Flexor
hallucis longus

Calcaneal
(Achilles')
tendon

Fibularis
brevis

Medial
malleolus

Lateral
malleolus

Tibialis
posterior

Calcaneus

Flexor
digitorum longus

Fibularis
brevis

Flexor
hallucis longus

Fibularis
longus

a

Gastrocnemius,
medial head

Gastrocnemius,
lateral head

Plantaris

Biceps femoris

Popliteus

Fibularis
longus

Soleus

Plantaris
tendon

Fibularis longus

Flexor
digitorum longus

Calcaneal
(Achilles')
tendon

Flexor
hallucis longus

Fibularis brevis

Tibialis
posterior

Calcaneus

Flexor
digitorum longus

Fibularis
brevis

Flexor
hallucis longus

Fibularis
longus

b

A The muscles of the right leg
Posterior view. The origins and insertions of the muscles are indicated
by color shading (red = origin, blue = insertion). The foot is shown in
a plantar-flexed position to better demonstrate the plantar tendons.

a The bulge of the calf is produced mainly by the triceps surae muscle
(= soleus plus the two heads of the gastrocnemius).
b Both heads of the gastrocnemius have been removed.

Gastrocnemius, medial head

Plantaris

Gastrocnemius, lateral head

Popliteus

Biceps femoris

Fibularis longus

Soleus

Tibialis posterior

Flexor digitorum longus

Flexor hallucis longus

Crural chiasm

Plantaris

Triceps surae

Plantar chiasm

Tibialis posterior

Fibularis brevis

Tibialis anterior

Flexor hallucis longus

Flexor digitorum longus

a

Gastrocnemius, medial head

Plantaris

Gastrocnemius, lateral head

Popliteus

Biceps femoris

Fibularis longus

Soleus

Tibialis posterior

Flexor digitorum longus

Flexor hallucis longus

Interosseous membrane

Fibularis brevis

Plantaris

Triceps surae

Tibialis posterior

Fibularis brevis

Tibialis anterior

Fibularis longus

Flexor hallucis longus

Flexor digitorum longus

b

B The muscles of the right leg

Posterior view. The origins and insertions of the muscles are indicated by color shading (red = origin, blue = insertion). The foot is shown in a plantar-flexed position to better demonstrate the plantar tendons.

a The triceps surae, plantaris, and popliteus muscles have been removed.

b All of the muscles have been removed.

513

21.7   The Tendon Sheaths and Retinacula of the Foot

Fibularis longus

Triceps surae

Tibialis anterior

Tibia

Extensor digitorum longus

Extensor hallucis longus

Fibularis brevis

Superior extensor retinaculum

Medial malleolus

Lateral malleolus

Inferior extensor retinaculum

Fibularis brevis

Tendon sheath

Fibularis tertius (variable)

Extensor hallucis brevis

Tuberosity of fifth metatarsal

Extensor digitorum brevis

Extensor digitorum longus

Abductor digiti minimi

Interossei

Extensor hallucis longus

A The tendon sheaths and retinacula of the right foot
Anterior view. The foot is plantar-flexed, with superficial fascia removed, to display the deep fascial bands—*retinacula*—that hold in place the tendon sheaths of the long foot extensors and flexors. The superior and inferior extensor retinacula retain the long extensor tendons, allowing efficient redirection of the forces generated by their muscles (tibialis anterior, extensor digitorum longus, extensor hallucis longus, and fibularis tertius) while preventing the tendons from rising away from the bones of the ankle when the foot is dorsiflexed. Similarly, the fibular retinacula, laterally, hold the fibular muscle tendons in place posterior to the lateral malleolus (see **B**, part **a**), and the flexor retinaculum retains the long flexor tendons behind the medial malleolus (see **B**, part **b**), preventing displacement of these tendons while enabling them to operate smoothly regardless of the orientation of the ankle joint.

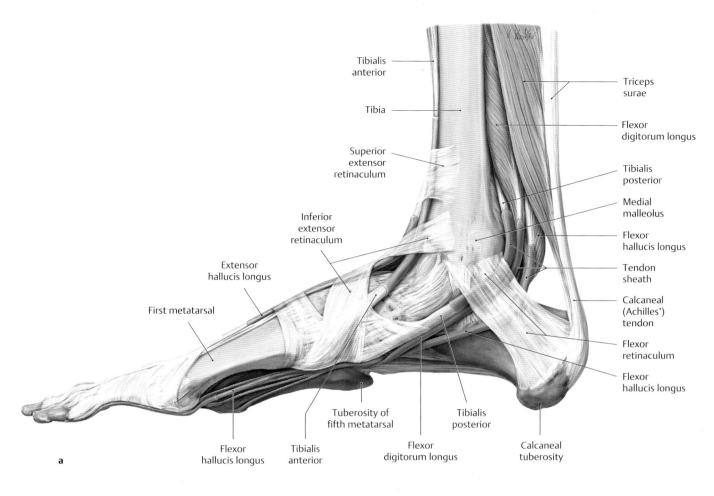

Tibialis anterior

Tibia

Triceps surae

Flexor digitorum longus

Superior extensor retinaculum

Tibialis posterior

Inferior extensor retinaculum

Medial malleolus

Flexor hallucis longus

Extensor hallucis longus

Tendon sheath

First metatarsal

Calcaneal (Achilles') tendon

Flexor retinaculum

Flexor hallucis longus

Flexor hallucis longus

Tibialis anterior

Tuberosity of fifth metatarsal

Tibialis posterior

Flexor digitorum longus

Calcaneal tuberosity

a

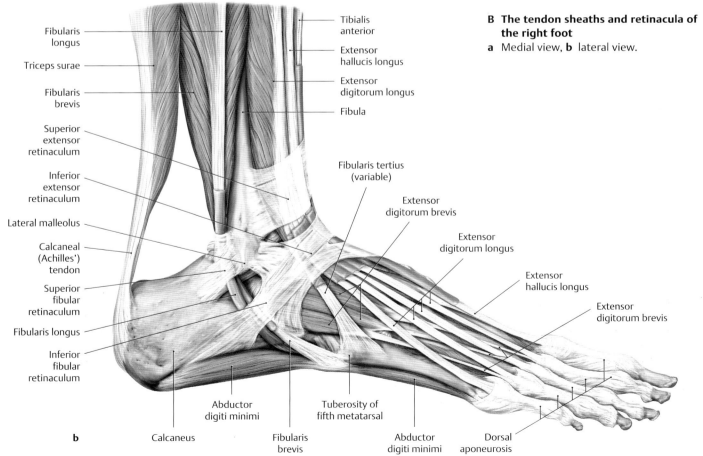

Fibularis longus

Triceps surae

Fibularis brevis

Superior extensor retinaculum

Inferior extensor retinaculum

Lateral malleolus

Calcaneal (Achilles') tendon

Superior fibular retinaculum

Fibularis longus

Inferior fibular retinaculum

Tibialis anterior

Extensor hallucis longus

Extensor digitorum longus

Fibula

Fibularis tertius (variable)

Extensor digitorum brevis

Extensor digitorum longus

Extensor hallucis longus

Extensor digitorum brevis

Abductor digiti minimi

Tuberosity of fifth metatarsal

Abductor digiti minimi

Dorsal aponeurosis

b

Calcaneus

Fibularis brevis

B The tendon sheaths and retinacula of the right foot
a Medial view, **b** lateral view.

21.8 The Intrinsic Foot Muscles from the Plantar View: The Plantar Aponeurosis and Superficial Layer

Superficial transverse metatarsal ligament

Transverse fascicles

Flexor hallucis brevis

Medial plantar septum

Abductor hallucis

Tibialis posterior

Flexor digitorum longus

Flexor hallucis longus

Calcaneal tuberosity

Flexor digiti minimi brevis

Third plantar interosseus

Tuberosity of fifth metatarsal

Abductor digiti minimi

Lateral plantar septum

Plantar aponeurosis

Fibularis longus

A The plantar aponeurosis of the right foot
Plantar view. The *plantar aponeu*rosis is a tough toponeurotic sheet that is thicker centrally than medially and laterally and blends with the dorsal fascia (not shown here) at the borders of the foot. Two sagittal expansions of the thick *central* aponeurosis (the medial and lat-

eral plantar septa) extend deep to the bones of the foot, defining the boundaries of three muscle compartments in the plantar region: the medial compartment, lateral compartment, and central compartment (not labeled here, see p. 494). The main function of the plantar aponeurosis is to give *passive* support to the longitudinal arch (see also p. 467).

Anular ligaments

Cruciform ligaments

Flexor
digitorum brevis

Flexor
hallucis longus

Lumbricals

Third plantar
interosseus

Flexor
hallucis brevis

Fourth dorsal
interosseus

Flexor digiti
minimi brevis

Flexor
digitorum brevis

Abductor
digiti minimi

Abductor
hallucis

Fibularis
longus

Tibialis posterior

Flexor
digitorum longus

Plantar aponeurosis
(cut edge)

Flexor
hallucis longus

Calcaneal tuberosity

B The short muscles of the right foot
Plantar view. The entire plantar aponeurosis, including the superficial transverse metacarpal ligament, has been removed.

Note the anular ligaments on the plantar side of the toes. Together with the oblique cruciform ligaments, they strengthen the tendon sheaths and help to hold the tendons in position.

21.9 The Intrinsic Foot Muscles from the Plantar View: Middle Layer

Flexor digitorum brevis

Flexor digitorum longus

Third plantar interosseus

Fourth dorsal interosseus

Flexor digiti minimi brevis

Abductor digiti minimi

Quadratus plantae

Fibularis longus

Flexor digitorum brevis

Plantar aponeurosis (cut edge)

Flexor hallucis longus

Adductor hallucis, transverse head

Lumbricals

Flexor hallucis brevis

Flexor digitorum longus

Tendon of insertion of fibularis longus

Abductor hallucis

Tibialis posterior

Flexor digitorum longus

Flexor hallucis longus

Calcaneal tuberosity

A The short muscles of the right foot
Plantar view. The plantar aponeurosis and flexor digitorum brevis have been removed.

Flexor
digitorum longus

Flexor
digitorum brevis

Abductor
digiti minimi

Plantar and
dorsal interossei

Opponens
digiti minimi

Flexor digiti
minimi brevis

Tuberosity of
fifth metatarsal

Fibularis brevis

Long plantar ligament

Quadratus plantae

Fibularis longus

Abductor
digiti minimi

Flexor
digitorum brevis

Plantar aponeurosis
(cut edge)

Flexor
hallucis longus

Lumbricals

Adductor hallucis,
transverse head

Flexor hallucis brevis,
medial and lateral meads

Adductor hallucis,
oblique head

Abductor hallucis

Tendon of insertion
of fibularis longus

Tendon of insertion
of tibialis posterior

Tibialis posterior

Abductor
hallucis

Flexor
digitorum longus

Flexor
hallucis longus

Calcaneal tuberosity

B The short muscles of the right foot
Plantar view. The plantar aponeurosis has been removed in addition to
the following muscles: flexor digitorum brevis, abductor digiti minimi,
abductor hallucis, quadratus plantae, the lumbricals, and the tendons
of insertion of the flexor digitorum longus and flexor hallucis longus.

Note that each of the four tendons of insertion of the flexor digitorum
brevis divides into two slips, and that the tendons of the flexor digitorum longus pass between these slips to insert on the distal phalanges.

519

21.10 The Intrinsic Foot Muscles from the Plantar View: Deep Layer and Origins and Insertions

Plantar ligaments

First through fourth lumbricals

Adductor hallucis, transverse head

Adductor hallucis, oblique head

Flexor digiti minimi brevis

Abductor digiti minimi

Third plantar interosseus

Fourth dorsal interosseus

Second plantar interosseus

Third dorsal interosseus

First plantar interosseus

Opponens digiti minimi

Flexor digiti minimi brevis

Tuberosity of fifth metatarsal

Long plantar ligament

Fibularis brevis

Quadratus plantae

Fibularis longus

Abductor digiti minimi

Flexor digitorum brevis

Plantar aponeurosis (cut edge)

Flexor hallucis brevis

First dorsal interosseus

Second dorsal interosseus

Abductor hallucis

Adductor hallucis, oblique head

Flexor hallucis brevis

Tendon of insertion of tibialis anterior

Tendon of insertion of fibularis longus

Tendon of insertion of tibialis posterior

Abductor hallucis

Talus

Calcaneus

A The short muscles of the right foot

Plantar view. All of the short foot muscles except for the dorsal and plantar interossei have been removed, leaving behind their origins and insertions.

Note the course of the tibialis posterior and fibularis longus tendons of insertion, both of which help to support the transverse arch of the foot.

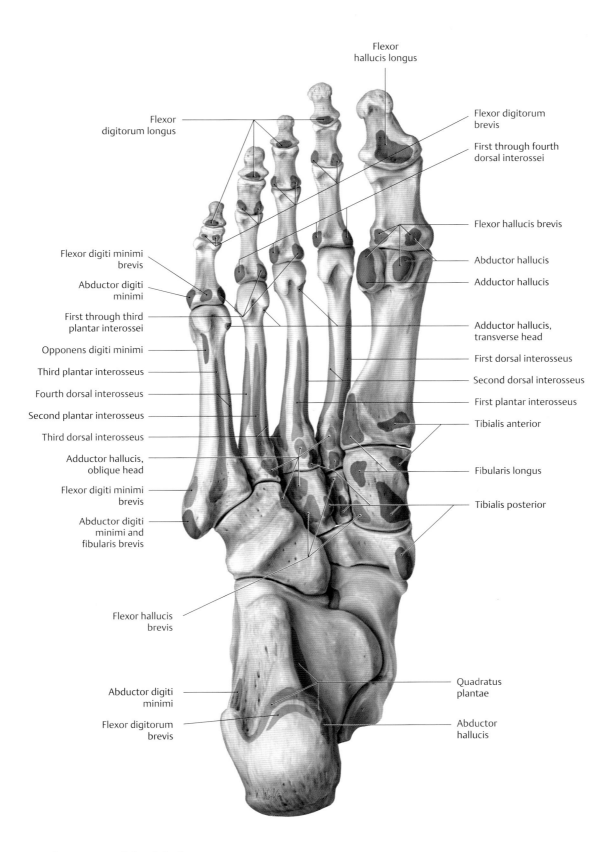

Flexor
hallucis longus

Flexor
digitorum longus

Flexor digitorum
brevis

First through fourth
dorsal interossei

Flexor digiti minimi
brevis

Abductor digiti
minimi

First through third
plantar interossei

Opponens digiti minimi

Third plantar interosseus

Fourth dorsal interosseus

Second plantar interosseus

Third dorsal interosseus

Adductor hallucis,
oblique head

Flexor digiti minimi
brevis

Abductor digiti
minimi and
fibularis brevis

Flexor hallucis
brevis

Abductor digiti
minimi

Flexor digitorum
brevis

Flexor hallucis brevis

Abductor hallucis

Adductor hallucis

Adductor hallucis,
transverse head

First dorsal interosseus

Second dorsal interosseus

First plantar interosseus

Tibialis anterior

Fibularis longus

Tibialis posterior

Quadratus
plantae

Abductor
hallucis

B Muscle origins and insertions of the right foot
Plantar view. The origins and insertions of the muscles are indicated by
color shading (red = origin, blue = insertion).

521

21.11 Cross-sectional Anatomy of the Thigh, Leg, and Foot

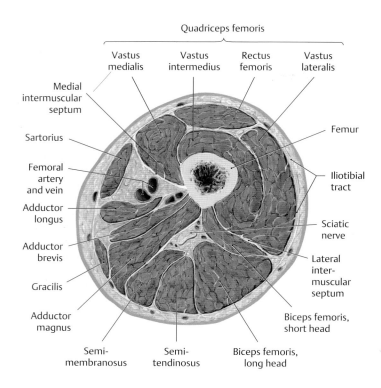

A Cross section through the right thigh
Proximal view. The level of the section is shown in **C**.

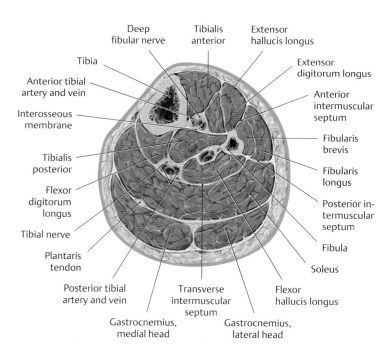

B Cross section through the right leg
Proximal view. The level of the section is shown in **C**.

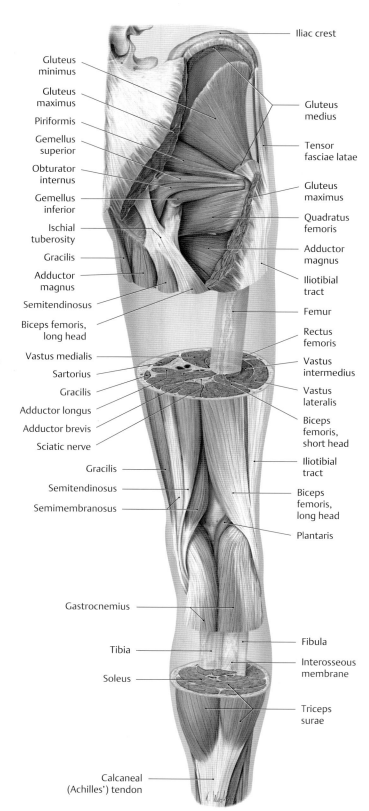

C "Windowed" dissection of the right lower limb
Posterior view. Portions of the gluteus maximus and medius have been removed (the removed cross sections are shown in **A** and **B**). The lower limb is one of the body regions most frequently examined by tomographic methods, and a knowledge of its cross-sectional anatomy is critically important in the identification of landmarks in both radiological and magnetic resonance (MR)–based images.

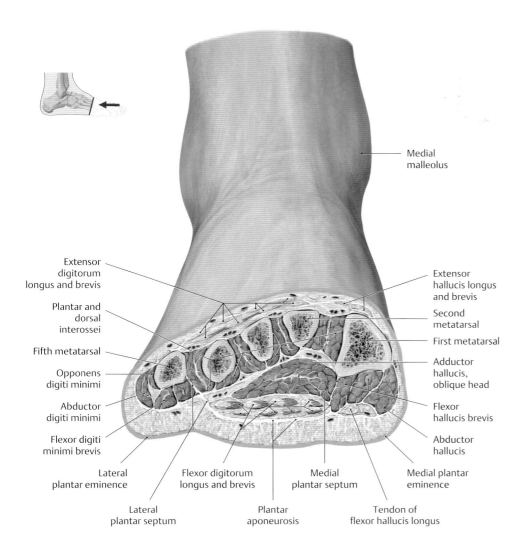

Medial
malleolus

Extensor
digitorum
longus and brevis

Plantar and
dorsal
interossei

Fifth metatarsal

Opponens
digiti minimi

Abductor
digiti minimi

Flexor digiti
minimi brevis

Extensor
hallucis longus
and brevis

Second
metatarsal

First metatarsal

Adductor
hallucis,
oblique head

Flexor
hallucis brevis

Abductor
hallucis

Lateral
plantar eminence

Flexor digitorum
longus and brevis

Medial
plantar septum

Medial plantar
eminence

Lateral
plantar septum

Plantar
aponeurosis

Tendon of
flexor hallucis longus

D Cross section through the right foot at the level of the metatarsals

View of the distal cut surface. The muscle compartments of the foot are formed mainly by the plantar aponeurosis, the medial and lateral plantar septa, and the deep plantar fascia (see also **E**). Foot injuries, such as fracture-dislocations of the tarsus and metatarsus, may lead to *compartment syndromes of the foot*. They are caused by increased tissue pressure in the affected compartment due to the local extravasation of blood. The raised pressure in the compartment leads to impaired venous drainage and diminished capillary perfusion, manifested clinically by swelling and pain. This leads in turn to neuromuscular dysfunction with circulatory compromise that may culminate in muscle necrosis (drawn from a specimen in the Anatomical Collection of Kiel University).

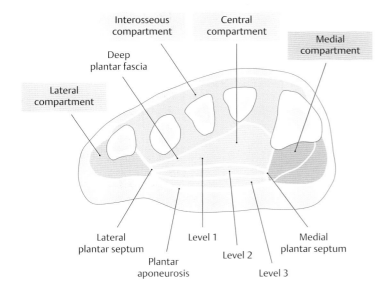

Interosseous
compartment

Central
compartment

Medial
compartment

Deep
plantar fascia

Lateral
compartment

Lateral
plantar septum

Level 1

Medial
plantar septum

Plantar
aponeurosis

Level 2

Level 3

E Location of the compartments of the foot

Schematic cross section through a right foot, distal view. The different muscle compartments are indicated by color shading.

F The four compartments of the foot and their muscular contents

(see also **E**)

Interosseous compartment
• Dorsal and plantar interossei

Medial compartment
• Abductor hallucis
• Flexor hallucis brevis
• Tendon of insertion of flexor hallucis longus

Lateral compartment
• Abductor digiti minimi
• Flexor digiti minimi brevis
• Opponens digiti minimi

Central compartment, consisting of three levels
• Level 1: adductor hallucis
• Level 2: quadratus plantae, lumbricals, and flexor digitorum longus tendons
• Level 3: flexor digitorum brevis

(after Mubarak and Hargens)

523

22.1 The Arteries

A Different segments of the arteries of the lower limb
a Right leg, anterior view; **b** right leg, posterior view. The different arterial segments are shown in different colors.

External iliac artery arises with the internal iliac artery from the common iliac artery and descends along the medial border of the psoas major through the lacuna vasorum (see p. 549). It becomes the femoral artery at the level of the inguinal ligament.
Femoral artery, the continuation of the external iliac artery, runs down the medial side of the thigh to the adductor canal, through which it passes from the anterior to the posterior side of the limb. On leaving the adductor hiatus, it becomes the popliteal artery.
Popliteal artery runs from the adductor hiatus through the popliteal fossa to the popliteus, dividing at the inferior border of that muscle into its terminal branches, the anterior and posterior tibial arteries.
Anterior tibial artery enters the extensor compartment of the leg at the upper border of the interosseous membrane and descends between the tibialis anterior and extensor hallucis longus. Distal to the extensor retinaculum, it continues onto the dorsum of the foot as the *dorsal pedal artery*.
Posterior tibial artery, the direct continuation of the popliteal artery, enters the flexor compartment of the leg and passes behind the medial malleolus. At that level it divides into its two terminal branches, the *medial* and *lateral plantar arteries* (the latter is shown in **D**), which continue onto the plantar side of the foot. The posterior tibial artery also gives rise to the fibular artery.

B Overview of the principal arteries of the lower limb
The arteries of the lower limb vary considerably in their origins and branching patterns (the main variants are reviewed in Chapter 5, Neurovascular Systems: Topographical Anatomy). The branches are listed in the order in which they arise from the parent vessels.

Branches of the external iliac artery
- Inferior epigastric artery
  - Cremasteric artery
  - Artery of the round ligament of the uterus
  - Pubic branch
- Deep circumflex iliac artery

Branches of the femoral* artery
- Superficial epigastric artery
- Superficial circumflex iliac artery
- Superficial external pudendal artery
- Deep external pudendal artery
- Deep artery of the thigh
  - Medial circumflex femoral artery
  - Lateral circumflex femoral artery
  - Perforating branches
- Descending genicular artery

Branches of the popliteal artery
- Medial and lateral superior genicular arteries
- Sural arteries
- Middle genicular artery
- Medial and lateral inferior genicular arteries
  Note that the paired superior and inferior genicular arteries form the *arterial anastomotic network* around the knee.

Branches of the anterior tibial artery
- Anterior tibial recurrent artery
- Anterior lateral malleolar artery
- Anterior medial malleolar artery
- Dorsal pedal artery
  - Lateral tarsal artery
  - Medial tarsal artery
  - Arcuate artery with the dorsal metatarsal arteries
    (→ dorsal digital arteries)

Branches of the posterior tibial artery
- Posterior tibial recurrent artery (arterial network of the knee)
- Fibular artery
  - Perforating branch
  - Communicating branch
  - Lateral malleolar branches
  - Calcaneal branches
- Medial malleolar branch
- Calcaneal branches
- Medial plantar artery
  - Superficial branch
  - Deep branch (→ deep plantar arch)
- Lateral plantar artery (→ deep plantar arch)
- Plantar metatarsal arteries
- Common plantar digital arteries

* Often referred to clinically as the superficial femoral artery.
→ = is continuous with
Note: In addition, the lower limb is supplied by branches of the internal iliac artery (e.g., the obturator artery).

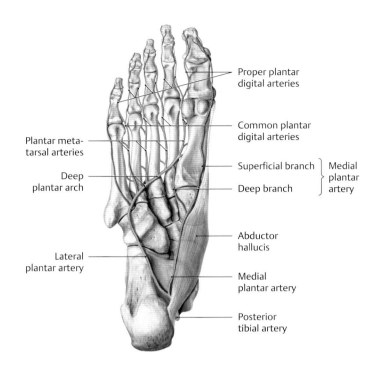

D **The arteries of the sole of the foot**
Right foot, plantar view.

Proper plantar digital arteries

Common plantar digital arteries

Plantar metatarsal arteries

Deep plantar arch

Superficial branch
Deep branch } Medial plantar artery

Lateral plantar artery

Abductor hallucis

Medial plantar artery

Posterior tibial artery

Abdominal aorta

Common iliac artery

Internal iliac artery

Superior and inferior gluteal arteries

External iliac artery

Inferior epigastric artery

External pudendal arteries

Deep circum-flex iliac artery

Superficial epigastric artery

Superficial circum-flex iliac artery

Piriformis

Lateral circum-flex femoral artery

Deep artery of thigh

Perforating arteries

Medial circumflex femoral artery

Femoral artery

Adductor canal and adductor magnus

Adductor hiatus

Descending genicular artery

Medial superior and inferior genicular arteries

Popliteal artery

Lateral superior and inferior genicular arteries

Anterior tibial recurrent artery

Interosseous membrane

Anterior tibial artery

Anterior lateral malleolar artery

Lateral tarsal artery

Arcuate artery

Anterior medial malleolar artery

Dorsal pedal artery

Dorsal metatarsal arteries

C **The arteries of the lower limb**
Right leg, anterior view with the foot in plantar flexion.

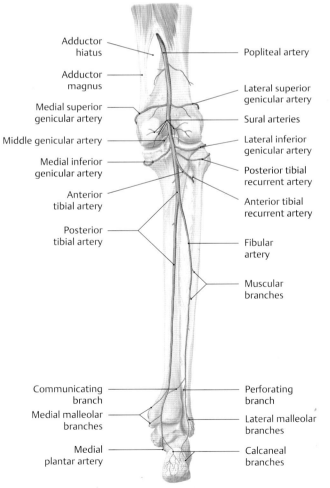

Adductor hiatus

Adductor magnus

Medial superior genicular artery

Middle genicular artery

Medial inferior genicular artery

Anterior tibial artery

Posterior tibial artery

Communicating branch

Medial malleolar branches

Medial plantar artery

Popliteal artery

Lateral superior genicular artery

Sural arteries

Lateral inferior genicular artery

Posterior tibial recurrent artery

Anterior tibial recurrent artery

Fibular artery

Muscular branches

Perforating branch

Lateral malleolar branches

Calcaneal branches

E **The arteries of the popliteal fossa and leg**
Right leg, posterior view.

525

22.2 The Veins

Inguinal ligament
Piriformis
Lateral circumflex femoral veins
Deep vein of thigh
Femoral vein
Adductor canal
Popliteal vein
Adductor hiatus
Anterior tibial veins
Small saphenous vein
Dorsal venous network of the foot

External iliac vein
Medial circumflex femoral veins
Great saphenous vein
Accessory saphenous vein
Adductor magnus
Genicular veins
Great saphenous vein

a

Popliteal vein
Small saphenous vein
Anterior tibial vein
Fibular veins
Small saphenous vein
Lateral malleolus

b

Plantar metatarsal veins
Plantar venous arch
Lateral plantar vein
Small saphenous vein

Posterior tibial veins

Plantar digital veins
Dorsal venous arch
Medial plantar vein
Great saphenous vein
Posterior tibial veins

c

A The deep and superficial veins of the right lower limb

a Thigh, leg, and dorsum of the foot, anterior view.

b Leg, posterior view.

c Sole of the foot, plantar view.

For clarity, only the most important veins are demonstrated here.

B Overview of the principal veins of the lower limb

The veins of the lower limb are subdivided into three systems: a superficial (epifascial) system, a deep (intermuscular) system, and a *perforating* system that interconnects the superficial and deep veins. The upright human body posture places an exceptional load on the veins of the lower limb, which must act against the force of gravity in returning the blood to the heart (the deep venous system handles approximately 85% of the venous return, the superficial veins approximately 15%). A series of venous valves help to maintain the normal superficial-to-deep direction of blood flow (compare **E**). Note that, for the sake of clarity, not all of the veins in the table below have been depicted in these illustrations.

Deep veins of the lower limb
- Femoral vein
- Deep vein of thigh
- Medial and lateral circumflex femoral veins
- Popliteal vein
- Sural veins
- Genicular veins
- Anterior and posterior tibial veins
- Fibular veins
- Dorsal and plantar metatarsal veins (see **Ac**)
- Plantar digital veins (see **Ac**)

Superficial lower limb veins
- Great saphenous vein
- External pudendal veins
- Superficial circumflex iliac vein
- Superficial epigastric vein
- Accessory saphenous vein
- Posterior arch vein
- Small saphenous vein (see **Cb**)
- Femoropopliteal vein (see **Cb**)
- Dorsal venous network (see **Ca**)
- Dorsal venous arch
- Plantar venous network
- Plantar venous arch

Perforating veins
Of the many perforating veins in the leg, three groups have the greatest clinical importance (see **E**):
- The Dodd group (medial side of the thigh, middle third)
- The Boyd group (medial side of the leg below the knee)
- The Cockett group (medial side of the distal leg)

C Superficial (epifascial) veins of the right lower limb

a Thigh, leg, and dorsum of the foot, anterior view.

b Leg, posterior view.

D Varices of the superficial leg veins

a Spider veins (tiny intradermal varices).

b Reticular varices (weblike dilations of small subcutaneous veins).

c Great saphenous varicosity.

d Small saphenous varicosity.

Varicose disease of the *superficial* leg veins is the most common *chronic* venous disease, affecting 15% of the adult population. Varicose veins can be classified as primary idiopathic varices (75%) or as secondary symptomatic varices. **Primary varices** generally result from degeneration of the vein wall leading to incompetence of the venous valves. **Secondary**

varices result from chronic occlusion of the *deep* venous system with incompetence of the perforator veins and a reversal in the direction of venous flow. Besides chronic conditions, there are also important *acute* diseases that may affect the superficial venous system (e.g., thrombophlebitis) and deep venous system (e.g., venous thrombosis).

E Clinically important perforating veins

Right leg, medial view. Numerous perforating veins interconnect the deep and superficial venous systems of the leg. Their venous valves normally prevent blood flow from the deep veins to the superficial cutaneous veins. The clinically important members of this system are located between the deep veins and the tributary region of the great saphenous vein:

- **Dodd veins:** located between the great saphenous vein and femoral vein at the level of the adductor canal.
- **Boyd veins:** located between the great saphenous vein and posterior tibial veins on the medial side of the proximal leg.
- **Cockett veins (I–III):** located between a curved branch of the great saphenous vein behind the medial malleolus (the posterior arch vein) and the posterior tibial veins. The Cockett veins on the medial side of the distal leg are of special clinical importance because of this region's susceptibility to ulceration.

22.3 The Lymphatic Vessels and Lymph Nodes

A The superficial lymphatic system of the right lower limb

a Anterior view, **b** posterior view. (The arrows indicate the main directions of lymphatic drainage.)

The lymph in the lower limb is drained by a superficial (epifascial) system and a deep (subfascial) system, similar to the arrangement in the arm. The largest lymph vessels, called collectors, basically follow the course of the superficial veins (great and small saphenous veins) and deep veins (popliteal vein, femoral vein) and are interconnected by anastomoses located mostly in the popliteal and inguinal regions. While the superficial lymph vessels primarily drain the skin and subcutaneous tissue, the deep system drains lymph from the muscles, joints, and nerves. The superficial lymphatics consist of an anteromedial bundle and a posterolateral bundle. The **anteromedial bundle** runs along the great saphenous vein to the superficial *inguinal* lymph nodes. It drains all of the skin and subcutaneous tissue of the lower limb except for the lateral border of the foot and a narrow strip on the calf. Those areas are drained by the **posterolateral bundle** (see **b**), which thus receives drainage from a considerably smaller region. The lymph in the posterolateral bundle first passes along the small saphenous vein to the superficial *popliteal* lymph nodes and then drains through the deep popliteal lymph nodes to the deep inguinal lymph nodes.

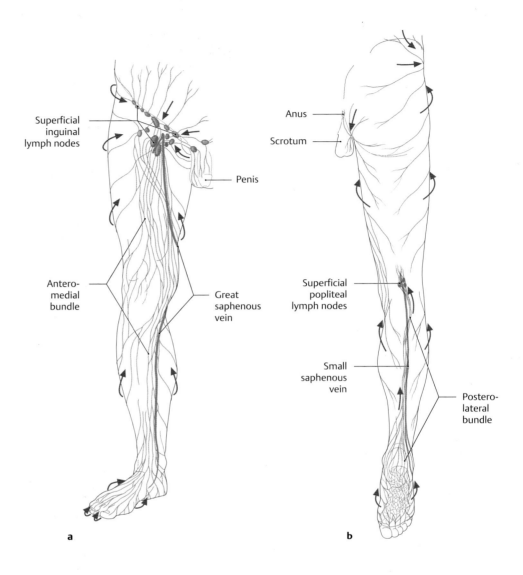

Superficial inguinal lymph nodes

Anus

Scrotum

Penis

Antero-medial bundle

Great saphenous vein

Superficial popliteal lymph nodes

Small saphenous vein

Postero-lateral bundle

a

b

B The deep lymph nodes of the inguinal region

Right inguinal region after removal of the cribriform fascia about the saphenous opening, anterior view. The veins and lymphatic system above the inguinal ligament are shown in light shading. The deep inguinal lymph nodes are located near the termination of the great saphenous vein, medial to the femoral vein. They are important because *all the lymph from the limb* filters through them before reaching the iliac lymph nodes. The largest lymph node of this group (*Rosenmüller's lymph node*) is also the highest, placed at the level of the femoral canal. The group of pelvic lymph nodes, which includes the external iliac nodes, begins just above the inguinal ligament.

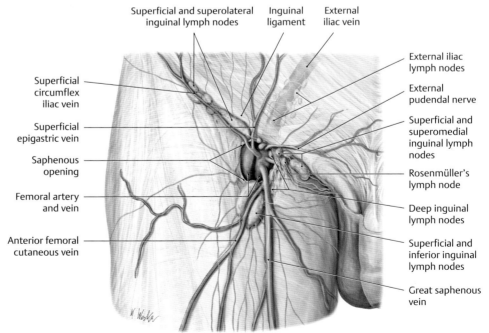

Superficial and superolateral inguinal lymph nodes

Inguinal ligament

External iliac vein

External iliac lymph nodes

Superficial circumflex iliac vein

External pudendal nerve

Superficial epigastric vein

Superficial and superomedial inguinal lymph nodes

Saphenous opening

Rosenmüller's lymph node

Femoral artery and vein

Deep inguinal lymph nodes

Anterior femoral cutaneous vein

Superficial and inferior inguinal lymph nodes

Great saphenous vein

Common iliac lymph nodes

- Receive drainage from:
  - Internal and external iliac nodes
- Drain mainly to:
  - Lumbar lymph nodes

External iliac lymph nodes

- Receive drainage from:
  - Deep inguinal lymph nodes
  - Urinary bladder, shaft and glans of penis, uterus
- Drain mainly to:
  - Common iliac lymph nodes

Superolateral lymph nodes

Superomedial lymph nodes

Inferior lymph nodes

Superficial inguinal lymph nodes

- Receive drainage from:
  - Skin of the limb (except the calf and the lateral border of the foot)
  - Abdominal wall below the umbilicus
  - Lower back
  - Gluteal region, bowel, anal region
  - External genitalia (in women, also the uterine fundus along the round ligament)
- Drain mainly to:
  - Deep inguinal lymph nodes

Deep popliteal lymph nodes

- Receive drainage from:
  - Leg
  - Foot
- Drain mainly to:
  - Deep inguinal lymph nodes

Lumbar lymph nodes

Inferior vena cava

Common iliac vein

External iliac vein

Inguinal ligament

Internal iliac vein

Internal iliac lymph nodes

- Receive drainage from:
  - Pelvic organs
  - Pelvic wall
  - Gluteal muscles
  - Erectile tissues
  - Deep perineal region
- Drain mainly to:
  - Common iliac lymph nodes

Deep iliac lymph nodes

- Receive drainage from:
  - Deep portions of the limb
- Drain mainly to:
  - External iliac lymph nodes

Great saphenous vein

Femoral vein

Superficial popliteal lymph nodes

- Receive drainage from:
  - Lateral border of foot
  - Calf
- Drain mainly to:
  - Deep popliteal lymph nodes

Popliteal vein

Small saphenous vein

C The lymph node stations and drainage pathways in the lower limb

Right limb, anterior view. The arrows indicate the main directions of lymph flow in the superficial and deep lymphatic systems.

Note: Lymph from the skin and subcutaneous tissues of the calf and the lateral border of the foot passes through the superficial and deep popliteal lymph nodes along the deep system of lymphatics *directly* to the deep inguinal lymph nodes. By contrast, lymph from the rest of the skin of the lower limb first drains through the anteromedial bundle along the great saphenous vein to the superficial inguinal lymph nodes (see also **A**).

The *superficial inguinal lymph nodes*, located on the fascia lata, consist of the following:

- Lymph nodes arranged parallel to the inguinal ligament (the superomedial and superolateral inguinal lymph nodes)
- Lymph nodes distributed vertically along the terminal segment of the great saphenous vein (the inferior inguinal lymph nodes)

These nodes first drain into the deep inguinal lymph nodes (see **B**) and then along the external iliac vein to the external and common iliac lymph nodes, finally reaching the lumbar lymph nodes.

Semi-membranosus

Popliteal artery and vein

Gastroc-nemius

Biceps femoris

Deep popliteal lymph nodes

Plantaris

Small saphenous vein

D The deep lymph nodes of the popliteal region

The popliteal fossa of the right leg, posterior view. Lymph from the deep lymphatics of the leg drains (through the deep popliteal nodes between the posterior knee joint capsule and popliteal vessels) along the femoral vein and then anteriorly through the adductor hiatus to the deep inguinal lymph nodes.

22.4 The Structure of the Lumbosacral Plexus

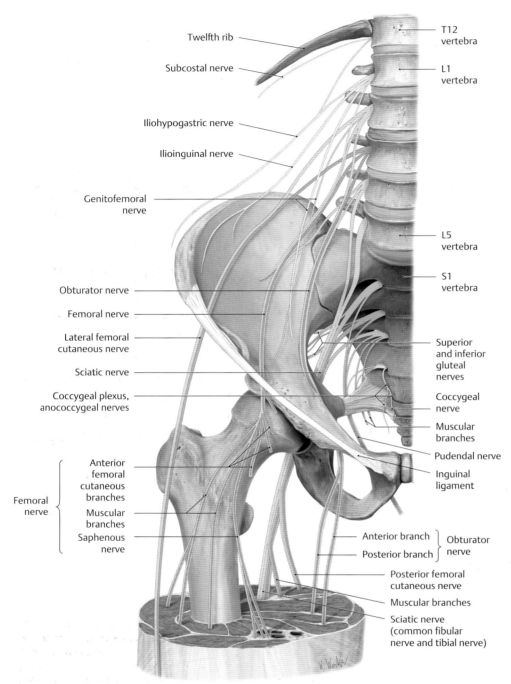

Twelfth rib

Subcostal nerve

Iliohypogastric nerve

Ilioinguinal nerve

Genitofemoral nerve

Obturator nerve

Femoral nerve

Lateral femoral cutaneous nerve

Sciatic nerve

Coccygeal plexus, anococcygeal nerves

Femoral nerve
- Anterior femoral cutaneous branches
- Muscular branches
- Saphenous nerve

T12 vertebra

L1 vertebra

L5 vertebra

S1 vertebra

Superior and inferior gluteal nerves

Coccygeal nerve

Muscular branches

Pudendal nerve

Inguinal ligament

Anterior branch ⎫ Obturator
Posterior branch ⎭ nerve

Posterior femoral cutaneous nerve

Muscular branches

Sciatic nerve (common fibular nerve and tibial nerve)

A The lumbosacral plexus and its branches
Right side, anterior view. For clarity, the muscles of the pelvis and lumbar spine have been removed. Lateral to the intervertebral foramina of the lumbar spine, the *ventral rami* of the first four *lumbar* spinal nerves (L1–L4) form the lumbar plexus and pass through the psoas major muscle. The smaller, muscular branches are distributed directly to the psoas major. The larger branches emerge from the muscle at various sites and pass sharply downward to reach the abdominal wall and thigh, except for the obturator nerve, which runs down the lateral wall of the lesser pelvis to the thigh. The ventral rami of the first four *sacral* spinal nerves (S1–S4) emerge from the anterior foramina of the sacrum and unite on the anterior surface of the piriformis with the anterior ramus of L5 to form the sacral plexus. The nerves from the sacral plexus are distributed to the back of the thigh, the leg, and the foot (after Mumenthaler).

B Spinal cord segments and nerves of the lumbosacral plexus
The lumbosacral plexus supplies sensory and motor innervation to the lower limb. It is formed by the ventral rami of the lumbar and sacral spinal nerves, with contributions from the subcostal nerve (T 12) and coccygeal nerve (Co1) (see **D**). The lumbosacral plexus is subdivided into the lumbar plexus and sacral plexus based on its distribution and topography.

Lumbar plexus (T12–L4)
- Iliohypogastric nerve (L1)
- Ilioinguinal nerve (L1)
- Genitofemoral nerve (L1, L2)
- Lateral femoral cutaneous nerve (L2, L3)
- Obturator nerve (L2–L4)
- Femoral nerve (L2–L4)
- Short, direct muscular branches to specific hip muscles

Sacral plexus (L5–S4)*
- Superior gluteal nerve (L4–S1)
- Inferior gluteal nerve (L5–S2)
- Posterior femoral cutaneous nerve (S1–S3)
- Sciatic nerve (L4–S3) with its two large branches:
  – Tibial nerve (L4–S3)
  – Common fibular nerve (L4–S2)
- Pudendal nerve (S2–S4)
- Short, direct muscular branches to specific hip muscles

* Often the sacral plexus is further subdivided into a sciatic plexus and a pudendal plexus. The main branch of the pudendal plexus, the pudendal nerve, supplies the skin and muscles of the pelvic floor, perineum, and external genitalia.

Iliohypogastric nerve

Ilioinguinal nerve

Genitofemoral nerve

Pudendal nerve

Obturator nerve

Lateral femoral cutaneous nerve

Femoral nerve

Inferior clunial nerves

Posterior femoral cutaneous nerve

Saphenous nerve

Sciatic nerve

Tibial nerve

Common fibular nerve

Deep fibular nerve

Tibial nerve

Superficial fibular nerve

Lateral sural cutaneous nerve and communicating branch

Sural nerve

Medial and lateral plantar nerves

C Topography of the lumbosacral plexus
Right lower limb, lateral view. The nerves of the lumbar plexus reach the lower limb *in front of* the hip joint and mainly supply the *anterior side of the thigh*, while the nerves of the sacral plexus descend *behind* the hip joint and innervate the *posterior side of the thigh*, most of the *leg*, and the entire *foot*.

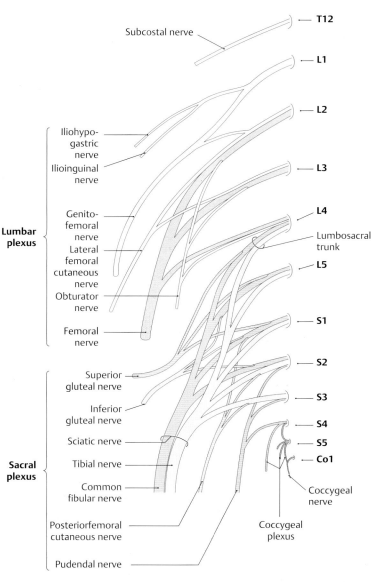

Subcostal nerve

T12

L1

L2

L3

L4

Lumbosacral trunk

L5

S1

S2

S3

S4

S5

Co1

Coccygeal nerve

Coccygeal plexus

Lumbar plexus

Iliohypo-gastric nerve

Ilioinguinal nerve

Genito-femoral nerve

Lateral femoral cutaneous nerve

Obturator nerve

Femoral nerve

Sacral plexus

Superior gluteal nerve

Inferior gluteal nerve

Sciatic nerve

Tibial nerve

Common fibular nerve

Posteriorfemoral cutaneous nerve

Pudendal nerve

D Structure of the lumbosacral plexus
The lumbar nerves combine to form the lumbar plexus, while the sacral nerves form the sacral plexus. A portion of the L4 anterior ramus and all of the L5 anterior ramus combine to form the lumbosacral trunk. This trunk combines with the sacral plexus to form the sciatic nerve. The last spinal nerve, the coccygeal nerve, emerges from the sacral hiatus. It unites with the anterior rami of S4 and S5 to form the coccygeal plexus (see p. 542).

531

22.5 The Nerves of the Lumbar Plexus: The Iliohypogastric, Ilioinguinal, Genitofemoral, and Lateral Femoral Cutaneous Nerves

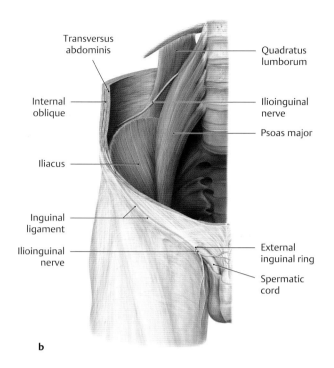

a

b

A Course of the iliohypogastric, ilioinguinal, genitofemoral, and lateral femoral cutaneous nerves after emerging from the lumbar plexus (after Mumenthaler).
Right lateral and posterior abdominal wall region, anterior view.

a The **iliohypogastric nerve** generally emerges with the ilioinguinal nerve (see **b**) at the lateral border of the psoas major and runs laterally and obliquely on the anterior surface of the quadratus lumborum. Approximately 3 to 4 cm past the lateral border of that muscle, it pierces the transversus abdominis and runs anteriorly above the iliac crest, passing between the transversus abdominis and internal oblique. After giving off several muscular branches to both of these muscles and a sensory lateral cutaneous branch to the skin of the lateral hip region, the terminal branch of the ilio-

hypogastric nerve courses medially, running parallel to the inguinal ligament. Above the external inguinal ring it pierces the aponeurosis of the external oblique muscle and supplies a sensory anterior cutaneous branch to the skin above the inguinal ligament.

b The **ilioinguinal nerve** generally courses with the iliohypogastric nerve (see **a**) on the quadratus lumborum but soon separates from it and runs at the level of the iliac crest to the lateral abdominal wall, which it pierces at a variable location. It runs medially at the level of the inguinal ligament between the transversus abdominis and internal oblique, supplying twigs to both muscles, and it distributes sensory fibers through the external inguinal ring to the skin over the symphysis and to the lateral portion of the labia majora or scrotum.

B Overview of the nerves of the lumbar plexus

Nerve	Segment	Innervated muscles	Cutaneous branches (to the region receiving sensory innervation, see **C** and pp. 534 and 535)
• Iliohypogastric nerve	L1	• Transversus abdominis, internal oblique (the inferior portions of each)	• Anterior cutaneous branch • Lateral cutaneous branch
• Ilioinguinal nerve	L1	• Transversus abdominis, internal oblique (the inferior portions of each)	• Anterior scrotal nerves in males, anterior labial nerves in females
• Genitofemoral nerve	L1, L2	• Cremaster in males (genital branch)	• Genital branch, femoral branch
• Lateral femoral cutaneous nerve	L2, L3		• Lateral femoral cutaneous nerve

• Obturator nerve (see p. 534)
  – Anterior branch
 	
  – Posterior branch
	L2–L4	• Obturator externus
		• Adductor longus, adductor brevis, gracilis, pectineus
		• Adductor magnus
			• Cutaneous branch

• Femoral nerve (see p. 535)	L2–L4	• Iliopsoas, pectineus, sartorius, quadriceps femoris	• Anterior cutaneous branches, saphenous nerve
• Short, direct muscular branches (see p. 534)	T12–L4	• Psoas major, quadratus lumborum, iliacus, intertransversarii lumborum	

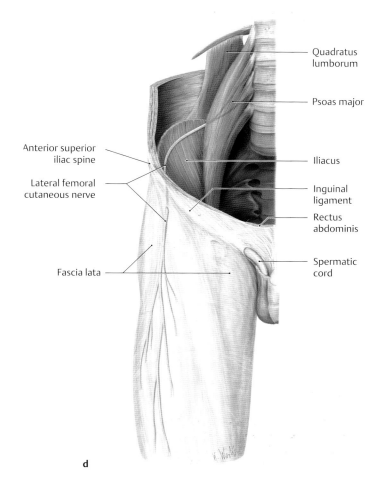

c

d

c The **genitofemoral nerve** pierces the psoas major and descends upon its anterior surface, dividing into its two terminal branches: the genital branch and femoral branch:

- The *purely sensory femoral branch* pierces the lacuna vasorum in the area of the saphenous opening (see p. 549) and becomes superficial, supplying the skin below the inguinal ligament in both sexes.
- The *mixed genital branch* runs in the spermatic cord in males. In females it initially passes through the inguinal canal accompanied by the round ligament of the uterus. In its further course it distributes sensory fibers to the scrotal skin in males and to the skin of the labia majora in females. It also supplies motor fibers to the cremaster muscle in males (see p. 176).

d The **lateral femoral cutaneous nerve** emerges from the lateral border of the psoas major and runs obliquely downward and laterally beneath the iliacus fascia toward the anterior superior iliac spine.

Medial to the iliac spine, the nerve leaves the pelvis through the lateral muscular compartment (see p. 549) and first runs beneath the fascia lata and then upon it to the skin of the anterior thigh, piercing the fascia approximately 2 to 3 cm below the anterior superior iliac spine. The nerve is susceptible to occasional mechanical injury at its site of emergence from the pelvis below the inguinal ligament, as it makes an approximately 80° angle at that site and is susceptible to stretching, especially on extension of the hip. The nerve also has only scant coverage by fatty tissue at that location. Stretch injuries are manifested by sensory disturbances (paresthesias) or pain in the *lateral* part of the thigh.

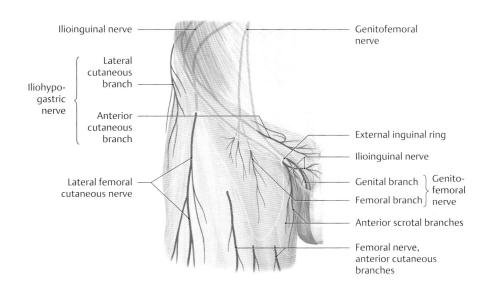

C Sensory innervation of the inguinal region and thigh
Right inguinal region of a male, anterior view. The territories of the various sensory nerves are indicated by different colors.
Note: Both the ilioinguinal nerve and the genital branch of the genitofemoral nerve pass through the external inguinal ring. The two nerves are frequently confused. The genital branch in males is located by first opening the spermatic cord. In females, the genital branch accompanies the uterine round ligament to supply the skin of the labia majora (see also **Ac**).

533

22.6 The Nerves of the Lumbar Plexus: The Obturator and Femoral Nerves

Obturator nerve

Obturator externus

Adductor brevis

Muscular branches

L2 vertebra

L4 vertebra

Linea terminalis

Pectineus

Anterior branch

Posterior branch

Adductor longus

Adductor magnus

Cutaneous branch

Gracilis

Cutaneous branch

B Sensory distribution of the obturator nerve
Right leg, medial view.

A Course of the obturator nerve
The right inguinal region and thigh, anterior view. The obturator nerve receives fibers from the L 2–L 4 spinal segments. After leaving the lumbar plexus, it descends behind and medial to the psoas major (not shown here) toward the lesser pelvis and enters the obturator canal (not shown here, see p. 558) below the linea terminalis, accompanied by the obturator vessels. Farther distally it distributes muscular branches to the obturator externus and subsequently divides into an anterior branch and a posterior branch. These branches continue distally, passing respectively anterior and posterior to the adductor brevis, and supply motor innervation to the rest of the adductor muscles (pectineus, adductor longus, adductor brevis, adductor magnus, adductor minimus, and gracilis). The anterior branch gives off a terminal, sensory cutaneous branch at the anterior border of the gracilis, which pierces the fascia lata to supply a palm-sized area of skin on the medial view of the distal thigh. In evaluating motor deficits that are associated with obturator nerve injuries (e.g., intrapartum or due to pelvic fractures), it is important to know that the femoral nerve contributes to the supply of the pectineus muscle, while the sciatic nerve helps to supply the adductor magnus.

Psoas major

Muscular branch

Iliacus

Inguinal ligament

Sartorius

Muscular branches

Rectus femoris

Quadriceps femoris

Vastus intermedius

Vastus lateralis

Rectus femoris

Vastus medialis

L1 vertebra

L4 vertebra

Iliopsoas

Muscular compartment

Femoral nerve

Anterior cutaneous branches of the femoral nerve

Pectineus

Saphenous nerve

Muscular branches

Vastoadductor membrane

Sartorius

Infrapatellar branch

Saphenous nerve

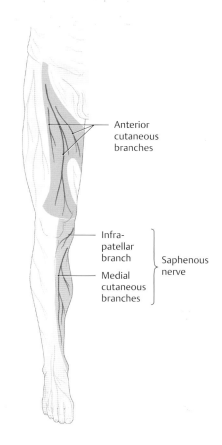

Anterior cutaneous branches

Infra-patellar branch

Medial cutaneous branches

Saphenous nerve

D Sensory distribution of the femoral nerve
Right leg, anterior view.

C Course of the femoral nerve

The right inguinal region and thigh, anterior view. As the largest and longest nerve of the lumbar plexus, the femoral nerve receives fibers from the second through fourth lumbar segments of the spinal cord. It supplies *motor* innervation to the iliopsoas, pectineus, sartorius, and quadriceps femoris muscles and *sensory* innervation to the skin of the anterior thigh, medial leg, and hindfoot (see **D**). The nerve, under cover of the psoas fascia, runs in a groove between the psoas major and iliacus to the medial muscular compartment while giving off branches to both muscles. Approximately 8 cm below the inguinal ligament, the femoral nerve divides into numerous cutaneous branches (anterior cutaneous branches) and muscular branches, as well as a long, terminal sensory branch that continues to the foot, the saphenous nerve. Initially, the saphenous nerve enters the adductor canal with the femoral vessels (below the vastoadductor membrane) but then leaves the canal through the vastoadductor membrane and passes with the sartorius toward the medial side of the knee. After giving off a sensory infrapatellar branch to the skin of the medial knee, it follows the great saphenous vein to the skin of the medial leg and foot.

535

22.7 The Nerves of the Sacral Plexus: The Superior Gluteal, Inferior Gluteal, and Posterior Femoral Cutaneous Nerves

A Nerves of the sacral plexus (part I)

(For nerves of the sacral plexus, parts II and III, see pp. 538 and 540.)

Nerve	Segment	Innervated muscles	Cutaneous branches
• Superior gluteal nerve	L4–S1	• Gluteus medius • Gluteus minimus • Tensor fasciae latae	
• Inferior gluteal nerve	L5–S2	• Gluteus maximus	
• Posterior femoral cutaneous nerve	S1–S3		• Posterior femoral cutaneous nerve – Inferior clunial nerves – Perineal branches (see **F** for sensory distribution)
• *Direct branches from the plexus:* – Nerve of piriformis – Nerve of obturator internus – Nerve of quadratus femoris	 S1, S2 L5, S1 L5, S1	 • Piriformis • Obturator internus • Gemelli • Quadratus femoris	

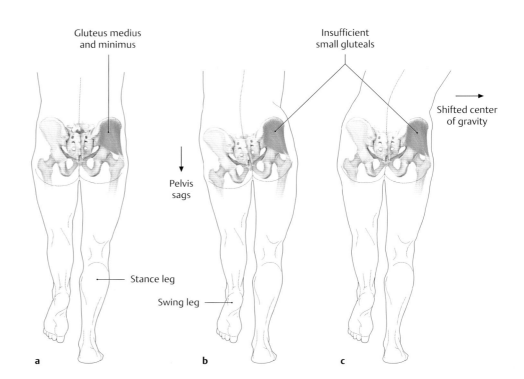

B Motor distribution of the superior gluteal nerve

Right hip region, lateral view. Accompanied by blood vessels with the same name, the superior gluteal nerve leaves the lesser pelvis through the greater sciatic foramen superior to the piriformis (see p. 554), runs in the intergluteal space, and supplies motor fibers to the small gluteal muscles (gluteus medius and minimus) and tensor fasciae latae.

C Clinical indicators of small gluteal muscle weakness: the Trendelenburg sign and the Duchenne limp

Lower half of body, posterior view.

a In normal one-legged stance, the small gluteal muscles on the stance side can stabilize the pelvis in the coronal plane.

b Weakness or paralysis of the small gluteal muscles (e.g., due to a faulty intramuscular injection causing damage to the superior gluteal nerve) is manifested by weak abduc-

tion of the affected hip joint and an inability to stabilize the pelvis in the coronal plane. In a positive Trendelenburg test, the pelvis sags toward the *normal* unsupported side.

c Tilting the upper body toward the affected side shifts the center of gravity onto the stance side, thereby elevating the pelvis on the swing side (*Duchenne limp*). With bilateral loss of the small gluteals, the patient exhibits a typical waddling gait.

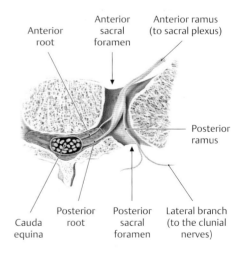

D Motor distribution of the inferior gluteal nerve

Right half of the pelvis, posterior view. The inferior gluteal nerve leaves the lesser pelvis with the sciatic nerve through the greater sciatic foramen inferior to the piriformis (see p. 554) and supplies numerous muscular branches to the gluteus maximus. Paralysis of the gluteus maximus causes little impairment of normal gait on even ground because the deficit is well compensated by the hamstrings (see p. 484). The affected patient is unable to run, jump, or climb stairs, however.

E Muscles that are supplied by direct branches from the sacral plexus

Right half of the pelvis, posterior view. The direct branches of the sacral plexus are listed in **A**.

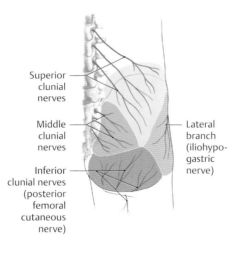

G Sensory innervation of the gluteal region

Right buttock, posterior view.

The gluteal region receives sensory innervation from portions of the sacral plexus and lumbar plexus (anterior rami of the spinal nerves) and also from posterior rami:

- From the sacral plexus: inferior clunial nerves (from the posterior femoral cutaneous nerve).
- From the lumbar plexus: the lateral branch of the iliohypogastric nerve.
- From posterior rami of the spinal nerves: the superior clunial nerves (posterior rami of L1–L3) and middle clunial nerves (posterior rami of S1–S3).

H An emerging sacral nerve

Horizontal section through the right half of the sacrum at the level of the sacral foramina. While the anterior ramus of a sacral nerve emerges from the sacrum through an *anterior* sacral foramen, the corresponding posterior ramus passes through the *posterior* sacral foramen to supply the skin of the buttock.

F Sensory distribution of the posterior femoral cutaneous nerve

Right lower limb, posterior view. Besides the skin of the posterior thigh, the posterior femoral cutaneous nerve distributes several branches to the skin of the gluteal sulcus (inferior clunial nerves), and its perineal branches supply the skin of the perineal region (darker shading indicates the exclusive area).

537

22.8 The Nerves of the Sacral Plexus: The Sciatic Nerve (Overview and Sensory Distribution)

A Nerves of the sacral plexus (part II)
The largest and longest of the peripheral nerves, the sciatic nerve, leaves the lesser pelvis through the greater sciatic foramen inferior to the piriformis and passes below the gluteus maximus to the back of the thigh. It divides into its two main branches, the tibial and common fibular nerves, at a variable level but generally before entering the popliteal fossa. The *muscular branches* of the sciatic nerve, however, can already be identified as consisting of a *fibular part* (Fib) and a *tibial part* (Tib) while still proximal to the bifurcation (see also p. 540). Injuries of the sciatic nerve may be caused by compression of the nerve at its emergence inferior to the piriformis (usually by extrinsic pressure, such as sitting). Other potential causes are misdirected intramuscular injections (in which the nerve is accidentally pricked), pelvic fractures, and surgical procedures (e.g., hip replacement).

Nerve	Segment	Innervated muscles	Cutaneous branches

Sciatic nerve	L4–S3	• Semitendinosus (Tib)
		• Semimembranosus (Tib)
		• Biceps femoris
		  – Long head (Tib)
		  – Short head (Fib)
		• Adductor magnus (Tib), medial part	

• Common fibular nerve	L4–S2		• Lateral sural cutaneous nerve • Fibular communicating branch
– Superficial fibular nerve		• Fibularis longus • Fibularis brevis	• Medial dorsal cutaneous nerve • Intermediate dorsal cutaneous nerve
– Deep fibular nerve		• Tibialis anterior • Extensor digitorum longus • Extensor digitorum brevis • Extensor hallucis longus • Extensor hallucis brevis • Fibularis tertius	• Lateral cutaneous nerve of the great toe • Medial cutaneous nerve of the second toe
• Tibial nerve	L4–S3	• Triceps surae • Plantaris • Popliteus • Tibialis posterior • Flexor digitorum longus • Flexor hallucis longus	• Medial sural cutaneous nerve (→ sural nerve) • Lateral calcaneal branches • Medial calcaneal branches • Lateral dorsal cutaneous nerve
– Medial plantar nerve		• Abductor hallucis • Flexor digitorum brevis • Flexor hallucis brevis, medial head • First lumbrical	• Proper plantar digital nerves
– Lateral plantar nerve		• Flexor hallucis brevis, lateral head • Quadratus plantae • Abductor digiti minimi • Flexor digiti minimi brevis • Opponens digiti minimi • Second through fourth lumbricals • First through third plantar interossei • First through fourth dorsal interossei • Adductor hallucis	• Proper plantar digital nerves

→ = is continuous with

Fibular communicating branch

Lateral sural cutaneous nerve

Medial dorsal cutaneous nerve

Intermediate dorsal cutaneous nerve

Superficial fibular nerve

Cutaneous branch of deep fibular nerve

a

B Sensory distribution of the sciatic nerve
Right leg. **a** Lateral view, **b** anterior view, **c** posterior view.

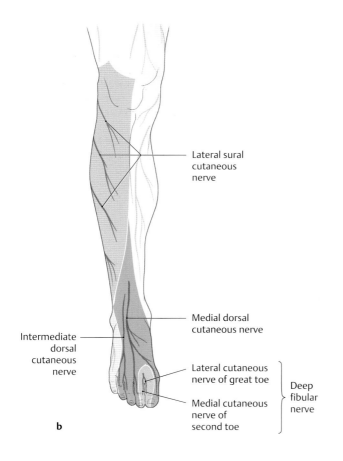

Lateral sural cutaneous nerve

Intermediate dorsal cutaneous nerve

Medial dorsal cutaneous nerve

Lateral cutaneous nerve of great toe

Medial cutaneous nerve of second toe

Deep fibular nerve

b

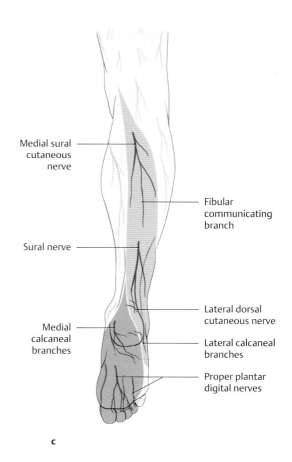

Medial sural cutaneous nerve

Sural nerve

Medial calcaneal branches

Fibular communicating branch

Lateral dorsal cutaneous nerve

Lateral calcaneal branches

Proper plantar digital nerves

c

22.9 The Nerves of the Sacral Plexus: The Sciatic Nerve (Course and Motor Distribution)

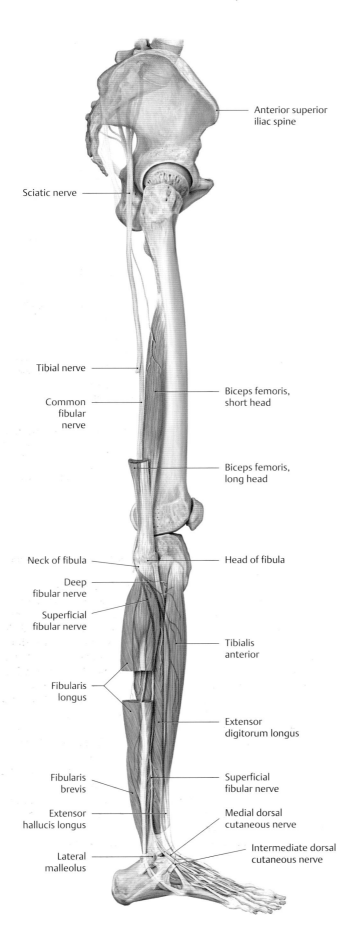

Anterior superior iliac spine

Sciatic nerve

Tibial nerve

Common fibular nerve

Biceps femoris, short head

Biceps femoris, long head

Neck of fibula

Deep fibular nerve

Superficial fibular nerve

Head of fibula

Tibialis anterior

Fibularis longus

Extensor digitorum longus

Fibularis brevis

Superficial fibular nerve

Extensor hallucis longus

Medial dorsal cutaneous nerve

Lateral malleolus

Intermediate dorsal cutaneous nerve

A Course and motor distribution of the sciatic nerve: the fibular part (common fibular nerve)

Right lower limb, lateral view. After giving off several muscular branches from its fibular part (to the short head of the biceps femoris), the sciatic nerve consistently divides in the lower third of the thigh into the tibial nerve and common fibular nerve. The common fibular nerve then follows the medial border of the biceps femoris to the head of the fibula and winds around the neck of the fibula to the front of the leg. Immediately after entering the fibularis longus, it divides into its two terminal branches, the *deep* fibular nerve and *superficial* fibular nerve. The superficial fibular nerve supplies the fibularis muscles and runs between the fibularis longus and fibula to the dorsum of the foot. The deep fibular nerve runs through the interosseous membrane to enter the extensor compartment. After supplying the tibialis anterior, extensor digitorum longus, and extensor hallucis longus, it runs in a groove between the tibialis anterior and extensor hallucis longus on the crural interosseous membrane, accompanied by the anterior tibial vessels, to the dorsum of the foot.

- If the nerve is damaged at the level of the fibular neck (a very exposed location!) before dividing into its two terminal branches, the result is weakness or paralysis of the anterior and lateral compartment muscles, resulting in foot drop with some inversion.
- If the nerve is damaged after dividing into its terminal branches, the result may be an isolated weakness or paralysis of the anterior compartment or the lateral muscles, depending on whether the deep fibular or the superficial fibular nerve is affected. Accordingly, the result may be weak dorsiflexion or weakness of eversion. An isolated lesion of the superficial fibular nerve generally affects only the sensory terminal branch, with pain involving the distal leg and dorsum of the foot. Gait disturbance will occur only with an isolated lesion of the deep fibular nerve (as in compartment syndrome caused by anterior compartment hemorrhage, see p. 567), resulting in foot drop and a "steppage gait." Increased flexion of the hip and knee joints is necessary to keep the toe from dragging the ground during the swing phase of gait.

Sciatic nerve

Sacro-
tuberous
ligament

Muscular
branches

Biceps femoris,
long head

Semi-
tendinosus

Adductor
magnus
(medial part)

Biceps femoris,
short head

Semi-
membranosus

Tibial nerve

Popliteal fossa

Tendinous arch
of soleus

Gastrocnemius

Soleus

Deep flexors

Deep flexor
tendons

Lateral
malleolus

Tibial nerve in
malleolar canal

a

Proper
plantar
digital
nerves

Lumbricals

Adductor
hallucis

Common
plantar
digital nerves

Tendon of
flexor hallucis
longus

Lateral plantar
nerve, super-
ficial branch

Muscular
branches

Abductor
digiti minimi

Base of fifth
metatarsal

Tendon
of flexor
digitorum
longus

Lateral
plantar nerve

Abductor
hallucis

Quadratus
plantae

Medial
plantar nerve

Flexor digitorum
brevis and plantar
aponeurosis

Tibial nerve

b

B Course and motor distribution of the sciatic nerve: the tibial part (tibial nerve)

a Right lower limb, posterior view; **b** right foot, plantar view. While still in the thigh, the tibial part of the sciatic nerve distributes several muscular branches to the semitendinosus, semimembranosus, biceps femoris (long head), and adductor magnus (medial part). After division of the sciatic nerve, the tibial nerve continues straight down through the center of the popliteal fossa and runs below the tendinous arch of the soleus muscle to the superficial and deep plantar flexors, which it supplies. In the deep posterior compartment, the tibial nerve continues distally in a neurovascular bundle with the posterior tibial vessels (not shown here) and passes through the tarsal tunnel, accompanied by the deep flexor tendons, to the plantar side of the foot (**b**). In passing through the tarsal tunnel, the tibial nerve divides into its two terminal branches (the lateral and medial plantar nerves), which supply all the muscles on the plantar side of the foot. Compression of the tibial nerve or its terminal branches at this site leads to an entrapment syndrome (= tarsal tunnel syndrome). This can result in pain and sensory disturbances affecting the sole of the foot or even palsies of the intrinsic foot muscles, particularly following severe nerve trauma in connection with a fracture of the tibial shaft or medial malleolus.

22.10 The Nerves of the Sacral Plexus: The Pudendal and Coccygeal Nerves

A Nerves of the sacral plexus (part III)

The pudendal nerve, the lowest branch of the sacral plexus, arises from a separate small plexus formed by the anterior rami of S1–S4; hence it is occasionally referred to as the *pudendal plexus*.

Nerve	Segment	Innervated muscles	Cutaneous branches
• Pudendal nerve (pudendal plexus)	S2–S4	• Pelvic floor muscles – Levator ani – Superficial transverse perineal – Deep transverse perineal – Bulbospongiosus – External anal sphincter – Urethral sphincter	• Inferior rectal nerves • Perineal nerves – Posterior labial nerves in females – Posterior scrotal nerves in males – Dorsal clitoral nerve in females
• Coccygeal nerve (coccygeal plexus)	S5–Co2	• Coccygeus	• Anococcygeal nerve (anterior rami) • Dorsal rami

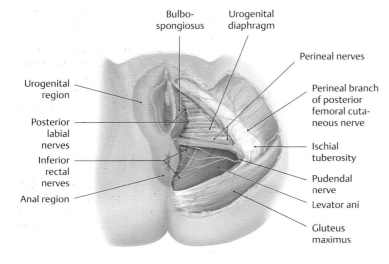

Bulbo-spongiosus · Urogenital diaphragm · Perineal nerves · Urogenital region · Perineal branch of posterior femoral cutaneous nerve · Posterior labial nerves · Ischial tuberosity · Inferior rectal nerves · Pudendal nerve · Anal region · Levator ani · Gluteus maximus

B The cutaneous branches of the pudendal nerve and its sensory distribution in the female

Lithotomy position, inferior view. The skin layers have been removed on the left side to demonstrate the terminal branches of the pudendal nerve in the ischioanal fossa (see p. 556). The area of cutaneous sensory innervation is color-shaded. Large portions of the urogenital region and anal region receive their sensory supply from the pudendal nerve. The skin area supplied by the pudendal nerve can be anesthetized during childbirth by infiltration anesthesia or a nerve block, enabling the obstetrician to perform and repair an episiotomy without pain (see p. 232). This can be done either by infiltrating the perineum between the anus and posterior fornix with a local anesthetic or by temporarily blocking the pudendal nerve with local anesthetic injected near the ischial spine (before the nerve has branched; see diagram in **C**).

Ischial tuberosity · Pudendal nerve · Ischial spine

C Technique of a left-sided pudendal nerve block

Lithotomy position, inferior view. The most common type of conduction anesthesia used in vaginal deliveries is the pudendal nerve block, which renders the perineum, vulva, and lower third of the vagina insensitive to pain. In the *transvaginal approach*, a special guide cannula is introduced into the vagina, and 10 mL of a local anesthetic solution is injected approximately 1 cm above and 1 cm lateral to the palpable ischial spine on each side. An injection at this site will block the pudendal nerve *before* it has entered the pudendal canal (Alcock's canal) and *before* it has divided into its terminal branches. Often the nerve block is administered at the end of the expulsion stage to relieve stretch pain in the perineal region (see p. 232).

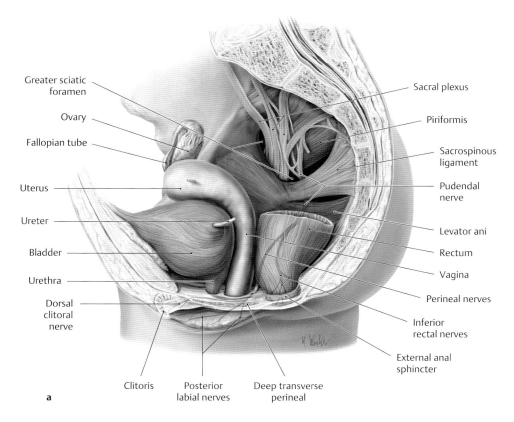

Greater sciatic foramen
Ovary
Fallopian tube
Uterus
Ureter
Bladder
Urethra
Dorsal clitoral nerve

Sacral plexus
Piriformis
Sacrospinous ligament
Pudendal nerve
Levator ani
Rectum
Vagina
Perineal nerves
Inferior rectal nerves
External anal sphincter

Clitoris   Posterior labial nerves   Deep transverse perineal

a

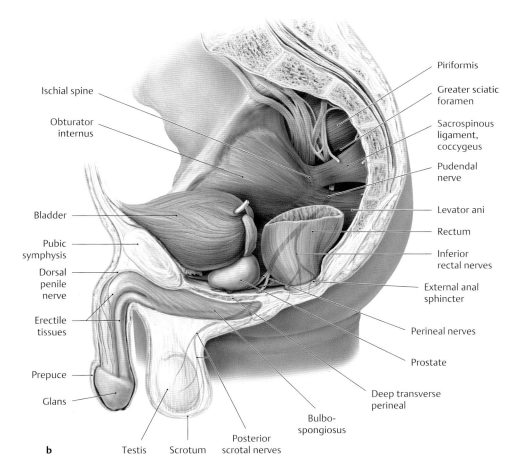

Ischial spine
Obturator internus
Bladder
Pubic symphysis
Dorsal penile nerve
Erectile tissues
Prepuce
Glans

Piriformis
Greater sciatic foramen
Sacrospinous ligament, coccygeus
Pudendal nerve
Levator ani
Rectum
Inferior rectal nerves
External anal sphincter
Perineal nerves
Prostate
Deep transverse perineal

Testis   Scrotum   Posterior scrotal nerves   Bulbo-spongiosus

b

D Course of the pudendal nerve and coccygeal nerve in the female and male

a Sagittal section through the female pelvis, left lateral view.
b Sagittal section through the male pelvis, left lateral view.

The **pudendal nerve** emerges from the lesser pelvis through the *greater* sciatic foramen. It then courses around the ischial spine and sacrospinous ligament and passes through the *lesser* sciatic foramen into the ischioanal (ischiorectal) fossa (see p. 556). It runs forward in the lateral wall of the fossa, embedded in a duplication of the obturator internus fascia (pudendal canal = Alcock's canal) and accompanied by the internal pudendal vessels (see p. 555). Below the symphysis it passes to the dorsum of the penis or the clitoris. The pudendal nerve gives off numerous *branches* from within the perineum:

* The *inferior rectal nerves* supply motor innervation to the external anal sphincter and sensory innervation to the skin around the anus.
* The *perineal nerves* distribute motor branches to the muscles of the perineum (see p. 162) and sensory branches to the skin of the posterior scrotum or labia majora and minora, to the skin of the penis or clitoris, and to the glans, prepuce, and erectile tissues.

Damage to the pudendal nerve (e.g., resulting from perineal injuries during childbirth) leads to loss of function of the muscles of the perineum, especially the sphincter muscles of the bladder and bowel, causing urinary and fecal incontinence. Pudendal nerve lesions can also lead to sexual dysfunction (e.g., male impotence).

The ventral rami of the fifth sacral nerve and the first or second coccygeal nerve form the **coccygeal nerve** (synonym: *coccygeal plexus*). This nerve and its terminal sensory branches, the anococcygeal nerves, pass along the anococcygeal ligament to supply the skin between the coccyx and anus.

23.1 Surface Anatomy and Superficial Nerves and Vessels: Anterior View

Anterior superior iliac spine

Tensor fasciae latae

Inguinal ligament

Adductor muscles

Rectus femoris

Vastus lateralis

Vastus medialis

Patella

Head of fibula

Tibial tuberosity

Tibia

Tibialis anterior

Gastroc-nemius

Lateral malleolus

Medial malleolus

Dorsum of foot

Tendon of tibialis anterior and extensor hallucis longus

Great toe

Second through fifth digits

A Surface anatomy of the right lower limb
Palpable *bony prominences* on the lower limb are reviewed on p. 409.

a   b   c

B The most common variants of the forefoot and toes (after Debrunner and Lelievre)
Three types of foot shape are distinguished based on the relative lengths of the first and second toes:

a The "Greek" type, in which the second toe is longer than the first.
b The square type, in which the first and second toes are of equal length.
c The "Egyptian" type, in which the first toe is longer than the second.

In the "Greek" type, the second metatarsal is generally longer than the metatarsal of the great toe. As a result, the head of the second metatarsal is often subject to painful overloading, especially when high heels are worn.

Dorsal venous network

Medial malleolus

Lateral malleolus

C The dorsal surface of the right foot
The superficial venous network is visible on the dorsum of the foot (compare with **D**).

E Radicular (segmental) cutaneous innervation pattern (dermatomes) in the right lower limb

As in the arm, the outgrowth of the lower limb during development causes the sensory cutaneous segments to become elongated and drawn out into narrow bands. The L4, L5, and S1 segments in particular move so far peripherally that they no longer have any connection with the corresponding segments of the trunk.

Note that the dermatomes of the lumbar trunk segments lie mostly on the front of the leg, while those of the sacral segments are mostly on the back of the leg (see p. 86). This can be of diagnostic importance in patients with a herniated disk, for example, in order to determine the level of the herniation (after Mumenthaler).

D Superficial cutaneous veins and nerves of the right lower limb

Anterior view. The dorsal venous network of the foot is drained by two large venous trunks (the great and small saphenous veins), which receive a variable pattern of cutaneous veins. While the small saphenous vein (see p. 547) enters the popliteal vein at the level of the popliteal fossa, the great saphenous vein extends up the medial side of the leg to a point just below the inguinal ligament, where it passes through the saphenous opening of the fascia lata to enter the femoral vein. The superficial veins of the lower limb are commonly affected by varicosity, causing them to become thickened, tortuous, and distinctly visible and palpable (see also p. 527).

F Pattern of peripheral sensory cutaneous innervation in the right lower limb

As in the arm, the sensory distribution in the lower limb corresponds to the branching patterns of the peripheral cutaneous nerves in the subcutaneous connective tissue. The territories of the individual peripheral nerves overlap, especially at their margins. Hence the clinically determined *exclusive area* of a particular cutaneous nerve (the area supplied by that nerve alone) tends to be considerably smaller than the *maximum area* that can be demonstrated anatomically. For this reason, the traumatic disruption of a nerve causes a complete loss of sensation (anesthesia) in the exclusive area but often will cause only diminished sensation (hypoesthesia) at the perimeter of that area.

Note that the sensory loss resulting from a peripheral nerve injury presents a completely different pattern from that caused by injury to a nerve root (see p. 88) (after Mumenthaler).

23.2 Surface Anatomy and Superficial Nerves and Vessels: Posterior View

a **b**

B Footprints (podograms) of the normal right foot in an adult
A podogram provides a graphic representation of the loads borne by the foot. Besides visual inspection of the sole of the foot, analysis of the podogram supplies the most useful information on the weight-bearing dynamics of the foot.

a Footprint created with an ink pad.
b Pressure podogram showing a normal weight-bearing pattern on the foot. The concentric lines indicate that the pressure is evenly distributed over all the major points of support. These three areas are clearly defined, while the intervening plantar arches bear essentially no weight (see p. 464).

A Surface anatomy of the right lower limb
The foot is in plantar flexion. (Palpable *bony prominences* on the lower limb are reviewed on p. 409.)

C The plantar surface of the right foot
The skin on the plantar surface of the foot serves as a sensory organ for contact with the ground, perceiving its consistency during stance and locomotion by means of receptors in the sole of the foot. Stresses acting on the heel pad and the balls of the great and little toes generate high local compressive forces at those sites, to which the subcutaneous connective tissue has adapted functionally by developing a system of *pressure chambers* (see p. 472).

Superior clunial nerves

Middle clunial nerves

Inferior clunial nerves

Posterior femoral cutaneous nerve

Obturator nerve, cutaneous branch

Saphenous nerve

Small saphenous vein

Calcaneal branches

Plantar cutaneous branches

Iliohypogastric nerve, lateral cutaneous branch

Lateral femoral cutaneous nerve

Medial sural cutaneous nerve (tibial nerve)

Lateral sural cutaneous nerve (common fibular nerve)

Sural nerve

Lateral dorsal cutaneous nerve

D The epifascial cutaneous veins and nerves of the right lower limb

Posterior view.

L2
L3
L4
L5

S5
S4
S3
S2
S1

L4
L5

E Radicular (segmental) cutaneous innervation pattern (dermatomes) of the right lower limb

As in the arm, the outgrowth of the lower limb during development causes the sensory cutaneous segments to become elongated into narrow bands. The L4, L5, and S1 segments in particular move so far peripherally that they no longer have any connection with the corresponding segments of the trunk.

Note that the dermatomes of the lumbar trunk segments lie mostly on the front of the leg, while those of the sacral segments are mostly on the back of the leg (see p. 86). This can be of diagnostic importance in patients with a herniated disk, for example, in order to determine the level of the herniation (after Mumenthaler).

Middle clunial nerves (S1–S3)

Inferior clunial nerves

Obturator nerve, cutaneous branch

Saphenous nerve

Sural nerve

Medial plantar nerve, cutaneous branch

Superior clunial nerves (L1–L3)

Iliohypogastric nerve, lateral cutaneous branch

Lateral femoral cutaneous branch

Posterior femoral cutaneous nerve

Common fibular nerve, lateral sural cutaneous nerve

Tibial nerve, medial sural cutaneous nerve

Lateral plantar nerve, cutaneous branch

F Pattern of peripheral sensory cutaneous innervation in the right lower limb

As in the arm, the sensory distribution in the lower limb corresponds to the branching patterns of the peripheral cutaneous nerves in the subcutaneous connective tissue. The territories of the individual peripheral nerves overlap, especially at their margins. Hence the clinically determined *exclusive area* of a particular cutaneous nerve (the area supplied by that nerve alone) tends to be considerably smaller than the *maximum area* that can be demonstrated anatomically. For this reason, the traumatic disruption of a nerve causes a complete loss of sensation (anesthesia) in the exclusive area but often will cause only diminished sensation (hypoesthesia) at the perimeter of that area.

Note that the sensory loss resulting from a peripheral nerve injury presents a completely different pattern from that caused by injury to a nerve root (see p. 88) (after Mumenthaler).

547

23.3 The Anterior Femoral Region Including the Femoral Triangle

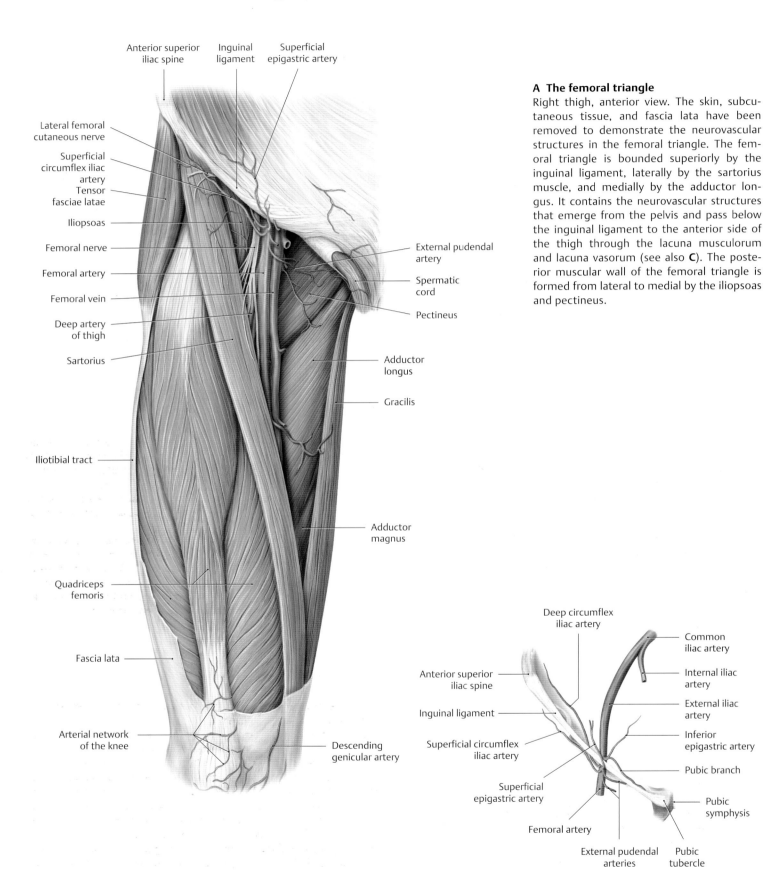

A The femoral triangle
Right thigh, anterior view. The skin, subcutaneous tissue, and fascia lata have been removed to demonstrate the neurovascular structures in the femoral triangle. The femoral triangle is bounded superiorly by the inguinal ligament, laterally by the sartorius muscle, and medially by the adductor longus. It contains the neurovascular structures that emerge from the pelvis and pass below the inguinal ligament to the anterior side of the thigh through the lacuna musculorum and lacuna vasorum (see also **C**). The posterior muscular wall of the femoral triangle is formed from lateral to medial by the iliopsoas and pectineus.

B The branches of the external iliac artery at its junction with the femoral artery in the region of the inguinal ligament

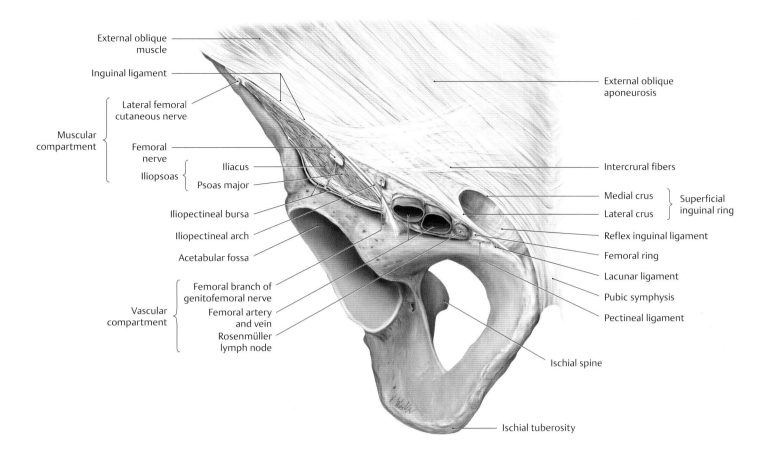

External oblique muscle

Inguinal ligament

Lateral femoral cutaneous nerve

Muscular compartment

Femoral nerve

Iliopsoas — Iliacus

Psoas major

Iliopectineal bursa

Iliopectineal arch

Acetabular fossa

Vascular compartment — Femoral branch of genitofemoral nerve

Femoral artery and vein

Rosenmüller lymph node

External oblique aponeurosis

Intercrural fibers

Medial crus — Superficial inguinal ring

Lateral crus

Reflex inguinal ligament

Femoral ring

Lacunar ligament

Pubic symphysis

Pectineal ligament

Ischial spine

Ischial tuberosity

C Inguinal region and the contents of the muscular and vascular compartments

Anterior view. The drawing shows a portion of the right hip bone and the adjacent anterior inferior abdominal wall with the superficial inguinal ring and the contents of the muscular and vascular compartments below the inguinal ligament. The site of emergence of the muscles and vessels, bounded by the inguinal ligament and the superior pelvic rim, is subdivided by the fibrous iliopectineal arch.

The **vascular compartment** is located medial to the iliopectineal arch and is traversed from lateral to medial by the femoral branch of the genitofemoral nerve, the femoral artery and vein, and the deep inguinal lymphatic vessels (only one lymph node is shown here). The part of the vascular compartment that lies medial to the femoral vein is called the *femoral ring*. The lymph vessels from the thigh pass through that

ring to enter the pelvis. The femoral ring is covered by a thin sheet of connective tissue called the femoral septum (not shown here), which usually contains a lymph node (the Rosenmüller node) belonging to the group of deep inguinal lymph nodes (see also p. 528).

The **muscular compartment** is lateral to the iliopectineal arch and is traversed by the iliopsoas muscle, femoral nerve, and lateral femoral cutaneous nerve.

Note the iliopectineal bursa located below the iliopsoas. It is the largest bursa of the hip region and communicates in 15% of cases with the joint cavity of the hip. For this reason, an inflammatory disease of the hip joint may incite inflammation of this bursa (bursitis). When inflamed, the iliopectineal bursa is frequently painful and swollen and may occasionally be mistaken for a neoplasm on MR images.

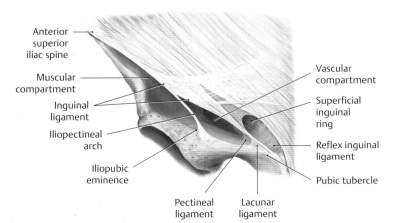

Anterior superior iliac spine

Muscular compartment

Inguinal ligament

Iliopectineal arch

Iliopubic eminence

Pectineal ligament

Lacunar ligament

Vascular compartment

Superficial inguinal ring

Reflex inguinal ligament

Pubic tubercle

D The connective-tissue and bony boundaries of the muscular and vascular compartments

Diagram of the right inguinal region, anterior view. The connective-tissue boundary between the muscular and vascular compartments is formed by the iliopectineal arch, a thickened band in the medial portion of the iliacus fascia. It extends between the inguinal ligament and the iliopubic eminence. The fibrous band that curves downward from the medial attachment of the inguinal ligament is called the lacunar ligament, which extends further medially as the pectineal ligament (Cooper's ligament) and runs along the superior pubic ramus. This sharp-edged ligament defines the medial boundary of the vascular compartment (femoral ring) and may entrap the hernial sac in patients with a femoral hernia (see p. 214). Above the inguinal ligament is the external (superficial) inguinal ring, which is the external opening of the inguinal canal (see p. 210). The muscular compartment is bounded laterally by the anterior superior iliac spine.

549

23.4 Arterial Supply to the Thigh

B Course of the profunda femoris artery and sites where the perforating arteries pierce the adductor muscles

a Right thigh, anterior view; **b** schematic longitudinal section through the adductor muscles at the level of the perforating arteries. The profunda femoris artery has approximately three to five terminal branches that pass from the front to the back of the thigh through the femoral insertions of the adductor muscles (= first through third perforating arteries) to supply the hamstring muscles (biceps femoris, semitendinosus, and semimembranosus). Generally, the arteries pierce the adductor muscles above and below the adductor brevis and just above the adductor hiatus. Ligation of the femoral artery proximal to the origin of the deep artery of the thigh is relatively well tolerated owing to a good collateral supply from branches of the internal iliac artery (superior gluteal artery and obturator artery).

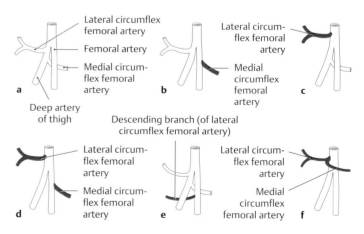

C Variants in the femoral artery branching pattern (after Lippert and Pabst)

a Usually the deep artery of the thigh and medial and lateral circumflex femoral arteries arise from the femoral artery by a common trunk (58% of cases, also shown in the other figures on this page).

b The medial circumflex femoral artery arises directly from the femoral artery (18% of cases).

c The lateral circumflex femoral artery arises directly from the femoral artery (15% of cases).

d The circumflex arteries arise separately from the femoral artery (4% of cases).

e The descending branch of the lateral circumflex femoral artery springs directly from the femoral artery (3% of cases).

f The circumflex arteries arise by a common trunk (1% of cases).

A Course and branches of the femoral artery

The femoral artery, the distal continuation of the external iliac artery, runs along the medial side of the thigh to the adductor canal, through which it passes to the back of the leg. After emerging from the adductor hiatus, it becomes the popliteal artery. In clinical parlance the femoral artery is often called the *superficial* femoral artery because of its superficial course down the front of the thigh, distinguishing it from the more deeply placed deep artery of the thigh that arises from it (see **D**).

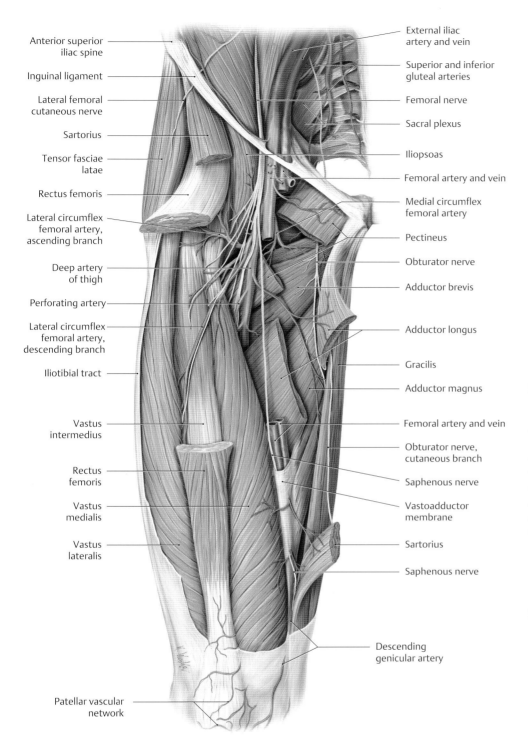

Anterior superior iliac spine

Inguinal ligament

Lateral femoral cutaneous nerve

Sartorius

Tensor fasciae latae

Rectus femoris

Lateral circumflex femoral artery, ascending branch

Deep artery of thigh

Perforating artery

Lateral circumflex femoral artery, descending branch

Iliotibial tract

Vastus intermedius

Rectus femoris

Vastus medialis

Vastus lateralis

Patellar vascular network

External iliac artery and vein

Superior and inferior gluteal arteries

Femoral nerve

Sacral plexus

Iliopsoas

Femoral artery and vein

Medial circumflex femoral artery

Pectineus

Obturator nerve

Adductor brevis

Adductor longus

Gracilis

Adductor magnus

Femoral artery and vein

Obturator nerve, cutaneous branch

Saphenous nerve

Vastoadductor membrane

Sartorius

Saphenous nerve

Descending genicular artery

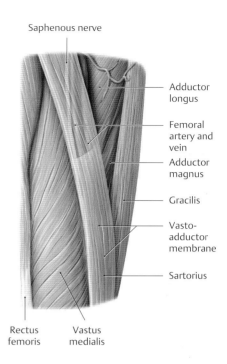

Saphenous nerve

Adductor longus

Femoral artery and vein

Adductor magnus

Gracilis

Vasto-adductor membrane

Sartorius

Rectus femoris

Vastus medialis

E The location of the adductor canal

Right thigh, anterior view. The saphenous nerve passes down the adductor canal on the anterior side of the thigh, accompanied by the femoral artery and vein. While both vessels continue toward the popliteal fossa through the adductor hiatus, the saphenous nerve pierces the vastoadductor membrane along with the descending genicular artery and passes to the medial side of the knee joint (see also **F**).

F The boundaries and contents of the adductor canal

Boundaries

• Adductor longus and magnus (posterior)
• Sartorius (medial)
• Vastoadductor membrane (anterior)
• Vastus medialis (lateral and anterior)

Contents

• Femoral artery
• Femoral vein
• Saphenous nerve   ⎫ Pierce the
• Descending   ⎬ vastoadductor
  genicular artery   ⎭ membrane

D The blood supply to the thigh from the profunda femoris artery

Right thigh, anterior view. The sartorius, rectus femoris, adductor longus, and pectineus muscles have been partially removed, along with the central portion of the femoral artery, to demonstrate the course of the deep artery of the thigh. For clarity, the veins have also been removed to the level of the external iliac vein. This dissection does not show the anterior abdominal wall or the pelvic and abdominal organs above the level of the inguinal ligament. While the branches of the medial and lateral circumflex arteries mainly supply blood to the hip joint and extensors and adductors of the thigh, the terminal branches of the deep artery of the thigh (the first through third perforating arteries, see **B**) on the medial side of the femur pass to the back of the thigh through gaps in the insertions of the adductor muscles land supply the hamstrings (biceps femoris, semitendinosus, and semimembranosus).

Note: The vastoadductor membrane is pierced by the descending genicular artery and saphenous nerve (see **E** and **F**).

551

23.5 The Gluteal Region: Overview of Its Vessels and Nerves

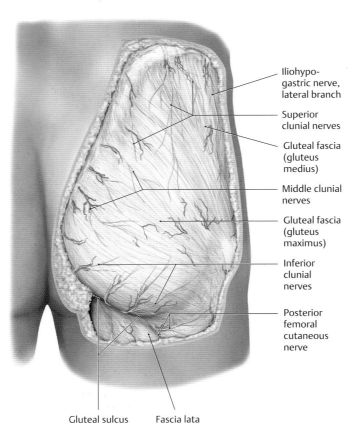

Iliohypo-
gastric nerve,
lateral branch

Superior
clunial nerves

Gluteal fascia
(gluteus
medius)

Middle clunial
nerves

Gluteal fascia
(gluteus
maximus)

Inferior
clunial
nerves

Posterior
femoral
cutaneous
nerve

Gluteal sulcus   Fascia lata

A The fasciae and cutaneous nerves of the superficial gluteal region

Right gluteal region, posterior view. The gluteal region is covered by the gluteal fascia, which is part of the fascia lata (although the term "fascia lata" strictly refers only to the part below the gluteus medius and maximus). The fascia covering the gluteus maximus forms septa-like invaginations between the muscle bundles. At the junction of the gluteal region with the back of the upper thigh is the gently curved gluteal sulcus, in which thickened fiber tracts of the fascia lata run transversely across the thigh at the level of the ischial tuberosity.

Note on surface anatomy: The oblique inferior border of the gluteus maximus (see **B**) *crosses* the gluteal sulcus. Its course, then, is not identical to that of the gluteal sulcus.

B The gluteal region and thigh with the fasciae removed

Right side, posterior view. With the fascia lata removed, the main trunk of the posterior femoral cutaneous nerve, which is subfascial over much of its course, can be traced into the popliteal fossa.

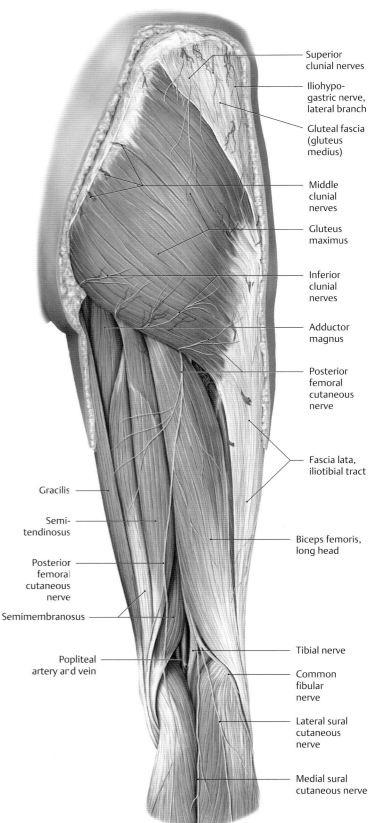

Superior
clunial nerves

Iliohypo-
gastric nerve,
lateral branch

Gluteal fascia
(gluteus
medius)

Middle
clunial
nerves

Gluteus
maximus

Inferior
clunial
nerves

Adductor
magnus

Posterior
femoral
cutaneous
nerve

Fascia lata,
iliotibial tract

Gracilis

Semi-
tendinosus

Biceps femoris,
long head

Posterior
femoral
cutaneous
nerve

Semimembranosus

Popliteal
artery and vein

Tibial nerve

Common
fibular
nerve

Lateral sural
cutaneous
nerve

Medial sural
cutaneous nerve

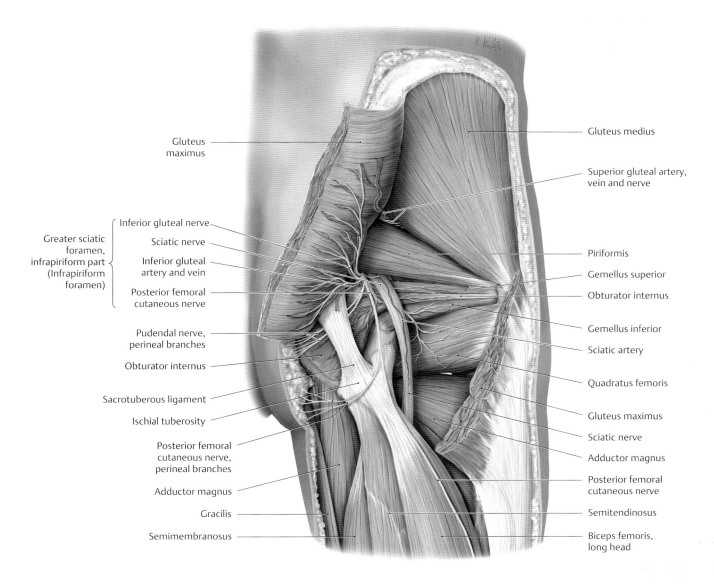

Gluteus maximus

Gluteus medius

Superior gluteal artery, vein and nerve

Greater sciatic foramen, infrapiriform part (Infrapiriform foramen)
- Inferior gluteal nerve
- Sciatic nerve
- Inferior gluteal artery and vein
- Posterior femoral cutaneous nerve

Piriformis

Gemellus superior

Obturator internus

Pudendal nerve, perineal branches

Gemellus inferior

Sciatic artery

Obturator internus

Quadratus femoris

Sacrotuberous ligament

Gluteus maximus

Ischial tuberosity

Sciatic nerve

Posterior femoral cutaneous nerve, perineal branches

Adductor magnus

Adductor magnus

Posterior femoral cutaneous nerve

Gracilis

Semitendinosus

Semimembranosus

Biceps femoris, long head

C The vessels and nerves of the deep gluteal region
Right side, posterior view, with the gluteus maximus partially removed. The neurovascular structures of the deep gluteal region traverse an extensive fatty and connective-tissue space below the gluteus maximus. The floor of this space is formed by the piriformis, obturator internus, gemellus superior, and quadratus femoris muscles. It communicates through the sciatic foramina with the connective-tissue spaces of the lesser pelvis and ischioanal fossa (not shown here). A useful topographic landmark is the piriformis, which extends from the pelvic surface of the sacrum through the greater sciatic foramen to the tip of the greater trochanter (see **A**, p. 554).

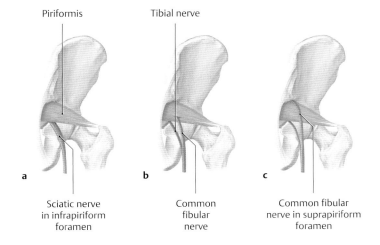

Piriformis

Tibial nerve

a

b

c

Sciatic nerve in infrapiriform foramen

Common fibular nerve

Common fibular nerve in suprapiriform foramen

D Variable course of the sciatic nerve in relation to the piriformis
(after Rauber/Kopsch)
a The sciatic nerve leaves the lesser pelvis inferior to the piriformis (almost 85% of cases).
b This variant illustrates a *high division* of the sciatic nerve (approximately 15% of cases). In this pattern the fibular division (common fibular nerve) and sometimes the posterior femoral cutaneous nerve pass through the piriformis muscle and may become compressed at that location, causing a "piriformis syndrome." Usually this term refers to the complaints that may develop following trauma to the gluteal region and are marked by severe gluteal pain. It is still uncertain whether these complaints are actually referable to the compression of sciatic nerve segments.
c In this variant the fibular part of the sciatic nerve leaves the lesser pelvis above the piriformis (rare, only about 0.5% of cases).

23.6 The Gluteal Region: The Sciatic Foramen and Sciatic Nerve

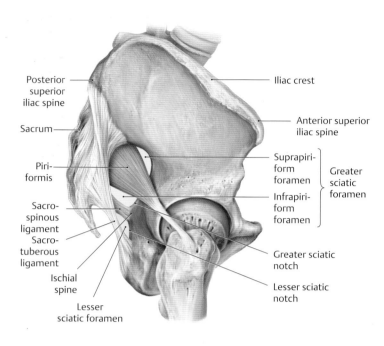

A Location of the greater and lesser sciatic foramina
Right hip bone, lateral view.

B The boundaries of the sciatic foramina and the structures that traverse them
The subgluteal connective-tissue space communicates through the sciatic foramina with the connective-tissue spaces of the lesser pelvis and the ischioanal fossa.

Foramen	Boundaries	Transmitted structures

• Greater sciatic foramen	• Greater sciatic notch
	• Sacrospinous ligament
	• Sacrum
		• *Suprapiriform portion*
		  – Superior gluteal artery and vein
		  – Superior gluteal nerve
		• *Infrapiriform portion*
		  – Inferior gluteal artery and vein
		  – Inferior gluteal nerve
		  – Internal pudendal artery and vein
		  – Pudendal nerve
		  – Sciatic nerve
		  – Posterior femoral cutaneous nerve

• Lesser sciatic foramen	• Lesser sciatic notch • Sacrospinous ligament • Sacrotuberous ligament	– Internal pudendal artery and vein – Pudendal nerve – Obturator internus

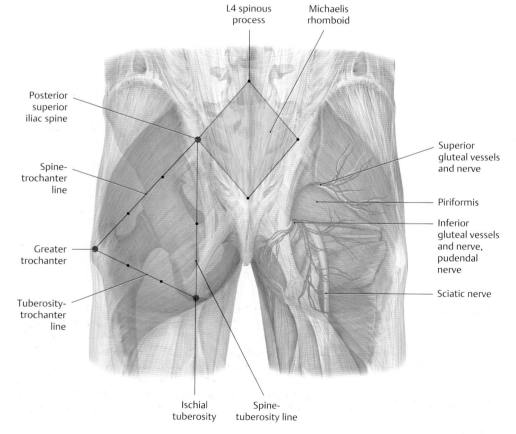

C Reference lines used for locating neurovascular structures in the gluteal region
Right and left gluteal regions, posterior view. The reference lines are drawn between the following points: the posterior superior iliac spine (lateral point of the Michaelis rhomboid), the ischial tuberosity, and the greater trochanter.

- **Spine-trochanter line:** The superior gluteal vessels emerge from the suprapiriform foramen between the middle and upper thirds of this line.
- **Tuberosity-trochanter line:** The sciatic nerve runs downward between the middle and medial thirds of this line.
- **Spine-tuberosity line:** The sciatic, inferior gluteal, and pudendal nerves and the inferior gluteal vessels emerge from the infrapiriform foramen at the midpoint of this line.

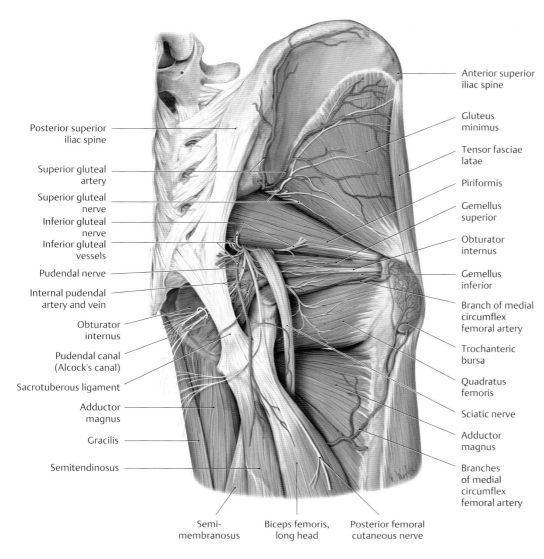

Posterior superior iliac spine

Superior gluteal artery

Superior gluteal nerve

Inferior gluteal nerve

Inferior gluteal vessels

Pudendal nerve

Internal pudendal artery and vein

Obturator internus

Pudendal canal (Alcock's canal)

Sacrotuberous ligament

Adductor magnus

Gracilis

Semitendinosus

Anterior superior iliac spine

Gluteus minimus

Tensor fasciae latae

Piriformis

Gemellus superior

Obturator internus

Gemellus inferior

Branch of medial circumflex femoral artery

Trochanteric bursa

Quadratus femoris

Sciatic nerve

Adductor magnus

Branches of medial circumflex femoral artery

Semi-membranosus

Biceps femoris, long head

Posterior femoral cutaneous nerve

D The vessels and nerves of the gluteal region and ischioanal fossa
Right gluteal region, posterior view, with the gluteus maximus and medius removed.
Note the course of the pudendal vessels and pudendal nerve in the lateral wall of the ischioanal fossa. They run in the pudendal canal (Alcock's canal), which is formed by the obturator internus fascia (see p. 478).

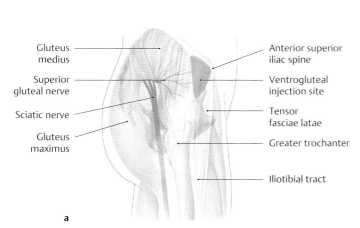

Gluteus medius

Superior gluteal nerve

Sciatic nerve

Gluteus maximus

Anterior superior iliac spine

Ventrogluteal injection site

Tensor fasciae latae

Greater trochanter

Iliotibial tract

a

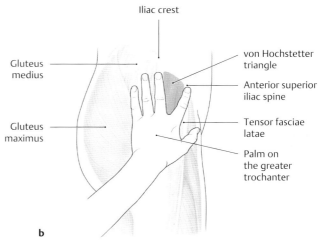

Iliac crest

Gluteus medius

Gluteus maximus

von Hochstetter triangle

Anterior superior iliac spine

Tensor fasciae latae

Palm on the greater trochanter

b

E Location of the sciatic nerve and superior gluteal nerves and their protection during intragluteal injections
Right gluteal region, lateral view.

a Two very important nerves are found in the gluteal region: the sciatic nerve and the superior gluteal nerve. To avoid jeopardizing these nerves during intramuscular injections, the needle should be inserted with the greatest possible safety margin with respect to these structures. Making the injection within the "von Hochstetter triangle" ensures that this safety margin is maintained.

b Locating the von Hochstetter triangle: The target site is located in the anterolateral gluteal region (accounting for the term "ventrogluteal injection"). To give an intramuscular injection on the right side, for example, place the palm of the left hand on the greater trochanter and the tip of the index finger on the anterior superior iliac spine. Keeping the hand in place, abduct the middle finger away from the index finger and introduce the needle perpendicular to the skin surface within the triangular zone between the two fingers and the iliac crest.

23.7   **The Ischioanal Fossa**

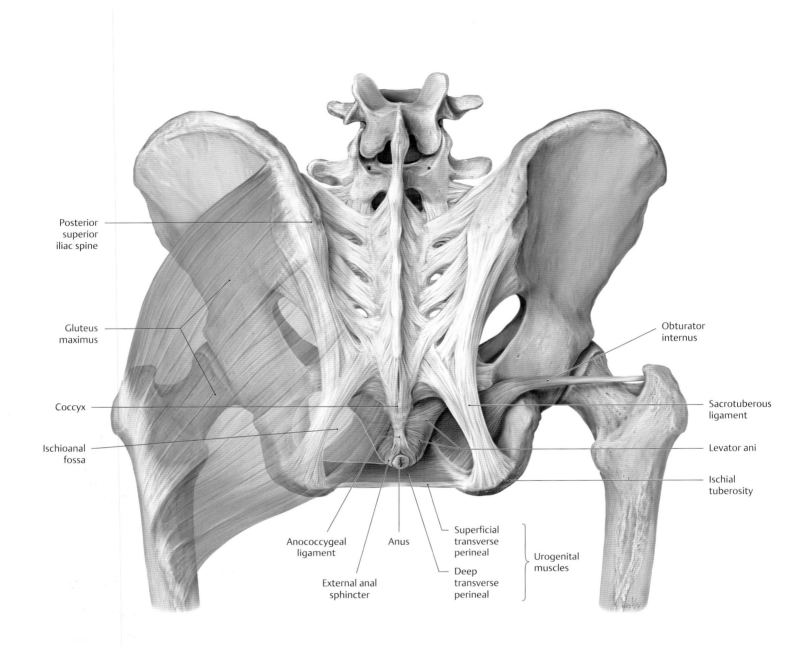

Posterior superior iliac spine

Gluteus maximus

Coccyx

Ischioanal fossa

Anococcygeal ligament

External anal sphincter

Anus

Superficial transverse perineal

Deep transverse perineal

Urogenital muscles

Obturator internus

Sacrotuberous ligament

Levator ani

Ischial tuberosity

A The muscular boundaries of the ischioanal fossa
Left and right gluteal region, posterior view. The ischioanal fossa is a pyramid-shaped space located lateral to the levator ani muscle on each side. The tip of the three-sided pyramid points toward the symphysis, and the base of the pyramid faces posteriorly. The ischioanal fossa is bounded by the following muscles:

- Superamedially by the levator ani
- Laterally by the obturator internus
- Inferiorly by the deep transverse perineal
- The entrance to the ischioanal fossa is bounded posteriorly by the gluteus maximus and sacrotuberous ligament.

The fatty tissue that occupies most of the ischioanal fossa (the fat pad of the ischioanal fossa) functions as a mobile pad that can slide downward and backward, for example, during bowel evacuation or during labor. It is traversed by the branches of the internal pudendal vessels and pudendal nerve (see **B**), whose trunks run in the pudendal, or Alcock's, canal; see **A**, p. 558.

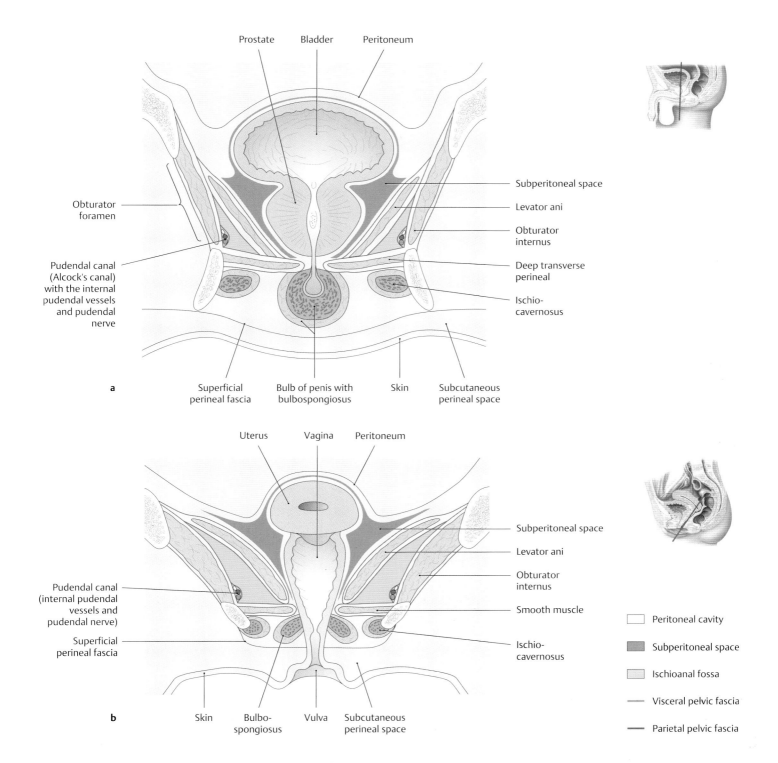

a

- Prostate
- Bladder
- Peritoneum
- Obturator foramen
- Pudendal canal (Alcock's canal) with the internal pudendal vessels and pudendal nerve
- Superficial perineal fascia
- Bulb of penis with bulbospongiosus
- Skin
- Subperitoneal space
- Levator ani
- Obturator internus
- Deep transverse perineal
- Ischio-cavernosus
- Subcutaneous perineal space

b

- Uterus
- Vagina
- Peritoneum
- Pudendal canal (internal pudendal vessels and pudendal nerve)
- Superficial perineal fascia
- Skin
- Bulbo-spongiosus
- Vulva
- Subcutaneous perineal space
- Subperitoneal space
- Levator ani
- Obturator internus
- Smooth muscle
- Ischio-cavernosus

Peritoneal cavity

Subperitoneal space

Ischioanal fossa

— Visceral pelvic fascia

— Parietal pelvic fascia

B The ischioanal fossa

a Coronal section through the male pelvis at the level of the prostate.

b Oblique coronal section through the female pelvis at the level of the vagina.

The pelvic organs make varying contributions to the shape of the peritoneal cavity and subperitoneal space, but they are not represented in the ischioanal fossa. While the peritoneal cavity is lined by the parietal peritoneum and the visceral peritoneum (on intraperitoneal organs such as the ovary), the subperitoneal space is lined by the pelvic fasciae (composed of parietal and visceral layers, see p. 183).

23.8 The Pudendal Canal and Perineal Region (Urogenital and Anal Region)

A Location of the pudendal canal (Alcock's canal) and the neurovascular structures it contains

Right half of the pelvis, medial view. All of the muscles have been removed except for the psoas major, piriformis, and obturator internus. For clarity, the individual veins are not shown. The pudendal canal is formed by the obturator internus fascia. It begins just below the ischial spine and courses in the lateral wall of the ischioanal fossa below the tendinous arch of levator ani, passing toward the pubic symphysis and the posterior border of the urogenital muscles (see p. 162). The neurovascular structures that are transmitted by the canal (the internal pudendal vessels, of which only the artery is shown, and the pudendal nerve, see **B**) exit the lesser pelvis through the greater sciatic foramen and enter the pudendal canal through the lesser sciatic foramen. They pass through the canal toward the pubic symphysis and the posterior border of the urogenital muscles.

Cauda equina

L5 vertebral body

Common iliac artery

Superior gluteal artery

Internal iliac artery

Sacral plexus

External iliac artery

Piriformis

Iliopsoas

Inferior gluteal artery

Obturator nerve

Internal pudendal artery, pudendal nerve

Obturator artery

Coccygeus

Ischial spine

Sacrospinous ligament

Obturator internus

Lesser sciatic foramen

Pubic symphysis

Levator ani

Femoral artery

Sacrotuberous ligament

Deep transverse perineal

Tendinous arch of levator ani

Internal pudendal artery, pudendal nerve in Alcock's canal

B Distribution of the pudendal nerve and internal pudendal vessels to the anus, perineum, and external genitalia

Gluteal region and ischioanal fossa on the right side, posterior view. The gluteus maximus and sacrotuberous ligament have been partially removed, and all fatty tissue has been removed from the ischioanal fossa to demonstrate the course of the pudendal nerve and the internal pudendal vessels. On their way through the pudendal canal (not shown here in order to display the course of the nerve and vessels below the sacrotuberous ligament), the various neural and vascular branches are successively distributed in a fan-shaped pattern to the anus, perineum, and external genitalia. It is very common in obstetrics to perform a pudendal nerve block by anesthetizing the pudendal nerve at the level of the ischial spine (i.e., before it branches into the inferior rectal, perineal, dorsal clitoral, and posterior labial nerves; see p. 542).

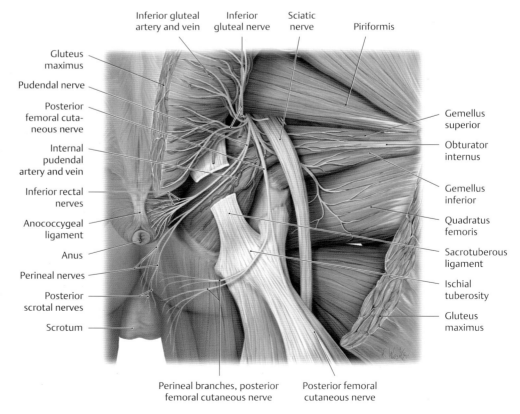

Inferior gluteal artery and vein

Inferior gluteal nerve

Sciatic nerve

Piriformis

Gluteus maximus

Pudendal nerve

Posterior femoral cutaneous nerve

Gemellus superior

Internal pudendal artery and vein

Obturator internus

Inferior rectal nerves

Gemellus inferior

Anococcygeal ligament

Quadratus femoris

Anus

Sacrotuberous ligament

Perineal nerves

Ischial tuberosity

Posterior scrotal nerves

Gluteus maximus

Scrotum

Perineal branches, posterior femoral cutaneous nerve

Posterior femoral cutaneous nerve

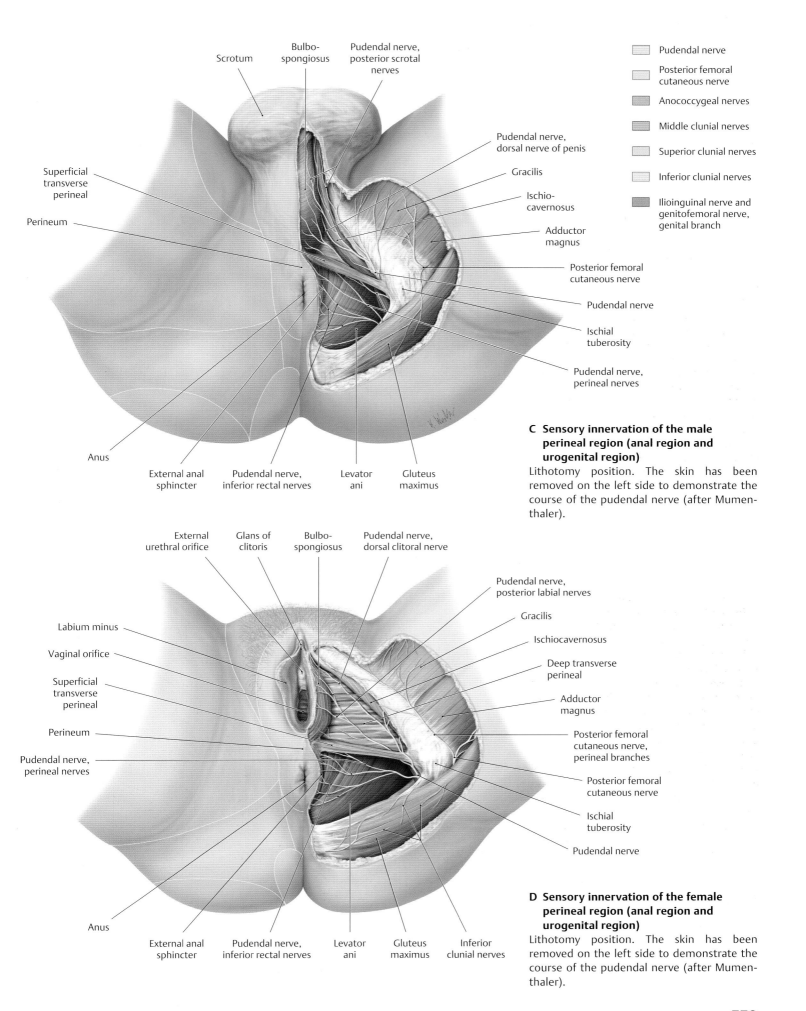

Scrotum

Bulbo-
spongiosus

Pudendal nerve,
posterior scrotal
nerves

Pudendal nerve,
dorsal nerve of penis

Gracilis

Ischio-
cavernosus

Adductor
magnus

Posterior femoral
cutaneous nerve

Pudendal nerve

Ischial
tuberosity

Pudendal nerve,
perineal nerves

Superficial
transverse
perineal

Perineum

Anus

External anal
sphincter

Pudendal nerve,
inferior rectal nerves

Levator
ani

Gluteus
maximus

Pudendal nerve

Posterior femoral
cutaneous nerve

Anococcygeal nerves

Middle clunial nerves

Superior clunial nerves

Inferior clunial nerves

Ilioinguinal nerve and
genitofemoral nerve,
genital branch

**C Sensory innervation of the male
perineal region (anal region and
urogenital region)**
Lithotomy position. The skin has been
removed on the left side to demonstrate the
course of the pudendal nerve (after Mumenthaler).

External
urethral orifice

Glans of
clitoris

Bulbo-
spongiosus

Pudendal nerve,
dorsal clitoral nerve

Pudendal nerve,
posterior labial nerves

Gracilis

Ischiocavernosus

Deep transverse
perineal

Adductor
magnus

Posterior femoral
cutaneous nerve,
perineal branches

Posterior femoral
cutaneous nerve

Ischial
tuberosity

Pudendal nerve

Labium minus

Vaginal orifice

Superficial
transverse
perineal

Perineum

Pudendal nerve,
perineal nerves

Anus

External anal
sphincter

Pudendal nerve,
inferior rectal nerves

Levator
ani

Gluteus
maximus

Inferior
clunial nerves

**D Sensory innervation of the female
perineal region (anal region and
urogenital region)**
Lithotomy position. The skin has been
removed on the left side to demonstrate the
course of the pudendal nerve (after Mumenthaler).

559

23.9 The Posterior Thigh Region and Popliteal Region

A The vessels and nerves of the posterior thigh

Right thigh, posterior view. To demonstrate the vessels and nerves in their course from the gluteal region down the back of the thigh to the popliteal fossa (see **C**), the skin and muscle fasciae have been removed, and the following muscles have been partially removed: gluteus maximus, gluteus medius, and biceps femoris. The semimembranosus has been retracted slightly medially to display the adductor hiatus (transmits the femoral artery and vein) (deeper neurovascular structures in the popliteal fossa are shown in **F**). The posterior femoral region receives most of its blood supply from branches of the profunda femoris artery (the first through third perforating arteries) and the deep branch (not shown) of the medial circumflex femoral artery. The proximal part of the sciatic nerve is supplied by the sciatic artery, which is a branch of the inferior gluteal artery, and its distal part is supplied by branches of the first through third perforating arteries.

B Sites of emergence of the perforating arteries on the back of the thigh

Right thigh, posterior view. All of the muscles have been removed except for the adductor magnus.

Note: The femoral artery enters the popliteal fossa through the adductor hiatus, thereafter becoming the popliteal artery.

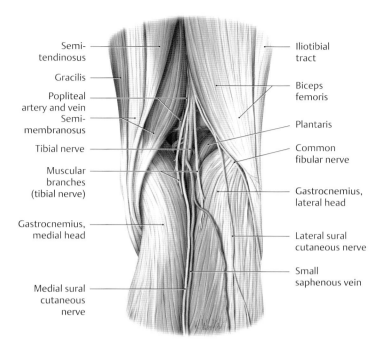

Semi-tendinosus

Gracilis

Popliteal artery and vein

Semi-membranosus

Tibial nerve

Muscular branches (tibial nerve)

Gastrocnemius, medial head

Medial sural cutaneous nerve

Iliotibial tract

Biceps femoris

Plantaris

Common fibular nerve

Gastrocnemius, lateral head

Lateral sural cutaneous nerve

Small saphenous vein

C The muscular boundaries of the popliteal fossa
Right popliteal fossa, posterior view. For clarity the skin, fasciae, and fat pads have been removed.

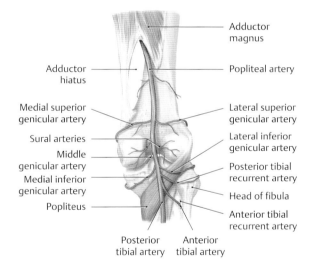

Adductor hiatus

Medial superior genicular artery

Sural arteries

Middle genicular artery

Medial inferior genicular artery

Popliteus

Posterior tibial artery

Adductor magnus

Popliteal artery

Lateral superior genicular artery

Lateral inferior genicular artery

Posterior tibial recurrent artery

Head of fibula

Anterior tibial recurrent artery

Anterior tibial artery

D Branches of the popliteal artery that course in the popliteal fossa
Right knee joint, posterior view. The popliteal artery begins at the outlet of the adductor canal and ends at the level of the popliteus muscle, where it divides into the anterior tibial artery and posterior tibial artery.

Popliteal artery

E Palpation of the popliteal artery in the popliteal fossa

Popliteal artery and vein

Sciatic nerve

Biceps femoris, long head

Gracilis

Semi-membranosus

Semi-tendinosus

Gastrocnemius, medial head

Subtendinous bursa of the medial gastrocnemius head

Middle genicular artery

Semimembranosus bursa

Oblique popliteal ligament

Tendon of insertion of semi-membranosus

Medial inferior genicular artery

Tibial nerve

Biceps femoris, short head

Common fibular nerve

Medial superior genicular artery

Lateral superior genicular artery

Plantaris

Gastrocnemius, lateral head

Lateral inferior genicular artery

Posterior tibial recurrent artery

Plantaris tendon

Popliteus

Soleus

Gastrocnemius

Triceps surae

F Deep neurovascular structures in the popliteal fossa
Right knee joint, posterior view. Portions of both heads of the gastrocnemius and portions of the hamstrings have been removed to demonstrate the course of the deep neurovascular structures in the popliteal fossa. Five vessels, some paired, branch from the middle portion of the popliteal artery to supply the knee joint (see **D**):

- Lateral and medial superior genicular arteries
- Middle genicular artery
- Lateral and medial inferior genicular arteries

One of these vessels, the middle genicular artery, pierces the joint capsule of the knee in the area of the oblique popliteal ligament and supplies the cruciform ligaments. The other vessels run forward on the medial and lateral sides to form the arterial network (articular rete) of the knee. The posterior and anterior tibial recurrent arteries contribute to the articular rete. The paired sural arteries supply the two heads of the gastrocnemius (see **D**, removed in **F**).
Note on the medial side the subtendinous bursa of the gastrocnemius, which consistently communicates with the joint cavity of the knee, and the bursa of the semimembranosus, which occasionally communicates with the bursa of the gastrocnemius head (this forms an extensive recess in the joint cavity of the knee, which may become abnormally enlarged to form a Baker cyst; see p. 442).

23.10 The Posterior Leg Region and the Tarsal Tunnel

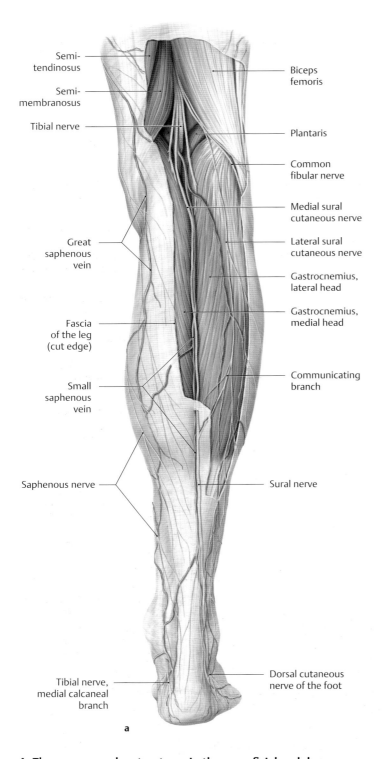

Semi-
tendinosus

Semi-
membranosus

Tibial nerve

Great
saphenous
vein

Fascia
of the leg
(cut edge)

Small
saphenous
vein

Saphenous nerve

Tibial nerve,
medial calcaneal
branch

Biceps
femoris

Plantaris

Common
fibular nerve

Medial sural
cutaneous nerve

Lateral sural
cutaneous nerve

Gastrocnemius,
lateral head

Gastrocnemius,
medial head

Communicating
branch

Sural nerve

Dorsal cutaneous
nerve of the foot

a

Semi-
tendinosus

Gracilis

Semi-
membranosus

Tibial nerve

Gastroc-
nemius

Tendinous arch
of soleus

Posterior tibial artery

Tibial nerve

Flexor digitorum
longus

Flexor hallucis
longus

Medial malleolus

Posterior tibial
artery

Tibial nerve

Flexor
retinaculum

Biceps
femoris

Plantaris

Common
fibular nerve

Popliteus

Popliteal artery
and vein

Soleus

Fibular
artery

Tibialis
posterior

Fibularis
brevis

Perforating
branch
Communi-
cating branch

Fibular
artery

Fibularis longus

Lateral malleolus

Calcaneal (Achilles')
tendon

Calcaneal rete

b

A The neurovascular structures in the superficial and deep posterior compartments

Right leg, posterior view.

a Neurovascular structures in the *superficial posterior compartment*: The superficial layer of the fascia of the leg ensheaths the triceps surae and has been partially removed proximally.

b Neurovascular structures in the *deep posterior compartment* after partial removal of the triceps surae and the deep layer of the fascia of the leg. The popliteal artery divides into the anterior and posterior tibial arteries at the distal border of the popliteus. The anterior

tibial artery pierces the interosseous membrane (not shown here, see **B**) and passes to the anterior side of the leg, entering the anterior compartment. The posterior tibial artery, accompanied by the tibial nerve, passes below the tendinous arch of the soleus into the deep posterior compartment, almost immediately gives off the fibular artery, and then continues distally behind the medial malleolus to the plantar side of the foot. The deep posterior compartment is one of four poorly distensible muscle compartments in the leg ("fibro-osseous canals"), which are potential sites for the development of a compartment syndrome following a vascular injury (see p. 567).

B The arteries of the leg
Posterior view.

C Typical branching pattern of the popliteal artery and variants (after Lippert and Pabst)

a Typical pattern: The anterior tibial artery arises from the popliteal artery behind the popliteus muscle, and the popliteal artery continues as the posterior tibial artery (i. e., the popliteal artery divides into an anterior and posterior tibial artery). Farther distally, the fibular artery branches from the posterior tibial artery.

b The anterior tibial artery and fibular artery arise *by a common trunk* from the popliteal artery behind the popliteus (4% of cases).

c The fibular artery arises from the anterior tibial artery (= fibulotibial trunk, 1% of cases).

d The fibulotibial trunk arises proximal to the popliteus (1% of cases).

e The anterior tibial artery arises from the popliteal artery proximal to the popliteus (1% of cases).

f The anterior tibial artery runs between the popliteus and the tibia (1% of cases).

D Palpation of the posterior tibial artery below the medial malleolus

E The neurovascular structures of the medial malleolar region
Right foot, medial view. The neurovascular structures pass from the deep flexor compartment to the plantar side of the foot through the tarsal tunnel, between the flexor retinaculum and medial malleolus. They are accompanied by the tendons of insertion of the long flexors (tibialis posterior, flexor digitorum longus, flexor hallucis longus) in their synovial sheaths.

Note the division of the posterior tibial nerve into the medial and lateral plantar nerves and the division of the posterior tibial artery into the medial and lateral plantar arteries within the malleolar canal. Compression of the nerves at this site can cause a medial or posterior tarsal tunnel syndrome (see p. 541).

23.11 The Sole of the Foot

A The plantar arteries and nerves of the foot (superficial layer)
Right foot, plantar view. The skin and subcutaneous tissue have been removed to demonstrate the plantar aponeurosis and superficial neurovascular structures.

B The plantar arteries and nerves of the foot (middle layer)
Right foot, plantar view, with the plantar aponeurosis and flexor digitorum brevis removed.

C The plantar arteries of the foot: possible variants
Right foot, plantar view. Any of four basic anatomic variants may be seen (after Lippert and Pabst):

a The deep plantar arch and the plantar metatarsal arteries arising from it are supplied entirely by the deep plantar branch of the dorsal pedal artery (53% of cases).

b The first through third plantar metatarsal arteries are supplied by the deep plantar branch of the dorsal pedal artery, the fourth plantar metatarsal artery by the deep branch of the lateral plantar artery (19% of cases).

c The first and second plantar metatarsal arteries sre supplied by the deep plantar branch of the dorsal pedal artery, the third and fourth metatarsal arteries by the deep branch of the lateral plantar artery (13% of cases).

d The deep plantar arch and the first through fourth plantar metatarsal arteries are supplied entirely by the deep branch of the lateral plantar artery (7% of cases).

564

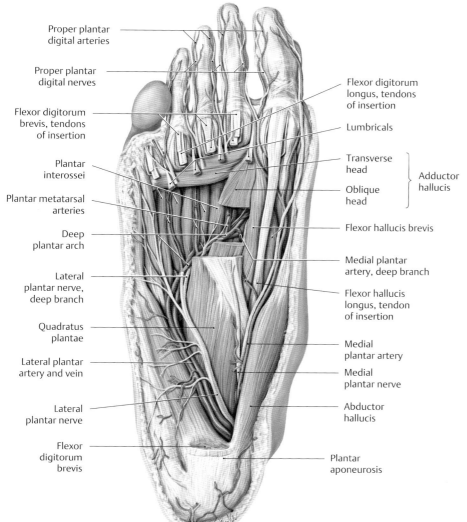

Proper plantar digital arteries

Proper plantar digital nerves

Flexor digitorum brevis, tendons of insertion

Plantar interossei

Plantar metatarsal arteries

Deep plantar arch

Lateral plantar nerve, deep branch

Quadratus plantae

Lateral plantar artery and vein

Lateral plantar nerve

Flexor digitorum brevis

Flexor digitorum longus, tendons of insertion

Lumbricals

Transverse head

Oblique head

} Adductor hallucis

Flexor hallucis brevis

Medial plantar artery, deep branch

Flexor hallucis longus, tendon of insertion

Medial plantar artery

Medial plantar nerve

Abductor hallucis

Plantar aponeurosis

D The plantar arteries and nerves of the foot (deep layer)

Right foot, plantar view. The plantar aponeurosis, flexor digitorum brevis, the tendons of flexor digitorum longus, and the oblique head of adductor hallucis have been removed to demonstrate the deep plantar arch and the deep branch of the lateral plantar nerve.

Note: The superficial branch of the lateral plantar nerve and the lateral plantar artery course in the *lateral plantar sulcus,* while the superficial branches of the medial plantar nerve and medial plantar artery course in the *medial plantar sulcus* (see **A**). The superficial branches of the medial and lateral plantar arteries help to supply the critically important pressure-chamber system in the sole of the foot (see p. 472).

E Overview of the plantar arteries of the foot

Right foot, plantar view.

The *deep plantar arch* is an arterial arcade in the sole of the foot that is formed by the deep plantar branch of the *dorsal pedal artery* and also by the deep branch of the *lateral plantar artery*. Often these two arteries that supply the deep plantar arch differ in size and thus make different contributions to the first through fourth plantar metatarsal arteries that consistently branch from the deep plantar arch (see **C**).

Proper plantar digital arteries

Common plantar digital arteries

Distal perforating branches

Plantar metatarsal arteries

Proximal perforating branches

Fifth plantar digital artery

Lateral plantar artery, deep branch

Lateral plantar artery

Medial plantar artery of great toe

Deep plantar branch (from dorsal pedal artery)

Superficial branch

Deep branch

} Medial plantar artery

Deep plantar arch

Medial plantar artery

Posterior tibial artery

23.12 The Anterior Leg Region and Dorsum of the Foot: Cutaneous Innervation

Patella

Head of fibula

Patellar ligament

Fibularis longus

Plane of section in C

Extensor hallucis longus

Extensor digitorum longus

Superficial fibular nerve

Fibularis brevis

Inferior extensor retinaculum

Lateral dorsal cutaneous nerve

Intermediate dorsal cutaneous nerve

Medial dorsal cutaneous nerve

Dorsal metatarsal arteries

Pes anserinus (insertion of sartorius, gracilis, and semitendinosus)

Gastrocnemius

Tibialis anterior

Muscular branches

Deep fibular nerve

Anterior tibial artery and vein

Soleus

Superior extensor retinaculum

Medial malleolus

Dorsal pedal artery

Extensor hallucis brevis

Tendon of extensor hallucis longus

Deep fibular nerve

A The neurovascular structures of the anterior compartment and dorsum of the foot

Right leg with the foot in plantar flexion, anterior view. The skin, subcutaneous tissue, and fasciae have been removed and the tibialis anterior and extensor hallucis longus muscles have been retracted to demonstrate the anterior tibial vessels (= anterior tibial artery and vein). The *anterior tibial artery* crosses beneath the tendon of the extensor hallucis longus at the junction of the leg with the dorsum of the foot. Below the extensor retinaculum it becomes the *dorsal pedal artery*, which runs lateral to the hallucis longus tendon on the dorsum of the foot, accompanied by the terminal branch of the *deep fibular nerve* (the site for taking the pedal pulse is shown in **E**). The *deep fibular nerve* may be compressed in its passage beneath the inferior extensor retinaculum (with sensory disturbances affecting the first and second toes).

Biceps femoris { Short head / Long head }

Lateral sural cutaneous nerve

Common fibular nerve

Head of fibula

Lateral sural cutaneous nerve

Gastrocnemius

Medial sural cutaneous nerve (tibial nerve)

Communicating branch

Soleus

Sural nerve

Fascia of the leg

Lateral malleolus

Lateral calcaneal branches

Iliotibial tract

Patella

Lateral tibial condyle

Anterior crural intermuscular septum

Deep fibular nerve

Superficial fibular nerve

Fibularis longus

Tibialis anterior

Extensor digitorum longus

Superficial fibular nerve

Medial dorsal cutaneous nerve   Intermediate dorsal cutaneous nerve

Deep fibular nerve, cutaneous branch

Lateral dorsal cutaneous nerve

B Division of the common fibular nerve into the deep and superficial fibular nerves

Right leg, lateral view. The origins of the fibularis longus and extensor digitorum longus have been excised below the head of the fibula and the lateral tibial condyle. After the *common fibular nerve* bifurcates in the proximal part of the lateral compartment, the *superficial fibular nerve* remains in the lateral compartment. The *deep fibular nerve* pierces the anterior intermuscular septum and descends with the anterior tibial vessels in the extensor compartment (**C** gives a sectional view of the compartments in the leg).

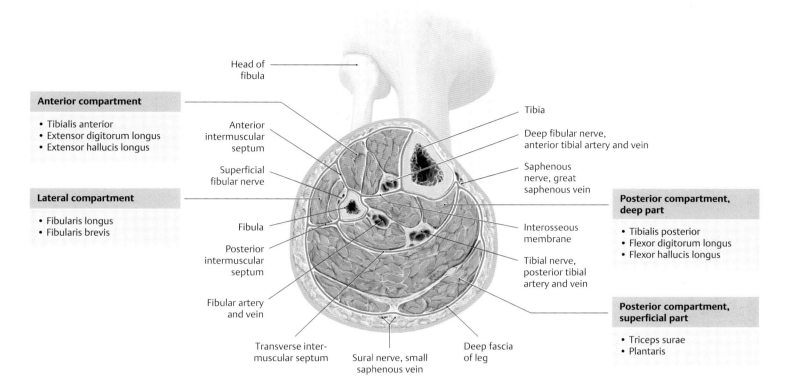

Anterior compartment

- Tibialis anterior
- Extensor digitorum longus
- Extensor hallucis longus

Lateral compartment

- Fibularis longus
- Fibularis brevis

Head of fibula

Anterior intermuscular septum

Superficial fibular nerve

Fibula

Posterior intermuscular septum

Fibular artery and vein

Transverse intermuscular septum

Sural nerve, small saphenous vein

Deep fascia of leg

Tibia

Deep fibular nerve, anterior tibial artery and vein

Saphenous nerve, great saphenous vein

Interosseous membrane

Tibial nerve, posterior tibial artery and vein

Posterior compartment, deep part

- Tibialis posterior
- Flexor digitorum longus
- Flexor hallucis longus

Posterior compartment, superficial part

- Triceps surae
- Plantaris

C The compartments and neurovascular structures in the leg
Cross section through a right leg one handwidth below the neck of the fibula, distal view (the level of the section is shown in **A**). The intermuscular septa and interosseous membrane, together with the superficial and deep layers of the fascia of the leg, define the boundaries of four distinct, poorly distensible fibro-osseous compartments in which the neurovascular structures descend through the leg. A rise in tissue pressure, which may result from conditions such as muscular edema or a fracture hematoma, can lead to neurovascular compression, inducing a local ischemia that can cause irreversible neuromuscular damage within a few hours (compartment syndromes such as the tibialis anterior syndrome). At greatest risk are the neurovascular structures of the deep posterior compartment (the posterior tibial artery and veins and the tibial nerve) and the anterior compartment (the anterior tibial artery and veins and the deep fibular nerve). Tibialis anterior syndrome is characterized in its acute stage by severe pain and an inability to dorsiflex the toes due to the unopposed action of the plantar flexors. This causes the toes to "claw up." Generally, the only effective treatment option at this stage is emergency incision of the fascia of the leg. This immediately decompresses the compartment and relieves the pressure on the vessels that supply the muscles.

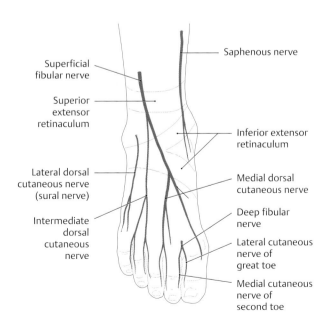

Saphenous nerve

Superficial fibular nerve

Superior extensor retinaculum

Inferior extensor retinaculum

Lateral dorsal cutaneous nerve (sural nerve)

Intermediate dorsal cutaneous nerve

Medial dorsal cutaneous nerve

Deep fibular nerve

Lateral cutaneous nerve of great toe

Medial cutaneous nerve of second toe

D The cutaneous nerves on the dorsum of the foot
Right foot, dorsal view.

Dorsal pedal artery

Anterior tibial artery

E Palpation of the pedal pulse
The dorsal pedal artery is palpable at the level of the navicular tuberosity, just lateral to the extensor hallucis longus tendon. In addition to determining regional skin temperature, checking the pedal pulse is an important step in the examination of patients with suspected lower limb arterial disease (one foot is markedly colder or paler than the other due to diminished blood flow). It is generally best to begin by palpating the femoral artery at the groin crease, then proceed distally to the popliteal fossa (popliteal artery), the medial malleolus (posterior tibial artery), and finally to the dorsum of the foot (dorsal pedal artery, which is the terminal branch of the anterior tibial artery). The palpable pulses should always be compared between the right and left sides. It should be noted that the pedal pulses may be difficult or impossible to palpate when peripheral edema is present, so it is best to examine the supine patient.

23.13 The Arteries of the Dorsum of the Foot

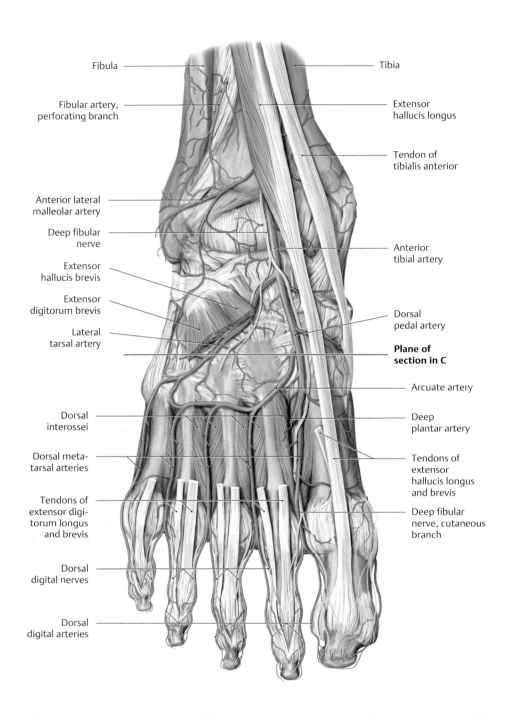

Fibula

Fibular artery, perforating branch

Anterior lateral malleolar artery

Deep fibular nerve

Extensor hallucis brevis

Extensor digitorum brevis

Lateral tarsal artery

Dorsal interossei

Dorsal meta-tarsal arteries

Tendons of extensor digitorum longus and brevis

Dorsal digital nerves

Dorsal digital arteries

Tibia

Extensor hallucis longus

Tendon of tibialis anterior

Anterior tibial artery

Dorsal pedal artery

Plane of section in C

Arcuate artery

Deep plantar artery

Tendons of extensor hallucis longus and brevis

Deep fibular nerve, cutaneous branch

A The dorsal arteries and nerves of the foot

Right foot in plantar flexion, dorsal view. The skin, subcutaneous tissue, and superficial and deep layers of the dorsal pedal fascia have been removed for clarity, along with the extensor digitorum longus tendons and the extensor digitorum brevis and extensor hallucis brevis muscles. Possible variants of the arteries are shown in **D**.

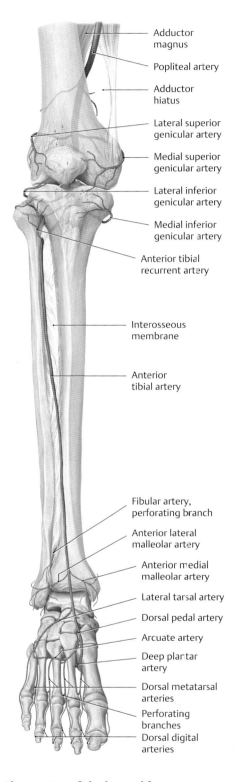

Adductor magnus

Popliteal artery

Adductor hiatus

Lateral superior genicular artery

Medial superior genicular artery

Lateral inferior genicular artery

Medial inferior genicular artery

Anterior tibial recurrent artery

Interosseous membrane

Anterior tibial artery

Fibular artery, perforating branch

Anterior lateral malleolar artery

Anterior medial malleolar artery

Lateral tarsal artery

Dorsal pedal artery

Arcuate artery

Deep plantar artery

Dorsal metatarsal arteries

Perforating branches

Dorsal digital arteries

B The arteries of the leg and foot

Right lower limb, anterior view.
Note: The dorsum of the foot is supplied mainly by branches of the anterior tibial artery.

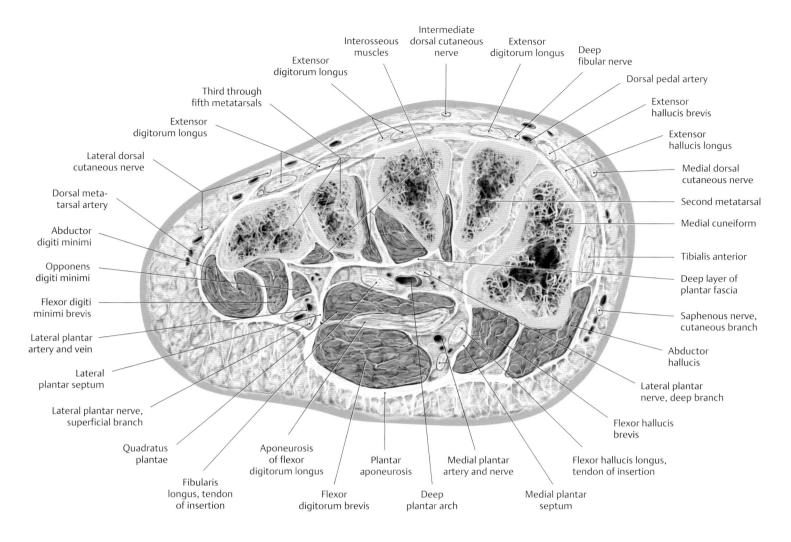

C The neurovascular structures in the sole of the foot
Cross section through the right foot at the level of the medial cunei-
form bone (the location of the section is shown in **A**), distal view (after
Rauber and Kopsch).

Note the deep layer of the plantar fascia, in which the deep neurovascular structures of the sole (the deep plantar arch and deep branch of
the lateral plantar nerve) are embedded in connective tissue that cush-
ions and protects them (for the arrangement of the pedal compartments, see p. 523).

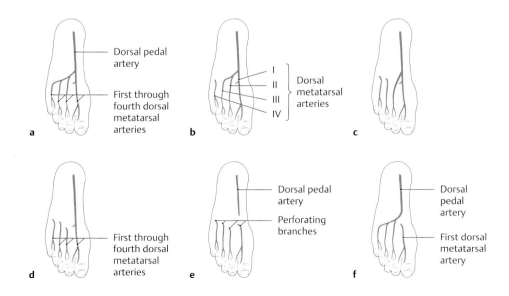

**D Variants in the dorsal arterial supply of
the foot** (after Lippert and Pabst)
a All of the dorsal metatarsal arteries arise
from the dorsal pedal artery (20% of cases).
b The fourth dorsal metatarsal artery is supplied by a perforating branch from the
plantar side of the foot (6% of cases).
c The third and fourth dorsal metatarsal arteries are supplied by perforating
branches from the plantar metatarsal
arteries (5% of cases).
d The first dorsal metatarsal artery is the only
branch of the dorsal pedal artery (40% of
cases).
e All of the dorsal metatarsal arteries are
supplied by perforating branches from the
plantar metatarsal arteries (10%).
f Only the first dorsal metatarsal artery is
supplied by a perforating branch (5%).

569

References

Agur AMR. Grants Anatomie. Lehrbuch und Atlas. Stuttgart: Enke; 1999

Bähr M, Frotscher M. Duus' Neurologisch-topische Diagnostik. 8th ed. Stuttgart: Thieme; 2003

Baumgartl F. Das Kniegelenk. Berlin: Springer; 1969

Bohndorf K, Imhof H, Fischer W. Radiologische Diagnostik der Knochen und Gelenke. 2nd ed. Stuttgart: Thieme; 2006

Chassard J, Lapiné C. Étude radiologique de l'arcade pubienne chez la femme enceinte. J Radiol Electrol 7 (1923), 113

Christ B, Wachtler F. Medizinische Embryologie. Wiesbaden: Ullstein Medical; 1998

Dauber W. Feneis' Bild-Lexikon der Anatomie. 8th ed. Stuttgart: Thieme; 1999

Debrunner AM. Orthopädie. Die Störungen des Bewegungsapparates in Klinik und Praxis. 2nd ed. Stuttgart: Hans Huber; 1985

Debrunner HU. Gelenkmessung (Neutral-0-Methode), Längenmessung, Umfangmessung. Bern: AO-Bulletin; 1971

Drews U. Taschenatlas der Embryologie. Stuttgart: Thieme; 1993

Echtermeyer V, Bartsch S. Praxisbuch Schulter. 2nd ed. Stuttgart: Thieme; 2004

Faller A. Anatomie in Stichworten. Stuttgart: Enke; 1980

Ficat P. Pathologie Fémoro-Patellaire. Paris: Masson; 1970

Földi M, Kubik S. Lehrbuch der Lymphologie. 3rd ed. Stuttgart: Gustav Fischer; 1993

Frick H, Leonhardt H, Starck D. Allgemeine und spezielle Anatomie. Taschenlehrbuch der gesamten Anatomie, Bd. 1 u. 2. 4th ed. Stuttgart: Thieme; 1992

Fritsch H, Kühnel W. Taschenatlas der Anatomie. Bd. 2. 7th ed. Stuttgart: Thieme; 2001

Gert SD, Liebman M. Basiswissen Neuroanatomie. 4th ed. Stuttgart: Thieme; 2003

Goerke K. Taschenatlas der Geburtshilfe. Stuttgart: Thieme; 2002

Graumann W, Sasse D. CompactLehrbuch Anatomie. Bd. 4. Stuttgart: Schattauer; 2005

Hansen K, Schliack K. Segmentale Innervation. 2nd ed. Stuttgart: Thieme; 1962

Hees H. Grundriss und Atlas der Mikroskopischen Anatomie des Menschen. Bd. 1. Zytologie und Allgemeine Histologie. 12th ed. Stuttgart: Gustav Fischer; 1996

Henne-Bruns D, Dürig M, Kremer B. Chirurgie. 2nd ed. Stuttgart: Thieme; 2003

Hepp WR. Radiologie des Femoro-Patellargelenkes. Bücherei des Orthopäden. Bd. 37. Stuttgart: Enke; 1983

Hilgenreiner H. Zur Frühdiagnose der angeborenen Hüftgelenksverrenkung. Med Klein 21 1925. Stuttgart: Hippokrates; 1981

Hochschild J. Strukturen und Funktionen begreifen. Bd. 1 u. 2. Stuttgart: Thieme; 1998 u. 2002

von Hochstetter A, von Rechenberg HK, Schmidt R. Die intragluteale Injektion. Stuttgart: Thieme; 1958

Hüter-Becker A, Schewe H, Heipertz W. Physiotherapie. Bd. 1. Biomechanik, Arbeitsmedizin, Ergonomie. Stuttgart: Thieme; 1999

Junghanns, H. Die funktionelle Pathologie der Zwischenwirbelscheibe als Grundlage für klinische Betrachtungen. Langenbecks. Arch Klin Chir 1951; 267: 393–417

Kahle W, Frotscher M. Taschenatlas der Anatomie. Bd. 1. Stuttgart: Thieme; 2001

Kapandji IA. Funktionelle Anatomie der Gelenke. Bd. 1–3. 2nd ed. Stuttgart: Enke; 1992

Kaufmann P. Reife Plazenta. In: Becker V, Schiebler TH, Kubli F, Hrsg. Die Plazenta des Menschen. Stuttgart: Thieme; 1981

Kilka HG, Geiger P, Mehrkens HH. Die vertikale infraklavikuläre Blockade des Plexus brachialis. Anästhesist 1995; 44: 339–344

Klinke R, Silbernagl S. Lehrbuch der Physiologie. 3rd ed. Stuttgart: Thieme; 2001

Koebke, J. Anatomie des Handgelenkes und der Handwurzel. Unfallchirurgie 1988; 14: 74–79

Konermann W, Gruber G. Ultraschalldiagnostik der Bewegungsorgane. Kursbuch nach den Richtlinien der DEGUM und der DGOOC, Buch und DVD. 2nd ed. Stuttgart: Thieme; 2006

Kristic, RV. General Histology of the Mammals. Berlin: Springer; 1985

Kubik S. Lymphsystem der oberen Extremität. In: Földi M, Kubik S, Hrsg. Lehrbuch der Lymphologie für Mediziner und Physiotherapeuten. Stuttgart: Gustav Fischer; 1989

Kummer, B. Biomechanik der Wirbelgelenke. In: Meinicke, FW. Die Wirbelbogengelenke. Stuttgart: Hippokrates; 1983

von Lanz T, Wachsmuth W. Praktische Anatomie. Bd. I/3 Arm. 2nd ed. Berlin: Springer; 1959

von Lanz T, Wachsmuth W. Praktische Anatomie. Bd. I/4 Bein und Statik. Berlin: Springer; 1972

Lehnert G. Dopplersonographische Diagnostik der erektilen Dysfunktion unter Anwendung des Papaverintests [Dissertation] Kiel: Universität Kiel, Medizinische Fakultät; 1995

Lelièvre J. Pathologie du Pied. 2nd ed. Paris: Masson; 1961

Lippert H, Pabst R. Arterial Variations in Man. München: Bergmann; 1985

Loeweneck H. Diagnostische Anatomie. Berlin: Springer; 1981

Lüllmann-Rauch R. Histologie. 2nd ed. Stuttgart: Thieme; 2006

Lundborg G, Myrhage R, Rydevik B. The vascularization of human flexor tendons within the digital synovial sheath region – structural and functional aspects. J Hand Surg 1977; 2: 417–427

Luschka, H. Die Halbgelenke des menschlichen Körpers. Berlin: Reiner; 1858

Masuhr KF, Neumann M. Neurologie. Duale Reihe. 4th ed. Stuttgart: Hippokrates; 1998

Matzen P. Praktische Orthopädie. 3rd ed. Stuttgart: J. A. Barth Verlag im Thieme Verlag; 2002

Meier G, Bauereis C, Maurer H, Meier Th. Interscalenäre Plexusblockade. Anästhesist 2001; 50: 333–341

Merk H, Jerosch J, Hrsg. Arthroskopie des Schultergelenks. Stuttgart: Thieme, 2000

Möller TB, Reif E. Taschenatlas der Röntgenanatomie. 2nd ed. Stuttgart: Thieme; 1998

Möller TB, Reif E. Taschenatlas der Schnittbildanatomie. Bd. 3: Extremitäten, Gelenke, Wirbelsäule. Stuttgart: Thieme; 2007

Mow VC, Hou JS, Owens JM. Biphasic and quasilinear viscoelastic theories for hydrated soft tissue. In: Mow JC, Ratcliffe A, Woo SL. Biomechanics of Diarthrodial Joints. Springer: New York; 1990. Vol. I: 215–260

Mubarak SJ, Hargens AR. Compartment Syndromes and Volkamn's Contracture. Philadelphia: W. B. Saunders; 1981

Mumenthaler M, Stöhr M, Müller-Vahl H. Läsion peripherer Nerven und radikuläre Syndrome. 8th ed. Stuttgart: Thieme; 2003

Netter FH. Farbatlanten der Medizin. Stuttgart: Thieme; 2000

Niethard FU, Pfeil J. Orthopädie. Duale Reihe. 5th ed. Stuttgart: Thieme; 2005

Niethard FU. Kinderorthopädie. Stuttgart: Thieme; 1997

Noback CR, Strominger NL, Demarest RJ. The Human Nervous System. 4th ed. Philadelphia: Lea & Febiger; 1991

O'Rahilly, Müller RF. Developmental Stages in Human Embryos. Carnegie Institution of Washington: Publication 637; 1987

Pauwels F. Eine neue Theorie über den Einfluss mechanischer Reize auf die Differenzierung der Stützgewebe (X). Beitrag zur funktionellen Anatomie und kausalen Morphologie des Stützapparates. Z Anat Entwickl Gesch 1968; 121: 478–515

Pauwels F. Atlas zur Biomechanik der gesunden und kranken Hüfte: Prinzipien, Technik und Resultate einer kausalen Therapie. Heidelberg: Springer; 1973

Petersen W, Tillmann B. Structure and vascularization of the cruciate ligaments of the human knee joint. Z Orthop 1999; 137: 31–37

Pette D. Das adaptive Potential des Skelettmuskels. Dtsch Z Sportmed 1999; 50: 262–271

Pette D, Staron RS. Transitions of muscle fiber phenotypic profiles. Histochem Cell Biol 2001; 115 (5): 359–379

Platzer W. Taschenatlas der Anatomie. Bd. 1. Stuttgart: Thieme; 1999

Platzer W. Atlas der topographischen Anatomie. Stuttgart: Thieme; 1982

Rauber A, Kopsch F. Anatomie des Menschen. Bd. 1–4. Stuttgart: Thieme; Bd. 1. 2nd ed. 1997; Bde. 2 u. 3 1987; Bd. 4 1988

Reiser M, Kuhn FP, Debus J. Radiologie. Duale Reihe. 2nd ed. Stuttgart: Thieme; 2006

Rockwood CA. Subluxations and dislocations about the shoulder. In: Rockwood CA, Green DP (eds). Fractures. Philadelphia: Lippincott; 1984: 722–985

Rohen, JW. Topographische Anatomie. 10th ed. Stuttgart: Schattauer; 2000

Rohen JW, Yokochi C, Lütjen-Drecoll E. Anatomie des Menschen. 4th ed. Stuttgart: Schattauer; 2000

Romer AS, Parson TS. Vergleichende Anatomie der Wirbeltiere. 5th ed. Hamburg und Berlin: Paul Parey; 1983

Rudigier J. Kurzgefasste Handchirurgie. 5th ed. Stuttgart: Thieme; 2006

Sadler, TW. Medizinische Embryologie. 10th ed. Stuttgart: Thieme; 2003

Scheldrup, EW. Tendon sheath patterns in the hand. Surg Gynec-Obestetr 1951; 93: 16–22

Schmidt HM, Lanz U. Chirurgische Anatomie der Hand. 2nd ed. Stuttgart: Thieme; 2003

Schumpelick V. Hernien. 4th ed. Stuttgart: Thieme; 2000

Schünke M. Funktionelle Anatomie–Topographie und Funktion des Bewegungssystems. Stuttgart: Thieme; 2000

Silbernagl S, Despopoulos A. Taschenatlas der Physiologie. 6th ed. Stuttgart: Thieme; 2003

Sökeland J, Schulze H, Rübben H. Urologie. 12th ed. Stuttgart: Thieme; 2002

Starck D. Embryologie. 3rd ed. Stuttgart: Thieme; 1975

Streater GL. Developmental horizons in human embryos: age group XI, 13–20 somites and age group XII, 21–29 somites. Contrib Embryol 1942; 30: 211–245

Tossy JD, Newton CM, Sigmond HM. Acromioclavicular separations: useful and practical classification for treatment. Clin Orthop 1963; 28: 111–119

Uhthoff HK. The Embryology of the Human Locomotor System. Berlin: Springer; 1990

Vahlensieck M, Reiser M. MRT des Bewegungsapparates. 3rd ed. Stuttgart: Thieme; 2006

Weber U, Greulich M, Sparmann M. Orthopädische Mikrochirurgie. Stuttgart: Thieme; 1993

Wiberg G. Roentgenographic and anatomic studies on the femoro-patellar joint. With special reference to chondromalacia patellae. Acta Orthop Scand 1941; 12: 319–410

Wiberg G. Studies on dysplastic acetabulum and congenital subluxation of the hip joint with special reference of the complication of osteoarthritis. Acta Chir Scand 1939; 83 (Suppl. 58)

Wolpert L, Beddington R, Brockes J et al. Entwicklungsbiologie. Weinheim: Spektrum; 1999

Index